Critical Care Nursing

Science and Practice

THIRD EDITION

EDITED BY

Sheila Adam
Chief Nurse, Homerton University Hospital NHS Foundation Trust, London, UK

Sue Osborne
Independent Consultant, formerly Sister in Critical Care, St George's Hospital, London, UK

John Welch
Consultant Nurse in Critical Care and Critical Care Outreach, University College London Hospitals, London, UK

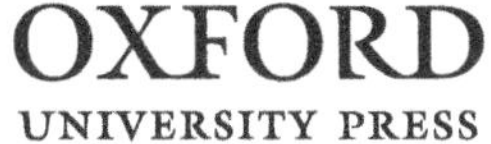

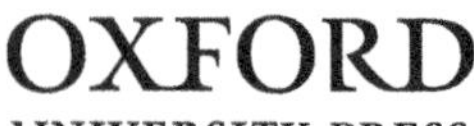

UNIVERSITY PRESS

Great Clarendon Street, Oxford, OX2 6DP,
United Kingdom

Oxford University Press is a department of the University of Oxford. It furthers the University's objective of excellence in research, scholarship, and education by publishing worldwide. Oxford is a registered trade mark of Oxford University Press in the UK and in certain other countries

First Edition published 1996
Second Edition published 2005
Third Edition published 2017

Published in the United States of America by Oxford University Press
198 Madison Avenue, New York, NY 10016, United States of America

British Library Cataloguing in Publication Data
Data available

Library of Congress Control Number: 2016951224

ISBN 978–0–19–969626–0

Preface to the third edition

Although it has taken longer to deliver than first anticipated, we have worked hard to make sure that the third edition of *Critical Care Nursing: Science and Practice* has developed and updated the key strengths and principles incorporated in both of the previous editions. The structure of the book has been altered to incorporate a new chapter on dealing with major incidents and pandemics, reflecting some of the challenges that have faced nurses working in critical care units across the globe. In addition, the support chapter around the technical elements of monitoring the patient has been subsumed into each of the appropriate chapters around care, reflecting our view that expertise is not subdivided into technical skills and caring principles but rather should be seen to form a common approach to delivering high quality care.

As before, our aim is to provide a text that will support nurses working across the continuum of critical care to deliver safe, knowledgeable, skilled, and compassionate care that is rooted in a strong evidence base. We believe passionately in the real difference that expert compassionate nursing care makes to the patient, their family, and the team as a whole, and we hope that this book provides a firm foundation to the development and retention of such precious expertise. We are grateful to our specialist chapter authors Sandra Fairley, Andrew Dimech, Deborah Dawson, and Claire Black who have contributed their highly advanced knowledge and skills to the book.

We would like to specifically thank and acknowledge the enormous support that we have received from our Medical Editor, Professor Mervyn Singer, who has read every word and offered invaluable advice and direction.

Sheila Adam, **Sue Osborne**, and **John Welch**

Contents

Abbreviations

AA arachidonic acid
ABG arterial blood gas
ACD active compression–decompression
ACE angiotensin-converting enzyme
ACh acetylcholine
AChE acetylcholinesterase
ACS abdominal compartment syndrome/acute coronary syndrome
ACT activated clotting time
ACTH adrenocorticotrophic hormone
ADH antidiuretic hormone
ADP adenosine diphosphate
AE adverse effect
AED automated external defibrillator
AF atrial fibrillation
AFE amniotic fluid embolism
AFLP acute fatty liver of pregnancy
AIDS acquired immunodeficiency syndrome
AKI acute kidney injury
ALI acute lung injury
ALL acute lymphatic leukaemia
ALS advanced life support
AMI acute myocardial infarction
AML acute myeloid leukaemia
ANA antinuclear antibody
ANCA antineutrophil cytoplasmic antibody
ANF atrial natriuretic factor
AP airway pressure
APACHE Acute Physiology And Chronic Health Evaluation
APC antigen-presenting cell
APTT activated partial thromboplastin time
ARDS acute respiratory distress syndrome/adult respiratory distress syndrome
AS aortic stenosis
ASDH acute subdural haematoma
AST aspartate transaminase
ATN acute tubular nerosis
ATP adenosine triphosphate
AV atrioventricular
BBB blood–brain barrier
BIS™ Bispectral Index monitoring
BiPAP bi-level positive airway pressure
BMT bone marrow transplant
BNP brain-type natriuretic peptide
BP blood pressure
bpm beats per minute
BPS Behavioural Pain Scale
BSA body surface area
CABG coronary artery bypass graft
CAPD continuous ambulatory peritoneal dialysis
cART combination antiretroviral therapy
CAUTI catheter-associated urinary tract infection
CAVH continuous arteriovenous haemofiltration
CBF cerebral blood flow
CBV cerebral blood volume
CCK cholecystokinin
CCU critical care unit/coronary care unit
ChE cholinesterase
CI cardiac index
CIM critical illness myopathy
CIMS clinical information management system
CIP critical illness polyneuropathy

CJD	Creutzfeldt–Jakob disease
CK	creatine kinase
CLL	chronic lymphatic leukaemia
CML	chronic myeloid leukaemia
$CMRO_2$	cerebral metabolic rate for oxygen consumption
CMV	controlled mechanical ventilation/ cytomegalovirus
CO	cardiac output
COP	capillary oncotic pressure
COPD	chronic obstructive pulmonary disease
CPAP	continuous positive airway pressure
CPK	creatine phosphokinase
CPOT	Critical Care Pain Observation Tool
CPP	cerebral perfusion pressure
CPR	cardiopulmonary resuscitation
CRBSI	catheter-related bloodstream infection
CRIMYNE	critical illness myopathy and neuropathy
CSDH	chronic subdural haematoma
CSF	cerebrospinal fluid
CSU	catheter specimen of urine
CSW	cerebral salt wasting (syndrome)
CT	computed tomography
CVA	cerebrovascular accident
CVC	central venous catheter
CVP	central venous pressure
CVR	cerebral vascular resistance
CVVH	continuous venovenous haemofiltration
CVVHD	continuous venovenous haemodialysis
CVVHDF	continuous venovenous haemodiafiltration
CXR	chest X-ray
DA	dopamine
DAI	diffuse axonal injury
DAMP	damage-associated molecular pattern
DBD	donation after brainstem death
DCD	donation after cardiac death
DDAVP	l-deamino-8-d-arginine vasopressin (desmopressin)
DI	diabetes insipidus
DIC	disseminated intravascular coagulation
DID	delayed ischaemic deficit
DIT	drug-induced thrombocytopenia
DKA	diabetic ketoacidosis
DMARD	disease-modifying anti-rheumatic drug
DNACPR	do not attempt cardiopulmonary resuscitation
DO_2I	oxygen delivery index
2,3-DPG	2,3-diphosphoglyceric acid
DTI	direct thrombin inhibitor
DSA	digital subtraction angiography
DVT	deep vein thrombosis
ECC	external chest compressions
$ECCO_2R$	extracorporeal carbon dioxide removal
ECG	electrocardiogram
ECMO	extracorporeal membrane oxygenation
ED	emergency department
EDH	extradural haematoma
EDV	end-diastolic volume
EEG	electroencephalogram
EF	ejection fraction
EMG	electromyography
ENT	ear, nose, and throat
ESR	erythrocyte sedimentation rate
ESV	end-systolic volume
$ETCO_2$	end-tidal carbon dioxide
ET(T)	endotracheal (tube)
EVLW	extravascular lung water
FAST	focused abdominal sonography for trauma
FDP	fibrin degradation product
FES	fat embolism syndrome

FFP	fresh frozen plasma/filtering face piece
FiO_2	fractionated inspired oxygen
FRC	functional residual capacity
FT_c	corrected flow time
FVC	forced vital capacity
GABA	gamma-aminobutyric acid
GAP	gravity-assisted positioning
GBS	Guillain–Barré syndrome
GCS	Glasgow Coma Score/Scale
GEDV	global end-diastolic volume
GFR	glomerular filtration rate
GH	growth hormone
GI	gastrointestinal
GIK	glucose–insulin–potassium
GM–CSF	granulocyte–macrophage colony stimulating factor
GPA	granulomatosis with polyangiitis
GPI	glycoprotein inhibitor
GRACE	Global Registry of Acute Coronary Events
GTN	glyceryl trinitrate
GUCH	grown-up congenital heart (disease)
HADS	Hospital Anxiety and Depression Scale
HAI	hospital-acquired infection
HAP	hospital-associated pneumonia
HASU	hyperacute stroke unit
Hb	haemoglobin
HB	heart block
HCM	hypertrophic cardiomyopathy
HCW	healthcare worker
Hct	haematocrit
HDL	high density lipoprotein
HDU	high frequency jet ventilation
HELLP	haemolysis, elevated liver enzymes, low platelet (syndrome)
HEPA	high efficiency particulate air
HFOV	high frequency oscillatory ventilation
HFV	high frequency ventilation
HHS	hyperosmolar hyperglycaemic states
HIT(S)	heparin-induced thrombocytopenia (syndrome)
HIV	human immunodeficiency virus
HL	Hodgkin's lymphoma
HLA	human leucocyte antigen
HME	heat and moisture exchanger
HOCM	hypertrophic obstructive cardiomyopathy
HPVG	hepatic venous pressure gradient
HR	heart rate
HRS	hepatorenal syndrome
hs-CRP	highly selective C-reactive protein
HSE	herpes simplex encephalitis
HSV	herpes simplex virus
5-HT	5-hydroxytryptamine
HUS	haemolytic–uraemic syndrome
HVHF	high volume haemofiltration
IABP	intra-aortic balloon pulsation/pump
IAH	intra-abdominal hypertension
IAP	intra-abdominal pressure
ICD	implantable cardioverter–defibrillator
ICH	intracerebral haematoma
ICP	intracranial pressure
ICS	intracellular space
ICU	intensive care unit
IDDM	insulin-dependent diabetes mellitus
IFN	interferon
Ig	immunoglobin
IHCA	in-hospital cardiac arrest
IHD	intermittent haemodialysis
IL	interleukin
IM	intramuscular
IMA	internal mammary artery

IMV	intermittent mandatory ventilation
INR	international normalized ratio
IO	inta-osseous
IPPB	intermittent positive pressure breathing
IPPV	intermittent positive pressure ventilation
IRDS	infant respiratory distress syndrome
IRIS	immune reconstitution inflammatory syndrome
ISS	Injury Severity Score/interstitial space
ITA	internal thoracic artery
ITBV	intrathoracic blood volume
ITP	idiopathic thrombocytopenic purpura
IV	intravenous
IVC	inferior vena cava
IVIg	intravenous immunoglobulin
IVS	intravascular space
JVP	jugular venous pressure
KPTT	kaolin partial thromboplastin time
KS	Kaposi's sarcoma
LAP	left atrial pressure
LDH	lactic dehydrogenase
LDL	low density lipoprotein
LDLT	live donor liver transplantation
LFPPV	low frequency positive pressure ventilation
LFT	liver function test
LiDCO™	lithium dilution cardiac output
LMA	laryngeal mask airway
LMW	low molecular weight
LMWH	low molecular weight heparin
LODS	Logistic Organ Dysfunction System
LPL	lipoprotein lipase
LPS	lipopolysaccharide
LV	left ventricle/left ventricular
LVEDP	left venticular end-diastolic volume
MAOI	monoamine oxidase inhibitor
MAP	mean arterial pressure
MARS	Molecular Adsorption Recycling System
MET	medical emergency team
MEWS	modified early warning score
MG	myasthenia gravis
MHC	major histocompatibility complex
MI	myocardial infarction
MIBG	meta-iodobenzylguanidine
MM	multiple myeloma
MODS	multiple organ dysfunction syndrome
MPAP	mean pulmonary artery pressure
MRAP	mean right atrial pressure
MRB	manual resuscitation bag
MRSA	methicillin-resistant *Staphylococcus aureus*
MS	mitral stenosis
MUD	matched unrelated donor
MUGA	multiple gated analysis (scan)
MV	minute volume
NAC	*N*-acetylcysteine
NAVA	neurally adjusted ventilatory assist
NE	norepinephrine (noradrenaline)
NG	nasogastric
NHL	non-Hodgkin's lymphoma
NHSCB	NHS Commissioning Board
NICE	National Institute for Health and Clinical Excellence
NIDDM	non-insulin-dependent diabetes mellitus
NIV	non-invasive ventilation
NK	natural killer (cells)
NOD	nucleotide oligomerization domain
NPE	neurogenic pulmonary oedema
NS	not significant
NSAID	non-steroidal anti-inflammatory drug
NSTEMI	non-ST-segment elevation myocardial infarction

O_2ER oxygen extraction ratio
OGD oesophagogastroduodenoscopy
PA pulmonary artery/pulmonary angiography
PACS picture archiving and communication system
P_aCO_2 artial pressure of arterial carbon dioxide
P_AO_2 partial pressure of alveolar oxygen
PADP pulmonary artery diastolic pressure
PAF platelet-activating factor
PAMP pathogen-associated molecular pattern
PAN polyarteritis nodosa
PAOP pulmonary artery occlusion pressure
PASP pulmonary artery systolic pressure
PAWP pulmonary artery wedge pressure
PCA patient-controlled analgesia
PCI percutaneous coronary intervention
PC-IRV pressure-controlled inverse ratio ventilation
PCP *Pneumocystis carinii* pneumonia
PCR polymerase chain reaction
PCV packed cell volume
PCWP pulmonary capillary wedge pressure
PD peritoneal dialysis
PE pulmonary embolism/plasma exchange
PEA pulseless electrical activity
PEEP positive end expiratory pressure
PEG percutaneous endoscopic gastrostomy
PEJ percutaneous endoscopic jejunostomy
PERT patient emergency response team
pH_i intramucosal pH
PICC peripherally inserted central catheter
PMNL polymorphonuclear leucocyte
PNH paroxysmal nocturnal haemoglobinuria
PP pulse pressure
PPE personal protective equipment
ppm parts per million
PPV pulse pressure variation
PRR pattern recognition receptor
PSV pressure support ventilation
PSVT paroxysmal supraventricular tachycardia
PT prothrombin time
PTFE polytetrafluoroethylene
PTH parathyroid hormone
PTSD post-traumatic stress disorder
PTT partial thromboplastin time
PV peak velocity
PVR pulmonary vascular resistance
RA right atrial
RAA renin–angiotensin–aldosterone (pathway)
RAP right atrial pressure
RAS reticular activating system
RCT randomized controlled trial
ROC receiver operating characteristic
ROM range of movement
ROS reactive oxygen species
RR respiratory rate
RRT renal replacement therapy
RSBI rapid shallow breathing index
rTPA (recombinant) tissue plasminogen activator
RTS Revised Trauma Score
RV right ventricle/right ventricular
RVDP right ventricular diastolic pressure
RVSP right ventricular systolic pressure
SA sinoatrial
SAH subarachnoid haemorrhage
SALT speech and language therapist
SAPS Simplified Acute Physiology Score
SBE subacute bacterial endocarditis
SBT spontaneous breathing trials
SCT stem cell transplantation

SCUF	slow continuous ultrafiltration
SD	standard deviation
SDD	selective decontamination of the digestive tract
SDH	subdural haematoma
SE	status epilepticus
SIADH	syndrome of inappropriate antidiuretic hormone
SID	strong ion difference
SIMV	synchronized intermittent mandatory ventilation
SIRS	systemic inflammatory response syndrome
SLE	systemic lupus erythematosus
SNOD	specialist nurse for organ donation
SOD	selective oropharyngeal decontamination
SOFA	Sepsis-related Organ Failure Assessment
S_aO_2	oxygen saturation of arterial blood
$S_{cv}O_2$	central venous oxygen saturation
$S_{jv}O_2$	jugular venous bulb oximetry
S_pO_2	peripheral oxygen saturation
S_vO_2	mixed venous oxygen saturation
STEMI	ST segment elevation myocardial infarction
SV	stroke volume
SVC	superior vena cava
SVR	systemic vacular resistance
SVT	supraventricular tachycardia
SVV	stroke volume variation
TAVI	transcatheter aortic valve implantation
TBI	traumatic brain injury
TBG	thyroxine-binding globulin
TCD	transcranial Doppler (ultrasonography
TENS	transcutaneous electrical nerve stimulation
TFPI	tissue factor pathway inhibitor
TIPS	transjugular intrahepatic portal systemic shunt
TISS	Therapeutic Intervention Scoring System
TLR	toll-like receptor
TMP	transmembrane pressure
TNF	tumour necrosis factor
tPA	tissue plasminogen activator
TRALI	transfusion-related acute lung injury
TRH	thyrotrophin-releasing hormone
TRISS	Trauma Score–Injury Severity Score
TSH	thyroid-stimulating hormone
TTP	thrombotic thrombocytopenic purpura
TXA_2	thromboxane A_2
UA	unstable angina
UFH	unfractionated heparin
uPA	urokinase-like plasminogen activator
UPS	uninterrupted power supply
UTI	urinary tract infection
VAC	vacuum-assisted closure
VAP	ventilator-associated pneumonia
VBL	variceal band ligation
VC	vital capacity
VC-IRV	volume-controlled inverse ratio ventilation
VF	ventricular fibrillation
VLDL	very low density lipoprotein
VMA	vanillylmandelic acid
VO_2I	oxygen consumption index
V/Q	ventilation/perfusion
VSD	ventricular septal defect
VT	ventricular tachycardia
vWF	von Willebrand factor
VZE	varicella zoster encephalitis
VZV	varicella zoster virus
WBPTT	whole blood partial thromboplastin time
WG	Wegener's granulomatosis
WPW	Wolff–Parkinson–White (syndrome)

Contributors

Sheila Adam, Chief Nurse, Homerton University Hospital NHS Foundation Trust, London, UK (Chapters 1, 2, 9, 15)

Claire Black, Clinical Specialist, Cardiorespiratory Physiotherapy, University College London Hospitals, London, UK (Chapter 4)

Deborah Dawson, Consultant Nurse Critical Care, St George's University Hospitals NHS FoundationTrust, London, UK (Chapter 1)

Andrew Dimech, Interim Divisional Clinical Nurse Director, The Royal Marsden NHS Foundation Trust, London, UK (Chapter 13)

Sandra Fairley, Clinical Nurse Specialist, Neurocritical Care, The National Hospital for Neurology and Neurosurgery, London, UK (Chapter 8)

Sue Osborne, Independent Consultant, formerly Sister in Critical Care, St George's Hospital, London, UK (Chapters 5, 11, 12, 14)

Mervyn Singer, Professor of Intensive Care Medicine, University College London, London, UK (Specialist adviser for all chapters)

John Welch, Consultant Nurse in Critical Care and Critical Care Outreach, University College London Hospitals, London, UK (Chapters 3, 4, 6, 7, 10, 16)

CHAPTER 1
The critical care continuum

Introduction and background

The focus of critical care has always been to improve outcomes in patients who become unwell due to a wide range of pathologies. These outcomes include not only survival but also the quality of life to which the patient can hope to return ('survivorship'). The initial development of critical care (or intensive care as it was then known) started with grouping patients into clearly identified separate geographical areas where they could be cared for and monitored to a far greater extent than was possible on a normal ward.

The roots are traced back to a large polio epidemic which affected Denmark in the 1950s. To deal with the many cases of respiratory failure, patients in a Copenhagen hospital were collected together to receive intensive round-the-clock multidisciplinary care involving physicians, nurses, and physiotherapists who developed more advanced skills to look after these sick patients. The patients underwent tracheostomy and positive pressure ventilation, and their haemodynamics and carbon dioxide levels were closely monitored, enabling prompt intervention as required. Outcomes improved dramatically as a consequence. However, the subsequent growth of intensive care units (ICUs) was fairly subdued until the 1960s when, especially in the USA, there was a big rise in their number in order to cope with patients after increasingly sophisticated, prolonged, and invasive surgery (ICS 2003).

As this separate speciality developed, segregation from other staff and wards increased. Patients were admitted to critical care areas from the wards, cared for by a separate group of highly expert staff, and, if they survived, returned to the wards with little or no ongoing follow-up from the critical care staff. The impetus behind the development of separate ICUs evolved from the need for skilled personnel, specific resources (such as ventilators and cardiac monitors), and adequate facilities (piped gases, larger bed areas). As critical care became more sophisticated, training of skilled staff became more complex and formal, and there was recognition of the need for competent, experienced, and technically capable staff.

Once the requirement for critical care became established, there was a gradual shift in culture so that patients who required these critical care skills (and this was often synonymous with requiring mechanical ventilation) were considered only to be those managed within the boundary walls of the designated critical care areas. As critical care has become more sophisticated, knowledge, skills, and expertise have increased. However, despite improvements in survival for many specific patient groups (such as those undergoing cardiac surgery), the mortality rate for patients who develop more complex multisystem disease, such as sepsis and multiple organ failure, remains high.

In the last few years, there has been a further shift in the culture of critical care in many countries, particularly Australia and the UK, which encompasses:

- earlier involvement of critical care expertise in a bid to prevent patient deterioration;
- ongoing follow-up of patients discharged to the ward from critical care to prevent readmission.

This has been variously named 'critical care without walls', the 'critical care continuum', and 'critical care outreach'. These initiatives are associated with an understanding that the patient requires access to critical care skills wherever they are cared for within the acute hospital setting (see Figure 1.1). As always, the aim is to improve the patient's chance of an optimal outcome, not just survival but the best possible quality of life. Although this is a complex multifaceted area to research, a study in Australia has shown significant differences in outcomes for those hospitals with mature rapid response teams which are a form of critical care outreach. Chen *et al.* (2014) demonstrated reductions in in-hospital cardiac arrests, mortality associated with arrests, and overall hospital mortality in a study of over 1,567,685 patients over a period of 7 years in four hospitals. Improvements were associated with mature response and escalation systems.

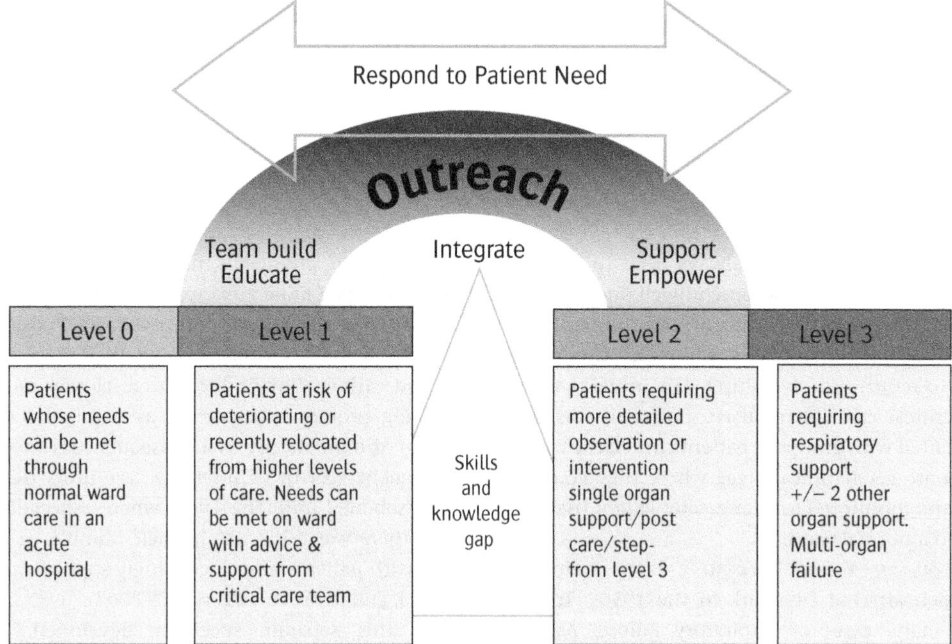

Figure 1.1 Model of critical care outreach.

Redefining the limits of critical care as a continuum from admission to rehabilitation

While no blockbuster drugs or other therapies have emerged over recent decades, there have nevertheless been significant improvements in outcomes for patients admitted to critical care. Although selective, the mortality rates of the placebo groups in large trials for septic shock and acute respiratory distress syndrome (ARDS) have fallen markedly, while the outcome prediction models used in large patient databases have needed several revisions to adjust for the better survival rates. This improvement should also be placed in the context of an ageing population with multiple comorbidities who would not have been considered suitable for critical care admission several decades ago, but are now generally accepted unless judged to be futile. Mortality rates still remain much higher than desired. However, in a significant proportion of cases, the underlying disease process (e.g. cancer) or the general fragility of the patient is the major determinant of outcome, with the acute decompensation requiring critical care admission representing the end-stage of this terminal course. Larger numbers of patients survive critical care only to die before they leave hospital or within the next 6–12 months after discharge.

Reasons for these improved figures are primarily related to (i) earlier identification and intervention for the deteriorating patient, (ii) better general care with, for example, greater efforts to prevent infection and pressure sores and to encourage mobilization and rehabilitation, and (iii) avoidance of injurious management strategies such as excessive ventilator-delivered tidal volumes, over-exuberant fluid resuscitation and over-sedation. Initiatives such as the Surviving Sepsis Campaign (education in early recognition and a bundle of protocolized responses for managing sepsis) (Rivers *et al.* 2001; Lyseng-Williamson and Perry 2002; Dellinger *et al.* 2013; ProCESS Investigators 2014) have been proposed—see section on 'Sepsis').

In effect, this is a continuum of critical care from the first contact with the patient to their discharge and, in some cases, beyond. Ghosh and Pepe (2009) suggest that critical care should be seen as a cascade supporting the need for a more seamless and interconnected continuum of patient care for a growing compendium of critical care conditions, starting in the pre-hospital and emergency department phases of management and continuing through ICU and rehabilitation services.

This new approach to improving the outcome of critically ill patients is a major factor in the need to expand the influence of critical care skills and responses outside the geographical area of the critical care environment itself. These positive initiatives to improve outcomes for the critically ill patient are not the only factor in the argument for expanding critical care skills and support. There is also an urgent need to manage more negative factors that have impacted on the existing system available in acute care for responding to critical illness.

Factors associated with the need for development of critical care support and expertise outside the critical care unit are numerous. Many have come about because of changes in methods of managing and delivering patient care as well as changes in education of staff. These factors include:

- increasing numbers of acutely ill patients in hospital (increased primary care interventions, day surgery, and reduced length of stay have reduced the number of less acutely ill inpatients);
- increasing comorbidity/multiple pathology and age of patients, as well as an increasing longevity of sufferers from chronic disease;
- decreased emphasis on acute illness in pre-registration education for nurses and doctors and increased emphasis on health education and prevention;
- decreased exposure to acutely ill patients during pre-registration education for nurses owing to supernumerary practice and increased time in college;
- increased workload for medical teams with less time for supervision of junior staff;
- an 'ivory tower' attitude in critical care staff resulting in decreased communication/sharing of knowledge and skills with ward staff;
- possible deskilling of ward staff, particularly in early recognition of deterioration, as sick patients are more frequently cared for in critical care units;
- transfer of routine observations such as temperature, heart rate, and blood pressure to healthcare assistants (untrained ward nursing staff), sometimes without proper supervision;

- a decline in the monitoring of respiratory rate by ward staff as a sensitive but non-specific marker of deterioration (Odell *et al.* 2002).

In a seminal study of the quality of care of patients prior to critical care admission, McQuillan *et al.* (1998) identified six factors (Box 1.1) associated with suboptimal care of acutely ill patients in general wards. Subsequent mortality was significantly higher ($p = 0.04$) in the group that received suboptimal care.

Some of these factors, particularly those requiring education, can be addressed by the development of critical care outreach services. Others, particularly cultural issues (such as 'coping' by junior staff without requesting senior help so as not to appear inadequate), require involvement and commitment to change by training bodies and professional groups as well as by healthcare institutions themselves. The development of better levels of supervision and immediate access to skilled resources for critically ill patients needs to be assisted by a combination of organizational, critical care, and interprofessional initiatives.

Box 1.1 Causes of suboptimal care in critically ill ward patients

Principal causes of suboptimal care

1. Failure of organization
2. Lack of knowledge
3. Failure to appreciate clinical urgency
4. Lack of experience
5. Lack of supervision
6. Failure to seek advice

Recategorized by system dysfunction

Process

1. Failure of organization
5. Lack of supervision

Education

2. Lack of knowledge
3. Failure to appreciate clinical urgency

Culture

4. Lack of experience
6. Failure to seek advice

Adapted from *British Medical Journal*, McQuillan, P. *et al.*, Confidential inquiry into quality of care before admission to intensive care, Volume 316, pp. 1853–7, copyright (1998) with permission from BMJ Publishing Group Ltd.

Limitations of cardiopulmonary resuscitation

Although considerable education, resources, and effort have been put into developing a fast and effective response to cardiac arrest, the outcome continues to be poor for patients who suffer an actual cardiac arrest, either as an inpatient or outside hospital. The most recent study of incidence and outcomes for adult in-hospital cardiac arrest (Nolan *et al.* 2014) shows a very similar picture to previous studies, with an overall incidence of of 1.6 arrests per 1000 hospital admissions and an unadjusted survival to hospital discharge rate of 18.4%. This study showed a major difference between outcomes of shockable (ventricular fibrillation (VF) or pulseless ventricular tachycardia (VT)) and non-shockable rhythms. Survival to hospital discharge was 49% in shockable rhythms but only 10.5% in non-shockable rhythms. The majority of arrests occurred in the latter group (72.3%) compared with 16.9% in the former. In a previous review of presenting rhythms and survival in 51,919 patients (Meaney *et al.* 2010), outcome for in-hospital arrests was 37% for VF/VT (shockable) arrhythmias. but only 12% for pulseless electrical activity (PEA) and 11% for asystole (Figure 1.2). Associations with increased survival included presenting with a VF

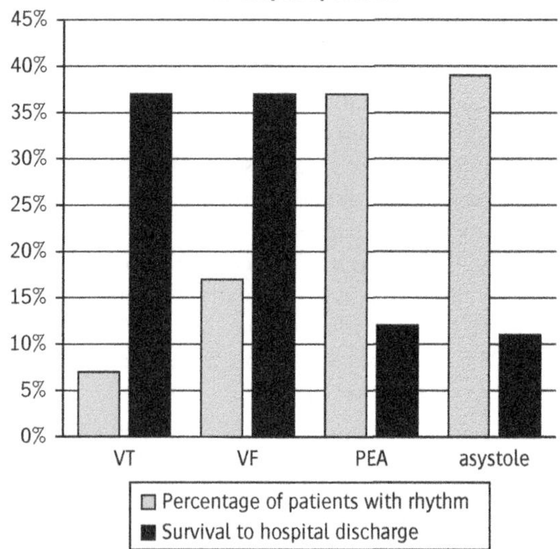

Figure 1.2 Type of cardiac arrest rhythm and survival to discharge in hospital patients.

Data from Meaney, P.A *et al.*, Rhythms and outcomes of adult in-hospital cardiac arrest, *Critical Care Medicine*, Volume 38, Issue 1, pp. 101–8, 2010, Lippincott Williams & Wilkins Inc.

or VT arrhythmia, having circulation restored within 3 min, and being under 70 years of age. Administration of epinephrine (adrenaline) was associated with a reduced likelihood of survival, perhaps because this is linked to longer periods of resuscitation.

There has also been little improvement in survival rates for out-of-hospital arrests. In a study of 5,505 patients, Herlitz *et al.* (2003) compared outcomes of patients who suffered an out-of-hospital cardiac arrest in 1980–1990 and in 1990–2000. Survival to hospital was 24% in both decades; of these, only 37% survived to hospital discharge in 1980–1990, and 35% in 1990–2000. Thus overall survival to discharge from hospital was approximately 8%, and this had not improved over the 20 years studied. Therefore it is important to look at prevention of such irreversible events by early recognition of deterioration with an appropriate and effective response.

Factors identified as being associated with survival following out-of-hospital arrest were:

- ventricular fibrillation/ventricular tachycardia (VF/VT) as the first recorded rhythm;
- witnessed arrest;
- bystander-initiated cardiopulmonary resuscitation (CPR);
- patient conscious at time of admission to hospital;
- sinus rhythm on admission to hospital.

Factors associated with worse outcomes were:

- asystole or pulseless electrical activity (PEA);
- chronic diuretic and oral hypoglycaemic medication.

Costs of CPR training programmes, as determined by Lee *et al.* (1996), were estimated at $406,605 per life saved and $225,892 per quality adjusted life year. These costs are likely to have increased significantly since the study was undertaken and remain a huge outlay for such a poor outcome. This suggests that other methods, primarily early detection and response, need to be explored and better utilized. The aim of early warning scores and call criteria (collectively known as 'track and trigger' mechanisms), along with support and education in managing acute deterioration, is to help general ward staff to identify patients who are deteriorating and initiate a response before a poor outcome event occurs.

Early recognition of clinical deterioration in patients

Pioneering work by Schein *et al.* (1990), Franklin and Mathew (1994), and Rich (1999) found that many ward patients who suffered a cardiorespiratory arrest had clear evidence of physiological deterioration in the hours prior to the event, particularly changes to respiratory rate and conscious level (see Box 1.2).

Rich (1999) also found variable response times to patient deterioration. Overall, nurses took a mean of 21.4 min to notify doctors of physiological deterioration. Patients who survived had a mean notification time of 14.3 min compared with 25.7 min for non-survivors (Tables 1.1 and 1.2). In view of the poor outcome associated with cardiac arrest, it makes sense to utilize early indicators as an opportunity to

Box 1.2 Signs of deterioration

- New changes in systolic blood pressure—alteration (up or down) >20 mmHg
- New heart rate changes to <45 or >125 beats per min (bpm)
- New ECG rhythm changes
- New respiratory rate to <10 or >30 breaths/min
- New complaints of chest pain or dyspnoea
- New changes in patient's mental status
- New critical laboratory values

Data from Rich, K., Inhospital cardiac arrest: pre-event variables and nursing response. *Clinical Nurse Specialist*, Volume 13, pp. 147–53, 1999, Wolters Kluwer Health Inc.

Table 1.1 Time taken by nurses to notify physicians about physiological changes prior to cardiac arrest

Variable	Mean (standard deviation) delay (min)
Overall mean time	21.4 (32.9)
Chest pain	7.3 (6.8)
Dyspnoea	10.5 (8.4)
ECG rhythm	22.3 (34.8)
Respiration	27.5 (32.0)
Blood pressure	28.4 (42.7)
Heart rate	31.0 (40.2)
Mental status	30.3 (34.2)

Data from Rich, K. Inhospital cardiac arrest: pre-event variables and nursing response. *Clinical Nurse Specialist*, Volume 13, pp. 147–53, 1999, Wolters Kluwer Health Inc.

Table 1.2 Evidence of deterioration prior to cardiac arrest

Authors	No of patients	Results
Schein *et al.* (1990)	64	8% survival after cardiac arrest 84% showed evidence of clinical deterioration
Franklin and Mathew (1994)	150	66% of patients had documented clinical deterioration prior to arrest
Rich (1999)	100	11% survival after cardiac arrest Physiological change noted in 60% up to 8 h prior to arrest

Data from Rich, K. Inhospital cardiac arrest: pre-event variables and nursing response. *Clinical Nurse Specialist*, Volume 13, pp.147–53,1999 Lippincott Williams & Wilkins Inc; Schein, R.M., Hazday, N., Pena, M., *et al.* Clinical antecedents to in-hospital cardiopulmonary arrest. *Chest*, Volume 98, pp. 1388–92, 1990, American College of Chest Physicians; Franklin, C., Mathew, J. Developing strategies to prevent in-hospital cardiac arrest: analysing responses of physicians and nurses in the hours before the event. *Critical Care Medicine*, Volume 22, pp. 244–7, 1994, Lippincott Williams & Wilkins Inc.

intervene more rapidly and prevent cardiac arrest from occurring. This may result in improved outcomes (Figure 1.2).

However, even with the introduction of a system to support recognition of acute deterioration and appropriate escalation and response, there is evidence that patients still do not receive the required response in a timely manner. One study of an early warning system response and escalation in a Danish hospital (Asger-Petersen *et al.* 2014) found that although 63% of patients received the correct level of monitoring, in 92% of patients there was a significant failure to follow the escalation requirements which encompassed everything from increasing the frequency of observations to calling the emergency team.

Hillman *et al.* (2001) and McGloin *et al.* (1999) examined antecedents to sudden death or critical care admission. Hillman *et al.* (2001) found that the most common physiological changes documented prior to death not preceded by cardiac arrest or critical care admission, were systolic blood pressure (BP) <90 mmHg and respiratory rate (RR) >36 breaths/min. Concern was frequently documented, but not reasons why appropriate intervention did not occur. This was also reported by McGloin *et al.* (1999), with tachypnoea (RR >25 breaths/ min), hypoxaemia (S_pO_2 <90%) and hypotension (systolic BP <100 mmHg) most commonly associated with admission to critical care and subsequent death.

In another study, Hodgetts *et al.* (2002) reported three positive associations for cardiac arrest, namely abnormal breathing, abnormal pulse, and abnormal systolic BP. Risk factors were weighted and showed that a score of 4 had 89% sensitivity and 77% specificity for cardiac arrest, while a score of 8 had 52% sensitivity and 99% specificity. All patients scoring >10 suffered a cardiac arrest. Parameters based on these findings have been developed into indicators of acute deterioration, and are accompanied by a didactic response usually requiring reaction from specified personnel within a set time frame (see Figure 1.3).

Lack of skills in recognition and response to critical deterioration in ward patients

Adequate levels of training to deal with critical deterioration are essential in order to deal with emergency situations, and a lack of training can lead to poor or ineffective responses. Smith and Poplett (2002) found that knowledge about recognizing and responding to acute situations, such as identfying complete airway obstruction or setting up high flow oxygen, was poor in the 108 junior medical staff questioned. As this group are the most likely to be called on to deal with such situations by ward nursing staff, it is vital that they should be able to intervene effectively. A systematic review of retention of knowledge and skills in advanced life support suggested that skills are lost in 6 months to 1 year, although knowledge may be retained for longer. This can be ameliorated by more frequent exposure to clinical situations (Yang *et al.* 2012).

Nurses often use personal experience to assess the patient's state (Cioffi and Markham 1997); however, Cioffi (2000) identified four specific findings most likely to alert nurses to patients requiring urgent intervention (see Box 1.3).

The combination of poor early recognition and lack of skill in responding to acute deterioration is likely to contribute to poor patient outcome. Education of healthcare staff in these important early warning signs is vital and must be a key component in their pre-registration curriculum. Equal emphasis is needed on the life-saving priorities of response which need to be taught using simulation in clinical skills areas.

Box 1.3 Specific findings associated with nurses activating the medical emergency team for 'worried or concerned'

- 'Not right' or 'unwell' declared by the patient or recognized by the nurse as a difference in the patient
- Colour, clamminess, and coldness with colour (quite pale, porcelain pale, pale dusky, and sort of grey) or draining colour
- Agitation
- Observations that were slightly abnormal or not unusual at all

Data from Cioffi, J., Recognition of patients who require emergency assistance: a descriptive study, *Heart & Lung*, Volume 29, pp. 262–8. 2000 Elsevier.

Early intervention could improve outcomes

It has been suggested that early recognition and aggressive intervention in a number of acute conditions (e.g. sepsis, pre-operative optimization, acute stroke, acute kidney injury) may be beneficial in preventing death and reducing the severity of illness after the patient is admitted to critical care. It is also likely that use of and compliance with a protocolized response such as the National Early Warning Score alleviates some of the requirement for retention of individual skills and knowledge.

Sepsis

Early studies in emergency care suggested that patient outcome could be improved by early and aggressive intervention. Rivers *et al.* (2001) randomized ED patients in severe sepsis and septic shock to receive either standard care or haemodynamic optimization with a central venous oximetry catheter and fluid/blood transfusion/inotropes following a specified resuscitation protocol for the 6 hours following presentation. This early aggressive intervention reduced mortality from 46.5% to 30.5%. However, a follow-up study to replicate this in 1341 patients across 39 emergency departments in the USA (ProCESS 2014) found no difference in outcome between early goal-directed therapy, standard protocolized therapy, and usual care. Adherence to the protocols was good, but did not produce a significant improvement associated with early goal-directed therapy. As there were more than 10 years between these studies it is possible that overall care has improved (Harrison *et al.* 2006), and the improved mortality seen in the Rivers study was a reflection of poorer overall care at the time.

There can be delays in responding to acute deterioration associated with sepsis in ward patients. In many cases acute deterioration is recognized, but it may take too long either to access the correct level of support and/or to transfer the patient to a critical care unit. Rivers *et al.* (2001) suggest that the transition to multi-organ failure and critical illness can be denoted as 'golden hours' during which definitive recognition and treatment can be of maximal benefit. This occurs regardless of whether the patient is on a general ward, in the emergency department, or in the intensive care unit.

Lundberg *et al.* (1998) found that onset of septic shock in a general ward patient was associated with a 5.5-fold increased risk of death compared with an onset in critical care. Review of the clinical course suggested that there were delays in specific responses in the general ward patients, such as intravenous fluid resuscitation and inotrope administration.

The introduction of the Surviving Sepsis Campaign in 2002 resulted in enhanced recognition of signs of sepsis and the development of a bundle of care (see Chapter 10 for more details). National adoption of the key elements in the sepsis bundle in the Netherlands have been shown to improve outcomes (van Zanten *et al.* 2014), with an improved adherence to the bundle and a decreased in-hospital mortality of 5.8% adjusted absolute mortality reduction over 3.5 years.

The most recent guidelines for improving survival from sepsis outline the key elements (shown in Box 1.4) as essential interventions (for details please refer to Chapter 10)

Peri-operative optimization

Multiple single-centre studies have shown that peri-operative haemodynamic optimization improves outcomes in a variety of surgical populations. For example, Wilson *et al.* (1999) studied 138 patients and compared the effects of pre-operative enhancement of oxygen delivery using fluid and inotropes against standard practice. This active treatment group required admission to critical care 4 hours prior to surgery, and for at least 12–24 hours post-operatively. They reported significant improvements in survival and length of hospital stay. Whether this benefit relates primarily to the targeting of oxygen delivery or to better overall care and attention to haemodynamics, breathing, pain relief, and mobilization is uncertain.

> **Box 1.4 Surviving Sepsis Campaign key interventions**
>
> **TO BE COMPLETED WITHIN 3 HOURS**
>
> (1) Measure lactate level
> (2) Obtain blood cultures prior to administration of antibiotics
> (3) Administer broad spectrum antibiotics
> (4) Administer 30 mL/kg crystalloid for hypotension or lactate 4 mmol/L
>
> **TO BE COMPLETED WITHIN 6 HOURS**
>
> (5) Apply vasopressors (for hypotension that does not respond to initial fluid resuscitation) to maintain a mean arterial pressure (MAP) of 65 mmHg
> (6) In the event of persistent arterial hypotension despite volume resuscitation (septic shock) or initial lactate 4 mmol/L (36 mg/dL):
> - measure central venous pressure (CVP)*
> - measure central venous oxygen saturation ($S_{cv}O_2$)*
>
> (7) Remeasure lactate if initial lactate was elevated*
>
> *Targets for quantitative resuscitation included in the guidelines are CVP of 8 mm Hg, $S_{cv}O_2$ of 70%, and normalization of lactate.
>
> Reproduced with permission from Dellinger, R.P., Levy, M., Rhodes, A., *et al.* Surviving Sepsis Campaign: International Guidelines for Management of Severe Sepsis and Septic Shock: 2012, *Critical Care Medicine*, Volume 41, Issue 2, pp. 580–637 Copyright © 2013 Society of Critical Care Medicine and the European Society of Intensive Care Medicine and Wolters Kluwer Health Inc.

Acute kidney injury

The incidence of acute kidney injury (AKI) has steadily increased globally due to a range of causes which vary depending on location (Lameire *et al.* 2013). Most recent estimates of in-hospital prevalence in the USA suggest that about 2% of patients develop AKI. Early recognition of incipient renal failure, particularly in the acute phase of illness, can often be managed with intravenous fluids targeted to physiological endpoints, such as mean arterial pressure, cardiac output, central venous pressure, and urine output (Lin *et al.* 2006). However, this needs to take place before resistant oligo-anuria has become established (Bagshaw *et al.* 2008). Nursing staff are uniquely placed to recognize early deterioration and to activate an appropriate response from their colleagues, but because traditional hierarchical methods of doing this (i.e. contacting a junior member of the medical or surgical staff) often result in delay, other forms of response which bring about immediate intervention have been set up.

Development of teams able to respond prior to cardiac arrest

Lee *et al.* (1995) in Liverpool, Australia, were the first to describe a team of this nature. Their medical emergency team (MET) consists of critical care medical and nursing staff who respond to calls from general ward staff based on a series of set criteria (Box 1.5). They reported decreases in the incidence of cardiac arrest (Buist *et al.* 2002, Bellomo *et al.* 2003) and a reduction in unanticipated admissions to intensive care (Bristow *et al.* 2000), but no clear evidence of a reduction in general hospital mortality (Bellomo *et al.* 2003). However, patients who suffered a cardiac arrest in the presence of the MET had a better chance of survival (Bellomo *et al.* 2003).

Moon *et al.* (2011) examined the impact of critical care outreach teams in the UK. Compared with the 4 years prior to the introduction of the teams and early warning scores, there was a halving of the cardiac arrest rate (0.2% vs 0.4% of adult hospital admissions). Furthermore, in-hospital mortality of patients admitted to critical care following cardiac arrest fell from 52% to 42%.

In Australia, Chen *et al.* (2014) compared in-hospital cardiac arrest (IHCA) rates and mortality in four hospitals; one had a mature rapid response system (RRS) in place and the other three introduced such a system in 2009–2010. Between 2002 and 2008, the mature RRS hospital demonstrated a reduction of >50% in the IHCA rate, a 40% lower IHCA-related mortality, and a 6% lower overall hospital mortality. Hospitals without an RRS up to 2008 showed a small improvement in these markers

> **Box 1.5 Criteria for calling the Medical Emergency Team**
>
> - Cardiorespiratory arrest
> - Threatened airway
> - Respiratory rate ≤5 breaths/min, ≥36 breaths/min
> - Pulse rate ≤40 bpm, ≥140 bpm
> - Systolic blood pressure ≤90 mmHg
> - Repeated or prolonged seizures
> - Fall in Glasgow Coma Score >2 points
> - Concern about patient status not detailed above
>
> Data from Lee, A., Bishop, G., Hillman, K., *et al.* The medical emergency team. *Anaesthesia and Intensive Care*, Volume 23, pp. 183–6, 1995, Anaesthesia and Intensive Care.

over the same time period. However, in their first year of RRS (2009), compared with 2008 the two hospitals achieved a 22% reduction in IHCA rate, a 22% reduction in IHCA- related mortality, and an 11% reduction in overall hospital mortality. During the same period, the mature RRS hospital showed no significant change in these outcomes, but in 2009 it still achieved a crude 20% lower IHCA rate and a 14% lower overall hospital mortality rate. There was no significant difference in 1-year post-discharge mortality for survivors of IHCA over the study period.

Introduction of teams such as these takes some time to develop full impact but can clearly contribute to significant improvement in reducing cardiac arrest incidence and improving outcomes.

Development of critical care outreach services

In the UK, the publication of two government reports—*Critical to Success* (Audit Commission 1999) and *Comprehensive Critical Care* (Department of Health 2000)—actively encouraged the establishment of critical care services that would support patients who were acutely ill outside the critical care unit (see Box 1.6). Over 100 of these critical care outreach services were set up in hospitals throughout England and Wales. However, with no central coordination and variable levels of funding, outreach services evolved locally with a wide variation in team personnel, hours of cover, call triggers and responses, and the level of education offered to other staff. Other countries such as Australia and the USA, worked on similar services such as METs and rapid response teams. The difference between a MET and the critical care outreach service is that while the former concentrates solely on pre-critical care admission, the latter covers both pre- and post-critical care admissions, as well as enhanced training for ward staff. An emphasis on education and support of staff outside the critical care area is vital in ensuring that patients who deteriorate throughout the hospital are recognized and managed in a timely and effective manner. Other countries, such as Canada, have followed suit more recently, developing critical care outreach services supported by state-wide initiatives.

In 2007 the UK National Institute for Health and Clinical Excellence (NICE) published guidelines for acutely ill patients in hospital (Figure 1.3). These recommended a minimum frequency of observation (12 hourly) for all acute hospital inpatients and specified which observations should be performed (Box 1.7).

The recommendations stipulated that a 'track and trigger' system should be used to enable a graded response. However, the organizational inconsistency described in the previous paragraph meant that nurses and doctors had to learn new systems when moving from one hospital to another. Recently a national version of an early warning system—the National Early Warning Score (NEWS)—has been developed (NEWS 2012), adoption of which is being encouraged nationwide (Table 1.3).

Evidence of the impact of these early recognition and response systems has grown. Ball *et al.* (2003) reported a 6% improvement in survival to hospital discharge and a significant reduction in critical care readmission, and Priestley *et al.* (2004) also showed better hospital mortality rates following the introduction of early warning systems and an outreach team. However, a systematic review by Esmonde *et al.* (2006) concluded that while individual studies suggested benefit, the overall body of evidence was equivocal owing to the small number of high quality studies available.

The maturity of the system (i.e. the length of time it has been in place) also appears to be influential. Calzavacca *et al.* (2010) found that unplanned ICU admissions and hospital mortality rates were significantly lower in the tenth year of a rapid response team service compared with the first year. Moon *et al.* (2011) and Chen *et al.* (2014) similarly demonstrated a significant impact on cardiac arrest incidence and survival

Box 1.6 Essential objectives of critical care outreach

- To avert admissions (to the ICU) by identifying patients who are deteriorating and either helping to prevent admission or ensuring that admission to a critical care bed happens in a timely manner to ensure the best outcome.
- To enable discharges from critical care by supporting the continuing recovery of discharged patients on wards and discharge from hospital.
- To share critical care skills with staff in wards and the community, ensuring enhancements for training opportunities and skills practice, and to use information gathered from the ward and community to improve critical care services for patients and relatives.

Reproduced from *Comprehensive Critical Care: A Review of Adult Critical Care Services*, Department of Health, 2000, pp. 14–15.

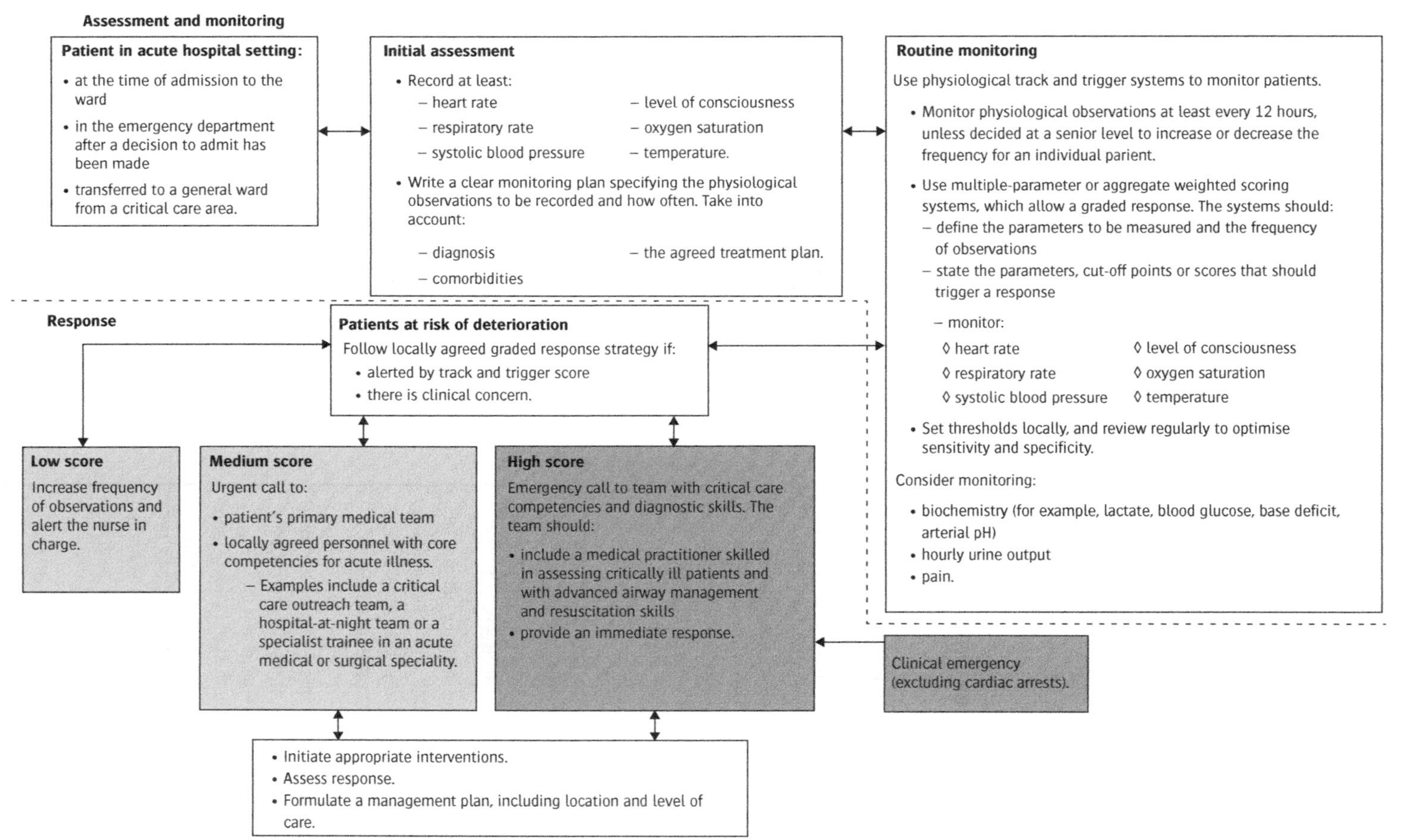

Figure 1.3 1-2-3 care pathway.

Reproduced with permission from National Institute for Health and Clinical Excellence (2007), CG 50 Acutely ill patients in hospital: recognition of and response to acute illness in adults in hospital. London: NICE. Accessed 23 May 2016 from http://www.nice.org.uk/CG50.

Box 1.7 Observations recommended by NICE for acute inpatients (minimum frequency 12-hourly)

- Respiratory rate
- Temperature
- Blood pressure
- Heart rate
- Oxygen saturation
- Level of consciousness

Reproduced with permission from National Institute for Health and Clinical Excellence (2007) CG 50 Acutely ill patients in hospital: recognition of and response to acute illness in adults in hospital. London: NICE. Accessed 23/05/2016 from http://www.nice.org.uk/CG50.

following development of a mature rapid response or critical care outreach service and early warning system.

Critical care outreach, rapid response, and early recognition of deterioration have now become an accepted part of good practice in England and Wales and form one component of the 2010 Care Quality Commission Standards to which all acute hospitals are required to adhere. This is mirrored in a number of other countries including Australia, the USA, and Canada (Peberdy *et al.* 2007). In view of the probable benefits of such services, they are now embedded as a gold standard requirement for every acute hospital.

Survival and follow-up after critical care

Critical care patients are two to three times more likely to die in the first year after discharge from critical care than an age-matched general population (Williams *et al.* 2008). They are also likely to suffer critical adverse events during their hospital stay following ICU discharge (McLaughlin *et al.* 2007). Therefore it is important that these patients receive additional support and care through follow-up and outreach services, and that outcomes from critical care are reviewed over the long term rather than at the point of discharge from either the intensive care unit or the hospital itself.

Age, comorbidity, and primary diagnosis have the strongest associations with poor long-term survival (Williams *et al.* 2008); management of comorbidities is probably the most significant of these factors as this is the most amenable to manipulation during the patient's critical care and hospital stay. Early studies identified that a significant proportion of patients die in hospital following discharge from critical care (Goldhill and Sumner 1998; Smith *et al.* 1999: Moreno and Agthé 1999). Those discharged while still requiring a high intensity of treatment and/or support fared much worse (Smith *et al.* 1999). While a proportion of these deaths are likely to reflect the underlying severity and terminal stages of a patient's illness, there are much less obvious reasons for a number of these cases.

The Stability and Workload Index for Transfer (SWIFT) score was developed using factors identified as being

Table 1.3 National Early Warning Score (NEWS)*

Physiological parameters	3	2	1	0	1	2	3
Respiration rate	≤8		9–11	12–20		21–24	≥25
Oxygen saturations	≤91	92–93	94–95	≥96			
Any supplemental oxygen		Yes		No			
Temperature	≤35.0		35.1 - 36.0	36.1–38.0	38.1–39.0	≥39.1	
Systolic BP	≤90	91–100	101–110	111–219			
Heart rate	≤40		41–50	51–90	91–110	111–130	≥131
Level of consciousness				A			V, P, or U

* The NEWS initiative flowed from the Royal College of Physicians NEWS Development and Implementation Group (NEWSDIG) report, and was jointly developed and funded in collaboration with the Royal College of Physicians, the Royal College of Nursing, the National Outreach Forum, and NHS Training for Innovation.

Reproduced from National Early Warning Score (NEWS), Royal College of Physicians. The original was produced in colour (http://www.rcplondon.ac.uk/sites/default/files/documents/national-early-warning-score-with-explanatory-text.pdf) linked to readmission and unexpected death in a study of 1131 medical ICU patients discharged to the ward:

- original admission from the ward
- length of stay >2 days and >10 days
- P_aO_2/FiO_2 ratio—the score increases as the ratio decreases
- Glasgow Coma Score—the score increases as the GCS decreases
- Last P_aCO_2 value >6 kPa (45 mmHg).

Patients scoring ≥15 on the day of discharge were considered to be at a significantly increased risk of readmission.[1]

Daly *et al.* (2001) used a logistic regression model to identify six variables associated with either an increased or reduced risk of dying following discharge from critical care (Table 1.4). A positive additional risk was associated with an increasing APACHE II score and a longer duration of critical care stay. Therefore it is possible to identify high risk patients at discharge and either prolong their stay in critical care or increase the level of support available to them after discharge. In practice, the demand for critical care beds often makes the former solution impossible, while the latter solution will depend on the provision of facilities such as step-down units or the use of a critical care outreach service.

Table 1.4 Variables for predictive discharge triage

Variable	Impact
Age	Positive
Chronic health points	Positive
Acute physiology points	Positive
Cardiac surgery	Negative
Length of ICU stay	Positive
Constant*	Negative

*Related to the methodology of the predictive model.

Variables selected by Daly *et al.* (2001) for discharge triage predictive model (either increased or reduced risk of death).

Adapted from Daly, K., Beale, R., Chang, R., Reduction in mortality after inappropriate early discharge from intensive care unit logistic regression triage model, *British Medical Journal*, Volume 322, pp. 1274–6. Copyright (2001) with permission from BMJ Publishing Group Ltd.

[1] Data from Gajic, O., Malinchoc, M., Comfere, T. The stability and workload index for transfer score predicts unplanned intensive care unit patient readmission: Initial development and validation. *Critical Care Medicine*, Volume 36, pp. 676–82, 2008. The Society of Critical Care Medicine and Lippincott Williams & Wilkins.

Timing of transfer has also been associated with poorer outcomes and a worse patient experience. Hanane *et al.* (2008) found that night-time discharge to a ward bed from intensive care was associated with a higher readmission rate and a longer length of hospital stay. Earlier studies (Goldfrad and Rowan 2000; Duke *et al.* 2004) have shown significantly increased mortality associated with night-time (22.00–07.30) discharges.

Readmission rates to critical care

A high unplanned readmission rate of patients to critical care during the same hospital stay is a useful indicator of poor follow-up and inappropriate or premature discharge from critical care areas. Readmission is associated with a fourfold risk-adjusted increase in probability of hospital mortality and a 2.5-fold increase in hospital stay (Kramer *et al.* 2012), so a reduction in such readmissions should be a major goal for the critical care outreach service.

A systematic review of the intensive care admission literature (Elliott *et al.* 2014) found that readmissions were most commonly associated with cardiovascular or respiratory problems and sepsis. Patients who were readmitted were older, had more comorbidities and non-surgical diagnoses, underwent emergency rather than elective surgery, and had higher illness severity and longer ICU lengths of stay. However, many factors affect the likelihood of readmission (Figure 1.4), and in some cases it is an important and appropriate early response to new deterioration.

Chen *et al.* (1998) reviewed the clinical features and outcomes of 236 patients readmitted to seven critical care units over a 13-month period. Patients with cardiovascular and respiratory problems were most likely to be readmitted for the same illness. In those patients developing new complications requiring readmission, 58% were respiratory in origin.

Post-critical care follow-up

Improvements in survival to discharge from intensive care and, ultimately, from hospital will significantly increase the number of patients facing longer-term problems associated with surviving critical illness. A systematic review of these complications (Desai *et al.* 2011) acknowledges that early rehabilitation and proactive management will enhance the patient's recovery and quality of life. Ongoing input from the critical care staff offers the patient, their family, and the ward staff better continuity in terms of general care, monitoring by critical-care-trained staff attuned to physiological deterioration, and improved exchanges of information

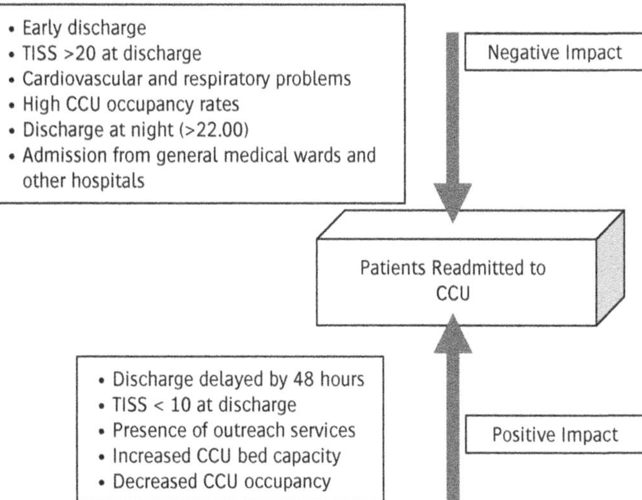

Figure 1.4 Factors affecting patient readmission to critical care.

and education of ward staff to help support these highly dependent patients.

The development of follow-up services post-critical care discharge is an important factor in reducing the risk of readmission. However, unless other factors are also addressed, these services will be unable to make a significant impact. Crucially, there is a need to ensure that patients are physiologically ready to move to a reduced level of monitoring, support, and intervention. As long as critical care bed capacity remains a major deciding factor determining discharge, it is unlikely that patients will always be discharged appropriately. Therefore it is vital that capacity should be sufficient to prevent early discharge likely to compromise a patient's potential for survival and the risk of developing new complications.

Problems for patients recovering from critical illness

Long-term physical and psychological effects are often associated with an episode of critical illness. The significant increase in mortality rate seen in the first year after critical care discharge does flatten off, but can remain a factor for the next 15 years (Williams *et al.* 2008). Many patients also experience well-recognized physical and neurocognitive problems after discharge which may impact significantly on their quality of life ('survivorship'). The proposed term for new or worsening problems in physical, cognitive, or mental health status associated with recovery from a critical illness is post-intensive care syndrome (Needham *et al.* 2012). Examples of these physical and psychological problems are given in Boxes 1.8 and 1.9.

Acquired muscle weakness is a significant factor in the long-term physical limitation of critical care patients. This is associated with the severity and

Box 1.8 Examples of physical problems after intensive care

- Recovering organ failure (e.g. lung, kidney, liver, etc.)
- Muscle wasting and weakness
- Reduced cough power
- Pharyngeal weakness
- Joint pain and stiffness (particularly shoulders)
- Numbness, paraesthesiae (peripheral neuropathy)
- Taste changes resulting in favourite foods being unpalatable
- Itching, dry skin
- Disturbances of sleep rhythm and pattern
- Waking at night, poor sleep, not rested
- Cardiac and circulatory decompensation
- Postural hypotension (autonomic neuropathy)
- Heart failure
- Reduced pulmonary reserve
- Breathlessness on mild exertion
- Increased work of breathing
- Disturbed sexual function
- Iatrogenic
- Tracheal stenosis (e.g. repeated intubations)
- Nerve palsies (needle injuries)
- Scarring (needle and drain sites)

Data from Griffiths, R.D., Jones, C., Practical aspects after intensive care. In: *Outcomes in Critical Care* (ed. S. Ridley), pp. 169–80, 2002, Butterworth-Heinemann, Oxford.

Box 1.9 Psychological problems following intensive care

- Depression
- Anger and conflict with the family
- Anxiety about recovery to normal state
- Panic attacks
- Fear of dying
- Guilt
- Recurrent nightmares
- Post-traumatic stress disorder

Data from Griffiths, R.D., Jones, C., Practical aspects after intensive care. In: *Outcomes in Critical Care* (ed. S. Ridley), pp. 169–80. 2002, Butterworth-Heinemann, Oxford

duration of the systemic inflammatory response, the length of critical care stay, and the duration of mechanical ventilation. Other possible causes include hyperglycaemia, hypo-albuminaemia, parenteral nutrition, corticosteroid administration, and neuromuscular blocking agents.

Clearly, early yet appropriate rehabilitation, including mobilization, is key to recovery (NICE 2009). A rehabilitation team consisting of a nurse, a therapist, and a healthcare assistant has been shown to positively impact on recovery and length of stay in hospital following critical care (Rooney 2013). Pharmacological methods of preventing atrophy or accelerating recovery, such as the use of testosterone or growth hormone, have had detrimental effects. Preliminary studies of the use of electrical muscle stimulation suggest that this is a possible non-pharmacological method of preventing muscle atrophy as it is a passive process not requiring patient effort or compliance (Puthucheary *et al.* 2010). However, discomfort may limit its widespread application.

NICE guidance on rehabilitation after critical illness (NICE 2009) suggests that multidisciplinary rehabilitation strategies after critical illness can aid physical recovery and help people cope with the physical and non-physical problems associated with critical illness. Their recommendations include the following elements of structured care.

- Healthcare professional(s) with the appropriate competencies should coordinate the patient's rehabilitation pathway.
- Ensure that short- and medium-term rehabilitation goals are reviewed, agreed, and updated throughout the pathway.
- Ensure delivery and support of a structured self-directed rehabilitation manual, when applicable.
- Liaise with primary/community care for functional reassessment 2–3 months after discharge from critical care.
- Ensure that information, including documentation, is communicated between hospitals, and to other hospital-based or community rehabilitation services and primary care services.
- Give patients the contact details of the appropriate healthcare professional(s) on discharge from critical care, and again on discharge from hospital.

Enhancing recovery

During the critical care stay

Knowledge of potential risk factors associated with long-term physical and psychological complications, and early intervention to prevent their occurrence, are vital to improve the quality of life of critical care survivors. Risk factors include an extended duration of ventilation, SIRS and sepsis, hyper- and hypoglycaemia, immobility and length of bed rest, systemic corticosteroids, age, pre-existing impairments in physical and cognitive function, previous psychiatric disorders, development of critical illness polyneuropathy, severity of illness, sedation, agitation, and delirum. Very few interventions have been clearly associated with minimizing the effects of these factors, but some research has identified limited positive effects.

Recommendations for enhancing recovery during the patient's critical care stay (NICE 2009) include the following.

- Early identification of patients at risk of developing physical and non-physical morbidity.
- Comprehensive clinical assessment.
- Agreement of short- and medium-term rehabilitation goals with the patient and their family/carer.
- Early commencement of rehabilitation including appropriate nutritional support, physiotherapy, and mobilization. There should be a structured individualized programme with appropriate levels of information for both patient and family/carer.

> **Box 1.10 Delusional memory and post-traumatic stress disorder**
>
> **Delusional memory**
>
> **Definitions**
>
> - A dream, nightmare, or hallucination experienced by the patient during their stay in critical care
> - A belief or memory of critical care that has been rejected as false by the patient
> - A belief or memory of events in critical care that is not shared by medical/nursing staff or family members present during the patient's stay
>
> **Post-traumatic stress disorder**
>
> **Definition**
>
> - Post-traumatic stress disorder (PTSD) is the development of characteristic symptoms after one or more traumatic events. Events that trigger PTSD involve experiencing a serious threat to one's own physical integrity, which is experienced with intense fear, horror, and helplessness. Diagnostic criteria for PTSD include a history of exposure to one or more traumatic events and symptoms from each of three symptom clusters: intrusive recollections, avoidant/ numbing symptoms, and hyper-arousal symptoms
>
> Data from Schelling, G., Stoll, C., Haller, M., *et al.* Health-related quality of life and posttraumatic stress disorder in survivors of the acute respiratory distress syndrome. *Critical Care Medicine*, Vol. 26, pp. 651–9, 1998, Lippincott Williams & Wilkins Inc.

Interventions and drugs known to be associated with long-term complications should be avoided or minimized if possible. These include corticosteroids, which can cause a steroid-induced myopathy (Hough *et al.* 2009), and neuromuscular blockers, which have been associated with polyneuropathy. Excessive use of sedation can increase the risk of post-traumatic stress disorder (see Box 1.10) as well as muscle atrophy. Delirium and hypoglycaemia are also associated with increased cognitive dysfunction (Girard *et al.* 2010, Duning *et al.* 2010) both during and after critical care.

Enhancing recovery following surgery

The enhanced recovery programme is designed to improve the process of surgical care by implementing a bundle of evidence-based pre-, intra-, and post-operative procedures that benefit patient outcomes and therefore reduce length of stay. The programme focuses on the inclusion of the patient as an active participant in their own recovery process. There are four elements to the programme:

- pre-operative assessment, planning, and preparation including patient education, enhanced nutrition, and physical assessment before admission
- reducing the physical stress of the operation by using minimally invasive surgery, local infiltration anaesthetic techniques (where applicable), and guided fluid management using Doppler or similar monitoring
- a structured approach to immediate post-operative and intra-operative management, including pain relief
- early mobilization with enhanced analgesic and physiotherapy support.

Impact has mainly been seen in orthopaedic and colorectal surgical interventions (Ibrahim *et al.* 2013)

This project by the NHS Institute in the UK is based on initiatives from a team in Denmark, led by Henrik Kehlet, working with colorectal patients. It includes the need for effective pre-operative assessment to enable optimization of organ function, and reducing the stress of the operation to improve patient recovery employing techniques such as regional anaesthesia, minimally invasive surgery, and normothermia (Wilmore and Kehlet 2001). Normothermia is associated with a threefold reduction in wound infection, a reduction in blood loss, a decrease in cardiac events, and improved patient comfort. Post-operative care includes a reduction in drains, nasogastric tubes, and urinary catheters, an increased level of mobilization, early and effective treatment of pain and nausea, and the initiation of oral intake 6 hours post-surgery. Positive outcomes for the patient include reduction in wound infection rates, earlier return home and lower levels of pain.

The transition from critical care to ward

Seamless transfer of care of patients from critical care to the ward requires preparation, communication, and information for the patient, ward staff, and allied health professionals including physiotherapists, dietitians, pharmacists, and speech and language therapists. Preparation should include careful identification and consideration of the needs of the patient through a comprehensive assessment (NICE 2009). Transfer will be discussed in more detail in Chapter 3.

Follow-up clinics

Critical care follow-up clinics first started in the UK in 1990 in Whiston Hospital, Liverpool (Griffiths and Jones 2002). A comprehensive review of long term problems post-critical care (Desai *et al.* 2011) identified physical, psychological, and cognitive impairment, as well as a reduction in quality of life and an increased requirement for healthcare in this group of patients. This often impacts on family members, with issues such as depression and disruption of lifestyle and employment.

Patients are seen in the clinic 2–6 months after discharge from hospital, allowing assessment of their physical and mental state. Questionnaires and a comprehensive assessment process support the identification of problems and the opportunity to refer to appropriate specialist support or treatment. The patient (and family) have the opportunity to raise issues and ongoing problems associated with their critical care stay and illness. For many, it is their only opportunity to discuss what happened to them during a period where they often have no memory, or a distorted memory, of events. Follow-up clinics also give critical care staff a more complete understanding of the effects of critical illness and the ability to see the patient's experience of critical illness as a whole. This provides very useful feedback about the positive or negative impacts of their interventions, and important learning points that can change practice.

Enhancing the care of critically ill patients throughout the continuum

Categorizing levels of patient need

A national UK expert group report (Department of Health 2000) recommended that patients should be categorized according to their level of need rather than their geographical location. These levels are defined in Table 1.5. A more detailed explanation and definitions was published by the UK Intensive Care Society (ICS) (Intensive Care Society 2002). The ICS definitions allow the demand for different levels of care to be assessed and quantified throughout the hospital, removing geographical location from being the defining factor in the patient's access to critical care skills.

Table 1.5 Levels of patient need

Level	
0	Patients whose needs can be met through normal ward care in an acute hospital
1	Patients at risk of their condition deteriorating, or those recently relocated from higher levels of care whose needs can be met on an acute ward with additional advice and support from the critical care team
2	Patients requiring more detailed observation or intervention including support for a single failing organ system or post-operative care, and those stepping down from higher levels of care
3	Patients requiring advanced respiratory support alone or basic respiratory support together with support of at least two organ systems—this level includes all complex patients requiring support for multi-organ failure

Reproduced from *Comprehensive Critical Care: A Review of Adult Critical Care Services*, Department of Health, 2000, p. 10.

Changes to ward nursing

The general level of skill for nursing acutely ill patients on the ward has reduced over the years for the following reasons:

- reduction in numbers of qualified nurses on the ward
- expanding demands on nursing time from other components of the role
- increasing dependence on unqualified staff to undertake patient observations
- increasing use of automated BP and O_2 saturation monitors by nursing assistants rather than qualified staff, with an accompanying reduction in awareness of their accuracy and limited use of alternative methods of patient assessment
- decreased teaching on acute care skills within the preregistration curriculum
- increased numbers of intensive and high dependency beds.

In an attempt to reverse this trend, outreach services from critical care have delivered increased levels of focused education for ward staff as well as assistance/

support for the care of the patient in the general ward. This is a change from the 'swoop and scoop' approach, where patients were only seen by critical care staff at a very late stage in their deterioration followed by immediate removal to a higher dependency area. The aim is to reduce the level of deskilling in general nurses that is considered responsible for some of the poor care delivery for dependent patients on the wards. An alteration in behaviour is evident, with increased use of respiratory rate monitoring in the wards, appropriate referral to outreach teams, and associated improved outcomes (Odell *et al.* 2002; Priestley *et al.* 2004).

However, nurses do not care for patients on their own. There is also clear evidence that medical staff working in general hospital wards have limitations which affect their ability to respond effectively to the acutely deteriorating patient on the ward (McQuillan *et al.* 1998; NCEPOD 2005). Therefore education needs to address the multiprofessional team; the use of clinical simulation training to enhance team working and develop appropriate responses has been shown to be highly effective.

Essential components of pre-ICU care, track and trigger systems for identification of patients with acute deterioration

To reduce the 'delay in recognition/failure to manage' acute illness of patients on the general ward there must be a system in place to support early recognition of deterioration and prompt intervention. Outreach services use warning signs of early patient deterioration, either in the form of indicators of physiological abnormality (e.g. RR >30 breaths/min) or as part of a scoring system (e.g. NEWS score—see Table 1.3). These markers (known as 'track and trigger' systems) alert the ward nursing and medical staff and also mandate a directed response (Box 1.11). Establishing such systems has become an accepted best practice for hospitals across England and Wales.

The outreach team response varies depending on how it is set up (Department of Health and Modernisation Agency, 2003). Many systems require a response within strictly defined time limits by the patient's own nursing and medical team. However, more commonly, a designated person or team will respond to the call, providing immediate access to expert critical care assistance.

The gold standard for an outreach service is likely to be a 24 hour/7 day team that can provide round-the-clock support for acutely ill patients on the ward.

Box 1.11 Example of a track and trigger system: Patient Emergency Response Team (PERT) call criteria

Patient Emergency Response Team call criteria

Call the outreach nurse if:

- respiratory rate <8 or >25 breaths/min
- oxygen saturation <90% on ≥35% inspired oxygen
- heart rate <50 or >125 bpm
- systolic BP <90 or >200 mmHg (or has dropped >40mmHg from baseline)
- sustained alteration in conscious level
- the patient looks unwell or you are worried about their clinical state.

Consider calling the outreach nurse and/or alert the patient's own doctor, and increase monitoring frequency if:

- urine output is <30ml/h for two consecutive hours
- hypoglycaemia continues despite glucose support.

It will be useful for the development of future services to compare the impact of different types of service set-up to establish the importance of having 24-hour cover. Similarly, attempts are being made to establish and validate the national track and trigger system (NEWS), identifying indicators and scores that are both adequately sensitive (to ensure patients are not missed) and specific (so that predominantly the right patients trigger a response).

Auditing the impact of pre-critical care intervention

All outreach services should incorporate data collection as part of their role. This allows evaluation of the impact of the service and provides a rich source of data for feeding back to hospital staff and improving services. To establish a global view of the effect of outreach, the following indicators should be considered, ideally on a rolling year-by-year basis, and certainly before and after any major structural change to the service:

1. Outreach team performance:
   - number of cardiac arrest calls per 1000 hospital admissions
   - number of critical care readmissions from the ward

- percentage of outreach calls requiring critical care admission
- length of stay, morbidity, and mortality associated with critical care admissions from general wards via outreach
- level of acute illness (using APACHE II and/or SAPS scores) in patients admitted to critical care via outreach
- number of facilitated and appropriate 'Do not attempt resuscitation' orders
- number of averted critical care admissions, and any impact on patient mortality and morbidity
- timing of critical care referral in relation to patient need and morbidity
- change in overall hospital mortality rates.

2. Ward staff performance:
   - number of cardiac arrest calls per ward, with unnoticed physiological deterioration in the hours prior to arrest
   - number of inappropriate arrest calls for patients in the terminal stages of their illness
   - incidence and frequency of observations recorded appropriately (e.g. respiratory rate)
   - assessed performance of specific skills such as suctioning of tracheostomies
   - attendance at outreach calls for patients by the patient's own team (collaborative working).

Components of care post-critical care

Relocation or transfer from the critical care environment can be extremely stressful for the patient and their family. Relocation stress is defined as 'a state in which an individual experiences physiological and/or psychosocial disturbances as a result of transfer from one environment to another' (Carpenito 1997). Components likely to influence the patient's perception of the transfer have been identified by McKinney (2002) and are detailed in Figure 1.5.

Conflicting evidence exists as to how significantly ward transfer impacts upon the patient. Compton (1991) and Odell (2000) found that patients seemed to view the transfer in fairly neutral terms, with anxiety about the reduction in levels of care being tempered by the positive aspect of being well enough to move. However, Hall-Smith *et al.* (1997) found that some patients described the experience as 'highly traumatic'. Brodsky-Israeli and Dekeyser Ganz (2011) found that transfer anxiety was associated with length of critical care stay and the amount of social support, and that women registered higher levels of anxiety than men.

Suggested interventions that may improve the transfer experience and reduce relocation stress include:

- pre-transfer preparation and teaching (Cutler and Garner 1995)
- use of written information as a leaflet or booklet for both patients and families (McKinney 2002; Paul *et al.* 2004)
- accentuation of the positive nature of transfer by critical care staff (McKinney 2002)
- good communication between ward staff and critical care staff with a visit to the patient in intensive care from a member of the ward staff prior to transfer (Hall-Smith *et al.* 1997).

Personal Factors

Coping Constraints
- Pain
- Fatigue
- Lack of control
- Frequent interruptions

Coping Resources
- Personal relationships (with family, carers, etc.)
- Problem-solving skills

Internal Demands
- Decreased physical health

Environmental Factors

External Constraints
- Noise
- Lack of privacy
- Unfamiliar setting
- Attachment or disconnection to machines/infusions

Demands
- Compliance with therapeutic interventions

Factors and events are seen as either benign or a potential stress according to the patient's personal beliefs and coping abilities

Figure 1.5 Components influencing patient perception of transfer to the ward.

Discharge planning and assessment for critical care patients

Development of a post-critical care follow-up service will allow these issues to be addressed and progressed, ensuring that the physical and psychological recovery of the patient is not impeded. A full assessment of the patient's physical and psychological needs should be carried out prior to transfer.

Progressing the patient's recovery in the ward

The recovering critical care patient will face many physical and psychological problems including:

1. **Muscle weakness and fatigue** Patients may lose up to 2% of their muscle mass per day because of the catabolic nature of their response to the illness. This may take up to a year to rebuild, and patients may have severely limited muscle power for the first few months, if not longer (Jones and Griffiths 2000). Ward staff are commonly unaware of this, and may inappropriately label patients as lazy, depressed, or unwilling to be independent unless an explanation is given.
2. **The after-effects of intubation/tracheostomy** Physical problems are commonly associated with artificial airways such as endotracheal and tracheostomy tubes. Suspected tracheal stenosis or tracheomalacia related to long-term or repeated intubation, and skin tethering related to poor healing of tracheostomies should be referred to ENT surgeons for early diagnosis and treatment.
3. **Swallowing difficulties and taste alterations** The involvement of speech and language therapists at this point will make a difference to the patient's safe recovery and early recognition of any long-term problem such as stricture formation. Taste alteration is common and can contribute to poor appetite.
4. **Breathlessness on mild exertion** Poor respiratory reserve can be associated with residual fibrosis from pulmonary infection or from cardiovascular limitations
5. **Altered sleeping patterns** Patients can have difficulty returning to their normal sleeping pattern and will often need naps during the day.
6. **Poor memory and lack of concentration** The ability to remember recent events may be affected by benzodiazepine or other sedative administration given during the patient's stay in critical care, but also to the underlying illness and its severity. There may have been a direct brain injury or secondary effects from sepsis, hypotension, or hypoxaemia. The ability to concentrate may also be affected and may take many months to recover. This can be very debilitating for patients, particularly if they have no memory of the severity of their illness (Griffiths *et al.* 1996). One proposed method of assisting with this has been the development of patient diaries (Bäckman and Walther 2001) which are used to record events (including photographs) on behalf of the patient, by either staff or family. However, a systematic review (Aitken *et al.* 2013) suggests that evidence for efficacy is limited at present.
7. **Nightmares, hallucinations, and delusional memories** (see Box 1.10). Up to 73% may have some kind of delusional memory at 2 weeks (Jones *et al.* 2001), while 33–60% (Russell 1999; Friedman *et al.* 1992) will have no memory of critical care after 2 months. Where delusional memory is combined with no memory of factual events, there is a significant likelihood of development of post-traumatic stress disorder (Jones *et al.* 2001).

Instituting a rehabilitation programme of exercise, information, and contact significantly improved SF-36 graded physical function scores in patients surviving critical care (Jones *et al.* 2003). However, giving the patients a discharge booklet alone did not affect the incidence of anxiety and depression (Jones and O'Donnell 1994). Patients should have ongoing follow-up, with the opportunity to discuss issues relating to their illness as well as their rehabilitation.

Components of a critical care follow-up clinic

Many survivors of critical illness have severe ongoing physical and psychological problems. The roots of these problems sit firmly within their critical care stay and should therefore be addressed by the same service; this not only allows the patient to have access to staff familiar with the environment and the patient's own experience but also allows the staff to develop a better understanding of the patient's ongoing issues and problems. The opportunity to research and learn about these issues can then be used to improve the way in which care is delivered and to lessen the adverse effects associated with critical illness.

In general, it is unlikely that patients who are admitted for short stays will need to attend a follow-up clinic. Most operate a cut-off system according to the length of time the patient has spent in a critical care unit (commonly ≥2 days or more). Although there is no evidence of a direct relationship between length of stay and long-term problems, it would seem likely that the longer the stay, the greater the impact on the patient and their family.

Follow-up clinics should have a multidisciplinary approach. Where possible a doctor, nurse, psychologist, physiotherapist, and dietitian should be involved. Many patients will not have returned to full health until at least 6 months after their discharge from hospital. Some never regain their previous state of health and their level of dependency may have risen significantly.

An important aspect of the clinic is to ensure that all staff are made aware of the patients' experiences while they were in the critical care environment. This can be both rewarding and educative for staff as they learn of the patients' progress and return to health, as well as developing an understanding of the way their actions are perceived or remembered by their patients, and how bad experiences can be remedied.

References and bibliography

Aitken, L.M., Rattray, J., Hull, A., *et al.* (2013). The use of diaries in psychological recovery from intensive care. *Critical Care*, **17**, 253.

Asger-Petersen, J., Mackel, J., Antonsen, K., Rasmussen, L.S. (2014). Serious adverse events in a hospital using early warning score. What went wrong? *Resuscitation*, **85**, 1699–1703.

Audit Commission (1999). *Critical to success—the place of efficient and effective critical care services within the acute hospital*. Report, Audit Commission, London.

Bäckman, C., Walther, S. (2001) Use of a personal diary written on the ICU during critical illness. *Intensive Care Medicine*, **27**, 426–9.

Bagshaw, S., Bellomo, R., Kellum, J. (2008) Oliguria, volume overload, and loop diuretics. *Critical Care Medicine*, **36**(Suppl.), S172–8.

Ball, C., Kirby, M., Williams, S. (2003). Effect of the critical care outreach team on patient survival to discharge from hospital and readmission to critical care: non-randomised population based study. *British Medical Journal*, **327**, 1014–18.

Bellomo, R., Goldsmith, D., Uchmo, S., *et al.* (2003). A prospective before-and-after trial of a medical emergency team. *Medical Journal of Australia*, **179**, 283–7.

Bristow, P.J., Hillman, K., Chey, T., *et al.* (2000). Rates of in-hospital arrests, deaths and intensive care admissions: the effect of a medical emergency team. *Medical Journal of Australia*, **173**, 236–40.

Brodsky-Israeli, M., Dekayser Ganz, F. (2011). Risk factors associated with transfer anxiety among patients transferring from the intensive care unit to the ward. *Journal of Advanced Nursing*, 67, 510–18.

Buist, M.D., Moore, C.E., Bernard, S.A., *et al.* (2002). Effects of a medical emergency team on reduction of incidence of and mortality from unexpected cardiac arrests in hospital preliminary study. *British Medical Journal*, **324**, 387–90.

Calzavacca, P., Licari, E., Tee, A., *et al.* (2010) Features and outcome of patients receiving multiple Medical Emergency Team reviews. *Resuscitation*, **81**, 1509–15.

Carpenito, L.J. (1997). *Handbook of Nursing Diagnosis*, p. 297. Philadelphia, PA: Lippincott Williams & Wilkins.

Chen, J.P., Ou, L., Hillman, K., *et al.* (2014). The impact of implementing a rapid response system: a comparison of cardiopulmonary arrests and mortality among four teaching hospitals in Australia. *Resuscitation*, 85, 1275–81.

Chen, L.M., Martin, C.M., Keenan, S.P. (1998). Patients readmitted to the intensive care unit during the same hospitalization: clinical features and outcomes. *Critical Care Medicine*, **26**, 1834–41.

Cioffi, J. (2000). Recognition of patients who require emergency assistance: a descriptive study, *Heart & Lung*, **29**, 262–8.

Cioffi, J., Markham, R. (1997). Clinical decision making: managing case complexity. *Journal of Advanced Nursing*, **25**, 265–72.

Compton, P. (1991). Critical illness and Intensive care: what it means to the client. *Critical Care Nurse*, **11**, 50–6.

Cutler, L., Garner, M. (1995). Reducing relocation stress after discharge from the intensive therapy unit. *Intensive and Critical Care Nursing*, **11**, 333–5.

Daly, K., Beale, R. Chang, R. (2001). Reduction in mortality after inappropriate early discharge from intensive care unit logistic regression triage model. *British Medical Journal*, **322**, 1274–6.

Dellinger, R.P., Levy, M., Rhodes, A., *et al.* (2013). Surviving Sepsis Campaign: International Guidelines for Management of Severe Sepsis and Septic Shock 2012, *Critical Care Medicine*, **41**, 580–637.

Department of Health (2000). *Comprehensive Critical Care. A Review of Critical Care Services*. Report, Department of Health, London.

Department of Health and Modernisation Agency (2003). *The National Outreach Report 2003*. Report, Department of Health, London.

Desai, S.V., Law, T.J., Needham, D.M. (2011). Long-term complications of critical care. *Critical Care Medicine*, **39**, 371–9.

Duke, G.J., Green, J.V., Briedis, J.H. (2004). Night-shift discharge from intensive care unit increases the mortality-risk of ICU survivors. *Anaesthesia and Intensive Care*, **32**, 697–701.

Duning, T., van den Heuvel, I., Dickmann, A., *et al.* (2010). Hypoglycemia aggravates critical illness induced neurocognitive dysfunction. *Diabetes Care*, **33**, 639–44.

Elliott, M., Worrall-Carter, L., Page, K. (2014). Intensive care readmission: a contemporary review of the literature. *Intensive and Critical Care Nursing*, **30**, 121–37.

Esmonde, L., McDonnell, A., Ball, C., *et al.* (2006). Investigating the effectiveness of critical care outreach services: a systematic review. *Intensive Care Medicine*, **32**, 1713–21.

Franklin, C., Mathew, J. (1994). Developing strategies to prevent in-hospital cardiac arrest: analysing responses of physicians and nurses in the hours before the event. *Critical Care Medicine*, **22**, 244–7.

Friedman, B., Boyee, W., Bekes, C. (1992). Long-term follow up of ICU patients. *American Journal of Critical Care*, **1**, 115–17.

Gajic, O., Malinchoc, M., Comfere, T. (2008). The stability and workload index for transfer score predicts unplanned intensive care unit patient readmission: initial development and validation. *Critical Care Medicine*, **36**, 676–82.

Girard, T.D., Pandharipande, P., Carson, S. *et al.*, (2010). Feasibility, efficacy, and safety of antipsychotics for intensive care unit delirium: the MIND randomized, placebo-controlled trial. *Critical Care Medicine*, **38**, 428–37.

Goldfrad, C., Rowan, K. (2000). Consequences of discharge from intensive care at night. *Lancet*, **355**, 1138–42.

Ghosh, R. and Pepe, P. (2009). The critical care cascade: a systems approach. *Current Opinion in Critical Care*, **15**, 279–83.

Goldhill, D.R., Sumner, A. (1998). Outcome of intensive care patients in a group of British intensive care units. *Critical Care Medicine*, **26**, 1337–45.

Griffiths, R.D., Jones, C. (2002). Practical aspects after intensive care. In *Outcomes in Critical Care* (ed. S. Ridley), pp. 169–80. Oxford: Butterworth-Heinemann.

Griffiths, R.D., Jones, C., Macmillan, R. (1996). Where is the harm in not knowing? Care after intensive care. *Clinical Intensive Care*, **7**, 144–5.

Hall-Smith, J., Ball, C., Coakley, J. (1997). Follow-up services and the development of a clinical nurse specialist in intensive care. *Intensive and Critical Care Nursing*, **13**(5), 243–8.

Hanane, T., Keegan, M., Seferian, E., *et al.* (2008). The association between nighttime transfer from the intensive care unit and patient outcome. *Critical Care Medicine*, **36**, 2232–7.

Harrison, D., Welch, C.A., Eddleston, J. (2006) The epidemiology of severe sepsis in England, Wales and Northern Ireland, 1996 to 2004: secondary analysis of a high quality clinical database, the ICNARC Case Mix Programme Database. *Critical Care*, **10**, R42.

Herlitz, J., Bång, A., Gunnarsson, J., *et al.* (2003). Factors associated with survival to hospital discharge among patients hospitalised alive after out of hospital cardiac arrest: change in outcome over 20 years in the community of Goteborg, Sweden. *Heart*, **89**, 25–30.

Hillman, K.M., Bristow, P.J., Chey, T., *et al.* (2001) Antecedents to hospital deaths. *Internal Medicine Journal*, **31**, 343–8.

Hodgetts, T.J., Kenward, G., Vlachonikolis, I.G., *et al.* (2002). The identification of risk factors for cardiac arrest and formulation of activation criteria to alert a medical emergency team. *Resuscitation*, **54**, 125–31.

Hough, C.L., Steinberg, K.P., Taylor Thompson, B.T., *et al.* (2009). Intensive care unit-acquired neuromyopathy and corticosteroids in survivors of persistent ARDS. *Intensive Care Medicine*, **35**, 63–8.

Ibrahim, M.S., Alazzawi, S., Nizam, I., Haddad, F.S. (2013). An evidence-based review of enhanced recovery interventions in knee replacement surgery. *Annals of the Royal College of Surgeons of England*, **95**, 386–9.

ICS Standards Committee (2003). *Evolution of Intensive Care in the UK Intensive Care Society*, pp. 3–4. Report, Intensive Care Society, London.

Intensive Care Society (2002). *Levels of Critical Care for Adult Patients*. Report, Intensive Care Society, London.

Jones, C., Griffiths, R.D. (2000). Identifying post intensive care patients who may need physical rehabilitation. *Clinical Intensive Care*, **11**, 35–8.

Jones, C., O'Donnell, C. (1994). After intensive care, what then? *Intensive and Critical Care Nurse*, **10**, 89–92.

Jones, C., Griffiths, R.D., Humphris, G., *et al.* (2001). Memory, delusions, and the development of acute posttraumatic stress disorder-related symptoms after intensive care. *Critical Care Medicine*, **29**, 573–80.

Jones, C., Skirrow, P., Griffiths, R., *et al.* (2003). Rehabilitation after critical illness: a randomised controlled trial. *Critical Care Medicine* **31**, 2456–61.

Kramer, A., Higgins, T.L., Zimmerman, J.E. (2012). Intensive care unit readmissions in U.S. hospitals: patient characteristics, risk factors, and outcomes. *Critical Care Medicine*, **40**, 3–10.

Lameire, N.H., Bagga, A., Cruz, D., *et al.* (2013). Acute kidney injury: an increasing global concern. *Lancet*, **382**, 170–9.

Lee, A., Bishop, G., Hillman, K., *et al.* (1995). The medical emergency team. *Anaesthesia and Intensive Care*, **23**, 183–6.

Lee, K., Angus, D., Abramson, N. (1996). Cardiopulmonary resuscitation: what cost to cheat death? *Critical Care Medicine*, **24**, 2046–52.

Lin, S.M., Huang, C.D., Lin, H.C., *et al.* (2006). A modified goal-directed protocol improves clinical outcomes in intensive care unit patients with septic shock: a randomized controlled trial. *Shock*, **26**, 551–7.

Lundberg, J.S., Perl, T.M., Wiblin, T., *et al.* (1998). Septic shock: an analysis of outcomes for patients with onset of hospital wards versus intensive care units. *Critical Care Medicine*, **26**, 1020–4.

Lyseng-Williamson, K.A., Perry, C.M. (2002). Drotrecogin alfa (activated). *Drugs*, **62**, 617–30.

McGloin, H., Adam, S., Singer, M. (1999). Unexpected deaths and referral to intensive care of patients on general wards. Are some cases potentially avoidable? *Journal of the Royal College of Physicians*, **33**, 255–9.

McKinney, A. (2002). Relocation stress in critical care: a review of the literature. *Journal of Clinical Nursing*, **11**, 149–57.

McLaughlin, N., Leslie, G.D., Williams, T.A., Dobb, G.J. (2007). Examining the occurrence of adverse events within 72 hours of discharge from the intensive care unit. *Anaesthesia and Intensive Care*, **35**, 486–93.

McQuillan, P., Pilkington, S., Allan, A., *et al.* (1998). Confidential inquiry into quality of care before admission to intensive care. *British Medical Journal*, **316**, 1853–7.

Meaney, P.A., Nadkarni, V.M., Kern, K.B., *et al.* (2010). Rhythms and outcomes of adult in-hospital cardiac arrest. *Critical Care Medicine*, **38**, 101–8.

Moon, A., Cosgrove, J.F., Lea, D., *et al.* (2011). An eight year audit before and after the introduction of modified early warning score (MEWS) charts of patients admitted to a tertiary referral intensive care unit after CPR. *Resuscitation*, **82**, 150–4.

Moreno, R., Agthé, D. (1999). ICU discharge decision-making: are we able to decrease post-ICU mortality? *Intensive Care Medicine*, **25**, 1035–6.

National Early Warning Score (2012). *Standardising the Assessment of Acute-Illness Severity in the NHS. Report of a Working Party.* London: Royal College of Physicians https://www.rcplondon.ac.uk/resources/national-early-warning-score-news.

NCEPOD (2005). *An Acute Problem. A Report of the National Confidential Enquiry into Patient Outcome and Death.* http://www.ncepod.org.uk/2005report/index.html

Needham, D., Davidson, J., Cohen, H., *et al.* (2012). Improving long-term outcomes after discharge from intensive care unit: report from a stakeholders' conference. *Critical Care Medicine*, **40**, 502–9

NICE (2007). *NICE Guideline CG50. Acute Illness in Adults in Hospital: Recognising and Responding to Deterioration.* http://www.nice.org.uk/guidance/cg50

NICE (2009). *Rehabilitation after Critical Illness*, p.19. http://www.nice.org.uk/nicemedia/live/12137/43526/43526.pdf

Nolan, J.P., Soar, J., Smith, G.B., *et al.* (2014). Incidence and outcome of in-hospital cardiac arrest in the United Kingdom National Cardiac Arrest Audit. *Resuscitation*, **85**, 987–92.

Odell, M. (2000). The patient's thoughts and feelings about their transfer from intensive care to the general ward. *Journal of Advanced Nursing*, **31**, 322–9.

Odell, M., Forster, A., Rudman, K., *et al.* (2002). The critical care outreach service and the early warning system on surgical wards. *Nursing in Critical Care*, 7, 132–5.

Paul, F., Hendry, C., Cabrelli, L. (2004). Meeting patient and relatives' information needs upon transfer from on intensive care unit: the development and evaluation of an information booklet. *Journal of Clinical Nursing*, **13**, 396–405.

Peberdy, M., Cretikos M., Abella, B.S., De Vita, M., *et al.* (2007). Recommended guidelines for monitoring, reporting, and conducting research on medical emergency team, outreach, and rapid response systems: an Utstein-style scientific statement. *Circulation*, **116**, 2481–500

Priestley, G., Watson, W., Rashidian, A., *et al.* (2004). Introducing critical care outreach: a ward-randomised trial of phased introduction in a general hospital. *Intensive Care Medicine*, **30**, 1398–1404.

ProCESS Investigators, Yealy, D.M., Kellum, J.A., Huang, D.T., *et al.* (2014). A randomized trial of protocol-based care for early septic shock. *New England Journal of Medicine*, **370**, 1683–93.

Puthucheary, Z., Harridge, S., Hart, N. (2010). Skeletal muscle dysfunction in critical care: wasting, weakness, and rehabilitation strategies. *Critical Care Medicine*, **38**(Suppl), S676–82.

Rich, K. (1999). Inhospital cardiac arrest: pre-event variables and nursing response. *Clinical Nurse Specialist*, **13**, 147–53.

Rivers, E., Nguyen, B., Havstad, S., *et al.* (2001). Early goal-directed therapy in the treatment of severe sepsis and septic shock. *New England Journal of Medicine*, **345**, 1368–77.

Rooney, A. (2013). Improving recovery with critical care rehabilitation. *Nursing Times*, **109**, 23–25.

Rosenberg, A.L., Hofer, T.P., Hayward, R.A., *et al.* (2001). Who bounces back? Physiologic and other predictors of intensive care unit readmission. *Critical Care Medicine*, **29**, 511–18.

Russell, S. (1999). An exploratory study of patients' perceptions, memories and experiences of an intensive care unit. *Journal of Advanced Nursing*, **29**, 783–91.

Schein, R.M., Hazday, N., Pena, M., *et al.* (1990). Clinical antecedents to in-hospital cardiopulmonary arrest. *Chest*, **98**, 1388–92.

Schelling, G., Stoll, C., Haller, M., *et al.* (1998). Health-related quality of life and posttraumatic stress disorder in survivors of the acute respiratory distress syndrome. *Critical Care Medicine*, **26**, 651–9.

Smith, G.B., Poplett, N. (2002). Knowledge of aspects of acute care in trainee doctors. *Postgraduate Medical Journal*, **78**, 335–8.

Smith, L., Orts, C.M., O'Neil, I., *et al.* (1999). TISS and mortality after discharge from intensive care. *Intensive Care Medicine*, **25**, 1061–5.

Stenhouse, C., Coates, S., Tivey, M., *et al.* (2000). Prospective evaluation of a modified early warning score to aid earlier detection of patients developing critical illness on a surgical ward. *British Journal of Anaesthesia*, **84**, 663.

van Zanten, A.R.H., Brinkman, S., Arbous, S., *et al.* (2014). Guideline bundles adherence and mortality in severe sepsis and septic shock. *Critical Care Medicine*, **42**, 1890–8.

Williams, T., Dobb, G., Finn, J., *et al.* (2008). Determinants of long-term survival after intensive care. *Critical Care Medicine*, **36**, 1523–30.

Wilmore, D.W., Kehlet, H. (2001). Management of patients in fast track surgery. *British Medical Journal*, **322**, 473–6.

Wilson, J., Woods, I., Fawcett, J., *et al.* (1999). Reducing the risk of major elective surgery, randomised controlled trial of preoperative optimisation of oxygen delivery. *British Medical Journal*, **318**, 1099–1103.

Yang, C.W., Yen, Z.S., McGowan, J.E., *et al.* (2012). A systematic review of retention of adult advanced life support knowledge and skills in healthcare providers. *Resuscitation*, **83**, 1055–60.

CHAPTER 2
The critical care environment

Introduction

The need for critical care was first recognized in the 1950s. The subsequent development and proliferation of these specialized areas of patient care was due to the following factors:

- the general advances in healthcare technology which occurred following the Second World War and the Korean War;
- the advent of mechanical ventilation, accelerated in response to the Copenhagen polio epidemic in 1952;
- the development of cardiac surgery with its requirement for intensive post-operative care.

As the speciality itself has progressed from these early beginnings, so too has the requirement for critical care units (CCUs), resulting in a demand that threatens to overwhelm provision.

The labour-intensive nature of the work and the need for specialist training has made the expansion of services both resource-consuming and very expensive. This has resulted in the recent development of a slightly different approach, known as comprehensive critical care or critical care outreach (see Chapter 1), which looks at responding to patient need in terms of their critical illness rather than their geographical location. This approach embraces the early recognition of patient deterioration in the ward area with a supportive response from teams with critical care skills, as well as providing continuation of support for patients who are discharged from the CCU. The specific goal in these patients is to prevent problems that may result in deterioration and readmission and reduce the demand on scarce, high resource intensive care beds. One aim of this approach is to reduce inappropriate admissions and to facilitate discharge, thus making CCU beds available for those patients who will benefit from them.

Therefore the patient should have access to appropriately skilled staff for the period of need rather than for only the period of their admission into a CCU (Department of Health 2000). The American Association of Critical Care Nursing (2015) underlined the need for certification in critical care as a benefit for patients, staff, and employers. However, access to specialist training and cost has meant that there are limited numbers of medical and nursing staff trained in critical care. This, together with the cost of such a resource, remains one of the factors limiting an increase in critical care beds.

Defining critical care

There are numerous definitions of critical care. The Intensive Care Society (ICS 2013) defines an intensive care unit as:

> . . . a specially staffed and equipped, separate and self-contained area of a hospital dedicated to the management and monitoring of patients with life-threatening conditions. It provides special expertise and the facilities for the support of vital functions and uses the skills of medical, nursing and other personnel experienced in the management of these problems. It encompasses all areas that provide Level 2 (high dependency) and/or Level 3 (intensive care) care as defined by the Intensive Care Society document *Levels of Critical Care for Adult Patients* (2009).

Most definitions are brief statements of the types of patients who would be admitted to critical care and do not provide a comprehensive picture of the work that is undertaken, nor do they contribute to an understanding of the service. However, there are useful common themes in determining the goals of critical care and using these to define the service.

Critical care exists to:

- provide care for severely ill patients with potentially reversible conditions
- provide care for patients who require close observation and/or specialized treatments that cannot be provided in the general ward
- provide care for patients with potential or established organ failure, most commonly the lungs
- reduce avoidable morbidity and mortality in critically ill patients.

In a comprehensive critical care approach, levels of care are used to define the patient's needs regardless of location (see Chapter 1).

There is still a need for a clearly defined critical care (or level 2/3 care) area where the skills of specialist personnel and technology can be successfully combined in the management and care of critically ill patients. It provides special expertise and the facilities for the support of vital functions and uses the skills of medical, nursing, and other personnel experienced in the management of these problems.

Which patients benefit from critical care?

Critical care should only be offered to those patients who are likely to receive real benefit for the following reasons.

- It can be physically distressing and potentially hazardous.
- It may be traumatic for patients emotionally, socially, and psychologically, and this combined cost should always be weighed against potential benefit.
- It is an expensive resource that has a major impact on other branches of healthcare when financial constraints are necessary.
- Critical care beds are limited. Data published in 2015 (HSCIC) identified 3,800 critical care beds in the UK—around 2.8% of total acute hospital beds. Comparisons of the number of critical care beds per head of population across a number of European countries, the USA, South Africa, China, and New Zealand found the highest number of beds in Gemany with 25 beds per 100,000 population and the lowest in the UK with fewer than four beds per 100,000 population (Murthy and Wunsch 2012).
- In a paper based on data from 2005, Wunsch *et al.* (2008) found a strong inverse correlation between hospital mortality rates and numbers of intensive care beds, suggesting that access to critical care that is not restricted by bed availability improves outcomes.

Identifying patients who will benefit from critical care

Predicting which patients will benefit from critical care is extremely difficult. Some categories of patients, e.g. haematological malignancy, previously had only limited access to critical care but turned out to have a similar (or even better) outcome than groups with unlimited access (Naik *et al.* 2001). Survival rates in the elderly are more likely to be dependent on level of frailty, chronic comorbidity, and cognitive function than on age per se, although this becomes an increasing independent factor over 75 years (Monkhouse 2013). Use of computerized prediction tools can only help to predict outcome risk and cannot determine which patients should be admitted and which should not.

The gradual broadening of groups likely to benefit from critical care has contributed to the increase in demand for these beds. While critical care bed numbers in England and Wales have risen significantly in the last 15 years, 35% of admissions stay for less than 24 h, usually for post-operative management (Hospital Episode Statistics 2015) (see Figure 2.1).

Holcomb *et al.* (2001) suggested that protocols and managed care would improve efficiency without necessarily needing to increase critical care bed numbers per se. The number of patients treated per critical care bed per year in England and Wales varies, but in 2013–2014 was on average 65 patients per bed, although this varies hugely depending on the type of critical care unit (Health and Social Care Information Centre 2015).

Some patients who are unlikely to benefit from critical care may be admitted either as a consequence of a medical/surgical intervention mishap, or in an emergency varies where the diagnosis and cause of the clinical deterioration is uncertain and refusal to admit would be inappropriate. Once the patient is in critical care and treatment has been instigated, moral and ethical dilemmas and family resistance can cloud the decision-making process in terms of continuing or escalating care. Where possible it is often advantageous to instigate care conferences involving the primary team, family, critical care staff, and other relevant parties to evaluate the benefits of ongoing critical care in a situation where survival is unlikely (this is discussed in more detail in Chapter 17).

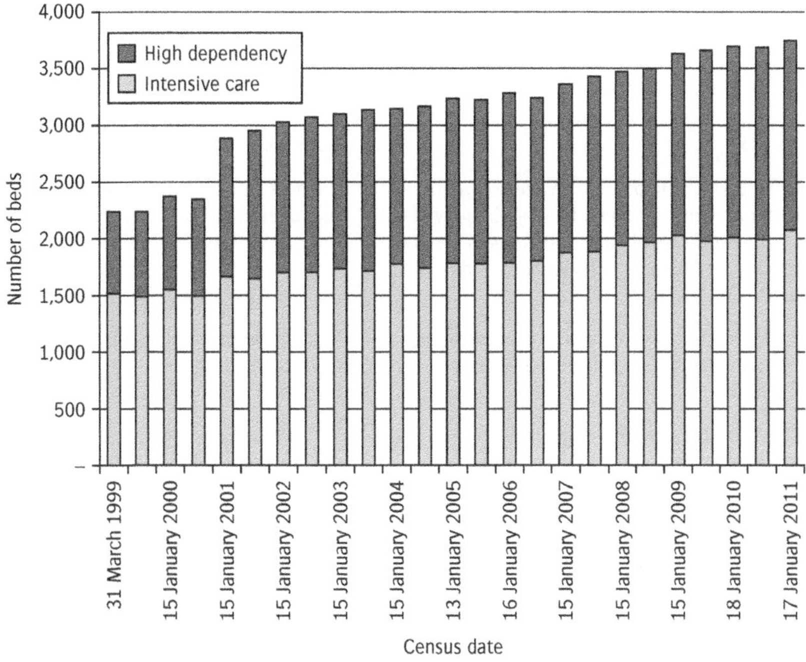

Figure 2.1 Increase in numbers of critical care beds in England and Wales 1999–2011.
Data from Hospital Episode Statistics (2011).

Admission guidelines

Units should have guidelines to direct appropriate utilization of critical care resources based upon evaluation of clinical priority and predicted benefit. A priority system model has been suggested by the American College of Critical Care Medicine (1999) which defines patients who will or will not benefit from critical care admission (Table 2.1). The dual purpose of this model is to support decisions on an individual patient need basis and to allow triage where bed availability is limited. Thirty-seven per cent of admissions to critical care in England and Wales are unplanned, meaning that, for many patients, decisions regarding admission are made under pressure.

Admission guidelines require an identified clinical lead, usually the consultant on call, to take responsibility regarding not only admission, but also discharge of patients to make space. UK guidelines for critical care admission (Department of Health 1996) suggest that the following factors should be considered prior to acceptance:

- little or no potential to reverse the illness
- presence of significant comorbidity
- stated or written preference against critical care.

If any of these factors are present, critical care should not be offered except under exceptional circumstances. Local policies may also include details of process and individual responsibilities for critical care consultants, the nurse in charge, and bed managers.

Discharge guidelines

Discharge is considered in the following circumstances, though the final decision will depend on associated factors such as level of care available on the wards, individual patient condition and needs, staffing, and expertise:

- the patient is stable and no longer requires active organ support
- the patient is no longer benefiting from the treatment available
- the patient (or family/partner) wish for transfer to palliative care facilities
- a persistent/permanent vegetative state is confirmed.

Details on planning for discharge and supporting/following up discharge are discussed in Chapter 1. Premature discharge is associated with increased morbidity, as is delay to discharge when medically fit (Garland and Connors 2013). This single-centre study found increasing improvement in survival with an odds ratio of 0.5 if delay was up to 20 h from the time the patient was declared medically fit. However, survival became increasingly poor if discharge was delayed beyond this, suggesting that many patients would benefit from up to a day longer in intensive care but do not benefit from prolonged delay to discharge.

Table 2.1 Priorities for admission of patients to critical care

Priority	Description	Example
1	Critically ill, unstable patients in need of intensive treatment and monitoring that cannot be provided outside the CCU. Usually these treatments include ventilator support, continuous vasoactive drug infusions, etc.	Patients with acute respiratory failure. Haemodynamically unstable patients.
2	Intensive monitoring is required and immediate intervention may be needed. No therapeutic limits are stipulated.	Patients with chronic comorbid conditions who develop acute severe illness which is potentially reversible.
3	Critically ill patients with a reduced likelihood of recovery because of underlying disease or the nature of their acute illness.	Patients with metastatic malignancy complicated by infection or airway obstruction.
4	Patients who are either (i) too well or (ii) too sick for critical care and therefore generally not appropriate for the CCU unless under highly specific circumstances. This may also apply to patients who have made a conscious decision not to undergo critical care	(i) Patients with low-level needs that can be met in the ward area with support such as mild congestive heart failure, stable/conscious drug overdose. ((ii) Patients with terminal irreversible illness such as unresponsive metastatic cancer, severe irreversible brain damage, or persistent vegetative state.

Good communication between critical care and ward staff regarding the patient's history and needs is essential. Different methods of ensuring this include the use of transfer documentation, planned visits by ward staff prior to transfer, and named links between critical care and ward nursing staff to facilitate queries. An outreach service will provide a link between the two areas.

The critical care unit as part of the hospital

The number of acutely ill patients in hospital has increased due to many social and disease-related factors (see Box 2.1). This has impacted considerably upon the level of dependency of patients nursed in general wards and has generated an increased demand for higher levels of care (see Figure 2.2). The continuum of enhanced levels of care now includes such areas as post-anaesthesia care units (24-hour recovery units), high dependency units, critical care units, step-down units, and progressive care units. None of these areas have been clearly defined and it is perhaps easiest to use the levels of care distinction (see Chapter 1) rather than this ill-defined group of titles.

Box 2.1 Factors increasing the number of acutely ill hospital in-patients

- Increasingly elderly population
- Increased survival in chronic disease
- Increased ability to treat, and therefore survival, in acute disease
- Increasing comorbidity
- Hospice/community facilities for dying patients
- Increasing expectations from service users
- Moves to treat less acute interventions in the community or as day surgery

Geographical location of the critical care unit

Ideally, the CCU should be situated in close proximity to the source of the patients and to the support services that are most frequently required (Valentin *et al.* 2011) (Figure 2.3). Transport between the source of

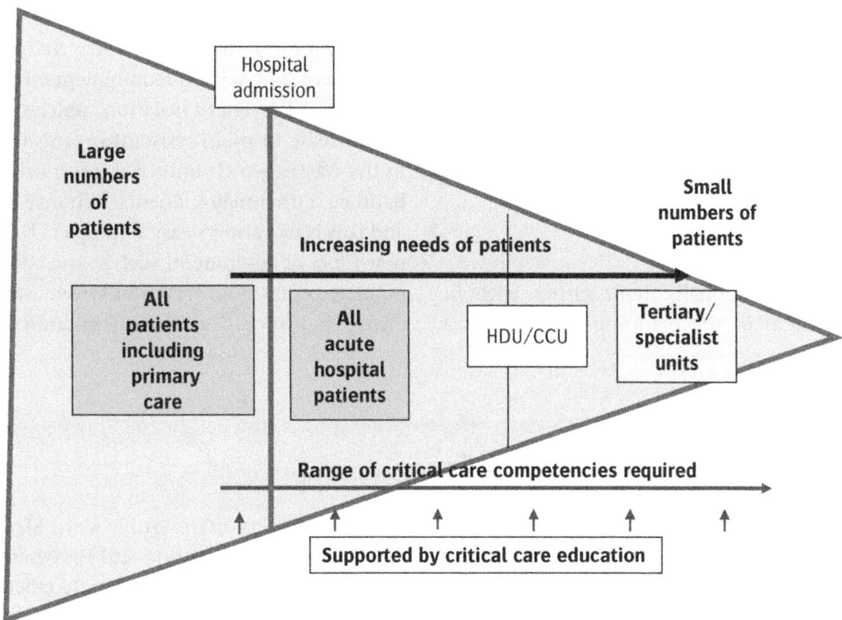

Figure 2.2 Modelling the patient continuum through hospital and critical care admission.

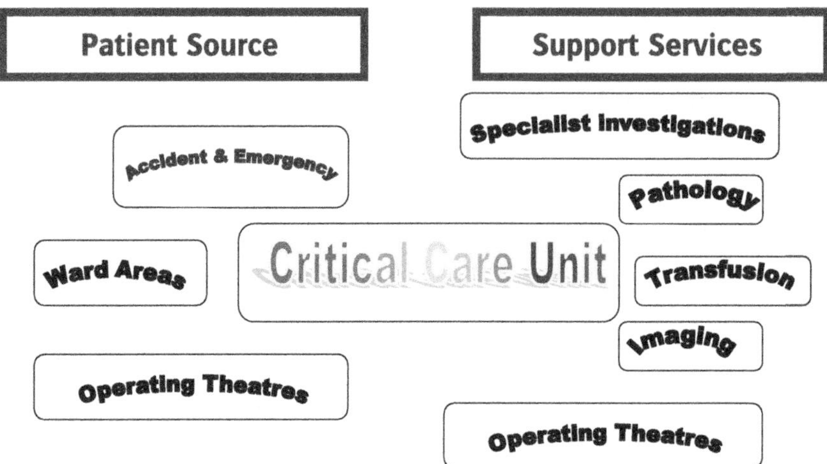

Figure 2.3 Location of critical care with reference to patient sources and support services.

patients or support services and the CCU should ideally be facilitated by the provision of dedicated lifts that are spacious enough to accommodate critically ill patients and the equipment and staff needed to accompany them.

Communications between these areas can be enhanced by direct telephone lines and/or intercom systems. The use of computerized reporting systems for records and results has reduced many of the difficulties of obtaining information from blood tests, but until digital imaging (picture archiving and communication system (PACS)) is available for all hospitals, the difficulties of access to X-ray films in the clinical area will remain.

Movement of patients from one area of the hospital to another during the acute phase of critical care can be a high risk procedure, so staff and equipment must be appropriate for the task (see Chapter 3 for further details).

The critical care unit

Many CCUs were traditionally built either without clinician involvement in the planning stages or as a compromise situation in an inappropriate area of the hospital. This increases the difficulties of working in the CCU environment and may add to risks to the patient, such as poor access to bed areas or insufficient space between beds adding to cross-infection risks.

CCUs must now be built to accepted standards. In the UK the Health Building Note Requirements (HBN 04-02) (Department of Health 2013) is a comprehensive document that gives clear guidelines on the size, components, distribution, facilities, and set-up of CCUs.

Planning a unit, which may take several years to build, requires a good deal of foresight in terms of future equipment and service requirements. For example, the number and design of isolation cubicles may depend on the increase in multi-resistant organisms or in changes in the way in which universal infection precautions are handled. Either may influence a change in requirements and this is not always easy to predict. The availability of new types of equipment, such as the addition of a computerized clinical information system, may also mean a change in bed space requirements and/or layouts.

General requirements for the design of a critical care unit

It has been suggested that the optimum working number of CCU beds is 8–15, or multiples thereof, based on a judgement that this number can be successfully managed by one consultant and their team (ICS 2013). This has been endorsed in recent recommendations from the Faculty of Intensive Care medicine (ICS 2013) and the European Society of Intensive Care Medicine (ESICM) (Valentin and Ferdinande 2011), where a minimum size of six beds (in order to operate efficiently) has also been suggested. It is likely that a unit with fewer than four beds, less than 200 admissions per year, or a bed occupancy <60% is not economical. It is also likely

Box 2.3 Disadvantages of open-plan bed areas in the CCU

- Less privacy for patients and relatives
- Increased risks of cross-infection
- The environment can be noisier with increased sensory overload

that sufficient numbers of admissions and therapeutic interventions are needed to ensure that the quality of staff competence and provision of specialist function is maintained.

Design

Most CCUs have a combination of open-plan areas and cubicles, with the recommended ratio being one or two cubicles per ten beds (Valentin and Ferdinande 2011, Department of Health 2013) (see Box 2.2). However, with the increasing number of multi-resistant organisms and an increase in neutropenic patients, both source and protective isolation needs have grown. Thus it is likely that one or two cubicles per six beds is nearer the requirement. Although expensive and difficult to staff, there are advantages to a 'single room for every patient' model in that infection risks may be reduced, noise is limited, and privacy can be maintained for both patient and family (see Box 2.3). Isolation rooms need to have negative/positive pressure capability and a lobby area for handwashing/donning personal protective equipment (PPE). Air filtration standards must meet the infectious diseases requirements, including the use of HEPA (high efficiency particulate air) filters and a minimum of six air changes per hour. However, some research suggests that automatic source isolation for methicillin-resistant *Staphylococcus aureus* (MRSA) may be unnecessary, as universal precautions are as effective in limiting its spread (Farr-Barry and Bellingan 2004, Cepeda *et al.* 2005).

Box 2.2 Advantages of open-plan bed areas in the CCU

- Easier observation of patients
- Faster mobilization of staff and equipment
- More economic to maintain bed areas/more effective use of resources such as staffing
- Improved staff support and motivation
- Patients may find the open areas more stimulating in the rehabilitation phase

Size of bed areas in the CCU

Recommendations for the size of CCU bed areas vary. The ESICM guidelines (Valentin and Ferdinande 2011) suggest a minimum of 20 m^2 for open-plan areas and 25 m^2 for cubicles, but the Health Building Note from the UK Department of Health (2013) recommends 25.5 m^2 for open plan and 30 m^2 for cubicles. There should be sufficient height (approximately 3 m) to accommodate pendant-style delivery of gases and other services and ceiling-mounted hoists. Sufficient room for the critical care team to move rapidly round the patient's bed, as well as space for additional technology such as haemofiltration and intra-aortic balloon pumps, is vital. In the rehabilitation phase, there must be space for the patient to sit out of bed and for family and friends to visit without feeling that they are compromising care or are in the way (see Box 2.4).

Safety in the CCU

While it is imperative that safety measures are adhered to in all parts of the hospital, there are significant additional factors which require heightened awareness in the CCU:

- a much greater abundance of electrical equipment located close to fluids and combustible gases
- the ubiquitous use of oxygen (a highly combustible gas)
- patients' dependence on a variety of technologies for life support.

These additional risks mean that all equipment should be checked prior to use for function and electrical safety and the following safety precautions should be followed.

- Any faults should be reported immediately and use of the equipment discontinued until the fault has been checked and repaired.
- All equipment should be regularly maintained.
- Accepted precautions for oxygen use should be scrupulously adhered to (i.e. no naked flames, antistatic flooring and footwear, increased atmospheric humidity, care when defibrillating, etc.).
- All staff should be aware of and be regularly updated in health and safety procedures, including the action required in the event of fire.

Box 2.4 Requirements for specific bed areas in the CCU

- Bed: mattress meeting needs of patients at high risk of developing pressure sores; electrically powered adjustment of patient position and bed height; tilt facility (Trendelenberg and reverse Trendelenberg); cot sides
- Patient monitoring facilities allowing continuous measurement of ECG, up to three transduced pressures, core and skin temperatures, arterial oxygen saturation, respiratory rate
- Ventilator, manual inflation bag with reservoir and oxygen supply, anaesthetic facemask, oropharyngeal airways, intubation equipment (if not on central trolley), humidifier or heat–moisture exchange (HME) system
- At least 28 electric sockets per bed, with half of these to be designated sockets with uninterrupted power supply (UPS)
- Up to four data outlets
- Powered ceiling-mounted pendants for location of data, power, gas, and vacuum outlets, emergency and nurse call systems, monitoring and computer systems, and some types of ventilator
- At least three oxygen points, two 4 bar compressed air points, and two vacuum outlets situated 1.5 m above the floor on a floor-, pendant-, or wall-mounted delivery system
- Provision for manual charting or computerized information systems
- Surfaces for preparation of infusions, drugs, and other interventions at an appropriate height
- Storage space for linen and minimal disposables such as syringes, oral care packs, gauze, dressings, etc.
- Storage space for patient's possessions and hygiene requirements

- Equipment should be available at each bedside in the event of mechanical or power failure (e.g. manual resuscitation bags, back-up oxygen cylinders). Torches and battery back-up equipment should be available.
- There should be the facility to turn off gas supplies and/or switch to a back-up system
- Evacuation equipment required in the event of a fire should be available at each bedside with fire mattresses in situ; all staff should be trained in their use.

Responsibility for patient safety rests equally with the organization and its employees. The organization is responsible for ensuring that procedures, equipment, and training are in place, and the employees are responsible for adhering to procedures, carrying out safety checks, and attending training.

Cleanliness and infection control

Hospital-acquired infections (HAIs) are a major problem. Approximately 9% of inpatients contract an HAI, and this is thought to contribute to around 5000 deaths per year in the UK. Critically ill patients are at high risk because of their compromised immune status and the large numbers of invasive procedures and devices which disrupt their defences. The most important and persistent source of cross-infection is probably unwashed hands (Fitzgerald *et al.* 2013, Pittet *et al.* 2000). In a study of missed opportunities for hand hygiene, Fitzgerald *et al.* (2013) found hand hygiene compliance to be 60% overall, but significantly less between the patient and the bedside trolley or computer (11% and 14% respectively). Hand hygiene and infection control practices are described in detail in Chapter 3. Specific design features, such as the availability and design of handbasins, will enhance the likelihood of handwashing, and positioning of hand gel dispensers will assist in their use (Scheithauer and Lemmen 2013).

Hand-basins should be available inside all single cubicles and just outside in the corridor for protective or source isolation. In open areas there should ideally be one hand-basin per bed. Each basin should have antiseptic scrub solutions, liquid soap, and alcohol gel. Towel dispensers should be kept supplied with towels, as wet hands are even more likely to act as vectors of infection if they become contaminated. Ideally, all taps should be elbow, foot, or sensor operated (Gould 1991).

The use and availability of protective disposable aprons, gloves, and eye/face protection are essential. Universal precautions should be followed by all staff; training in this and care bundles aimed at reducing specific infection risks such as ventilator-acquired pneumonia (VAP) should be part of all staff education (see Chapter 3 for more details).

Storage areas for drugs, fluids, and disposables should be close to the patient area but enclosed so that vector transmission is limited. A storage space designated for all cleaning materials and equipment within or in close proximity to the CCU is essential. Floors should be swept and mopped at least daily, and patient areas and equipment damp-dusted on a daily basis to reduce dust. There should be agreed protocols within the unit for the cleaning of bed areas following patient discharge. There should also be protocols to determine protective and source isolation procedures which every member of staff needs to be aware of.

National guidance and cleaning standards should be followed, e.g. The national specifications for cleanliness in the NHS: a framework for setting and measuring performance outcomes (e.g. Department of Health 2007).

Staff facilities

Critical care is a demanding working area and a staff rest room with facilities for making refreshments and snacks is essential. The consistently warm air-conditioned environment can be very dehydrating and staff (as well as some patients) will need access to cooled water throughout their shifts. Staff facilities must be separate from any patient food preparation area.

Staff also require a changing area with showering facilities to ensure that uniforms are not worn to and from work, thus transferring organisms to the home / community environment or vice versa. Even with a daily change of uniform, home washing of uniforms is rarely adequate for all organisms and this may allow further cross-exposure for patients who are vulnerable.

Other necessary staff areas are an office for general use with computer and small library facilities, a teaching area, and a room for on-call medical staff. The extension of the European working time directive to doctors in training from 2003 and the ruling that 'on-call' time is counted as working hours has meant the introduction of shift systems for many medical staff. This has obviated the need for bedroom availability for junior staff, though in many European countries consultants are resident on-call so overnight facilities should be provided for them.

Visitor facilities in the CCU

Visitors need a general waiting room which should be apart from the main unit to avoid observation of any potentially disturbing situations. The room should have toilets, telephones, and refreshment facilities and be decorated in a relaxed and informal style. In some cases, relatives require a room in which to stay overnight, and this should be available as near as possible to the unit. A room for private discussions with staff or used as a quiet area after hearing bad news or bereavement is also useful; again, this should be decorated in a soothing and relaxed style.

General decor in the CCU

Decoration should promote a relaxed and restful atmosphere for patients, staff, and visitors. It should be painted in a colour scheme that does not camouflage spillages as well as being appropriate to a restful mood, such as cool or neutral colours, and should be easily washable (Chambers and Bowman 2011). Any paintwork, especially on the ceiling, should be a matt rather than a gloss finish to avoid reflection and the glare that can be associated with it.

Wall-mounted clocks that are in easy view of the patient should be placed in every bed area so that patients in the rehabilitation phase can orientate themselves to time. All materials should be fire resistant.

Noise

Noise levels can be very high (sometimes exceeding 100 decibels (dB)), with averages of between 50 and 60 dB, mainly due to equipment alarms and constant activity. This can contribute significantly to sensory overload for the patient (see Chapter 3). The noises most likely to disturb patients include monitor alarms, patient admissions, conversations amongst staff, waste removal, and vacuum cleaning (Akansel and Kaymakci 2008). Walls and floors should use sound-absorbing materials so that transmission is limited as much as possible. Curtains or partitions between bed spaces should be of sufficient density to reduce the levels of transmitted general noise (Department of Health 2013). Decibel levels should be kept below 40 dB in the day and 30 dB at night. Management of equipment to reduce the incidence of false alarms can decrease the number of alerts and the overall level of sound (Schmid *et al.* 2013). Telephones need to be in a position where they can be heard and answered by staff, but this can cause considerable disturbance to patients. Cordless phones are ideal if staff are not in the immediate vicinity of the telephone or to enable patients to speak to callers. Waste bins should be fitted with silent closure mechanisms.

There has been debate over the safety of mobile phones in the CCU area as the signal was thought to cause artefactual alarm conditions in some equipment (Clifford *et al.* 1994). However, these fears have largely been allayed. There is a potential risk if the phone is very close to medical equipment (probably within a metre). Walkie-talkies are more liable to cause interference and thus should not be used close to medical equipment.

One of the major contributors to noise levels on the unit are the equipment alarms. Setting appropriate alarm parameters and responding immediately to alarms should be part of the principles of monitoring in the unit.

Lighting

It is desirable for CCUs to have windows allowing in natural daylight to assist in maintaining diurnal rhythms and to improve staff and family mood (Chambers and Bowman 2011). If the unit is situated on a lower floor with windows, there must be the facility to ensure privacy and provide shade. This can best be achieved by using blinds layered between glass or solar-tinted glass, as blinds and curtains external to the glass can be a source of cross-infection unless removed and washed between each patient.

Light levels have a significant impact on a number of biological processes, hormone secretion (e.g. cortisone and melatonin), and general alertness. Modulation of general immune function is also associated with exposure to light (Castro *et al.* 2011). Light affects the patient's mood and ability to recover as well as impacting on the performance of staff. Light levels are measured in lux or footcandles. Light levels <1 lux are about the brightness of moonlight and levels >32,000 lux are equivalent to a bright sunny day.

Good quality general lighting (recommended illumination of around 1600 lux) is important for staff performance. Either dimmer control or night lighting (recommended illumination 100–200 lux) should be provided in all areas (Ferdinande 1997). Additional examination lights and operating theatre style lights may be required for procedures.

Back-up emergency lighting in the event of electricity mains power failure is essential.

Storage, utility, and technical areas

Many CCUs have inadequate storage space for the large volumes of equipment, disposables, fluids, and drugs which must be immediately available in the area. Top-up services restocking CCU two or three times daily are one solution to this problem, but this is labour intensive and can be costly.

As the need for more readily available diagnostic/interventional equipment increases (e.g. echocardiography, bronchoscopy, ultrasound) more equipment needs to be situated within the CCU itself, and this places an additional demand on available storage space.

Utility areas should be separated into clean (treatment, preparation and storage of drugs, IV, and haemofiltration fluids, and equipment for procedures) and dirty (disposal of soiled linen and clinical waste, and sluice facilities). If possible, disposal of soiled linen and clinical waste from dirty utility areas should not pass through the unit.

Designated space is required for technical support, cleaning, repair, and maintenance of equipment. Ideally, this should be situated close to the equipment storage areas.

Testing facilities near the patient should be available for arterial blood gases, electrolytes, and glucose, and perhaps for other measures such as coagulation screens.

Emergency equipment

A defibrillator, drugs, and resuscitation equipment should be available in a central location in every CCU (see Box 2.5). They should be mobile and easily accessible. Intubation equipment may be kept either in a central location or at the bedside.

CCUs with cardiothoracic surgical patients should have equipment available for emergency thoracotomy (see Chapter 5), including diathermy and extra suction as well as a thoracotomy pack, internal defibrillation paddles, and drains.

Use of computerized clinical information management systems (CIMS)

The volume of data collected and interpreted by nurses in critical care has grown over the last 10 years. The level and sophistication of monitoring now available for all aspects of patient function has also increased. The development of computerized systems to manage this level of information has become increasingly accepted as a means of releasing nursing time to allow increased patient care. However, a systematic review of studies of time spent on documenting and on direct patient care had equivocal results, with only four studies finding increased direct patient care and decreased documentation time and 58 studies finding either no difference

Box 2.5 **Equipment requirements for a level 3 CCU**

Monitoring and documentation

Monitors with display capability for at least two or three waveforms, ECG, SpO_2, $ETCO_2$, respiratory rate, and 12-lead ECG

- Cardiac output capability
- Co-oximeter blood gas analyser with capability for measuring electrolytes, lactate, and blood glucose
- Computerized clinical information system
- Respiratory support

Patient-responsive third-generation ventilators

- CPAP and NIV devices
- Fibre-optic bronchoscope

Renal support

- Renal replacement therapy devices

Radiology

- Portable X-ray machine
- Digital X-ray system or viewer

Cardiovascular support

- Multiple infusion pumps (3–6)
- Syringe pumps (4–10)
- Defibrillator and external pacing device
- Pacing boxes and flotation pacing catheters

Nutritional support

- Enteral nutrition pumps
- Access to kitchen for snacks/oral diet

Miscellaneous

- Range of electronic beds according to patient's pressure risk, equipped with bedside rails, and dripstands
- Warming/cooling mattresses
- Fans or air conditioning
- Blood warmers
- Blood refrigerator
- Hoists and support chairs
- Commodes/urinals and bedpans
- Dressing trolleys
- Storage for drugs, equipment, cleaning facilities, linen

NIV, non-invasive ventilation; $ETCO_2$, end-tidal CO_2; CPAP, continuous positive airway pressure.

(five studies) or increased documentation (three studies) (Mador and Shaw, 2009)

These systems are designed to collect information from any electronic equipment capable of exporting data in a digital format and then transposing it into either graphical or numerical displays. These displays can be customized to suit the individual unit and then form an electronic patient record, which includes demographic, physiological, biochemical, physical, and interventional information.

However, the use of a CIMS has many more potential advantages than simply releasing the nurse from charting observations. The system may provide prompts and reminders as well as flagging up errors or triggering drug delivery. Some systems can detect a deterioration in the patient's physiology and notify the

Box 2.6 Advantages of CIMS

- Direct collection of information from monitoring systems
- Immediate access to unit policies and protocols through an intranet
- Development of prompts or reminders for care needs, e.g. two-hourly mouth care
- Automated identification of patient deterioration
- Electronic prescribing with error prompts
- Sharing of information across the professions—use of a multiprofessional record
- Reduction of repetitious note-recording, e.g. diagnosis recorded in the physician assessment is automatically transferred to other records such as daily problem lists, physiotherapy assessments, etc
- Immediate access to other electronic databases such as the hospital formulary and drug information
- Direct transfer of laboratory results into current patient records via computerized results services
- Retrieval of stored data is easier to access for audit, benchmarking, and research

Box 2.7 Disadvantages of CIMS

- Major requirements for training of both permanent and temporary staff.
- Confidentiality of patient records must be protected by a password system involving logging in and out of patient records. This must be managed by senior staff.
- Direct data collected must still be validated by staff, otherwise erroneous readings will be collected as true. For example, if the arterial line transducer is on the floor, the systolic reading will be much higher than in reality.
- Equipment data must have the capacity to feed directly into the CIMS, e.g. ventilators and infusion pumps as well as monitors.
- Staff must be confident in the system and its reliability.

caregiver of this trend. This deterioration may be far more subtle than a physiological value simply hitting a threshold that triggers an alarm, such as a BP monitor. Several physiological variables may be automatically integrated.The CIMS also provides a huge repository for audit and research, allowing data to be retrospectively interrogated to assess quality improvements, temporal changes in complication rates and outcomes, etc. (see Boxes 2.6 and 2.7).

Setting up a CIMS requires a huge investment of time and resource. However, the benefits identified, including rapid retrieval of data for audit, clinical decision support, and improved record-keeping for medico-legal purposes (Harmworth and Still 2002), make it worth the outlay.

Staffing

The number, variety and skills of the staff required in a CCU will reflect the level and activity of the unit. There are five main groups of staff:

- nursing (largest in number)
- medical
- allied health professionals
- administrative and clerical staff
- cleaning and portering staff.

In some CCUs, the nurses, medical staff, and administrative staff may be the only group permanently attached to the unit. Members of the various allied health professional groups will respond to referrals or provide a rotating cover service. However, in larger units there will be designated allied health professionals who will also be permanently attached (see Box 2.8). This has many advantages in terms of collaborative working, expertise, and sharing of skills and competencies.

Box 2.8 **Allied health professionals**

- Physiotherapists
- Pharmacists
- Radiographers
- Dietitians
- Speech and language therapists
- Medical physics technicians
- Occupational therapists
- Social workers

Nursing staff

There has been considerable debate over the numbers of nurses required to staff CCUs, and in particular over the nurse-to-patient ratio. While a full debate is not possible in this text, there are a number of issues worth considering.

1. The number of acutely ill patients in hospital is growing as methods of treatment change and the emphasis on primary healthcare increases. The number of patients surviving into old age, with an increasing likelihood of comorbidity, and the number of chronically ill patients surviving past middle age have all dramatically increased the workload associated with in-hospital nursing care. This means that patients in general wards are sicker and require more care, and are more likely to require critical care. The demand for critical care has also increased as more interventions/operative procedures have taken place on patients with complex comorbidity.
2. The number of qualified nurses available to deliver care has decreased, and is likely to decrease further as the effects of significant cuts in training places are felt.
3. The costs of staffing are high, and there are major financial implications to the institution of continuing to support such a high level of qualified nurse staffing
4. The average age of nurses is increasing. More than 25% of the nursing population are predicted to reach retirement age in the next 10 years (NMC 2002).

The implication of this is that there will be insufficient nurses available to maintain the current level of staffing in CCU. However, with a flexible approach to working with patients at different levels of need, it may be possible to continue to provide the highest quality of care within these limitations.

Staffing numbers in the CCU

Although the generally accepted gold standard in the UK for ventilated patients is one qualified nurse to one patient, there has been an increasing recognition that this is not sustainable in every situation. A more flexible approach which takes into account the competence of the nurse, the needs of the individual patient, and the availability of additional support staff is needed.

A common standard for staffing in critical care developed by all the UK critical care nursing associations (Bray *et al.* 2010) identifies the following requirements for delivering safe, high quality critical care nursing.

1. Every patient must have immediate access to a registered nurse with a post-registration qualification.
2. Ventilated patients should have a minimum of one nurse to one patient.
3. The nurse-to-patient ratio should not fall below one nurse to two patients.
4. The level of care needs required by each patient should equate to the skills and knowledge of the registered nurse delivering and/or supervising that care.
5. Units should employ flexible working patterns as determined by unit size, activity, case mix, and the fluctuating levels of care for each patient to ensure patient safety and care delivery.
6. A supernumerary clinical coordinator, who is a senior critical care qualified nurse, will be required for larger and geographically diverse units of more than six beds. The clinical coordinator's role is to ensure that effective, safe, and appropriate care is delivered each shift by managing and supporting staff and patients, and acting as a communicator and liaison between the rest of the multidisciplinary team.
7. When setting staffing levels, the layout of beds and use of siderooms/cubicles must be taken into account to ensure safe patient care.
8. Ongoing education for all nursing staff is of principal importance to ensure knowledgeable and competent care. Clinical educator posts should be utilized to support this practice.
9. Nursing assistants (NAs), also known as healthcare assistants (HCAs), play a key role in assisting registered nurses to deliver direct patient care and in maintaining patient safety (BACCN 2003). These roles should be developed to meet the demands of both patients and the unit. However, the registered nurse remains responsible for the assessment, planning, delivery, and evaluation of patient care.

10. The role of the assistant practitioner (AP) is not so well established, but individuals with this increased level of training can provide direct patient care under the supervision of a registered nurse, who will remain responsible for the assessment, planning, and evaluation of patient care. The effectiveness of the role of APs requires further evaluation and research.
11. Administrative staff should be employed to ensure that registered nurses are free to give direct patient care, and to support the unit and staff with essential data collection.

Although several studies have shown an association between patient outcome and the ratio of trained nurses to patients in critical care (Numata *et al.* 2006), these have all been observational without risk adjustment for illness severity. Impact on morbidity (e.g. infectious complications, length of weaning, and length of stay) has also been demonstrated and may be more representative of the effect of levels of nurse staffing. There is a minimum number of nurses below which the patient's recovery is put at risk, but this remains difficult to determine because of the number of confounding factors involved.

Nursing roles

The vast majority of nurses will be competent critical-care-trained nurses, delivering direct care at the bedside to the patient and supporting the patient's family and friends. There is a need for a shift leader or coordinator (the nurse in charge) and, frequently in larger units, another nurse to act as general support to junior or newly appointed nurses, provide meal breaks without compromising patient safety, and facilitate other organizational issues. The nurse in charge is responsible for the standard of patient care during his/her shift.

The continuing need for training in critical care skills means that a proportion of nurses will be novices or advanced beginners learning these skills while providing direct care as part of a structured critical care training course. They require supervision by the nurse in charge or other designated trained critical care nurse.

A number of units employ nursing assistants who are trained to assist the registered nurses in the delivery of nursing care. They may also have a stocking and cleaning responsibility.

The overall direction of the nursing staff will require a nurse manager/leader. In small units, one person can fulfil this role but in larger units the size of the task will require a manager and a professional/clinical lead as separate roles (Table 2.2).

The nursing establishment comprises a significant proportion of the overall unit budget and therefore must be managed efficiently and cost effectively. Maintenance

Table 2.2 Comparison of CCU manager, nurse consultant, and clinical nurse specialist roles

CCU manager	Nurse consultant	Clinical nurse specialist
Responsibility for delivery of the service	Responsibility for leadership and development of the nursing service	Responsibility for delivery of high quality nursing care
Responsibility for the budget	Responsibility for overall direction and participation in teaching and education	Responsibility for delivery of teaching and education
Responsibility for recruitment and retention process	Responsibility for strategies for recruitment and retention	Responsibility for delivery of strategies for recruitment and retention
Delivery of appraisal and IPR process*	Ensures appraisal and IPR occurs appropriately	Participates in appraisal and IPR
Deals with complaints and manages risk issues	Ensures that bench-marking, audit, and standard setting occur	Carries out benchmarking, audit, and standard setting
Manages staff	Leads on research.	Carries out research, may lead on it
	Develops/trials into new methods of delivering the service	
	Acts in a consultative role to the hospital trust on critical care nursing issues	

*IPR, individual performance review.

of standards of nursing care must be balanced with staffing requirements and the dependency of the patients admitted.

Education of nursing staff in the CCU

A balance is necessary in the nursing establishment between the number of fully trained critical care nurses and those who are in training. Units who train students on a post-registration general critical care course will require at least 50% of their staff to have undertaken the course in order to provide an adequate number of supervisors, mentors, and facilitators.

Critical care nurses must be appropriately trained and educated so that they possess the necessary level of knowledge, skills, and confidence to deliver safe and effective care to critically ill patients and their families (BACCN 2010). Critical Care courses are delivered by higher education providers (universities), and the course content and assessments will vary according to the institution. A position statement on curriculum content from the European Federation of Critical Care Nursing Associations (EFCCNA) outlines the recommended content (Box 2.9).

Multi-centre research looking at the impact of rates of specialist certification amongst nursing staff in surgical intensive care units found that higher numbers of specialist trained nurses significantly impacted on the incidence of central-line-associated bloodstream infections (Boyle *et al.* 2014). Mean rates of nurses with specialist certificates were 30.8% across 178 intensive care units. Other nurse-related outcomes such as pressure ulcers were not affected by the level of specialist education.

Box 2.9 Recommendations for nursing critical care course contents

- Anatomy and physiology
- Pathophysiology
- Pharmacology
- Clinical (physical) assessment
- Illnesses and alternations of vital bodily functions
- Medical indications and prescriptions with resulting nursing care responsibilities
- Psychological, social, and spiritual aspects
- Use and application of technology
- Patient and family education
- Legal and ethical issues
- Multicultural issues
- Plans of care and nursing interventions
- Clinical examination and diagnostic reasoning
- Hygiene and microbiology
- Health promotion and safety standards
- Professional and nursing roles in critical care
- Evidence-based multidisciplinary care
- Appropriate use of current research findings
- Information technology
- Communication and interpersonal skills

Reproduced from *Position Statement on Post-registration Critical Care Nursing Education within Europe*, European Federation of Critical Care Nursing Associations (EFCCNA), 2004. http://www.efccna.org/downloads/Position%20statement%20on%20education%20EfCCNa.pdf

Collaborative working and patient safety

There is a strong link between the way the intensive care team work and the safety of the patients. Failure of communication is a frequent source of error. A systematic review of literature around teamworking associated with a strong safety culture (Dietz *et al.* 2014) identified good communication as a key feature in high functioning teams as well as the need to focus on transition-orientated tasks. One of the few organizational features associated with benefit for both patient outcome and staff satisfaction is the process of collaborative working originally described by Baggs *et al.* (1997). Collaborative working was described as 'nurses and physicians cooperatively working together, sharing responsibility for solving problems and making decisions to formulate and carry out plans for patient care'. It depends on a multiprofessional approach to the patient's problems and needs which is coordinated (usually by the medical consultant) on the ward rounds.

Despite this recognition more than 20 years ago, discrepancies still remain. Perceptions between specific groups of staff about the quality of cooperation may differ. Thomas *et al.* (2003) surveyed 320 nurses and physicians working in eight US CCUs and found that nurses reported that, relative to physicians, it was difficult to speak up, disagreements were not appropriately resolved, more input into decision-making was needed, and nurse input was not well received. Nathanson *et al.* (2011) found a similar discrepancy when comparing junior medical staff perceptions of collaboration with those of the nursing staff. This difference was thought to be due to professional culture and a nursing focus on the patient's social history and the higher level of personal involvement. The researchers suggested that there was a need for multiprofessional training focusing on communication and teamworking.

An ethnographic systematic review of studies (Paradis *et al.* 2013) suggested that safety is improved by:

- enhancing relational elements amongst the team such as clarifying roles, improving the flow of information, and enhancing work relations and family relationships
- mapping workflows to identify error prone points and generating solutions to improve safety
- providing a space where clinicians can bond to improve both the work climate and emotional well-being
- including all stakeholders in the development of protocols, particularly around the transfer of responsibility for new technology and including the discussions of evidence on which they are based.

There is a clear relationship between all of these elements and a collaborative approach which supports a culture of safety and improvement.

In many cases collaborative working is facilitated by the presence of CCU-based teams of medical staff ('closed' rather than 'open' unit organization). A structured handover is essential as the patient's needs are complex, the number of professionals involved is large, and the potential risks of failing to pass on essential information are high. This type of working is supported by a multiprofessional patient record which is contributed to by all staff. The separation of notes by medical, nursing, physiotherapy, and other health professionals leads to duplication, confusion, and decreased communication.

If the written record cannot be completed as a common document, there is a strong need for regular handover and meetings to enhance verbal communication between professions. The larger the unit, the more important this becomes.

Medical staff

Each team of medical staff should be led by a consultant trained in critical care medicine who provides overall direction and supervision of care, as well as teaching, for junior medical staff, management, and leadership. It has been suggested that a full-time intensivist can reduce mortality rates and improve efficiency (Faculty of Intensive Care Medicine/Intensive Care Society 2013, Pronovost *et al.* 2002). The UK Faculty of Intensive Care Medicine and the Intensive Care Society recommend that the CCU is consultant led at all times (Faculty of Intensive Care Medicine/Intensive Care Society 2013). The number of medical staff should be related to the number of beds and patient workload. A member of the medical team should be resident or immediately available 24 hours a day.

The European Society for Intensive Care Medicine (ESICM) has developed a programme of training to ensure that all medical staff working in intensive care across Europe are trained to the same level (ESICM 2006). The competencies required include:[1]

(1) resuscitation and initial management of the acutely ill patients
(2) diagnosis—assessment, investigation, monitoring, and data interpretation
(3) disease management
(4) therapeutic interventions/organ system support in single or multiple organ failure
(5) practical procedures
(6) peri-operative care
(7) comfort and recovery
(8) end-of life care
(9) Paediatric care
(10) transport
(11) Patient safety and systems management
(12) Professionalism

They recommend that training in critical care should be at the higher professional training level for those wishing to make a career in the specialty. In common with some other European countries (e.g. Spain, Switzerland), critical care in the UK has achieved specialty status recognition and it is possible to train solely in critical care. The Faculty of Intensive Care Medicine has recently been established in the UK with a programme of training which ensures that specialist trainees will develop the right skills and experience. This can be 'stand-alone' or linked to another specialty such as anaesthesia, nephrology, or emergency medicine.

The ESICM also offers a remote access training programme (PACT) and a European Diploma of Intensive Care Medicine. Doctors who have trained for at least two years in critical care and four to five years in their basic speciality are eligible to apply.

1 Data from The CoBaTrICE Collaboration. Development of core competencies for an international training programme in intensive care medicine, *Intensive Care Medicine*, Volume 32, pp. 1371–83, 2006, Springer-Verlag.

References and bibliography

Adhikari, N., Fowler, R., Bhagwanjee, S., Rubenfeld, G. (2010). Critical care and the global burden of critical illness in adults. *Lancet*, **375**, 1339–46.

Akansel, N., Kaymakçi, S. (2008). Effects of intensive care unit noise on patients: a study on coronary artery bypass graft surgery patients. *Journal of Clinical Nursing*, **17**, 1581–90.

American Association of Critical-Care Nurses (2015). AACN scope and standards for acute and critical care nursing practice. http://www.aacn.org/wd/practice/docs/scope-and-standards-acute-critical-care-2015.pdf.

American College of Critical Care Medicine (1999). Guidelines for ICU admission, discharge and triage. *Critical Care Medicine*, **27**, 633–8.

Angus, D., Kelley, M.A., Schmitz, F.J., *et al.* (2000). Current and projected workforce requirements for care of the critically ill and patients with pulmonary disease. Can we meet the requirements of an aging population? *Journal of the American Medical Association* **284**, 2762–70.

BACCN (British Association of Critical Care Nurses) (2003). Health care assistants' role, function and development: results of a national survey. *Nursing in Critical Care*, **8**, 141–8.

BACCN (British Association of Critical Care Nurses) (2010). Standards for nurse staffing in critical care. http://icmwk.com/wp-content/uploads/2014/02/nurse_staffing_in_critical_care_2009.pdf.

Baggs, J.G., Schmitt, M.H., Mushlin, A.I., *et al.* (1997) Nurse–physician collaboration and satisfaction with the decision-making process in three critical care units. *American Journal of Critical Care*, **6**, 393–9.

Boyle, D.K., Cramer, E., Potter, C., *et al.* (2014) The relationship between direct-care RN specialty certification and surgical patient outcomes. *Association of Operating Room Nurses Journal*, **100**, 511–28.

Bray, K., Wren, I., Baldwin, A., *et al.* (2010). Standards for nurse staffing in critical care units determined by the British Association of Critical Care Nurses, the Critical Care Networks National Nurse Leads, Royal College of Nursing Critical Care and In-flight Forum. *Nursing in Critical Care*, **15**, 109.

Castro, R., Angus, D.C., Rosengart, M.R. (2011). The effect of light on critical illness. *Critical Care*, **15**, 218.

Cepeda, J., Whitehouse, T., Cooper, B., *et al.* (2005). Isolation of patients in single rooms or cohorts to reduce spread of MRSA in intensive-care units: prospective two-centre study. *Lancet*, **365**, 295–304

Chambers, M., Bowman, K. (2011). Finishes and furnishings: considerations for critical care environments. *Critical Care Nursing Quarterly*, **34**, 317–31.

Clifford, K.J., Joyner, K.H., Stroud, D.B., *et al.* (1994). Mobile telephones interfere with medical electrical equipment. *Australasian Physics, Engineering Science and Medicine*, **17**, 23–7.

Department of Health (1996). *Guidelines on Admission to and Discharge from Intensive Care and High Dependency Units*. Report, Department of Health, London.

Department of Health (1999). *Making a Difference*. Report, Department of Health, London.

Department of Health (2000). *Comprehensive Critical Care: A Review of Adult Critical Care Services*, p. 10. Report, Department of Health, London.

Department of Health (2007). *National Specifications for Cleanliness in the NHS: A Framework for Setting and Measuring Performance Outcomes*. Report, Department of Health, London

Department of Health (2013). *Critical Care Units*, Health Building Note (HBN) 04-02, Department of Health, London.

Dietz, A.S., Pronovost, P.J., Mendez-Tellez, P.A., *et al.* (2014). Systematic review of teamwork in the intensive care unit. What do we know about teamwork, team tasks, and improvement strategies? *Journal of Critical Care*, **29**, 908–14.

EFCCNA (European Federation of Critical Care Nursing Associations) (2004). Position statement on post-registration critical care nursing education within Europe. http://www.efccna.org/downloads/Position%20statement%20on%20education%20EfCCNa.pdf

ESICM (European Society of Intensive Care Medicine) (2006). The CoBaTrICE Collaboration Development of core competencies for an international training programme in intensive care medicine. *Intensive Care Medicine*, **32**, 1371–82.

Faculty of Intensive Care Medicine/Intensive Care Society (2013). *Core Standards for Intensive Care Units*. http://www.ficm.ac.uk/sites/default/files/Core%20Standards%20for%20ICUs%20Ed.1%20(2013).pdf

Farr-Barry, M., Bellingan, G. (2004). Pro/con clinical debate: isolation precautions for all intensive care unit patients with methicillin-resistant *Staphylococcus aureus* colonization are essential. *Critical Care*, **8**, 153–6.

Ferdinande, P. (1997). Recommendations on minimal requirements for intensive care departments. Task Force of the European Society of Intensive Care Medicine. *Intensive Care Medicine* **23**, 226–32.

FitzGerald, G., Moore, G., Wilson, A.P.R. (2013). Hand hygiene after touching a patient's surroundings: the opportunities most commonly missed. *Journal of Hospital Infection*, **84**, 27–31.

Garland, A., Connors, A.F. (2013). Optimal timing of transfer out of the intensive care unit. *American Journal of Critical Care*, **22**, 390–7.

Goldfrad, C., Rowan, K. (2000). Consequences of discharge from intensive care at night. *Lancet*, **355**, 1138–42.

Gould, D. (1991). Nurses' hands as vectors of hospital-acquired infection: a review. *Journal of Advanced Nursing*, **16**, 1216–25.

Harmworth, A., Still, B. (2002). Procurement and implementation of a clinical information system within an intensive care unit. *Care of the Critically Ill*, **18**, 11–13.

Health and Social Care Information Centre (2015). *Hospital Episode Statistics. Adult Critical Care in England—April 2013 to March 2014*. http://digital.nhs.uk/catalogue/PUB17343/adul-crit-care-data-eng-apr-13-mar-14-rep.pdf.

Holcomb, B.W., Wheeler, A.P., Ely, E., *et al.* (2001). New ways to reduce unnecessary variation and improve outcomes in the intensive care unit. *Current Opinion in Critical Care* **7**, 304–11.

ICS (Intensive Care Society) (2013). *Standards for Intensive Care Units*. Report, Intensive Care Society. London. http://www.ics.ac.uk/ics-homepage/guidelines-and-standards/

Mador, R., Shaw, N. (2009). The impact of a Critical Care Information System (CCIS) on time spent charting and in direct patient care by staff in the ICU: a review of the literature. *International Journal of Medical Informatics*, **78**, 435–45.

Monkhouse, D. (2013). Advances in critical care for the older patient. *Reviews in Clinical Gerontology*, **23**, 118–30.

MHRA (Medicines and Health Care Regulatory Agency) (2004). *Guidelines For Mobile Communications Systems*. Report, Department of Health, London.

Murthy, S., Wunsch, H. (2012). *Critical Care*, 16, 218.

Naik, P., Morris, E., Mackinnon, S., *et al.* (2001). Do critically ill patients with haematological malignancy survive intensive care and beyond? *Proceedings of the ICS Conference, London*, p. 89. London; Intensive Care Society.

Nathanson, B.H., Henneman, E.A., Blonaisz, E.R., *et al.* (2011). How much teamwork exists between nurses and junior doctors in the intensive care unit? *Journal of Advanced Nursing*, **67**, 1817–23.

National Patient Safety Agency (2007). *The National Specifications for Cleanliness in the NHS: a Framework for Setting and Measuring Performance Outcomes*,. pp 24–31. Report, National Patient Safety Agency, London. http://www.nrls.npsa.nhs.uk/resources/patient-safety-topics/environment/?entryid45=59818

NMC (Nursing and Midwifery Council) (2002). *Statistical Report 2001–2*. Report, Nursing and Midwifery Council, London.

Numata, Y., Schulzer, M., van der Wal, R., *et al.* (2006). Nurse staffing levels and hospital mortality in critical care settings: literature review and meta-analysis. *Journal of Advanced Nursing*, **55**, 435–48.

Paradis, E., Myles, L., Gropper, M.A., *et al.* (2013). Interprofessional care in intensive care settings and the factors that impact it: results from a scoping review of ethnographic studies. *Journal of Critical Care*, **28**, 1062–7.

Pittet, D., Hugonnet, S., Harbarth S., *et al.* (2000). Effectiveness of a hospital-wide programme to improve compliance with hand hygiene. *Lancet*, **356**, 1307–12

Pronovost, P., Angus, D., Dorman, T., *et al.* (2002). Physician staffing patterns and clinical outcomes in critically ill patients: a systematic review. *Journal of the American Medical Association*, **288**, 2151–62.

Scheithauer, S., Lemmen, S.W. (2013). How can compliance with hand hygiene be improved in specialized areas of a university hospital? *Journal of Hospital Infection*, **83**(S1), S17–22.

Schmid, F., Goepfert, M.S., Reuter, D.A. (2013) Patient monitoring alarms in the ICU and in the operating room. *Critical Care*, **17**, 216.

Thomas, E.J., Sexton, J.B., Helmreich, R.L. (2003). Discrepant attitudes about teamwork among critical care nurses and physicians. *Critical Care Medicine*, **31**, 956–9.

Valentin, A., Ferdinande, P. (2011). *ESICM Working Group on Quality Improvement. Recommendations on basic requirements for intensive care units: structural and organisational aspects.* http://www.esicm.org/data/upload/files/Intensive%20care%20medicine%202011%20Valentin-1.pdf

Wunsch, H., Angus, D., Harrison D., *et al.* (2008). Variation in critical care services across North America and Western Europe. *Critical Care Medicine*, **36**, 2787–93.

CHAPTER 3

The patient within the critical care environment

Introduction

Critical illness is extremely stressful, as is having treatment in the critical care unit. This fact has sometimes been overlooked by caregivers, but the significant contribution of iatrogenic stress towards poor outcomes is now widely understood. Commonplace problems such as shortness of breath, anxiety, pain, confusion, and disturbed sleep can be highly distressing, as are the side effects of many of the interventions used and the environment in general. The body mounts a wide range of compensatory responses to stress which are generally adaptive and can even feel positively stimulating in the short-term, but severe or prolonged stress can induce responses that develop into a destructive spiral of decompensation. Furthermore, alterations in either the internal or external environment cause both physical and psychological responses; the individual's emotional condition is inextricably linked with their physical state.

While any illness is stressful, those serious enough to require critical care greatly intensify the physical and psychological challenges that the patient and family must face. Each patient is a thinking, feeling person with an unique history. However, the critical care environment, with its complex equipment and vivid displays of physiological data, can create an impression that patients are simply collections of organs with varying levels of dysfunction. One patient described critical care as 'rooted in the minute analysis of charts and the balancing of chemicals, not so much in the warmth of human contact' (Watt, 1996). In these circumstances, the importance of a holistic approach to care cannot be overemphasized, otherwise essential patient needs and problems will be forgotten or neglected. Much of the skill required for effective nursing in critical care relates to the need to integrate all of the diverse information available about a given patient, to view any change in their condition in context rather than in isolation, and to deliver care tailored to the individual.

This chapter will set out the priorities of care for critically ill patients, and will discuss their common needs and problems, as well as those of their families. Two concepts are particularly important to the understanding of the critically ill patient: homeostasis and stress.

Homeostasis

Homeostasis (from the Greek *homoios*, similar, and *sta*, stand) represents the body's attempts to maintain crucial aspects of its internal environment, such as pH, temperature, and electrolytes, within a tightly controlled range. Multiple complex corrective mechanisms are triggered when the levels of key physiological variables become progressively abnormal. For example, serum acid–base balance is usually maintained with a pH between 7.35 and 7.45. Any deviations activate a series of compensatory changes in respiratory, metabolic, and renal functions in order to restore or maintain the pH at its normal level (see Chapters 4 and 7.)

Unfortunately, many critically ill patients deteriorate to a point where the intrinsic compensatory mechanisms cannot restore homeostasis. In these cases, extrinsic interventions, i.e. critical care therapies, are required to re-establish normal physiological functioning or at least acceptably abnormal values that allow a level of functioning compatible with life and ultimate recovery. An important insight in recent years is that aggressive attempts to normalize abnormal values are often detrimental. Therefore lower values of blood pressure and oxygen saturation and higher values of carbon dioxide are now tolerated to prevent harm arising from treatments—in these instances, catecholamines and increased tidal volumes—used to correct these aspects of abnormal physiology.

Manipulation of abnormal clinical variables must be performed by critical care staff as the therapies used have no negative feedback mechanisms in themselves, and so can only be effectively regulated with careful monitoring and analysis of clinical data. For example, when using an intravenous infusion of potassium chloride to treat hypokalaemia, periodic blood samples must be taken to monitor the response, with further doses given (or not) according to the results. Not all physiological derangements are easily managed, and some will prove to be untreatable. Nonetheless, working to maintain homeostasis—or at least restore it to an acceptable level—is one of the most important aspects of caring for the critically ill. Supporting the failing organ systems allows time for the organs to recover from the initial insult(s) that brought the patient into critical care in the first place.

Stress

All patients are stressed to a greater or lesser degree during critical illness, and the responses to stress can place a considerable extra burden on failing body systems. Tolerance of stress varies between individuals, but there is always a limit to the stress that any person can withstand. Some stressors cannot be reduced or eliminated, but there are also some inherent stressors in the critical care environment which can be relieved by appropriate measures, for example by providing sufficient understandable information so that patients can make sense of their surroundings. The stressors identified in Box 3.1 have features that can be managed with nursing interventions.

There are several models of stress that highlight important concepts and provide insights into patients' responses to critical illness (Cuesta and Singer 2012).

Box 3.1 Stressors reported in studies of mechanically ventilated patients

- Dyspnoea/air hunger
- Tension/anxiety/stress
- Fear
- Pain/discomfort
- Agony/panic/frustration
- Fatigue
- Inability to talk
- Confusion/bewilderment/altered level of consciousness
- Anger/hostility
- Depression
- Insecurity/uncertainty
- Mastery alterations
- Sleeplessness
- Hope alterations
- Negative mood
- Secretions
- Self-efficacy alterations
- Suctioning

Adapted with permission from Thomas L.A., Clinical management of stressors perceived by patients on mechanical ventilation, *AACN Clinical Issues*, Volume 14, Issue 1, pp. 73–81, Copyright © 2003 Wolters Kluwer Health Inc.

These include the general adaptation syndrome and the transactional model of stress.

1. **The general adaptation syndrome** Hans Selye (1936[1], 1946) described a general adaptation syndrome of systemic reactions that occur when there is prolonged exposure to 'diverse nocuous agents'. As described, these reactions are 'independent of the nature of the damaging agent' and have effects including enlargement of the adrenal gland, atrophy of the spleen and lymphoid tissue, and gastric ulceration. Selye postulated that these responses happened in three stages:
   (a) an alarm (or 'shock') reaction—a transient phase that cannot be sustained.
   (b) resistance or adaptation ('contra-shock') producing either a successful adaptation to the stressor or progression to phase (c)
   (c) exhaustion—which can eventually lead to death.

   Later researchers highlighted the importance of the wider environment and individual choices in both creating disease and stress, and potentially modifying the response (e.g. Sterling 2004). This approach is described by the term allostasis or 'stability through change' (Sterling 2004). An allostatic response can be a positive stimulating experience. However, an excessive 'allostatic overload' is harmful, occurring either when the stress response to a severe acute insult requires more energy than the body possesses, or when the patient is subject to a long-term stress-related condition which can only be effectively managed by changes in lifestyle or behaviour (McEwen 2005).
2. **The transactional model of stress** The transactional model particularly emphasizes the significance of different patterns of information processing and personal interpretations of the nature of a given event, as well as individuals' beliefs about their ability to manage a situation. Stress is created when there is a mismatch between perceived demands and the perceived ability to meet those demands (Lazarus and Folkman 1984). External factors (e.g. noise levels, bright light, etc.) and individual factors (e.g. fatigue and anxiety) all affect the ability to cope with a stressor.

Physical responses to stress

The limbic system—a rim of cortical tissue surrounding the hilum of the cerebral cortex and other related deep structures—facilitates the relay of emotional states to the endocrine system. It connects with the cerebral cortex to transmit social and emotional influences, and also connects with the hypothalamus for control of endocrine activity. Therefore hypothalamic activation of sympathetic nervous activity and adrenaline secretion is stimulated via the limbic system (see Figure 3.1).

Although stress reactions are generally appropriate and adaptive as short-term responses to injury, these same mechanisms are harmful over extended periods. Continued breakdown of protein stores causes muscle wasting and fatigue, while suppression of the inflammatory response leads to super-infection, inhibition of tissue granulation prevents healing, and increased extracellular fluid volumes produce fluid shifts and oedema. Nurses have a key role in reducing or even eliminatating extraneous stressors so that their patients can adapt and respond appropriately to injury while minimizing the complications associated with protracted stress.

[1] Republished as Selye (1998).

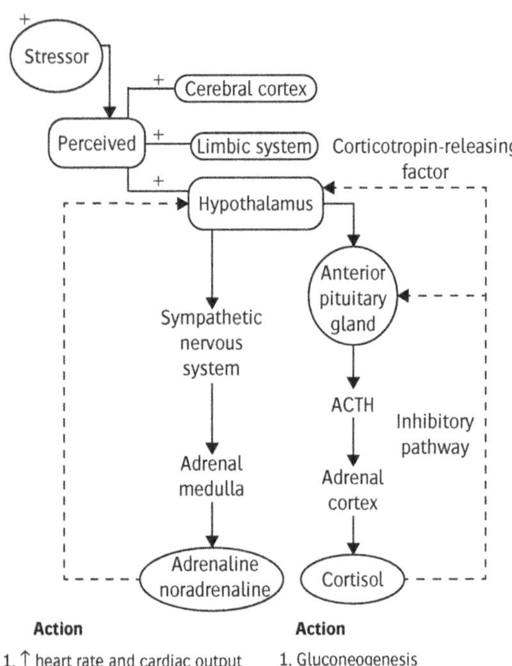

Figure 3.1 Stress, the hormonal response (↑= increase).

Non-physical aspects of stress: disturbed mood, anxiety, and fear

Critical care patients are at significant risk of disturbed mood. Numbers vary greatly in published reports, partly because different methods of measurement are used. One recent UK study of high acuity critical care patients showed that 28% suffered significant problems of this type, including anger, anxiety, depression, and confusion (Wade *et al.* 2012). Various predisposing influences may play both positive or negative roles, including many drugs commonly given in critical care, e.g. benzodiazepines, inotropes, vasopressors and corticosteroids (Wade *et al.* 2012).

Anxiety is a particular issue. Anxiety is a state of increased arousal with disequilibrium, or tension related to apprehension about possible harm. Some individuals can utilize personal coping mechanisms to manage such feelings, but many will also need the help and support of members of the critical care team as well as family members if these are available. A review of 15 published studies from various critical care units found that patients mostly experience moderate levels of anxiety, but some suffer severe anxiety with scores higher than the norm for neuropsychiatric patients (Perpiñá-Galvañ and Richart-Martinez 2009). Unfortunately, these conditions are often under-recognized and under-treated by critical care staff (Rincon *et al.* 2001). Symptoms can include:

- feelings of numbness or detachment
- lack of emotional responsiveness
- reduction in awareness of the environment
- derealization (a sense of one's surroundings being unreal)
- depersonalization (a sense of one's self being unreal)
- amnesia.

Anxiety can result from any stress perceived to threaten personal security and self-determination, and can lead to feelings of real fearfulness—a state of apprehension and distress causing sympathetic arousal. Assessment of anxiety in the critical care patient can be very difficult, particularly when verbal communication is not possible and the nurse depends mainly on subjective interpretation of non-verbal cues. In such cases, tools such as the Faces Anxiety Scale can be used, although this method assumes that the patient is able to indicate which of five different drawings of faces most accurately reflects their mood: (see Figure 3.2) (McKinley *et al.* 2004).

Response to anxiety and fear

The physiological response to anxiety and fear is sympathetic arousal: increased circulating catecholamines, raised heart rate, blood pressure, and respiratory rate, dilated pupils, dry mouth with decreased saliva production, and peripheral and splanchnic vasoconstriction. Changes in behaviour are aimed at managing the stressor, with each person's behavioural responses depending on their background, culture, and social conditioning. Many stressors associated with critical illness, such as physical discomfort, the prospect of pain, disability, and death, isolation, and loss of family support, cannot be completely eliminated so patients very often need assistance to cope. Various strategies can be used:

- Creation of a therapeutic environment, with minimization of extraneous sound, and construction of a routine of day–night differentiation/wake–sleep cycles.

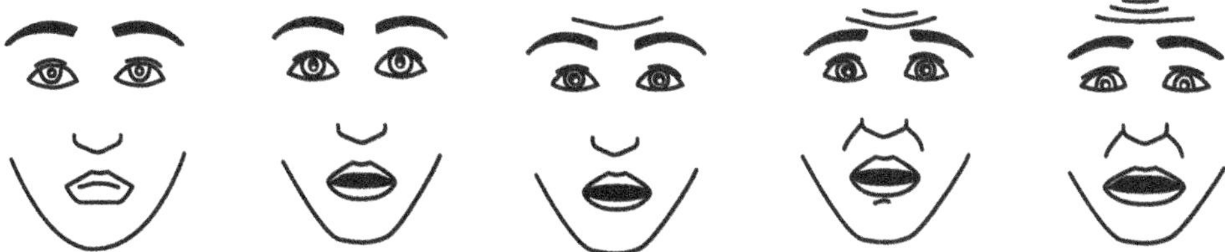

Figure 3.2 The Faces Anxiety Scale.

Reproduced with permission from Sharon McKinley, Katherine Coote, Jane Stein-Parbury, Development and testing of a Faces Scale for the assessment of anxiety in critically ill patients, *Journal of Advanced Nursing*, Volume 41, Issue 1, pp.73–79, Copyright © 2003 John Wiley and Sons.

- Support and augmentation of the patient's intrinsic coping mechanisms.
- Communication of caring and understanding of the patient through attentiveness, tone of voice, touch, etc.
- Provision of information repeatedly and in enough detail for the patient to understand what is happening.
- Making every effort to enable the patient to communicate by any possible means, and use of communication aids.
- Encouragement and support of relatives in reassuring patients and reiterating information. Generally, the nurse should enable relatives to have as much time with the patient as possible without unduly fatiguing him/her.
- Use of music therapy of the patient's liking—particularly with slower tempos—to create a relaxing atmosphere (Bradt *et al.* 2010). Chlan *et al.* (2013) studied ventilated patients who were alert and able to participate in their own care and who were enabled to play music whenever they chose. They found reduced anxiety levels and sedation requirements when compared with similar patients receiving standard care (see also Box 3.2).

Sensory imbalance and disorientation

Sensory imbalance or disorientation occurs when the level of sensory stimuli received by the individual is either too great or too little to be recognizable or meaningful. Five main types are described (e.g. Clifford 1985), and all can apply to patients in critical care:

(1) reduction of the amount and variety of stimuli
(2) monotony of indistinct meaningless stimuli
(3) isolation, either physical or social

Box 3.2 Assisting coping mechanisms for anxiety

Patient's own mechanisms

- Denial
- Rationalization
- Substitution of positive for negative thoughts
- Retention of control (often via the nurse) of aspects of care and the environment (e.g. position, personal hygiene, lighting)

Nursing interventions

- Unrestricted family visiting
- Biofeedback
- Empathetic touch
- Encouragement to verbalize fears
- Ensuring adequate pain relief
- Increase the patient's sense of control of aspects of care/environment, (e.g. lighting, temperature, timing of wash, meals, etc.)
- Arrange for spiritual counselling
- Teach relaxation techniques
- Ameliorate environmental stressors
- Remain with the patient
- Offer meditation techniques
- Positive feedback for coping techniques
- Give appropriately worded and timed information
- Play music
- Therapeutic touch
- Speak calmly and slowly
- Administration of anxiolytic

Data from Frazier SK, Moser DK, Daley LK, *et al.*, Critical care nurses' beliefs about and reported management of anxiety. *American Journal of Critical Care*, Volume 12, Issue 1, pp. 19–27, 2003, American Association of Critical-Care Nurses.

(4) confinement, immobilization, or restriction of movement
(5) excessive sensory input.

Types 1–4 will cause sensory deprivation and type 5 will cause sensory overload. Causes of sensory alteration of types 1–4 are believed to include:

- loss of caring touch (although there may be an overload of procedural touch)
- confinement (due to invasive devices and other equipment) and sedation
- isolation (either physical or social)
- limited visual stimuli.

Common causes of type 5 sensory alteration include:

- continuous high noise levels due to equipment alarms, telephones, buzzers, staff conversation, etc. (see Box 3.3)
- the loss of meaningful sounds and other environmental stimuli that would help the patient orientate him/herself
- many unfamiliar and often incomprehensible sounds
- frequent uninvited touch and invasion of personal space
- constant lighting (i.e. a lack of diurnal phasing of light levels).

The nurse has an important part to play in the prevention or alleviation of sensory imbalance, as many of the interventions initiated or controlled by nurses have tangible effects on the patient's sensory load. Every effort should be made to limit the impact of the technologically oriented environment, with appropriate use of support from family and friends, alternative therapies, explicit appreciation of noise levels, and therapeutic nursing interventions. Failure to alleviate this can contribute to patients experiencing altered perceptions and even acute delusional states (see Box 3.4).

Strategies that assist in optimizing the patient's response to sensory stimuli include:

- assessing the patient for predisposing factors (see Boxes 3.5 and 3.6)
- where possible, providing pre-operative visits and information to elective admission patients to reduce anxiety associated with the unknown
- giving repeated frequent orientation to time, place, person, and events
- establishing an appropriate day–night differentiation and markers of daily routine such as morning toilet, meals, etc.
- making the patient comfortable for the night with attention to analgesia, sedation, positioning,

BOX 3.4 Definitions of altered perception precipitated by sensory imbalance

- Illusion: a false interpretation of external (usually auditory or visual) stimuli
- Hallucination: a false sensory perception occurring without external stimulus
- Delusion: a fixed irrational belief not consistent with cultural mores which may include persecutory, grandiose, nihilistic, or somatic ideas

Box 3.3 Noise in critical care

The World Health Organization recommends that average hospital sound levels should not exceed 35dB. However, a recent study found average sound levels of over 45dBA in UK ICUs, with frequent peaks above 85dBA occurring during both day and night (Darbyshire and Young 2013). Nonetheless, it is possible to reduce sound levels within the ICU; Kahn *et al.* (1998) found that most noise came from talking, which could be significantly decreased by staff education and feedback. Other measures, such as switching bleeps and mobile phones to vibrate mode, are also useful.

Box 3.5 Predisposing factors to sensory imbalance

- Alcohol/drug addiction
- Previous cerebral damage
- Psychological illness
- Chronic cardiovascular, respiratory, metabolic, or renal disease
- Increasing age
- Previous episodes of delirium
- Previous psychological stressors

Box 3.6 Pharmacological agents implicated in sensory imbalance

- Anticholinergics (e.g. atropine)
- Anticonvulsants (e.g. phenytoin)
- Barbiturates
- Penicillin and cephalosporins
- Corticosteroids
- Opoids (e.g. morphine)
- Benzodiazepines
- Digoxin

warmth, and reduced light (eye-shades can be useful adjuncts)

- limiting and clustering interventions during the night to allow periods of at least 90 min of uninterrupted sleep (this is the typical length of a normal complete sleep period (Kamdar *et al.* 2012a))
- reducing unnecessary 'meaningless' noise, and providing earplugs when needed
- using large clocks and calendars within the patient's sight
- introducing the patient to staff entering their bed space
- having formal greeting and leave taking from the nurse caring for the patient on each shift
- using family photos and familiar objects from home to create a less hostile environment
- encouraging involvement of family members in conversation, obtaining information about topics of interest to the patient, and including the patient in conversation
- ascertaining the patient's likes and dislikes
- playing music appropriate to the patient's taste (Bradt *et al.* 2010)
- using television, radio, newspapers, magazines, and conversation to provide meaningful stimulation
- including caring touch in communicating with the patient
- ensuring that the patient can see out of windows and that natural light is used as much as possible
- providing explanations and information on the critical care environment to assist the patient in interpretation and understanding
- encouraging autonomy in self-care, where possible, with explanations and information so that the patient can participate in decisions about daily care.

Disturbance of diurnal (circadian) rhythm

Humans possess a 24-hour cycle that is resistant to change. Prolonged disruption of this cycle can be very damaging (see Box 3.7). It is an unfortunate feature of the critical care environment that treatments and care activities must continue round the clock. This makes the patient highly vulnerable to interruptions of sleep and diurnal rhythm. However, the nurse should consider whether all interventions are truly necessary; Le *et al.* (2012) studied 1831 night-time nursing interventions performed on 200 patients and found that one in seven actions could have been safely omitted. As well as patient care activities, noise and light, mechanical ventilation, medications (particularly sedatives), pain, anxiety, stress, severity of illness, and pre-existing disease (e.g. chronic pulmonary obstructive disease) all contribute to sleep disturbance (Andersen *et al.* 2013). These disturbances result in:

- severely broken sleep—a striking recent study using polysomnography monitoring found that critical care patients averaged just 3 min sleep without waking (Elliott *et al.* 2013);
- a disproportionate loss of rapid eye movement (REM) sleep—REM sleep was observed in just two of 21 patients in one study (Gehlbach *et al.* 2012)
- loss of the restorative phase (slow-wave deep sleep) of non-REM sleep.

Reported effects of sleep disturbance include:

- anxiety (perhaps due to episodes of sympathetic activity when sleep is frequently disrupted (Meerlo *et al.* 2008)) and depression
- respiratory disorders (e.g. reduced endurance of respiratory muscles and response to hypercapnia)

Box 3.7 Functions of sleep

- Mental restoration
- Anabolic processes:
  - protein synthesis is inhibited by cortisol, glucagon, and catecholamines which reach their highest level during the day
  - during sleep, energy expenditure can be diverted towards protein synthesis
  - growth hormone (which stimulates protein and RNA synthesis and amino acid uptake) reaches peak secretion rates during slow-wave sleep

- circulatory disturbances (e.g. episodes of hypertension during awakening at night)
- generalized fatigue
- disruption of immune function (e.g. decreased natural killer cell activity)
- metabolic and hormonal abnormalities (e.g. increased cortisol and catecholamine levels)
- increased energy expenditure and negative nitrogen balance
- cognitive dysfunction and delirium (Kamdar *et al.* 2012a).

There are various methods that nurses can use to limit the detrimental effects of 24-hour care.

- Assessment of the patient's sleep pattern by observing sleep–wake states overnight.
  - When asked to assess patients' sleep patterns, nurses' judgements were accurate 82% of the time (Edwards and Schuring 1993), allowing for early recognition of potential problems. However, nurses may also over-estimate patients' own views of their quality of sleep (Kamdar *et al.* 2012b).
- Be conscious of environmental noise from both equipment and staff, and aim to minimize unnecessary noise, particularly at night.
- Use sound-absorbing and sound-masking methods (Xie *et al.* 2008) or, probably more easily, employ earmuffs or earplugs to promote sleep (van Rompaey *et al.* 2012).
- Provide protected periods of uninterrupted sleep lasting at least 90 min.
- Carry out only vital observations and interventions at night.
- Avoid procedures likely to add to patient stress in the early hours of the morning (when the levels of secretions of cortisol and other stress-related hormones are lowest).
- Ensure that pain relief and other comfort needs, such as warmth, comfortable positioning, reassurance, are all addressed prior to sleep.

Although sedation from benzodiazepines, narcotic analgesics, propofol, and other agents can produce sleep-like behaviours, their effects are not always that of true sleep. Benzodiazepines and narcotics supress REM and slow-wave sleep and therefore may not provide the usual physiological benefits associated with sleep (Kamdar *et al.* 2012a).

Critical care delirium

Delirium is an acute fluctuating syndrome of brain dysfunction characterized by disturbance of consciousness (e.g. reduced awareness, decreased attention) and disturbance of cognition (memory deficits, disorientation, disordered language), or by perceptual disturbance resulting from a a general medical condition or substance intoxication, rather than being due to dementia (American Psychiatric Association 2013).

There are two subtypes of delirium, both of which are frequently seen in critical illness. **Hypoactive delirium** is manifest when the patient becomes withdrawn, lethargic, and apathetic, sometimes to the point of complete unresponsiveness. It very often passes unrecognized in the critical care patient. **Hyperactive delirium** is what is more typically thought of as critical care delirium. The patient exhibits significant agitation and emotional lability, sometimes leading to refusal of care and disruptive behaviours such as shouting, removal of invasive devices, attempts to leave, and even violence.

The numbers of critical care patients diagnosed with delirium vary greatly, with prevalence reported to range from 20% to over 80%, and incidence from 22% to 83% (Vasilevskis *et al.* 2012). Differences in patient populations and diverse approaches to treatment account for much of the variability, but inconsistent definitions of delirium and study design are also factors.

It is likely that there is significant under-recognition of delirium because of poor awareness of the syndrome, and a lack of clarity about diagnosis. However, delirium is important; it is associated with increased complications and morbidity (e.g. self-extubation), increased length of stay, and increased mortality (Zhang *et al.* 2013). The routine use of assessment tools such as the Confusion Assessment Method-ICU (CAM-ICU) (Ely *et al.* 2001) allow early identification of delirium, treatment, and monitoring of progress.

Over 100 factors have been suggested as possible influences on the development of delirium (Vasilevskis *et al.* 2012). These risk factors can be grouped as follows (van Rompaey *et al.* 2009):

- patient characteristics (e.g. age, alcohol use)
- chronic pathology (e.g. pre-existing cognitive impairment, long- term respiratory or circulatory conditions (particularly hypertension)
- acute illness (e.g. severity of illness, length of stay, drug treatments)
- environmental factors (e.g. isolation, lack of natural light).

Many studies suggest that elderly patients are most likely to develop delirium. While the presence of pre-existing cognitive impairment is reported to be significant, so is the severity of illness (Vasilevskis *et al.* 2012). Unfortunately, these are features that cannot be changed.

However, there is potential to adjust drug treatments for patients at risk/already suffering from delirium, with attention to sedative and analgesic regimens being especially important. Benzodiazepine use is particularly correlated with delirium, with opoids also frequently found to be risk factors (Vasilevskis *et al.* 2012).

Management of delirium

Checking for delirium should be a routine part of the nursing assessment on every shift, at least for patients with the risk factors listed in the previous section, or those receiving advanced respiratory or cardiovascular support, or intravenous sedative or opoid drugs (Barr *et al.* 2013). The CAM-ICU tool (Ely *et al.* 2001) or the Intensive Care Delirium Screening Checklist (Bergeron *et al.* 2001) are recommended assessment methods (Barr *et al.* 2013).

Patients at risk of or actually diagnosed with delirium can be helped with the techniques previously described aimed at enabling coping with anxiety and fear, optimizing the response to sensory stimuli, and limiting the detrimental effects of 24-hour care. In addition, early mobilization of critically ill patients decreases the occurrence and severity of delirium; this includes programmes of passive exercises for unresponsive patients as well as active assisted and active exercises when possible (Schweickert *et al.* 2009).

Communication

Communication is a universal need but a great challenge in critical care. Normal channels of communication are disrupted by sedation, opiates, endotracheal and tracheostomy tubes, altered consciousness; and fear. The inability of ventilated patients to communicate is frequently reported to be a source of great distress (Karlsson *et al.* 2012; Samuelson 2011); and is also a cause of frustration for nurses (Happ *et al.* 2011). Therefore one of the most vital skills required of a critical care nurse is the ability to facilitate effective therapeutic communication and always to be aware of the potential impact of all verbal and non-verbal interactions. This requires patience, motivation, a perception of the patient as an individual, and perseverance in providing appropriate levels of understanding and response. Interviews with 100 patients who had previously been unconscious revealed that they had often heard, understood, and responded emotionally to what was being said around them and to them, even when it was believed that they were unaware (Lawrence 1995). Seven categories of verbal communication have been described (Elliott and Wright 1999):

- procedural/task intentions
- orientational information
- reassurance
- apologies/recognition of discomfort
- efforts to elicit a response
- intentional and unintentional distraction (humour, singing, and light-hearted references),
- social conversation with colleagues while recognizing the patient's presence; with most observed communications being brief, reflecting the difficulties of continuing communication for both patients and staff.

The barriers to communication experienced by critical care patients have been described by Börsig and Steinacker (1982).

- Psychical and psychologically conditioned causes—previous psychiatric illness, and psychiatric disturbance related to the critical care environment.
- Socially conditioned causes—hospitalization and unfamiliar environments, use of jargon, ethnic differences, social isolation.
- Chemically conditioned causes—drugs such as sedatives, narcotics, and muscle relaxants.
- Environmental causes—sensory deprivation, sensory overload, isolation, and contact with the normal outside world.
- Organic and therapeutic causes—fatigue, breathlessness, presence of endotracheal or tracheostomy tubes, neuropathy, head injury, and other aspects of illness or treatment.

Communication difficulties can invoke feelings of frustration, anxiety, and fear (Happ *et al.* 2011). There are many methods and aids which can be utilized to assist patients in communicating (see Boxes 3.8 and 3.9).

An essential adjunct to identifying and using the most appropriate methods of communication for an individual patient is the crucial requirement to document this information for other members of the multidisciplinary team. The patient's feelings of isolation and alarm can and should be reduced through effective communication by all members of staff.

Patients' perceptions of their critical illness

As just described, the patient's ability to communicate in the critical care unit is very often seriously restricted. Staff may only become aware of key problems during the recovery phase—or later. Some understanding of the problems facing the critically ill can be gained by listening to survivors' accounts of their experiences. Follow-up studies have shown that critical care patients often have

Box 3.8 Strategies for communicating effectively with critically ill patients: speech, writing, symbols, mime, touch

- Assess the patient's ability to see, hear, touch, respond, understand, use sign language, speak.
- Identify the most appropriate communication device(s) according to patient ability.
- In pre-operative visits prepare the patient for communication difficulties. Agree gestures for minimal communication and document them.
- Use positive feedback such as smiling, nodding attentively, and giving the patient full attention.
- Use touch as a means of communicating to the patient that they have attention and empathy.
- Orientate the patient to time and place, and identify who is speaking to them.
- Use appropriate questions: open questions for the patient who is able to speak/communicate more fully; closed questions for patients who can only gesture and nod.
- Include the patient's visitors and family in planning methods of communication.

little or no recollection of their stay, although memories may be more common in the modern era of critical care as lower doses of sedative and narcotic drugs are being used (Samuelson *et al.* 2006). Those patients who have remembered their stay have described several important issues (Cox *et al.* 2009; Cutler *et al.* 2013; Karlsson *et al.* 2012; Roberts *et al.* 2007; Samuelson 2011; Watt 1996). The main themes from these reports are outlined in the following sections, together with suggestions for limiting the effects of specific problems.

Box 3.9 Communication devices

- Passy–Muir valve
- Devices using ability to suck or press to alter indicators on a screen
- Pen/pencil and paper
- Lip-reading
- Alphabet board
- Touch
- Symbol board/book
- Mime/gesture/facial expression
- Computer
- Eye contact
- Magic writer
- Electronic communicator (e.g. Lightwriter)

Presence of endotracheal tube and discomfort

Patients describe the presence of an endotracheal tube (ETT) as very uncomfortable, particularly during turning or movement. Oral ETTs can give rise to a continuous gagging sensation, although this may help keep the mouth moist by stimulating saliva. Nasal ETTs are usually felt to be more comfortable, as long as the process of intubation does not damage the nasal passages.

- Meticulous mouth care is essential.
- Support of the tube during movement or turning is essential to prevent further discomfort.
- Friction/pressure damage can be caused by securing tapes and other devices used to prevent movement of the ETT, so it is important to inspect the face/neck on every shift for any mucosal or skin injury. There are a range of commercial products and methods of securing tubes and padding the skin that can be useful. (See Chapter 4, 'Specific nursing care of the intubated patient: securing the tube').

Disconnection from the ventilator

Patients who undergo long-term respiratory support can develop a psychological dependence on the ventilator. Disconnection from the ventilator has been described as a terrifying experience with what feels like intolerable periods passing before reconnection occurs. Such feelings can be modified by confidence—or lack of confidence—in the staff caring for the patient.

Ventilator and other machine alarms are also a source of distress. Patients are often unable to identify whether alarms emanate from equipment connected to them or from equipment attached to other patients. Alarms allowed to continue for too long a period of time can cause considerable stress.

- A level of trust and confidence must be developed between the patient and their nurse.
- Disconnection from the ventilator should only be performed after full explanation to the patient and reassurance that it will not continue any longer than necessary.
- Ventilator alarms should be cancelled as quickly as possible, and their causes and remedies explained to the patient.

Communication

Patients express great frustration at their inability to speak or communicate in other ways, and are very appreciative of persistent efforts by nursing staff to understand them.

- Communication with and by the patient should be given a high priority; a determination to understand is valued by patients.
- Individual patient assessment is essential; defective vision or hearing, illiteracy, cognitive impairment or learning disability, or lack of familiarity with the language spoken in a particular critical care unit are all possible problems that can be addressed when identified from the patient assessment, the history, or from talking to the family.
- Developing the ability to lip-read patients who cannot vocalize is a very useful skill that can reduce distress.
- Use appropriate adjuncts for communication, such as boards with letters, words, phrases or pictures that can be pointed to/indicated with the eyes (e.g. Patak *et al.* 2006), or written on.
- When it is safe in terms of the requirements for ventilatory support, aim to enable at least short spells when patients with a tracheostomy can try to vocalize, with tracheostomy cuff deflation and use of a one-way speaking valve if possible (Grossbach *et al.* 2011). If the ventilator is configured appropriately (e.g. by switching to a mode which can compensate for cuff deflation and leak), some types of speaking valve can be placed in the ventilator circuit itself, allowing the patient to speak with a background level of ventilatory support.
- More technological solutions, such as electronic larynxes, are available in some centres.

The importance of touch

Patients describe gaining great comfort from human touch, and from hand-holding in particular. It is an important indicator to the patient that they are cared for (Henricson *et al.* 2009).

- Use hand-holding and touch to communicate caring and comfort, and tactile relaxation methods such as progressive muscle relaxation and massage where appropriate (Richards 1998).

Staff noise and talking at the bedside

The high sound levels associated with the critical care environment have already been discussed. While some patients find a level of background noise comforting, many find it difficult to sleep and are generally bothered by noise. In particular, radios played at high volumes, 'staff chatter', and 'nurses who raise their voices unnecessarily when talking to patients' are mentioned as disturbing phenomena.

- Aim to keep background noise levels low.
- Use a normal level of speech when talking to patients, unless it is known that their hearing is impaired.
- Do not play radios loudly unless it is music known to be enjoyed by specific patients.
- Reduce sound levels at night.

Sensory deprivation and temporal disorientation

Many patients report an inability to distinguish the passage of time. They find high levels of fluorescent lighting unpleasant and appreciate natural daylight where possible.

- Where possible, patients—especially long-term patients—should be nursed where natural light is available. Alternatively, light sources that simulate natural light can be used.
- Methods of marking the time and the day should be used (see earlier).

Dreams and hallucinations

Patients commonly refer to dreams and/or hallucinations that they have experienced during their critical care stay (Roberts *et al.* 2006). Themes of imprisonment, torture, depersonalization and even death have been described (Magarey and McCutcheon 2005). These impressions may not be unreasonable rationalizations of some experiences in critical care, but obviously create a frightening and distressing perception of the critical care unit.

- It can be difficult to help the patient in such situations.
- Touch, verbal reassurance, comfort, and communication may help.
- Having factual memories or awareness of the critical care environment can help patients to understand and deal with altered perceptions of reality (Roberts *et al.* 2007). Use of diaries that summarize details of the patient stay can be useful, even when these are given to the patient as late as a month after discharge. One randomized trial showed that this intervention reduced subsequent post-traumatic stress (Jones *et al.* 2010).

Transition to the ward

Many patients who have spent a lengthy period in critical care express great fear of transfer to the ward (Field *et al.* 2008; Cypress 2013). They feel that the loss of an individual nurse caring for them means that they may suffer neglect while they are still unable to perform all their care needs themselves.

- Use of a step-down care facility to bridge the gap between critical care unit and general ward may be of help.
- Effective liaison and communication between critical care and ward staff can smooth the transition. Detailed handover is essential. A visit from key ward staff to the patient on the critical care unit prior to transfer may also be of benefit. After discharge to the ward, follow-up from a critical care outreach service (where available) allows a continuing critical care perspective for a period (Park *et al.* 2003), and reduces the risk of readmission (Niven *et al.* 2014).
- Appropriately timed discharge in normal working hours is also important.

Pain experience

Patients identify pain as one of the biggest stressors associated with critical care; many say that the management of their pain was inadequate (Joffe *et al.* 2013), and that communicating their pain was difficult. It is a nursing responibility to:

- regularly assess for pain and discomfort using an appropriate tool (see later)
- evaluate the efficacy of analgesia and other methods of pain relief when administered
- be aware of the place of alternative methods such as warmth, massage, imagery, etc.

Supporting and maintaining patient/family relationships

The term 'family' includes all those who provide the patient's intimate social support structure. Problems affecting family relationships when a member is critically ill are caused by:

- loss of normal communication and interaction
- high stress related to the patient's illness
- anxiety about the patient's outcome
- in emergency admissions, the shock of a sudden acute critical illness and removal of the patient from their family role
- the threat to family stability and the loss of normal family rituals and day-to-day routine.

Families' needs when a relative is in critical care have several typical components which nurses should appreciate (Verhaeghe *et al.* 2005).

- Cognitive needs—regularly updated, accurate, and understandable information about the patient and their care is seen as particularly important, while failure to give adequate information is a significant cause of dissatisfaction (Hunziker *et al.* 2012).
- Emotional and social needs—providing hope, without being unrealistic, and giving comfort and all opportunities to be with or near the patient are highly valued (while any loss of confidence in the competence and caring of nurses is a significant problem (Hunziker *et al.* 2012).
- Practical issues—family members can neglect their own basic needs (e.g. by not eating properly or getting enough rest), but nurses can help by reminding them that it is crucial that they care for themselves so that they can most effectively help in caring for the patient.

Jamerson *et al.* (1996) described the types of behaviour and a model of family experience in critical care (Table 3.1) which strongly highlights the need for information.

Modern critical care departments generally assume that care of patients' families is an integral part of the service, with family-centred care embedded into polices and everyday practices (Henneman and Cardin 2002). Nonetheless, it may not be possible to completely satisfy all family needs, particularly with regard to absolute clarity about the patient's prognosis. Family support can be time consuming and emotionally draining, but it is an essential part of enhancing the patient's coping mechanisms and morale, and is one of the most important aspects of nursing the critically ill patient. Overall, the aim should be to establish a positive supportive relationship with the family. Various principles and practices of effective care of the family have been described (e.g. Henneman and Cardin 2002).

- Care of the family should be a multidisciplinary responsibility, but it is generally most effectively coordinated by nursing staff as they are the constant presence at the bedside.
- Systems that promote continuity of care, such as primary nursing and primary team nursing, enable staff to get to know the patient's family and appreciate their particular needs.
- The family should be given detailed updates of the patient's condition, progress, and, where possible,

Table 3.1 A model of family experiences in critical care

Category	Definition	Possible nursing interventions
Hovering	Initial stress, confusion, and uncertainty in family members	Individual: • anticipate need for information and provide it • orientate families to critical care environment/routine • assess any previous experiences in critical care • provide empathy and advocacy for the family Organizational: • provide volunteers, pastoral care, or ancillary staff to provide information on patient status.
Information seeking	Active gathering of information about the patient	Individual: • anticipate information needs and supply regular updates • include the family in discharge planning Organizational: • provide message board for communication and exchange of information • provide printed orientation booklet and ensure distribution to all patients' families • where possible, provide materials via website • post visiting hours
Tracking	Process of observing, analysing, and evaluating the patient's care	Individual: • provide fundamental nursing care as well as high-technology care • treat families with respect and dignity • maintain flexible open communication • assign consistent caregiver(s) whenever possible Organizational: • provide privacy in facilities/environment • provide in-service training to develop and maintain nursing knowledge and skills
Garnering resources	The acquisition of resources to meet the family's needs	Individual: • allow individualized, flexible visiting • assess the need for a family gatekeeper • provide open honest communication • collaborate with family regarding treatment and discharge plans. • allow families to assist with non-technical care Organizational: • provide a waiting environment with comfort items and diversionary activities • supply phones when needed • identify areas for solitude

Adapted from *Heart and Lung*, Volume 25, Issue 6, Jamerson PA, Scheibmeir M, Bott MJ, *et al.*, The experiences of families with a relative in the intensive care unit, pp. 467–74 copyright © 1996 with permission by Mosby-Year Book Inc. published by Elsevier Inc.

prognosis, usually at least once a day (Verhaeghe *et al.* 2005).

- A standard approach must be sought from all staff, with constant intercommunication about any contacts with the family.
- A common record should be kept of all approaches by staff to the family.
- Questions should be answered honestly.
- Where possible, the family should be included in planning and carrying out the patient's non-therapeutic care.
- The family should have encouragement and education in communicating, touching, and caring for the patient.
- The strengths and weaknesses within the family's coping mechanisms should be identified. Support

should be aimed at accentuating strengths and moderating or diminishing weaknesses (see Box 3.10).

- The family should generally have open access to the patient but be encouraged to take time away from him/her in order to have time to themselves and rest when necessary.
- In the case of the longer-term critically ill patient, the family may need encouragement and assistance to resume a modified form of daily life.
- The whole multidisciplinary team should monitor family members for signs of failure to cope, overwhelming stress, and exhaustion.

BOX 3.10 Family support network

- Nursing staff
- Medical staff
- Social work department
- Spiritual support
- Extended family, friends, neighbours
- Specialist support groups
- Community workers (e.g. family doctor, district nurse)

Models of care

Critical care nursing tends to focus on the importance of the physical state of the patient as this forms the basis for admission, and the barriers to communication in the critical care unit mean that the patient as a person can be difficult to get to know. Information regarding important personal features other than physical status is often only obtainable indirectly from relatives or friends.

However, although the nurse frequently works in acute situations where non-physical aspects must take second place, the priorities will change in other circumstances, and it is important that physical functions give way to psychological or social needs where it is appropriate and beneficial to the patient. One of the benefits of a well-structured framework of care lies in the ability to switch emphasis when needed.

Priorities of care

Best critical care nursing practice strives to prevent, or at least reduce, the severity of the complications of critical illness by employing close observation and monitoring of the patient and skilled interpretation of all the available data so that timely and effective therapies can be administered whenever possible. While the importance of psychological and social support for patients in critical care cannot be underestimated, the hierarchy of human need means that the initial focus must be on those factors that are potentially life-threatening. A structured framework should be used to assess, clarify, and prioritize patient needs, and to guide any necessary interventions and evaluations of effectiveness. Consideration in turn of the fundamental A–B–C–D–E aspects of care is one useful method, i.e. appraising the following.

- **A**irway: with establishment and maintenance of airway patency (using airway adjuncts or advanced airways when necessary, removal of pulmonary secretions, etc.).
- **B**reathing: ensuring adequacy of oxygenation and ventilation etc.
- **C**irculation: assessing blood volume and pressures; perfusion of brain, heart, lungs, kidneys, gut and other organs; control of bleeding, haematology, etc.
- **D**isability: checking the level of consciousness, and the factors that affect it (systemic and also localized neurology), including the need for analgesia and/or sedation.
- **E**xposure: hands-on, head-to-toe, front and back examination, and review of everything else, with consideration of wounds and drains together with review of blood test results etc.

Treatment strategies in critical illness can be prioritized using this schema, which has the additional benefit that it will be familiar to colleagues trained in advanced life support and similar systems. Further detail can then be obtained by review of the following.

- **F**luid and electrolyte balance, fluid input, urine output.
- **G**astrointestinal function: nutritional needs; elimination.
- The **H**istory and holistic overview of the patient as a person (and their sociocultural background).

- Infection and infection control issues, microbiology—and personal hygiene.
- Lines and other invasive devices—utility and risks.
- Medications.
- Nursing and multidisciplinary teamwork: ensuring that the staff resource is sufficient for the patient's severity of illness and the physical demands of care.
- Psychology (cognition, communication, and mood)—and the Plan of care and Prognosis in the short, medium, and longer term (after Hillman *et al.* 2002; Welch 2014).
- Relatives and loved ones.

Nursing philosophy

More sophisticated models can be used to frame a wider impression of the patient, to reflect a particular philosophy or approach to care, and to express a view of the specific role of nurses in the service (Shirey 2008; McCrae 2012). Whichever method is used, there must be explicit definitions of the patient's problems and a clear statement of measurable therapeutic goals. There is great benefit in developing a shared vision or philosophy within the department, and in agreeing how core values will be demonstrated in practice (Warfield and Manley 1990) (see Figure 3.3).

The objective is to be able to comunicate:

- the values and goals of the staff
- a synopsis of how the staff view the patient and their needs,
- the environment in which care is delivered
- any other significant external issues which might affect the delivery of care.

For example, stated values could include stressing the primary importance of patient safety and well-being, ensuring that the kindness an individual would want for their own loved ones is always offered, emphasizing the importance of effective teamworking, and having systems in place to achieve continuous improvement (University College London Hospitals

- I/we believe the purpose of critical care is ....
- I/we believe my/our purpose in critical care is ....
- I/we believe this purpose can be achieved by ....
- I/we believe the factors that inhibit or enable this purpose to be achieved include ....
- I/we believe critically ill care patients need ....
- I/we believe the nurse-patient relationship is about ....
- I/we believe I/we can help a critically ill patient ....
- I/we believe critically ill patients' families/relatives/significant others value ....
- I believe that what makes an effective team is ....
- As a member of the critical care team, I/we most value ....
- As a member of the critical care team, I need the critical care team leader(s) to ......
- I/we believe the work environment for staff should be ....
- I/we believe individuals learn best when ....
- Other values and beliefs that are important to me are ....

Having agreed core values, it needs to be decided how these will be genuinely reflected in everyday practice, and what simple measures can be used to provide assurance that patient care is routinely based on such principles.

Figure 3.3 Values clarification: example questions to ask of staff to prompt discussion and articulation of common values in the department.

Adapted from Warfield C, Manley K, Developing a new philosophy in the NDU, *Nursing Standard*, Volume 4, Issue 41, pp.27–30 Copyright © 1990. With permission from the Royal College of Nursing.

NHS Foundation Trust 2013). This last point is neatly captured in the phrase:

> everyone in healthcare really has two jobs when they come to work . . . to do their work and to improve it
>
> (Batalden and Davidoff 2007).

The most effective critical care units are founded on multidisciplinary teamworking, so it is important that the philosophy is compatible with the vision of other team members.

Bedside emergency equipment

A key task for the nurse taking over the care of the patient is ensuring that essential emergency equipment is available at the bedside and is functioning properly. Unit-wide emergency equipment, such as intubation equipment, defibrillators, and pacing systems, should be checked by a designated nurse on each shift. The following equipment and the skills to use it provide a minimum standard of safety for emergency events and will at least allow the nurse to maintain a patient's vital functions until help arrives. The bedside nurse should complete these checks at the beginning of each shift and whenever they take over the care of a patient.

1. Equipment for airway protection
   - Check that the suction equipment is functioning by occluding the end of the suction tubing and ensuring that a vacuum pressure builds up (see Chapter 4 for details).
   - Ensure that the correct size suction catheters are available for the size of the patient's endotracheal or tracheostomy tube (see Chapter 4).
   - If closed suction systems are used, check the connections and the entire length of the plastic sleeve for patency, and then clear the catheter with normal saline injected through the irrigation port to ensure function.
   - An oropharyngeal (Guedel) airway of a size appropriate to the patient (usually 2–3 for women and 3–4 for men) and an oral suctioning device (Yankauer sucker) should also be available.
2. Equipment for support of the patient's breathing
   - Check that the manual bag–valve system/self-inflating resuscitator is functioning and leak-free by occluding the end of the valve outlet with the valve screwed tight. The bag should inflate without air escaping.
   - Any nurse responsible for a ventilated patient should be competent to perform manual ventilation using a bag–valve system/resuscitator, as this is the only method of ensuring adequate ventilation and oxygenation if the ventilator or gas supply fails. It may also be necessary to ventilate the patient manually in the event of emergency evacuation.
   - Check that the bag has the correct attachment to allow ventilation, and that it is attached to an oxygen (not air) delivery system. There should be a catheter mount if the patient is intubated, and an anaesthetic facemask should be available if the patient is not intubated or in case of accidental extubation.
   - Check any portable oxygen cylinders to ensure that they are at least half full.
3. Equipment for support of the patient's circulation
   - Check that the arterial or non-invasive blood pressure monitoring system is functional and accurate. Ensure that transducers are placed at the correct height (see Chapter 5).
   - Every nurse caring for a patient should be competent in performing chest compressions in the event of a cardiac arrest (see Chapter 6). The cardiac arrest call button should be in close proximity and functioning, with help also available within easy calling distance.
   - In almost all critical care patients some form of intravenous access should be available and patent.
   - Other additional checks of drug infusions and fluids will also be necessary to ensure that the patient is receiving what is prescribed. Checks specific to treatments such as renal replacement therapy (see Chapter 7) should also be performed.

Common core problems for patients in the critical care environment

Many patient problems are a result of general physiological and psychological responses to critical illness and the nature of the critical care environment, and therefore are experienced by the majority of patients. These are listed in Table 3.2. These common core problems are discussed in this chapter if they constitute a global problem

Table 3.2 **Common core problems for intensive care patients**

Problem	Chapter
Airway maintenance	Chapter 4
Support of ventilation	Chapter 4
Support of circulation	Chapter 5
Fluid balance	Chapter 7
Nutrition	Chapter 9
Elimination	Chapter 9
Pain relief and sedation	Chapter 3
Communication	Chapter 3
Anxiety/fear	Chapter 3
Maintenance of sensory balance	Chapter 3
Support of the family	Chapter 3
Alterations in diurnal rhythm	Chapter 3
Prevention of the effects of limited mobility	Chapter 3
Personal hygiene	Chapter 3

or in the specific chapters listed if they appertain to a particular body system.

Pain relief and sedation

The experience of pain is a complex phenomenon involving social, cultural, emotional, psychological, and physiological components. Pain is aggravated in critical illness by:

- anxiety and fear, agitation and delirium
- difficulty in communicating
- the fact that life-saving priorities may complicate or displace administration of pain relief and sedation (e.g. by limiting medications such as opoids when hypotension is present).

Patients' recollections of critical care show that their greatest concerns are very often related to pain (Joffe *et al.* 2013). Even being positioned comfortably is felt to be problematic much of the time. Pain contributes to stress, and can increase confusion and delirium as well as decreasing the ability to manage other stressors. Pain is also a significant cause of sleeplessness (Andersen *et al.* 2013).

Pain is often inadequately assessed in the critical care unit. Patients' inability to communicate effectively and the associated tendency to underestimate analgesic requirements are key issues (Joffe *et al.* 2013). Other factors, including workload (Park *et al.* 2001) and the local culture (Glynn and Ahern 2000), have also been cited.

Physiology of pain

Ensuring patient comfort and freedom from pain are priorities in critical care. The sensation of pain is caused by noxious stimuli resulting from the release of products of tissue damage. These products include bradykinins, histamines, prostaglandins, and hydrogen ions. These are also associated with other pathologies, such as systemic inflammation and sepsis. They act by binding to nerve receptors and depolarizing the nerve membrane, thus initiating an action potential and impulse generation in nociceptive fibres. These impulses can produce both spinal (reflex) and central responses (see Figure 3.4 for pain pathways).

Pain is perceived at thalamic and forebrain levels and constitutes both sensory and reactive components. The thermal threshold is used as a determinant of sensory pain threshold and is remarkably constant in humans

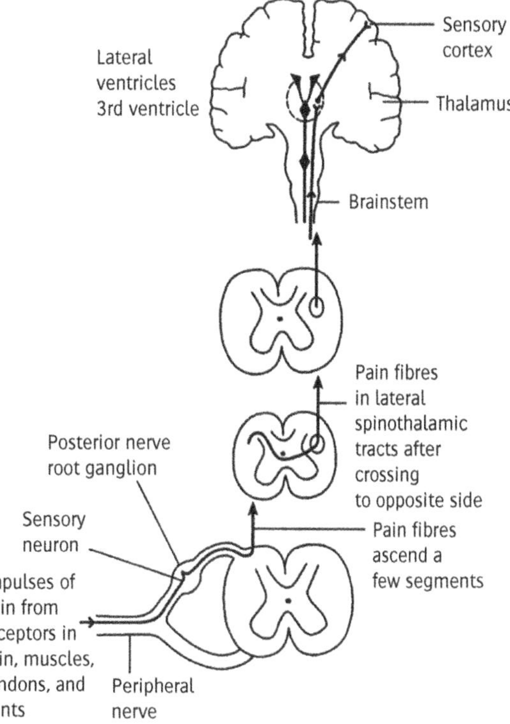

Figure 3.4 Diagram of pain pathways

Reproduced from Verran B, Aisbitt P, *Neurological and Neurosurgical Nursing*, Edward Arnold, 1988 published by Taylor and Francis.

(at 44–45°C). However, the reaction to that sensation varies from person to person. The perception of pain by an individual is affected by many factors including the specific pathophysiology, culture, the environment, personal experience, and mood. In other words, the meaning any individual attaches to the pain they perceive affects their response.

Another component of the individual response to pain is the functioning of the endogenous opioid (endorphin release) system which modulates the perception of pain to varying degrees. Endorphin release probably occurs in response not only to pain but also to hypertension and hypoglycaemia, and to stress, fear, and restraint. Many of these elements occur in critical illness and therefore, if they are well managed, may allow at least some opportunities for reducing perceived pain. Unfortunately, it is impossible to measure or manipulate levels of endogenous opioids, so the patient's expressed response is the only means available to guide how much analgesia is required.

There are several theories of pain perception that reflect the complexity of the phenomenon. The gate control theory, originally described by Melzack and Wall (1965), postulated that the perception of pain transmitted by small-diameter nerve fibres (which carry pain stimuli) can be inhibited by stimulation of large-diameter nerve fibres (which carry innocuous information about touch, pressure, etc). The proposed mechanism is as follows.

1. Small-diameter fibres inhibit modulation by specialized tissue and excite cells which act as activators of central transmission of sensory and emotional aspects of pain. Therefore they 'open the gate'.
2. Large-diameter fibres inhibit the excitatory cell activity and 'close the gate' to pain.
3. Higher central nervous system processes can influence the gate control via inhibitory messages to the spinal cord.

The gate control theory provides a plausible explanation for the effects of some alternative methods of pain management, e.g. simple rubbing or massage, or use of transcutaneous electrical nerve stimulation (TENS) which preferentially stimulates large-diameter fibres that then inhibit, to varying degrees, central transmission of pain stimuli.

Assessment of pain

At least half of critical care patients do not have their pain well controlled (e.g. Chanques *et al.* 2007). The numbers may well be higher; even routine procedures such as tracheal suctioning, manipulation of invasive devices, wound care, and changes of position have been found to be highly distressing and poorly managed (Puntillo *et al.* 2004). Failures of pain control are often attributed to communication difficulties, although it has been shown that concerted effort and the use of formalized methods of assessment can overcome many presumed barriers (Ahlers *et al.* 2008). Using a structured method of assessment and a standardized approach to pain management that includes reassessment after any intervention to evaluate its effectiveness improves patient outcomes (Skrobik and Chanques 2013). Barr *et al.* (2013) recommend the Behavioural Pain Scale (BPS) and the Critical Care Pain Observation Tool (CPOT) as the best methods for assessing pain in patients unable to self-report, provided that their motor function is preserved.

When verbal and non-verbal communications are impossible, physiological signs of pain, such as tachycardia and hypertension, and other responses, such as sweating and lacrimation, may still be recognized. Unfortunately, these signs and symptoms have many causes and are subject to a range of influences that make precise interpretation difficult.

Methods of pain relief

1. **Analgesia** Opoid analgesics (e.g. morphine, fentanyl, alfentanil, remifentanil) remain the mainstay of pain relief for critical care patients. When patients are mechanically ventilated using non-physiological modes, these drugs have the additional advantage of blunting respiratory drive. Continuous intravenous infusions produce a relatively consistent analgesia which can be titrated to patient response. Doses will depend on age, weight, haemodynamic status, and clinical effect. Intravenous boluses—small doses, delivered relatively slowly—prior to any unpleasant procedure provide increased analgesic effect in the short term. In the latter stages of a patient's critical care stay, other methods of administration may be used, particularly the enteral route and, for fentanyl, the transdermal route.
2. **Regional analgesia** Epidural analgesia is most advantageous following upper abdominal and chest surgery, when coughing, deep breathing, and mobility are facilitated. The epidural catheter is inserted between T7 and T10 for abdominal and thoracic pain, or at Ll–2 or L2–3 for lower abdominal and pelvic pain. Analgesia can then be delivered either as a constant infusion or as boluses.
3. **Transcutaneous electrical nerve stimulation (TENS)** Large-diameter afferent nerve fibres are

stimulated by a low-level electric current, thus selectively inhibiting transmission of pain signals via small-diameter nerve fibres. The value of this method in critical care seems to be limited and may only reduce pharmacological analgesic requirements, rather than providing complete pain relief.

4. **Nitrous oxide** Inhalation of a gas consisting of 50% nitrous oxide and 50% oxygen (Entonox) can provide good analgesic effects, although it should only be used for short-term pain relief as bone marrow depression may occur after 36 hours. Its primary use is to provide pain relief for patients who are breathing spontaneously and are able to use the demand valve delivery system for analgesia during unpleasant procedures. It can also be delivered via a rigid oxygen mask, albeit with a reduced concentration of nitrous oxide. It is possible to deliver the gas through a positive pressure ventilator, but this requires special adaptation of the circuit.
5. **Localized warmth and/or cooling** Application of local heat using warming pads or warmed bags of fluid can help relieve aching or muscular spasm pain. Alternatively, topical cooling using permeable gel dressings or cool (but not iced) dressings can relieve some of the pain associated with burns.
6. **Relaxation techniques** Methods such as progressive muscle relaxation and massage may have a role in pain management (e.g. by reducing muscle tension) and also provide other benefits such as decreasing anxiety and promoting sleep (Tracy and Chlan 2011). Braun *et al.* (2012) studied the effects of massage therapy on patients in the days after elective cardiac surgery, and found that treated patients reported significant reductions in both pain and anxiety compared with those who were not treated.
7. **Effective communication between staff and patients** Attention to the need for information and personal factors identified by patients (or their families) regarding the nature of their pain and any anxieties can assist in decreasing the 'distress' factor associated with pain perception and therefore increase the ability to tolerate pain.
8. **Patient-controlled analgesia (PCA).** Some critically ill patients are able to control their pain with a PCA infusion pump. The pump is set to administer a specific dose of analgesia with a pre-set period of time which must elapse before the next dose can be delivered. Most PCA pumps record the number of actual patient demands for a dose of analgesia against the number of delivered doses. This allows assessment of the efficacy of the set dose of analgesia.

Sedation in the critically ill

The purposes of sedation in critical care are:

- facilitation of mechanical ventilation
- obtundation of the physiological response to stress (e.g. reduction of tachycardia, hypertension, raised intracranial pressure)
- relief of discomfort and distress, anxiety, and agitation
- facilitation of therapeutic or diagnostic procedures
- promotion of sleep (when appropriate)
- management of acute confusional states
- prevention of awareness during therapeutic paralysis with neuromuscular blocking agents.

Assessment of sedation

Assessment of the patient's level of sedation should be performed at regular intervals (i.e. hourly during the day) using a structured sedation scoring system. The Richmond Agitation–Sedation Scale (a scale ranging from the situation of the patient being unarousable, to combative/violent and all points in between) and the Sedation–Agitation Scale are recommended (Barr *et al.* 2013). The aim is generally for the patient to be aware but calm and cooperative, while also feeling comfortable and able to sleep at appropriate times

Drug therapy

Opioid drugs have anxiolytic and euphoric effects as well as analgesic properties. They are often used in conjunction with sedative drugs to provide a combination of pain relief, drowsiness, and, when necessary, respiratory depression.

Sedative drugs

See Table 3.3 for an overview.

1. **Benzodiazepines** Benzodiazepines are sedative anxiolytics which promote amnesia, and when combined with opiates can significantly reduce recall of unpleasant events. They also potentiate analgesic efficacy (thus reducing analgesic requirements: In addition, benzodiazepines act as anticonvulsants, muscle relaxants, and in prophylaxis of alcohol withdrawal.

When required, reversal of benzodiazepine respiratory and central depressant effects can be achieved in most patients using the competitive benzodiazepine receptor antagonist flumazenil. Care must be taken in these situations to continue to observe the patient following administration of flumazenil because of its short half-life and the danger of re-sedation.

Table 3.3 Sedative drugs

Drug	Bolus dose	IV infusion rate	Elimination half-life	Notes/cautions
Midazolam	2.5–5.0 mg	0.5–6.0 mg/h	2–7 h extended after prolonged infusion	Respiratory depression especially in the elderly. Hepatic and renal dysfunction prolongs action. About 10% of patients are slow metabolizers. ↓ SVR, ↑ HR, and ↓ BP effects increased in volume depletion, the elderly, and cardiac disease. Delirium and paradoxical confusion/agitation with withdrawal symptoms in long-term use.
Propofol	10–20 mg	1.0–4.0 mg/kg/h	3–12 h	Negative inotropic effect. Significant ↓ BP especially with hypovolaemia or CVS dysfunction. Decreased clearance may occur in the elderly and in renal dysfunction. Seizures have been reported.
Dexmedetomidine		0.7 mcg/kg/h, then 0.2–1.4 mcg/kg/h	Distribution half-life 6 min; terminal elimination half-life 2 h	Sedates without respiratory depression, so enables of ETT toleration while still allowing awareness. ↓ HR (not to be used in second/third degree HB), ↓ BP. Analgesic effects.
Clonidine	50 mcg (up to 250 mcg 8 hourly)	50 mcg/kg/h, then 0.2–1.4 mcg/kg/h	10–20 h	To be used for no more than 3 days (sudden withdrawal effects). ↓ HR, ↓ BP. Analgesic effects.
Haloperidol	2.5–5.0 mg	0.5–6.0 mg/h	12–38 h	Minimal respiratory depression. May prolong QT interval (with risk of torsades de pointes), ↓ BP.
Ketamine	1.0–2.0 mg/kg, additional doses 0.5 mg/kg	3.0–10.0 mg/kg/min	2-4 h	Minimal respiratory depression unless large doses. ↑ HR and ↑ catecholamine stimulation. Nightmares and hallucinations. Analgesic effects.

SVR, systemic vacular resistance; HR, heart rate; BP, blood pressure; CVS, cardiovascular system; ETT, endotracheal tube; HB, heart block.
Data from Paw, H. and Shulman, R., *Handbook of Drugs in Intensive Care*,(5th edn). 2013, Cambridge University Press.

Benzodiazepines have been widely used for sedation in critical care for many years, but may have undesirable side effects including accumulation (particularly with renal or liver impairment) and prolonged sedation (especially in elderly patients), as well as being associated with the development of delirium. Consequently, other agents (e.g. propofol and dexmedetomidine) are now recommended as preferred agents for sedation (Barr *et al.* 2013).

2. **Propofol** Developed as an anaesthetic induction agent, propofol is used in continuous infusion for critical care sedation. It has a rapid action and allows rapid awakening when stopped, though it can accumulate with prolonged use. Propofol should be administered with caution in patients with impaired cardiovascular function (e.g. hypovolaemia or severe sepsis) as it has vasodilator and negative inotropic properties which can cause significant hypotension. It can also cause fat overload (hypertriglyceridemia) as it is dissolved in lipid. Propofol is not licensed for use in children, but is still sometimes used in some paediatric centres.

3. **Dexmedetomidine** Dexmedetomidine is a relatively new short-acting selective α_2 agonist which provides mild to moderate sedation, reduces anxiety and agitation, and can decrease the requirement for analgesia, all without significant respiratory depression. Therefore dexmedetomidine may be used in

a range of situations, for example as an alternative to propofol to facilitate comfortable non-invasive ventilation (without respiratory depression), or to aid the cessation of benzodiazepine sedation and the last stages of weaning from invasive ventilation. In two multicentre trials, dexmedetomidine reduced the duration of mechanical ventilation when compared with midazolam, and improved the ability to communicate when compared with both midazolam and propofol (Jakob *et al.* 2012). Nonetheless, dexmedetomidine can have cardiovascular effects, specifically bradycardia (so should not be used with patients suffering from second- or third-degree heart block) and hypotension.

4. **Clonidine** Clonidine is also an α_2 agonist with both sedative and analgesia enhancing properties, usually used short term (for no more than 3 days), for example to manage withdrawal from infusions of opoid drugs. Potential side effects are bradycardia and hypotension.
5. **Haloperidol** Haloperidol is a butyrophenone derivative typically used to manage agitation and also delirium in critical care, although there is no strong evidence that it is an effective treatment for delirium (Barr *et al.* 2013). It has much less of a respiratory depressant effect than other sedatives, but can prolong the QT interval (with a risk of torsades de pointes) and cause hypotension (particularly in hypovolaemia). It also has known extrapyramidal effects (e.g. Parkinson-like symptoms).
6. **Ketamine** Ketamine is an anaesthetic and sedative agent which also has potent analgesic properties. It directly stimulates the myocardium and sympathetic nervous system but has little effect on respiration, although it reduces airway resistance by its action on β-receptors. It can be used in unstable critically ill patients, particularly asthmatics who benefit from its bronchodilator effects. Its use is associated with distressing and unpleasant nightmares which may be exacerbated by external irritants such as noise, touch, etc. Thus it should be used with benzodiazepines or other agents that provide an amnesic effect.
7. **Isoflurane (desflurane, sevoflurane)** Isoflurane, desflurane, and sevoflurane are inhalational anaesthetic agents used for short-term sedation. Isoflurane has been shown to allow a shorter time to extubation than midazolam, although without any difference in quality of sedation, haemodynamics, or duration of ICU stay. There are technical difficulties with the use of these agents because of the need to modify the ventilator circuit and to use scavenging equipment.

Muscle relaxants (paralysing agents, neuromuscular blockers)

There are four major indications for the use of muscle relaxants:

(1) facilitation of endotracheal intubation
(2) assisting the use of certain ventilatory modes (e.g. inverse ratio ventilation)
(3) prevention of activity associated with high levels of oxygen consumption (e.g. shivering) in patients with very poor respiratory function and high oxygen requirements
(4) reducing muscle spasm associated with tetany.

Muscle relaxants should only be given to patients who are either intubated or about to be intubated, and should also only be used in conjunction with adequate sedation to avoid the terror of conscious paralysis. Levels of sedation should be regularly assessed by reducing or discontinuing the paralysing agent to allow that assessment. Atracurium, rocuronium, and vecuronium are least likely to be associated with adverse cardiovascular effects and are favoured for haemodynamically unstable patients (see Table 3.4).

Malignant hyperthermia is a rare genetic disorder which can be precipitated by the use of muscle relaxants (mostly suxamethonium) usually in combination with an inhalational anaesthetic. The patient rapidly becomes pyrexial and develops severe muscle rigidity, with gross metabolic derangements as a result of abnormal cellular calcium metabolism. Treatment consists of stopping the muscle relaxant, aggressive cooling, and possibly administering IV dantrolene (though this is contentious).

The key to successful sedation of critically ill patients is regular assessment using a recognized sedation scoring system and titration of sedative doses according to agreed unit protocols, with effective pain control a particular and primary priority—the so-called 'analgesis first' approach. Kress *et al.* (2000) found that daily interruption of sedation until patients were awake was associated with significant reductions in duration of mechanical ventilation and ICU length of stay. This approach became standard practice in many units. However, a recent multi-centre trial, where standard practice was protocolized light sedation, found no additional benefit with daily interruptions of sedation; in fact, such interruptions meant that more sedation was given overall (Mehta *et al.* 2012).

Table 3.4 Muscle relaxants (neuromuscular blockade)

Drug	Bolus dose	Elimination half-life	Notes/cautions
Atracurium	0.6 mg	Approximately 20 min	Anaphylaxis has been reported. Adequate sedation is essential. Accumulation of metabolite may cause seizures. Breakdown delayed in hypothermia and acidosis.
Rocuronium	0.60 mg/kg, then 0.15 mg/kg as needed	1.2–1.4 h	Anaphylaxis has been reported.
Vecuronium	100 mcg/kg, then 20–30 mcg/kg as needed	0.5–1.3 h	Anaphylaxis and prolonged effects reported. Renally excreted, so use with caution in kidney dysfunction.
Suxamethonium	For rapid sequence induction for tracheal intubation: 1.0–1.5 mg/kg, then 0.25–0.50 mg/kg as needed	2–3 min	Can cause hyperkalaemia, so contraindicated in patients with existing elevated serum potassium. Must be stored in refrigerator.

Data from Paw, H. and Shulman, R., *Handbook of Drugs in Intensive Care* (5th edn). 2013, Cambridge University Press.

Bispectral index monitoring (BIS™)

Bispectral index monitoring is an objective method of monitoring awareness using a processed signal electroencephalogram (EEG) which is measured on a scale of 0–100, where 0 is a flat-line EEG and 100 is fully awake (Figure 3.5). It has mainly been used in the operating theatre, but may have some value in critical care, particularly when assessing underlying sedation levels in patients receiving muscle relaxants. However, it remains poorly validated in ICU populations so its use is not widespread. There are some problems with this type of monitoring, as there may be spurious values associated with muscle movement and critical illness encephalopathy.

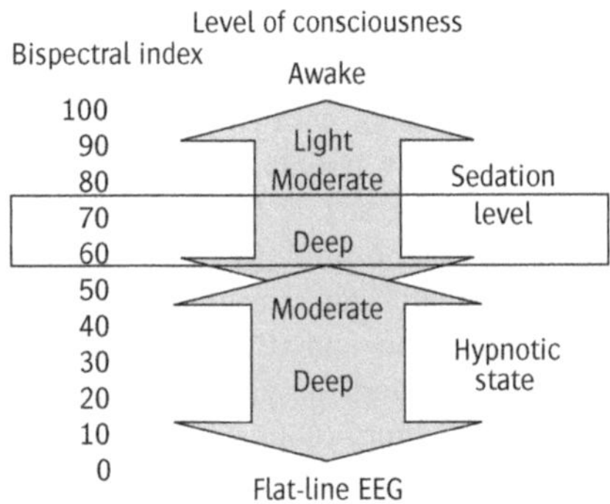

Figure 3.5 Bispectral index monitoring (BIS™) scale indicating level of consciousness.

Personal hygiene

Mouth care

In the healthy mouth rapidly proliferating squamous epithelial cells form a lining from the inside of the lips to the oropharynx. These cells are vulnerable to the effects of low blood flow, malnutrition, and drug toxicity, and are therefore particularly at risk in critical illness. The risk is increased by the loss of normal cleaning mechanisms and the presence of an oral endotracheal (ET) tube pressing on fragile tissue. Other contributory factors include the following.

- Decreased or absent oral fluid intake.
- Dehydration of the buccal mucosa related to inhalation of dry gases, systemic dehydration, stress, and tachypnoea (which tends to increase mouth breathing).
- Decreased salivary stimulation due to loss of food as a stimulating factor and increased sympathetic arousal.
- Increased likelihood of impacts from other factors such as antibiotic therapy, kidney dysfunction, vitamin deficiency, or xerostomic drugs (e.g. catecholamines).
- Decreased host defence mechanisms, and therefore an increased risk of mouth infection, particularly with Candida species, herpes simplex virus, and *Streptococcus viridans*. Microbiological deposits in the mouth are also implicated in promoting infective processes at other sites, including

ventilation-associated pneumonia and infective endocarditis.

- Inability to maintain own oral hygiene.
- Continued formation of plaque and debris on teeth whether or not the patient is eating or drinking. Plaque formation can also lead to gingivitis.
- Oral ET tube impeding full assessment and access to the oral cavity.

Assessment and management of oral hygiene and preventive care

The general principles of effective oral hygiene, based on a regular regimen of gentle debridement and moisturization of oral tissue, are set out in this section. It should be noted that each patient's specific needs should be appraised with an individualized daily assessment. Prendergast *et al.* (2013) have produced a useful illustrated guide to systematic oral examination and the implementation of an oral care protocol (see also Table 3.5).

- The lips, mucus membranes, tongue, teeth and gums should be inspected at least twice daily (usually as a prelude to teeth brushing).
- The oral mucosa should be cleaned with dampened oral swabs and moisturized four-hourly, more often if the patient is intubated or the mouth is in particularly poor condition.
- The teeth should be brushed with a small soft toothbrush and a small blob of toothpaste for a minimum of two minutes twice a day, using a systematic approach (back to front, inside/outside) to ensure that all accessible surfaces are brushed (Prendergast *et al.* 2012). Non-foaming toothpaste may make it easier to remove residual material after brushing.
- Excessive fluid can be removed from the mouth with a Yankauer suction device.
- Artificial saliva may be useful for a persistently dry mouth.
- Following toothbrushing, gentle debridement of any coating of the tongue should be performed. This may also be done with the toothbrush, although use of a purpose-made tongue scraper has been recommended (Prendergast *et al.* 2013).
- Toothbrushes and other equipment should be cleaned and stored in clean dedicated containers between use.
- The lips should be protected from drying out with petroleum jelly.
- Dentures should be removed overnight when they should also be cleaned and soaked.
- Adequate fluid hydration of the patient will help with xerostomia.
- Oral candida should be treated with nystatin mouthwash.

Table 3.5 Assessment of the oral cavity

Oral cavity	Normal	Abnormal	Intervention
Mucosa	Pink, moist, intact, smooth	Reddening, ulceration, other lesions	Hydration, cleaned and moisturized at least four-hourly, analgesic gel for ulceration.
Tongue	Pink, moist, intact, papillae present	Coated, absence of papillae with smooth shiny appearance, debris, lesions, crusted, cracks, blackened	Hydration, moisturization/neutral mouthwashes at least four-hourly, gentle debridement with toothbrush/tongue scraper as needed.
Lips	Clean, intact, pink	Dry skin, cracks, reddened, encrusted, ulcerated, bleeding	Hydration, protection using petroleum jelly
Saliva	Watery, white, or clear	Thick, viscous, absent, bloodstained	Hydration, use of artificial saliva
Gingiva (gums)	Pink, moist, firm	Receding, overgrowing, oedematous and reddened, bleeding,	Toothbrushing at least twice daily with small soft brush.
Teeth	White, firm in sockets, no debris, no decay	Discoloured, decayed, debris present, unstable	Toothbrushing at least twice daily with small soft brush. Dental assessment.

Data from: Crosby C, Method in mouth care. *Nursing Times*, Volume 85, Issue 35, pp. 38-41. 1989, EMAP Publishing Ltd; Richardson A, A process standard for oral care. *Nursing Times*, Volume 83, Issue 32, pp. 38-40. 1987, EMAP Publishing Ltd.

Eye care

The healthy eye is protected from dehydration and infection by the production of tears and by the so-called tear film that covers the eyes. The tear film is made up of three layers, an outer lipid layer, a middle water-based layer, and an inner mucilaginous layer. Each layer has a specific purpose: the outer layer retards fluid evaporation and prevents overflow of tear film; the middle layer contains oxygen, electrolytes, and proteins, including antibacterial agents; and the inner layer aids wetting of the cornea. The normal rate of production of tears by the lacrimal gland is about 1–2 μL/min with tears spread over the surface of the cornea by the blink reflex.

Critical care patients are susceptible to ocular disorders, such as dry eyes and exposure keratopathy (drying of the cornea, affecting ≤60% of patients), chemosis (conjunctival swelling, affecting ≤80%), and microbial keratitis (Grixti *et al.* 2012).

These eye problems are due to the following.

1. Reduced or absent ability to blink.
2. Incomplete lid closure (causing by drying of the cornea, with the potential for epithelial erosions and corneal ulceration as well as increased risk of infection).
3. Decreased tear production as a side effect of certain drugs including atropine, phenothiazines, and tricyclic antidepressants.
4. Decreased resistance to infection as well as the potential for cross-infection from respiratory pathogens. This may be related to poor technique when suction catheters are withdrawn from the ET or tracheostomy tube and moved across the eyes so that droplets containing micro-organisms fall onto the cornea (Parkin *et al.* 1997). This problem may be alleviated by use of a closed suction system. Cross-infection can also occur if the same container of eyedrops or ointment is used to treat both eyes (Hernandez and Mannis 1997).
5. Increased likelihood of orbital oedema due to the increased intrathoracic pressures generated by positive pressure ventilation, and concomitant decreased venous return. These effects are exacerbated if the patient is nursed flat, or if tape securing an ET or tracheostomy is tied too tightly. Dependent areas of the body are affected, with fluid forced into the periocular tissues and conjunctival membrane.
6. Dehydration reduces tear production.
7. Misplaced high flow oxygen delivery sysyems, nebulizer drug delivery devices, or continuous positive airway pressure equipment can propel gas into the eyes with drying and contamination effects.

Management of the eyes and eye problems

Effective eye care is based on regular assessment (at least twice daily), cleansing, moistening, and lubrication of the surface of the eye as required, and ensuring that the eyes are completely closed or, if that is not possible, that any exposed tissue is protected.

1. Assess the following aspects to determine the required frequency of intervention:
   - the patient's ability to close their eyelids, identifying if:
     - the eyelids are completely closed (or not)
     - there is conjunctival exposure (i.e. the white of the eye is visible)
     - the cornea is exposed
   - patient position
   - the patient's hydration status
   - the condition of the cornea—look for evidence of infection (purulent or crusting exudate), clouding, haemorrhage, etc.
   - evidence of discharge
   - any relevant drug therapies.
2. Use sterile water for cleansing (so-called normal saline disrupts the normal tear film structure and increases the rate of evaporation as its sodium chloride content is significantly greater than that of body fluids).
3. If corneal wetting is inadequate, administer artificial tears (e.g. hypromellose) at least two- to four-hourly; a liquid paraffin ointment may be given if required, particularly if the conjunctiva or cornea is exposed.
4. If open or partially open, the eyelids can often be closed manually, but if the corneal surface remains exposed, closure or protection of the eye surfaces must be achieved by other means. Closure with hypoallergenic tape, covering the eyes with gauze, transparent hydrogel, or polyethylene film are amongst the methods used in different institutions (Rosenberg and Eisen 2008; Kam *et al.* 2013). Taping the eyes is a widely used technique but has the potential to damage delicate tissue and may be seen as unsightly by the patient's family. Hydrogel placed over the eyes was found to be the most common method used in a recent survey of ICUs in England (Kam *et al.* 2013) but it is actually not licensed for this purpose. Creation of a 'moisture chamber' (e.g. with a layer of polyethylene film ('cling film')) that covers the eyes,

extending beyond the orbits and eyebrows, and is taped to the face) has been shown to preserve the corneal epithelium more effectively than lubrication alone, and may become the method of choice in future (Rosenberg and Eisen 2008).

5. Care should be taken when withdrawing suction catheters to avoid droplet transference of respiratory organisms to the corneal surface. Bacterial keratopathy is associated with poor suction technique and the use of open suction systems (Parkin *et al.* 1997).
6. If the eye is discharging or obviously infected take a swab for microbial culture and sensitivity and apply appropriate topical antibiotic drops or ointment as prescribed.

Prevention of problems associated with urinary catheterization

Most critically ill patients are catheterized to allow close monitoring of urinary output. However, the presence of a urinary catheter is associated with several problems.

Problems to be addressed

Increased risk of urinary tract infection

One in seven of infections in the critical care unit are infections of the urinary tract (UTIs) (Vincent *et al.* 2009), usually in patients with indwelling urinary catheters (Shuman and Chenoweth 2010). UTIs occur for the following reasons.

- The trauma associated with insertion of the catheter which creates breaks in mucosal integrity allowing bacterial colonization.
- Contamination during insertion and afterwards due to poor handwashing/hygiene procedures.
- Bypassing of the normal defence mechanisms of the urethra.
- Use of larger than necessary catheters which may cause pressure on the urethral wall and ischaemia.
- Use of larger than necessary balloons which may cause pressure on the bladder wall and an increase in residual urine.
- Obliteration of the natural urethral mucosal cleansing which occurs during normal voiding when the flow of urine discourages migration of pathogens.
- Susceptibility to infection is generally increased in critical illness.
- The critical care environment has an increased level of pathogenic bacteria. Many catheterized patients develop bacteriuria within 48 hours.

Trauma and discomfort associated with the presence of the catheter

This is due to:

- use of larger than necessary catheters and larger than necessary balloons
- movement/dragging of the catheter.

Blockage of the catheter from debris or blood

This is due to:

- poor urinary flow, allowing debris to collect in the bladder
- urinary tract infection producing large amounts of debris

Management of problems associated with urinary catheterization

The Royal College of Nursing (2012) has produced a comprehensive guide to urinary catheter care, albeit not specific to critical care patients. The key principles of care are summarized below.

- There should be strict asepsis for catheter insertion.
- Handwashing must take place prior to any manipulation of the catheter.
- A closed urinary drainage system should be maintained with minimal manipulation of any part.
- Unimpeded urinary flow should be maintained with no reflux. The tubing and drainage bag should be carefully positioned to ensure continuous gravity-aided flow, i.e. ensure that the tubing is not kinked or looped.
- There must be strict asepsis for collection of catheter specimens of urine (CSUs) through the specimen port. (NB: the drainage system should never be disconnected for this.)
- Bladder irrigation should be avoided unless absolutely necessary. If required, and where possible, irrigation should be done via the specimen port rather than by disconnecting the drainage system.
- Use the smallest size catheter that will drain adequately. This is usually 12–14 Ch (with an external diameter of 4–4.5 mm).
- A 10 ml balloon catheter should be used, except immediately after bladder or prostatic surgery when a larger balloon may be necessary for haemostatic purposes.
- Attach the catheter to the inner aspect of the thigh and support the tubing so as to prevent drag (Fisher 2010). A range of securement devices are available.

- Carry out meatal cleansing with soap and water daily, or more frequently if necessary. There is no evidence to support the use of antiseptic solutions for cleansing (Royal College of Nursing 2012).
- Ensure that the catheter material used is appropriate to the likely length of catheterization, i.e. polytetrafluoroethylene (PTFE) for medium-term use up to 4 weeks, and hydrogel or silicone elastomer for use up to 12 weeks. Patients with a latex allergy should only have a pure silicone catheter.
- Ensure that the foreskin does not remain retracted, as this can cause a painful phimosis.
- The use of antiseptic- or antimicrobial-impregnated catheters may be considered for particularly high risk patients or if there is an especially high incidence of catheter-associated UTIs; however, the evidence for the value of these devices is mixed (Schumm and Lam 2008; Pickard *et al.* 2012).
- The catheter should be removed as soon as it is possible for the patient to manage their urinary function without it.

Effects of restricted mobility

Most critically ill patients have only limited movement or cannot move themselves at all, and so will remain in a static position, which may be flat-lying if the patient is unstable, unless moved by the nurses. Even in the recovery phase, patients are often too weak to move themselves and may remain in one position for much longer than they should. Therefore the effects of immobility are a major problem for the critically ill patient, and prevention of the complications of immobility can make the difference between eventual recovery or otherwise. The quality of life of critical care survivors may also be reduced if these potential problems are not managed.

The effects of restricted mobility include the following.

Increased risk of chest infection

Risk factors include:

- basal collapse
- increased secretions
- decreased sputum clearance
- ventilation to perfusion (V/Q) mismatch secondary to atelectasis, dependent lung oedema, and alterations due to positioning.

Lung volumes (functional residual capacity (FRC) and residual volumes) are reduced when lying supine because of the rise in the diaphragm resulting from the change in position of the abdominal contents. Impaired ability to cough, decreased ciliary movement, and weak thoracic muscles cause stasis and pooling of secretions. In addition, production of alveolar surfactant may be impaired during periods when the patient is flat. The V/Q ratio of is also altered in supine, lateral, and prone positions.

Increased risk of deep vein thrombosis and peripheral oedema

Underlying factors include:

- decreased venous return
- venous stasis
- increased coagulability.

Loss of muscle movement means that the normal pumping mechanism returning venous blood to the heart is reduced. Blood pooling occurs, which increases intracapillary hydrostatic pressure and leads, in turn, to increases in the movement of fluid through the capillary membrane into the interstitial tissue. The loss of fluid from the intravascular compartment increases the viscosity of the blood, causing further stasis and an increased risk of platelet aggregation and coagulation.

Neuromuscular dysfunction

Critical illness myopathy and polyneuropathy are early complications of immobilization that can rapidly and drastically reduce both respiratory and limb muscle strength (Latronico and Bolton 2011). These processes are further accelerated by the catabolic nature of most critical illnesses. Respiratory muscle weakness leads to difficulty with weaning from mechanical ventilation, while loss of strength of thigh and calf muscles, in particular, can mean that a very lengthy convalescence is required to restore normal function (Herridge *et al.* 2011).

Joint stiffness and contractures

Over a third of patients with a critical care stay ≥14 days develop clinically significant joint contractures (Clavet *et al.* 2008). The main risk lies with flexion, as flexor muscles are stronger than extensors. Common sites include plantar flexor, shoulder, hand, hip, and knee joints. Passive exercise programmes to maintain the normal range of movement are commonly performed by nurses and physiotherapists with the goal of preventing muscle shortening, although currently there is no definitive evidence of benefit (Katalinic *et al.* 2010).

Demineralization and loss of density in the long bones

Loss of weight-bearing pressure within the long bones results in decreased osteoblastic (bone-forming and repair) activity. Osteoclastic (bone destruction) activity continues, resulting in a loss of bone density and, ultimately, osteoporosis. Hypercalcaemia and hypercalciuria are also seen within 1–2 days of immobility and have been associated with prolonged immobility even when there is adequate calcium intake.

Peripheral nerve injury

The particular risk is ulnar nerve injury due to incorrect positioning. Pronation of the forearm in the supine position traps the ulnar nerve in the cubital tunnel and flexion of the elbow in this position adds further pressure on the ulnar nerve.

Increased risk of pressure ulcers

This is damage to skin and the underlying tissue due to pressure on dependent areas and an inability to change position when required. Development of pressure ulcers is a function of the level of pressure exerted and the length of time it is exerted; the higher the pressure, the less time is required for a sore to develop. The most vulnerable areas are the tissues over bony prominences including the sacrum, coccyx, ears, and heels (see Box 3.11). Generic risk factors, which often feature in critical illness, include (National Pressure Ulcer Advisory Panel & European Pressure Ulcer Advisory Panel 2009):

- reduced oxygenation/circulation
- inadequate nutrition
- skin status (including moisture)
- old age.

Critically ill patients are particularly vulnerable to pressure ulcers; incidence rates of 10–41% have been reported (Cooper 2013). Various risk factors have been described in critical care populations, including:

- (im)mobility
- friction/shear

Box 3.11 Prevention of pressure ulcers

The SSKIN framework provides a practical approach for prevention of pressure ulcerss.

Surface

- Patients with multiple risk factors should be prophylactically placed on a high specification (not standard foam) mattress on admission. Placing pillows under the calves allows the heels to be suspended away from the mattress surface. Purpose made pressure relieving boots are also available to prevent heel tissue injury.

Skin inspection

- Top-to-toe and back-and-front skin inspection should take place at least once per shift.

Keep Moving

- Critically ill patients should be proactively turned at least two- three-hourly, placed on alternate sides to avoid the supine position and minimize pressure on 'at risk' areas.
- Very few patients are genuinely 'too sick' to move or turn.

Incontinence

- Urine, faeces, or perspiration increase the risk of skin injury, particularly to the perineum, buttocks, groin, inner thighs, and other skin folds.
- The skin should be kept clean and dry, and barrier creams used to protect the skin from excessive moisture.
- A bowel management system may be needed to prevent faeces causing further damage and to allow skin healing.

Nutrition

- Poor nutritional status (and dehydration) is associated with increased risk of pressure ulcers. Nutritional requirements should be assessed as soon as possible after admission and a nutrition plan to meet those needs formulated.

- catecholamines (Cox 2011)
- renal replacement therapy
- mechanical ventilation (Nijs *et al.* 2009)
- acuity of illness/presence of comorbidities
- faecal incontinence
- anaemia
- length of stay (Theaker *et al.* 2000).

All critical care patients should have full top-to-toe and back-and-front-inspections of all skin surfaces at least twice daily, and two- to four-hourly or more frequently if very high risk or significant pressure damage has occurred. Identification and classification of any pressure ulcers can guide subsequent care:

Grade 1—non-blanchable erythema (redness) of intact skin

Grade 2—partial thickness skin loss

Grade 3—full thickness skin loss

Grade 4—full thickness tissue loss (with visible bone or muscle).[2]

Relief of pressure by frequent (e.g. two-hourly) changes of position is an essential component of nursing care of the critically ill. Very few patients are genuinely too unstable to be turned for very long periods (Brindle *et al.* 2013). Nonetheless, other methods of pressure relief are often required, such as special low pressure or alternating pressure support surfaces.

Increased risk of urinary tract infection

Supine positioning results in the renal pelvis filling with urine before drainage via the ureter occurs, and this urinary stasis can act as a focus for bacterial growth and the formation of renal calculi. There will also be an accumulation of urine in the bladder in the supine position due to filling of the dependent portion of the bladder prior to drainage via the urethra; this may be relieved by urinary catheterization. There may be an increase in urinary pH (i.e. it is less acidic) because of increased calcium and phosphate excretion. This will tend to increase infection risk. Other risk factors include (Bagshaw and Laupland 2006):

- immunocompromise
- the presence of a urinary catheter—and duration of catheterization
- length of stay
- female gender
- systemic antimicrobial therapy.

Increased incidence of nephrolithiasis (kidney stones)

This is due to increased urinary calcium excretion related to bone degeneration. Hypercalcaemia occurs as a result of degeneration of bone from disuse (see earlier), which produces an increase in renal excretion of calcium and phosphate from the first week of bed rest. This can continue for up to 5 weeks.

Decreased gut motility and constipation

Muscle wasting and loss may include the muscles controlling excretion (diaphragm, abdominal muscles, and levator ani). Reduced gut motility may occur as a result of loss of stimuli such as the presence of food passing through the oesophagus.

The degree of bowel dysfunction is related to the severity of illness, a direct result of the illness (e.g. with spinal injuries, acute polyneuropathy (e.g. Guillain–Barré) syndrome), use of opiate, sedative, and paralysing agents, haemodynamic instability, and loss of muscle function due to muscle wasting.

Management of problems due to restricted mobility

Frequent changes of position are essential in preventing many of the complications associated with immobility. This is not always possible for reasons such as adverse changes in ventilation/perfusion ratios related to shunting in certain positions, significant haemodynamic instability, and spinal or pelvic trauma. In these situations other goals may take priority, but ensuring awareness of the many problems caused by immobility should ensure that patients are moved whenever possible. The following points are important for optimal care of the critically ill.

- Regular turning and repositioning of the patient.
- Knowledge of the correct alignment and positioning of limbs to prevent joint injury.
- Use of specialist beds and mattresses which relieve pressure over susceptible points and spread the pressure load.
- Regular systematic head-to-toe and back-and-front inspection of skin integrity, with particular attention to the high risk dependent areas
- Whenever possible, a schedule of active isotonic limb and full range of movement (ROM) exercises to

[2] Data used with the permission of the National Pressure Ulcer Advisory Panel 2009.

maintain muscle strength and joint mobility. When patients cannot participate in active exercise, passive limb movements and exercises with the aim of maintaining joint mobility may be beneficial.
- Chest physiotherapy, use of adequate humidification, etc. (see Chapter 4).
- Monitoring of bowel function.
- Early commencement of feeding (especially enteral).
- Scrupulous attention to infection control measures.
- Early and frequent mobilization.

Prevention of the complications associated with immobility may not necessarily alter patient outcome, but may contribute significantly to the rate of rehabilitation and the degree of morbidity following discharge.

Infection risks in intensive care

Critically ill patients tend to have compromised host defence mechanisms and an increased susceptibility to infection; over half of the critical care patients in the multinational EPIC II study were being treated for infection (Vincent *et al.* 2009). Many of these infections are acquired as a result of the invasive therapies routinely used in critical illness,for example ventilator-associated pneumonia (VAP), vascular catheter-related bloodstream infection (CRBSI), urinary catheter-associated urinary tract infection (CAUTI), and surgical site infection (Majumdar and Padiglione 2012). Invasive devices facilitate colonization by nosocomial organisms and greatly increase vulnerability to infection.

Critical care patients are also subjected to resistant strains of bacteria that have been created by excessive or inadequately managed antibiotic usage in critical care units over many years (Varley *et al.* 2009). In addition, antibiotics reduce indigenous bacterial flora, allowing overgrowth of other organisms and development of opportunistic infections such as invasive fungal disease (Martin and Yost 2011; Muskett *et al.* 2011). See Box 3.12 for a summary of potential influences on infection in critical care.

Box 3.12 Summary: potential influences on infection in critical care

Patient-related problems
- Invasive procedures and monitoring
- Patient positioning (e.g. leading to aspiration of gastric contents)
- Abnormal humoral immunity
- Abnormal phagocytic function
- Abnormal antibody function
- Genetic factors (Wong 2012)

Environment-related problems
- Cohorting of many high risk patients in one area
- High usage of antibiotics encouraging growth of resistant bacteria, fungal infection, etc
- Poor infection control, e.g. inadequate hand hygiene
- Insufficient nurses: review of 12 studies found a trend towards or association between lower nurse–patient ratios and problems such as increased cross-infection (Penoyer 2010)

Ventilator-associated pneumonia (VAP)

The term VAP refers to a new episode of pneumonia in a ventilated patient at least 48 hours after intubation (or acute tracheostomization) (Hunter 2012). Risk factors implicated in the development of this type of nosocomial pneumonia include (Hunter 2012):

- the presence of an ET tube (the standard tube is said to be inherently flawed (Zolfaghari and Wyncoll 2011)
- chronic ill health, particularly chronic pulmonary disease (history of smoking)
- malnutrition
- use of H_2 (histamine receptor) antagonists used to prevent stress ulceration (see Chapter 9)
- use of antibiotics
- prolonged upper abdominal or thoracic surgery
- impaired upper airway reflexes such as the cough reflex
- advanced age and obesity
- supine body position
- enteral nutrition
- duration of ventilation.

Mechanisms of infection include (Hunter 2012):

- contamination of inspired gas (e.g. respiratory therapy equipment)
- spread from contiguous (neighbouring) infected tissue
- blood-borne spread from distant infections on tricuspid valve vegetations
- oropharyngeal and gastric colonization with transmission to the trachea, probably by aspiration.

Aspiration is the most frequent cause of infection in ventilated patients. ET tubes provide protection from large volume aspiration but may actually facilitate transfer of tiny amounts of aspirate (microaspiration) by preventing closure of the vocal cords and bypassing the cough reflex (Zolfaghari and Wyncoll 2011). The presence of enteral feed in the stomach and the resultant rise in gastric pH may also be related to overgrowth of bacteria and an increase in aspiration pneumonia, although an overall benefit of enteral feeding in critically ill patients is generally accepted (Seron-Arbeloa *et al.* 2013). Supine body positioning is also implicated in aspiration; Drakulovic *et al.* (1999) reported a significant decrease in VAP when patients were nursed in a semi-recumbent position rather than supine. Subsequently, elevation of the head of the bed has been widely adopted as a key component of the bundle of care processes recommended to prevent VAP (Resar *et al.* 2005). However, concerns have been raised about the quality of evidence supporting this approach (e.g. Niël-Weise *et al.* 2011).

Practices aimed at prevention of VAP are essential, as identification and treatment of the causative organism can be difficult and ineffective. VAP that develops in the first few days of ventilation is most often caused by bacteria including *Haemophilus* species (Gram-negative), *Streptococci* species (e.g. *Streptococcus pneumoniae*) (Gram-positive), and *Staphylococcus aureus* (Gram-positive), which are usually antibiotic sensitive (Hunter 2012). Cases that occur later on are more likely to be due to drug-resistant bacteria including *Pseudomonas* species (e.g. *Pseudomonas aeruginosa*) and *Acinetobacter* species (both Gram-negative), and methicillin-resistant *Staphylococcus aureus* (MRSA) (Hunter 2012).

Vascular access devices

These comprise central venous catheters, peripheral venous and arterial cannulae, and pulmonary artery flotation catheters (see Box 3.13).

> **BOX 3.13 Routes of infection in vascular access devices**
>
> - Hub contamination leading to transfer of organisms down the cannula
> - Connections between the giving set and cannula such as three-way taps
> - Site contamination
> - Thrombosis of the cannula, providing a medium for organism growth

Any vascular access device provides a portal of entry for microorganisms into the circulation. Local and systemic infections can occur even with peripheral cannulae, especially if the device is inserted or cared for in suboptimal conditions, for example in an emergency (Chittick and Sherertz 2010).

Infections related to vascular access devices are most often caused by migration of skin flora from the insertion site along the catheter so that the tip is colonized, or direct contamination of the catheter or catheter hub during manipulation by staff, or connection to other devices that are contaminated (O'Grady *et al.* 2011).

There is conflicting evidence as to the infection rates associated with multi-lumen as opposed to single-lumen central venous catheters, with some studies reporting no difference while others report significant differences (Dezfulian *et al.* 2003). This variation may be related to the heterogeneity involved in the study populations, with some studies using non-randomized samples. When higher-quality studies were examined in a meta-analysis by Dezfulian *et al.* (2003), there was no significant difference in catheter-related bloodstream infection. This is thought to be due to other advantages of multiple lumens such as decreased need for manipulation and use of multiple connection devices, and the reduction in the number of invasive procedures required.

There are several types of needle-less system that can be used to access venous catheters without breaking the circuit which also reduce the risk of harm (to staff) from needlestick injuries. Some of these devices have been associated with increased catheter-related bloodstream infection rates; the split septum type is reported to be the preferred device (Btaiche *et al.* 2011).

Preventative measures

Ventilator-associated pneumonia

1. Ventilator and circuits:
    - use of heat and moisture exchangers (HMEs), with bacterial filters, rather than water bath humidifiers.
    - regular change of ventilator circuits and manual ventilation systems—at least every 48 hours if HMEs are not used.
    - scrupulous handwashing and use of gloves prior to endotracheal suctioning
    - use of disposable nebulizers or scrupulous washing and drying of reusable nebulizers between use
    - use of closed suction catheter systems (American Association for Respiratory Care 2010).

2. The patient:
   - regular changes of position from semi-recumbent to left and right lateral to enable maximum basal lung expansion.
   - regular chest physiotherapy (see Chapter 4).

Various other measures have been advocated for the prevention of VAP (see Chapter 4, Box 4.14). The five principles of the 'Ventilator Bundle' set out by the US Institute for Healthcare Improvement (http://www.ihi.org) and adopted by the UK NHS Patient Safety First programme (http://www.patientsafetyfirst.nhs.uk) are:

- patient positioning as near as possible to 45°
- daily 'sedation holds'—or simply light sedation—and assessment of readiness to extubate
- oral decontamination
- stress ulcer prophylaxis as appropriate
- venous thromboembolism prophylaxis.

However, the utility of these measures in preventing ventilator-associated adverse events has been questioned in recent years; indeed, the effectiveness of the bundle approach itself has not been tested in a randomized controlled trial (O'Grady *et al.* 2012). It may even be that some of these elements have potential for harm; for example, the practice of sedation holds may increase the total amount of sedation given—and nursing workload—without reducing time on the ventilator or ICU stay (Mehta *et al.* 2012), while stress ulcer prophylaxis has been linked to increased infection rates (Plummer *et al.* 2014).

The key point is that each patient's specific risk factors must be assessed and both benefits and potential adverse effects of treatments considered if **individualized** evidence-based care is to be provided.

Vascular catheter-related bloodstream infections

Multiple studies (e.g. Bion *et al.* 2013) have shown that ensuring consistent use of a standard set of interventions when placing and then managing central venous catheters (CVCs) reduces bloodstream infections. These measures include:

- using strict hand hygiene, and then wearing a sterile gown and gloves, cleaning the skin with chlorhexidine in alcohol, and positioning full barrier sterile drapes for CVC insertion;
- thereafter, inspecting the site (and considering if the CVC could be removed) at least daily, and using aseptic methods when accessing the device (Bion *et al.* 2013).

Urinary tract infections

The most important preventative measure is to avoid urinary catheterization unless absolutely essential, but this strategy is very difficult to achieve in the critical care unit where monitoring of renal function and urine production is essential for most patients. If catheterization is performed, the possibility of removal should be considered as early as possible. The principles of care of the catheterized patient have already been described.

Some of the points noted earlier and other key aspects of care of the critically ill have been incorporated into the acroynym FASTHUG (Vincent 2005): **F**eeding, **A**nalgesia, **S**edation, deep vein **T**hrombosis prophylaxis, **H**ead-of-bed elevation, stress **U**lcer prevention, and **G**lucose control. This mnemonic provides the basis of a useful checklist of issues to be regularly reviewed and optimized. Extra components have been added in some critical care units.

Hand hygiene

The main preventable route of transmission of nosocomial infection is via the hands of healthcare staff (Allegranzi and Pittet 2009), and the single most important factor in preventing transmission is scrupulous hand hygiene (Tschudin-Sutter *et al.* 2010). Environmental factors such as positioning of wash-basins with easy access from each bed area and providing enough wash-basins to allow unrestricted access are important in supporting hand-washing. Use of alcohol-based handrubs is recommended for regular hand antisepsis (Tschudin-Sutter *et al.* 2010). These handrubs can be widely distributed, for example in individual containers attached to staff uniforms or in dispensers at the bedside. Visual and auditory prompts to engage in hand hygiene procedures, as well as education programmes tailored to critical care practice and regular audits with feedback on performance can be effective in improving compliance (Mazi *et al.* 2013). The recommended schedule of hand hygiene procedures is that they should occur (Sax *et al.* 2007):

(1) before patient contact
(2) before clean and aseptic procedures
(3) after body fluid exposure risk
(4) after patient contact
(5) after contact with patient surroundings.

Individual unit policies may vary; however, essential measures aimed at reducing nosocomial infections in critical care are set out in Box 3.14.

Box 3.14 Essential measures for limiting infection in the critical care environment

- Strict adherence to local infection control policies
- Handwashing/use of alcohol rub between patient contacts
- Use of aprons and gloves for patient contact (universal precautions)
- Maintaining a 30–45° semi-recumbent position to reduce aspiration
- Maintaining staffing ratios appropriate to patient need/workload
- Strict aseptic technique for dressings, line insertions, invasive procedures, etc.
- Limitation of manipulation of IV lines, urinary catheters, dressings
- Policy of immediate removal of IV lines if infection is suspected
- Infection control standards/protocols for staff
- Feedback from microbiology regarding infection rates
- Avoidance of antacid ulcer prophylaxis and H_2 blockers in combination
- Avoidance of endotracheal intubation, wherever possible, by use of non-invasive respiratory support
- Adherence to a locally defined antimicrobial policy

Transfer of critically ill patients

Secondary transfer refers to transfer from or within a hospital setting to another centre. These journeys may entail either accompanying a patient from one critical care unit to another, or going out from a specialist critical care unit to pick up a patient from another facility. Movement of critically ill patients inevitably involves some risk; adverse events have been reported in 34% of transfers notwithstanding that 70% of these events were judged to be potentially avoidable, for example failures to provide sufficent oxygen or batteries in some journeys (Ligtenberg *et al.* 2005). Analysis of 759 critical care patients subjected to non-clinical transfer found that their critical care length of stay was 3.2 days longer than matched patients who were not transferred, although their mortality was no higher (Barratt *et al.* 2012).

Effective risk management in these situations should be a team effort, but the nurse caring for an individual patient has a particular responsibility for ensuring the safety of their patient. Transfer of critically ill patients requires careful planning and preparation, suitable equipment, and the deployment of appropriately trained competent staff (Intensive Care Society 2011).

Suggested procedure

A comprehensive guide to safe transport of the critically ill is available from the UK Intensive Care Society (2011). This includes pre-transport checklists which help to clarify the level of potential risk and to decide whether or not a particular patient is stable for transport and ready to be moved, as well as descriptions of the competencies required by different staff and what equipment will be needed. The key principles are as follows.

- Transfers should be managed by experienced, suitably qualified, and trained personnel.
- The equipment used should be designed for transport with reliable performance and battery back-up.
- Monitoring should consist of a minimum of pulse oximetry, end-tidal CO_2, ECG, invasive or non-invasive blood pressure, and temperature.
- Staff should be familiar with the equipment used.
- The patient should be stabilized prior to transfer.
- If it is likely that intubation or other invasive or aggressive manoeuvres might be needed, these procedures should be performed before transfer.
- Ideally, dedicated transport teams should be utilized to stabilize and then transfer patients.
- The patient's infective status should be checked in order that adequate precautions can be taken in the event of problems such as MRSA.

Care prior to and during transport

1. Ensure patient safety prior to and during transfer:
    - check all equipment for functioning, battery life, and functioning alarm systems
    - set up and use appropriate individualized alarm settings

- ensure that all staff transferring the patient are familiar with all equipment including emergency equipment.

2. Stabilize the patient prior to transfer and monitor the patient during transfer (see Table 3.6). Any patient with respiratory problems should be assessed prior to the journey by an experienced intensivist or anaesthetist to assess the possible need for intubation and elective ventilation prior to transfer. If the patient is not intubated, patients at risk should be accompanied by someone experienced in emergency intubation.
3. Notification of relatives: ensure relatives are aware of the reason for transfer, the approximate journey time, the details of the receiving hospital, and the name of the receiving consultant. If possible, provide a copy of the unit information booklet for the patient's relatives and, if necessary, supply directions.
4. Collection of copies of documentation. The following are needed: notes, X-rays and scans, diagnostic reports, charts, nursing documentation, and drug prescription chart. A synopsis of the relevant history, key problems and treatments given, any significant incidents, and nursing care given should be produced by the transferring hospital.
5. Arrangements for transfer (these should be completed only when the patient is approaching readiness for transfer):
   - Notify ambulance control, and the police if necessary.
   - Inform the receiving hospital immediately prior to departure of an estimated time of arrival (NB: inter-hospital transfer by helicopter or aircraft is a specialized procedure which should only be carried out by trained teams).

Table 3.6 Preparing the critically ill patient for transfer

Problem	Prior to transfer	During transfer
Airway and O_2 requirements	ABGs. CXR. Insert, secure chest drains as needed. Intubate if necessary. Chest physiotherapy and suction.	Portable ventilator (if ventilation is needed/likely to be needed). Pulse oximetry and end-tidal carbon dioxide monitoring for ventilated patients. Portable suction and catheters. Oxygen supply with at least one hour over calculated requirements. Mapleson C/Waters circuit or manual bag–valve system with self-inflating resuscitator.
Cardiovascular support	Insert and secure any venous/arterial access devices needed, ensuring at least two venous access devices available. Correct any electrolyte or pH abnormalities (as far as possible). Set up supportive drug infusions with adequate supplies for maximum calculated requirements. Check temperature. Insert pacing wire if needed.	ECG and BP monitoring system. Continuous drug infusions via battery-operated pumps. Portable defibrillator and emergency drugs available. Adequate bed linen for patient.
Maintenance of fluid balance	Insert urinary catheter. Set up required infusions. Consider need for nasogastric tube.	Carry appropriate fluid for infusions and extra fluid in case emergency fluid resuscitation is needed. Maintain urinary and nasogastric drainage during transfer.
Patient anxiety	Inform patient, and relatives, of reasons for transfer, the destination, and approximate journey time. Take time to answer questions. Introduce transfer team to patient.	Continue to reassure the patient and inform them of progress. Ensure the patient is secure and comfortable on the trolley.
Pain control and sedation	Assess patient's pain. Ensure adequate supplies of analgesia for journey. Set up analgesic/sedative infusions as needed.	Regularly reassess pain and sedation.
Miscellaneous	Assess pressure areas. Insert wound drains. Stabilize fractures as required.	Transfer on pressure-relieving mattress as appropriate. Carry adequate drainage containers.

Elective versus emergency admissions to critical care

Most critical care units admit a mixture of elective and emergency admissions. Preparation for these two types of patients is different and their needs, and prognosis, will also differ.

Elective patients

Admissions are usually post-operative but may occasionally be pre-operative, for example for haemodynamic optimization.

1. The patient is usually prepared for admission. They may have visited the critical care area and should have been given some information by nursing and/or medical staff. Thus the elective patient has the opportunity to gain some understanding of critical care and to develop coping mechanisms that may help manage the stresses inherent in the environment. It is likely that relatives will also have some prior information and may have met critical care staff before the admission.
2. The admission is usually only for a short period (often just overnight), so the effects of close observation and monitoring, ventilation, the general environment, and sensory disturbance are likely to be minimal.
3. Recovery is usually swift unless complications occur; the patient may have relatively limited recollection of the time spent in the critical care unit because of the effects of anaesthesia, analgesia, and sedation.

Overall, elective admissions are much less vulnerable to the problems associated with critical care, especially if adequate efforts are made to prepare them.

Emergency admissions

1. The very nature of the crises which precipitate emergency admission generally mean that these patients tend to be more severely ill and have a worse prognosis. Patient scoring systems such as the Acute Physiology and Chronic Health Evaluation (APACHE) carry weightings which reflects these risk factors (see Chapter 16). Unexpected life-threatening events induce stress and often profound shock in both patients and relatives.
2. Lack of preparation increases fear and decreases the ability of the patient to cope with the stresses of the critical care environment. Therefore they are more vulnerable to the problems associated with critical care.
3. Recovery is frequently less certain and more prolonged, although this varies with the cause of admission.

Strategies to reduce stress in patients and families

1. Detailed and repeated information giving is essential. It is difficult to process information or retain it when distressed or shocked, so it is important not to overload patients or relatives with too much information at one time.
2. Support is often limited to relatives at the beginning of an admission to critical care as circumstances can make it impossible to establish effective two-way communication with the patient straight away. However, efforts to provide information to the patient should continue, with reassurance that all necessary care and treatment is being given.
3. Alternative support agencies for both relatives and patients should be considered and used where appropriate.

The dying critical care patient

Critical care is associated with high mortality rates which vary from week to week but typically average about 20% (Scottish Intensive Care Society Audit Group 2013). In some cases—often emergencies—death occurs relatively soon after admission to the unit and there is little time to prepare either the patient or the family. More often, death occurs after a number of days and is more of an expected outcome. In a few patients, it becomes evident that the continuation of treatment and/or more interventions are both distressing for the patient and futile. The ethics of decisions regarding withdrawal of treatment are discussed in Chapter 16; however, the care of the dying patient and his/her family is set out here.

Withdrawal of treatment

Once it has been decided that further interventions will not benefit the patient, the priorities change to focusing on care and comfort. It should be stressed to the family that this does not mean any reduction in the standard of care the patient will receive.

Before this point, analgesia and sedation may have been used to limit cardiovascular side effects when important but uncomfortable treatments such as suction and physiotherapy are performed to improve the likelihood of recovery. Once a decision is taken to withdraw or limit further interventions, care—as opposed to cure—becomes the priority; the patient's physical and psychological needs should supersede any other considerations. Analgesia should be given at doses that ensure pain relief, and distressing interventions such as suction should be limited to the minimum required to maintain patient comfort.

Comfort, psychological care, and support are paramount, not only for the patient but also for the patient's family. Where the patient is able to respond, any decisions on pain relief, movement, personal hygiene, and comfort should be discussed with them.

Use of alternative methods of pain relief and managing anxiety should be considered. The patient may feel that they would prefer to be alert and able to communicate with their family as long as possible. In this case, they may choose to accept a certain amount of (bearable) pain in order to avoid the drowsiness and disorientation associated with increased quantities of analgesia.

Supporting the family/friends of the dying patient

The phrases 'family' and/or 'friends' will be used as a label for all those with relationships of significance to the patient. Kirchhoff *et al.* (2002) described some of the significant issues that families and friends experience during dying and death in the critical care unit.

- A feeling of uncertainty pervades the end-of-life experience of patients' families.
- Family members can be torn between what are seen as choices between what medical technology may offer and what they know about the patient's wishes.
- Family members feel a responsibility to protect the patient.
- Families' information about patients is often inadequate.
- Effective communication with staff is the best remedy for uncertainty.
- Families need adequate opportunies to say goodbye to the patient.

The key principles that should guide caring for family/friends of a dying patient are as follows (Kirchhoff *et al.* 2002).

- Ensuring effective provision of information (i.e. information that is consistent, clear, and objective) and ongoing communication.
- Family/friends should be supported in 'letting go' and saying goodbye to the patient.
- The patient's family/friends should be helped in managing the two alternating processes that occur in order to make sense of traumatic events: (1) intrusive experiencing and re-experiencing of the traumatic event and (2) protective denial.

Breaking the news of impending death

Ideally, a senior member of the medical staff who is familiar with the patient and their family/friends should lead the process, particularly if a discussion of the medical care will be needed. A member of the nursing staff should be present and, if appropriate, other professional support such as the chaplain, a counsellor, or a member of the hospital palliative care/end-of-life care team.

The setting should be private, set up with enough comfortable chairs for all involved to have easy eye contact, be available for as long as may be necessary, and be away from the commotion of the busy critical care unit.

Details may have to be repeated a number of times. The family/friends are usually distressed and often unable to take in and retain much information. They may need reassurance regarding concerns about the patient's comfort and what he/she may have suffered. Individual spiritual needs/values should be addressed (organ donation is dealt with in Chapter 8).

Supporting the family in coping with death

The news that the patient is dying will usually end any hope that the family may have had. Hearing their greatest fears explicitly articulated can be a trigger for an acute crisis; it is often only at this point that family members or friends feel able to really express their feelings and show how severely distressed they are. Responses range from grief to denial and anger, with physical manifestations that may include fainting or collapse. Some people use denial as a coping mechanism and will be unable to accept what is said to them. Such responses may seem inappropriate and may not be helpful to the family member or friend; staff will need to assess the individual to determine whether further reinforcement of the reality at this time is the right thing to do or whether it would be better to pause the process for a period. Anger may also be expressed as a response to the situation and should be dealt with using understanding and tact.

Communication

Frequent communication and information within an open and honest relationship between staff and the family/friends are important aspects of support. Any interaction with the family/friends may include cues for help, information, and support, so watching and listening is as vital as saying the right things at the right time. Use of non-verbal communication—touch, facial expression, sitting with the family—is comforting and expresses empathy. Sometimes, it may be helpful to simply sit in silence, and it is useful for the nurse to become comfortable with this.

Participation in care of the patient

This should be discussed with the family/friends as well as the patient where possible, and areas of care which are appropriate should be defined. Support and encouragement as well as education and direction in the delivery of care should be given. Examples include:

- mouth care
- massage
- hair washing and brushing
- reading to the patient
- positioning limbs
- caressing and holding
- helping to take oral fluids.

Steinhauser *et al.* (2000) found that dying patients rated freedom from pain, being at peace with God, the presence of the family, being mentally aware, knowing that treatment choices were being followed, having their finances in order, feeling that life was meaningful, being able to resolve conflicts, and being able to die at home as most important to them. Patients also rated periods of lucidity that enabled preparation for death as almost as important as the relief of pain.

Continuity of care

The family/friends should not have to keep forming new relationships with members of staff they do not know at this stage. It is important to provide continuity of care from a few nurses who are known to the family and who may have some affinity with them. This will help the family to feel supported and may relieve some of their stress. However, it is likely to increase the stress that these specific nurses experience and they may well require extra support from those in charge or their peers.

Establishing delivery of care to suit the patient, family, and friends

The nurse should discuss with the family whether they prefer privacy with the patient or the company of the nurse, and should arrange care accordingly. If the family prefer privacy, the nurse should withdraw from the immediate area but reassure the family that he/she is readily available should they or the patient need him/her.

The family/friends should also be approached as to whether they wish to be present at the patient's death and if there is anyone else they would wish to be there (e.g. the chaplain or their own minister). This information should be recorded and communicated clearly to all those looking after the patient so that whenever death occurs the wishes of the family/friends can be met.

If the family/friends have expressed the desire to be present at the patient's death, every effort should be made to ensure that they are informed in time for them to reach the hospital if they are not already present. Many people experience guilt associated with bereavement, and failing to arrive in time to be with their loved one at their death can only add to this.

The patients' family/friends should be supported in deciding how they wish to organize the interim time. They may all wish to stay or they may take it in turns to remain with the patient until death is near.

Assuring and improving quality of care

Nelson *et al.* (2006) have proposed a set of measures that can be used as an indicator of quality of palliative care in critical care and as a means to highlight deficiences and then improve, suggesting that:

- by day 1 of the admission, the key decision-makers, any advance directive, and resuscitation preference should have been identified, information leaflet(s) should have been provided, and the patient's pain should have been systematically assessed and managed
- by day 3, social work support and spiritual support should have been offered
- by day 5, at the latest, an interdisciplinary family meeting should have been conducted.

After death has occurred

Interventions that can help the bereaved to eventually come to terms with their loss include:

- viewing the body after death—this generally facilitates grief and ultimate acceptance of the loss
- avoidance of euphemisms for death
- providing opportunities to return to bereavement support groups either specific to the critical care unit or generically within the healthcare service.

If there is a follow-up counselling service available, this further help should be offered.

Clear details should be given of what is required for registering the death and arranging removal of the body by the undertakers. Ideally, there should be an information sheet with these details to give to the family. If not, the nurse should make sure these are written down.

The effect of caring for the dying patient on the nurse

The quality of care the patient and family receive in the critical care unit will have a major impact on their lives, not only at the time but also for many years afterwards. It is an essential part of the caring function of nursing to ensure that their experience is as benign as is possible in the circumstances. However, the experience of death is stressful for staff as well. It is a significant part of work in critical care, so staff have to develop, and often be helped to develop, coping mechanisms of one kind or another. Critical care staff feel that patient death is easier to manage if it is believed that good care has been given (Shorter and Stayt 2010).

Peer support can be important but can also work negatively for some individuals. The culture in the department is an important factor. An open accepting environment where staff feel able to express their feelings will help coping. Team feeling and concern for coworkers is supportive; indeed, there is also evidence that organizations that emphasize training and teamworking have better clinical outcomes (West *et al.* 2006). Support groups and networks based in the unit or the hospital can provide a useful external release and, depending on how they are organized, have the added advantage of being confidential.

Junior staff are more likely to be stressed than experienced senior staff (Kincey *et al.* 2003) so particular attention should be paid to effective mentorship, clinical supervision, and support for this group of staff. There will always be variation in how well individuals cope; senior staff should be vigilant about signs of stress in colleagues and intervene when necessary for those vulnerable to the stress of caring for dying patients.

References and bibliography

Ahlers, S.J., van Gulik, L., van der Veen, A.M., *et al.* (2008). Comparison of different pain scoring systems in critically ill patients in a general ICU. *Critical Care*, **12**, R15.

Allegranzi, B., Pittet, D. (2009). Role of hand hygiene in healthcare-associated infection prevention. *Journal of Hospital Infection*, **73**, 305–15.

American Association for Respiratory Care (2010). Endotracheal suctioning of mechanically ventilated patients with artificial airways. *Respiratory Care*, **55**, 758–64.

American Psychiatric Association (2013). *Diagnostic and Statistical Manual of Mental Disorders* (5th edn). Arlington, VA: American Psychiatric Publishing.

Andersen, J.H., Boesen, H.C., Skovgaard Olsen, K. (2013). Sleep in the Intensive Care Unit measured by polysomnography. *Minerva Anestesiologica*, **79**, 804–15.

Bagshaw, S.M., Laupland, K.B. (2006). Epidemiology of intensive care unit-acquired urinary tract infections. *Current Opinion in Infectious Diseases*, **19**, 67–71.

Barr, J., Fraser, G.L., Puntillo, K., *et al.* (2013). Clinical practice guidelines for the management of pain, agitation, and delirium in adult patients in the intensive care unit. *Critical Care Medicine*, **41**, 263–306.

Barratt, H., Harrison, D.A., Rowan, K.M., *et al.* (2012). Effect of non-clinical inter-hospital critical care unit to unit transfer of critically ill patients: a propensity-matched cohort analysis. *Critical Care*, **16**, R179.

Batalden, P.B., Davidoff, F. (2007). What is 'quality improvement' and how can it transform healthcare? *Quality & Safety in Health Care*, **16**, 2–3.

Bergeron, N., Dubois, M.J., Dumont, M., *et al.* (2001). Intensive Care Delirium Screening Checklist: evaluation of a new screening tool. *Intensive Care Medicine*, **27**, 859–64.

Bion, J., Richardson, A., Hibbert, P., *et al.* (2013). 'Matching Michigan': a 2-year stepped interventional programme to minimise central venous catheter-blood stream infections in intensive care units in England. *BMJ Quality & Safety*, **22**, 110–23.

Börsig, A., Steinacker, I. (1982). Communication with the patient in the intensive care unit. *Nursing Times*, **78**(Suppl), 1–11.

Bradt, J., Dileo, C., Grocke, D. (2010). Music interventions for mechanically ventilated patients. *Cochrane Database of Systematic Reviews*, **12**, CD006902.

Braun, L.A., Stanguts, C., Casanelia, L., *et al.* (2012). Massage therapy for cardiac surgery patients—a randomized trial. *Journal of Thoracic and Cardiovascular Surgery*, **144**, 1453–9.

Brindle, C.T., Malhotra, R., O'Rourke, S., *et al.* (2013). Turning and repositioning the critically ill patient with hemodynamic instability: a literature review and consensus recommendations. *Journal of Wound Ostomy and Continence Nursing*, **40**, 254–67.

Btaiche, I.F., Kovacevich, D.S., Khalidi, N., *et al.* (2011). The effects of needleless connectors on catheter-related bloodstream infections. *American Journal of Infection Control*, **39**, 277–83.

Chanques, G., Sebbane, M., Barbotte, E., *et al.* (2007). A prospective study of pain at rest: incidence and characteristics of an unrecognized symptom in surgical and trauma versus medical intensive care unit patients. *Anesthesiology*, **107**, 858–60.

Chittick, P., Sherertz, R.J. (2010). Recognition and prevention of nosocomial vascular device and related bloodstream infections in the intensive care unit. *Critical Care Medicine*, **38**(Suppl), S363–72.

Chlan, L.L., Weinert, C.R., Heiderscheit, A., *et al.* (2013). Effects of patient-directed music intervention on anxiety and sedative exposure in critically ill patients receiving mechanical ventilatory support: a randomized clinical trial. *JAMA*, **309**, 2335–44.

Clavet, H., Hébert, P.C., Fergusson, D., *et al.* (2008). Joint contracture following prolonged stay in the intensive care unit. *Canadian Medical Association Journal*, **178**, 691–7.

Clifford, C. (1985). Helplessness: a concept applied to nursing practice. *Intensive Care Nursing*, **1**, 19–24.

Cooper, K.L. (2013). Evidence-based prevention of pressure ulcers in the intensive care unit. *Critical Care Nurse*, **33**, 57–66.

Cortese, D., Capp, L., McKinley, S. (1995). Moisture chamber versus lubrication for the prevention of corneal epithelial breakdown. *American Journal of Critical Care*, **4**, 425–8.

Cox, C.E., Docherty, S.L., Brandon, D.H., *et al.* (2009). Surviving critical illness: acute respiratory distress syndrome as experienced by patients and their caregivers. *Critical Care Medicine*, **37**, 2702–8.

Cox, J. (2011). Predictors of pressure ulcers in adult critical care patients. *American Journal of Critical Care*, **20**, 364–75.

Cremasco, M.F., Wenzel, F., Zanei, S.S., *et al.* (2013). Pressure ulcers in the intensive care unit: the relationship between nursing workload, illness severity and pressure ulcer risk. *Journal of Clinical Nursing*, **22**, 2183–91.

Cuesta, J.M., Singer, M. (2012). The stress response and critical illness: a review. *Critical Care Medicine*, **40**, 3283–9.

Cutler, L.R., Hayter, M., Ryan, T. (2013). A critical review and synthesis of qualitative research on patient experiences of critical illness. *Intensive & Critical Care Nursing*, **29**, 147–57.

Cypress BS (2013). Transfer out of intensive care: an evidence-based literature review. *Dimensions of Critical Care Nursing*, **32**, 244–61.

Darbyshire, J.L., Young, J.D. (2013). An investigation of sound levels on intensive care units with reference to the WHO guidelines. *Critical Care*, **17**, R187.

Dennis, C.M., Lee, R., Woodard, E.K., *et al.* (2010). Benefits of quiet time for neuro-intensive care patients. *Journal of Neuroscience Nursing*, **42**, 217–24.

Dezfulian, C., Lavelle, J., Nallamothu, B.K., *et al.* (2003). Rates of infection for single-lumen versus multilumen central venous catheters: a meta-analysis. *Critical Care Medicine*, **31**, 2385–90.

Drakulovic, M.B., Torres, A., Bauer, T.T., *et al.* (1999). Supine body position as a risk factor for nosocomial pneumonia in mechanically ventilated patients: a randomised trial. *Lancet*, **354**, 1851–8.

Edwards, G.B., Schuring, L.M. (1993). Pilot study: validating staff nurses' observations of sleep and wake states among critically ill patients, using polysomnography. *American Journal of Critical Care*, **2**, 125–31.

Elliott, R., Wright, L. (1999).Verbal communication: what do critical care nurses say to their unconscious or sedated patients? *Journal of Advanced Nursing*, **29**, 1412–20.

Elliott, R., McKinley, S., Cistulli, .P, *et al.* (2013). Characterisation of sleep in intensive care using 24-hour polysomnography: an observational study. *Critical Care*, **17**, R46.

Ely, E.W., Margolin, R., Francis, J., *et al.* (2001). Evaluation of delirium in critically ill patients: validation of the Confusion Assessment Method for the Intensive Care Unit (CAM-ICU). *Critical Care Medicine*, **29**, 1370–9.

European Pressure Ulcer Advisory Panel & National Pressure Ulcer Advisory Panel (2009). *Prevention and Treatment of Pressure Ulcers: Quick Reference Guide*. Report, National Pressure Ulcer Advisory Panel, Washington, DC.

Field, K., Prinjha, S., Rowan, K. (2008). 'One patient amongst many': a qualitative analysis of intensive care unit patients' experiences of transferring to the general ward. *Critical Care*, **12**, R21.

Fisher, J. (2010). The importance of effective catheter securement. *British Journal of Nursing*, **19**, S14–8.

Frazier, S.K., Moser, D.K., Daley, L.K., *et al.* (2003). Critical care nurses' beliefs about and reported management of anxiety. *American Journal of Critical Care*, **12**, 19–27.

Freedman, N.S., Gazendam, J., Levan, L., *et al.* (2001). Abnormal sleep/wake cycles and the effect of environmental noise on sleep disruption in the intensive care unit. *American Journal of Respiratory and Critical Care Medicine*, **163**, 451–7.

Gehlbach, B.K., Chapotot, F., Leproult, R., *et al.* (2012). Temporal disorganization of circadian rhythmicity and sleep–wake regulation in mechanically ventilated patients receiving continuous intravenous sedation. *Sleep*, **35**, 1105–14.

Glynn, G., Ahern, M. (2000). Determinants of critical care nurses' pain management behaviour. *Australian Critical Care*, **13**, 144–51.

Grixti, A., Sadri, M., Edgar, J., *et al.* (2012). Common ocular surface disorders in patients in intensive care units. *The Ocular Surface*, **10**, 26–42.

Grossbach, I., Stranberg, S., Chlan, L. (2011). Promoting effective communication for patients receiving mechanical ventilation. *Critical Care Nurse*, **31**, 46–60.

Happ, M.B., Garrett, K., Thomas, D.D., *et al.* (2011). Nurse–patient communication interactions in the intensive care unit. *American Journal of Critical Care*, **20**, e28–40.

Henneman, E.A., Cardin, S. (2002). Family-centered critical care: a practical approach to making it happen. *Critical Care Nurse*, **22**, 12–19.

Henricson, M., Segesten, K., Berglund, A.L., *et al.* (2009). Enjoying tactile touch and gaining hope when being cared for in intensive care—a phenomenological hermeneutical study. *Intensive & Critical Care Nursing*, **25**, 323–31.

Hernandez, E.V., Mannis, M.J. (1997). Superficial keratopathy in intensive care unit patients. *American Journal of Ophthalmology*, **124**, 212–16.

Herridge, M.S., Tansey, C.M., Matté, A., *et al.* (2011). Functional disability 5 years after acute respiratory distress syndrome. *New England Journal of Medicine*, **364**, 1293–1304.

Hillman, K.M., Bishop, G., Flabouris, A. (2002). Patient examination in the intensive care unit. In *Yearbook of Intensive Care and Emergency Medicine* (ed. J.L. Vincent). Berlin: Springer-Verlag.

Hunter, J.D. (2012). Ventilator associated pneumonia. *BMJ*, **344**, e3325.

Hunziker, S., McHugh, W., Sarnoff-Lee, B., *et al.* (2012). Predictors and correlates of dissatisfaction with intensive care. *Critical Care Medicine*, **40**, 1554–61.

Intensive Care Society (2011). *Guidelines for the Transport of the Critically Ill Adult* (3rd edn). Report, Intensive Care Society, London.

Jakob, S.M., Ruokonen, E., Grounds, R.M., *et al.* (2012). Dexmedetomidine vs midazolam or propofol for sedation during prolonged mechanical ventilation: two randomized controlled trials. *JAMA*, **307**, 1151–60.

Jamerson, P.A., Scheibmeir, M., Bott, M.J., *et al.* (1996). The experiences of families with a relative in the intensive care unit. *Heart & Lung*, **25**, 467–74.

Joffe, A.M., Hallman, M., Gélinas, C., *et al.* (2013). Evaluation and treatment of pain in critically ill adults. *Seminars in Respiratory and Critical Care Medicine*, **34**, 189–200.

Jones, C., Bäckman, C., Capuzzo, M., *et al.* (2010). Intensive care diaries reduce new onset post traumatic stress disorder following critical illness: a randomised, controlled trial. *Critical Care*, **14**, R168.

Kahn, D.M., Cook, T.E., Carlisle, C.C., *et al.* (1998). Identification and modification of environmental noise in an ICU setting. *Chest*, **114**, 535–40.

Kam, K.Y.R., Haldar, S., Papamichael, E., *et al.* (2013). Eye care in the critically ill: a national survey and protocol. *Journal of the Intensive Care Society*, **14**, 150–4.

Kamdar, B.B., Needham, D.M., Collop, N.A. (2012a). Sleep deprivation in critical illness: its role in physical and psychological recovery. *Journal of Intensive Care Medicine*, **27**, 97–111.

Kamdar, B.B., Shah, P.A., King, L.M., *et al.* (2012b). Patient–nurse interrater reliability and agreement of the Richards–Campbell sleep questionnaire. *American Journal of Critical Care*, **21**, 261–9.

Karlsson, V., Bergbom, I., Forsberg, A. (2012). The lived experiences of adult intensive care patients who were conscious during mechanical ventilation: a phenomenological–hermeneutic study. *Intensive & Critical Care Nursing*, **28**, 6–15.

Katalinic, O.M., Harvey, L.A., Herbert, R.D., *et al.* (2010). Stretch for the treatment and prevention of contractures. *Cochrane Database of Systematic Reviews*, **9**, CD007455.

Kincey, J., Pratt, D., Slater, R., *et al.* (2003). A survey of patterns and sources of stress among medical and nursing staff in an intensive care unit setting. *Care of the Critically Ill*, **19**, 83–7.

Kirchhoff, K.T., Walker, L., Hutton, A., *et al.* (2002). The vortex: families' experiences with death in the intensive care unit. *American Journal of Critical Care*, **11**, 200–9.

Kress, J.P., Pohlman, A.S., O'Connor, M.F., *et al.* (2000). Daily interruption of sedative infusions in critically ill patients undergoing mechanical ventilation. *New England Journal of Medicine*, **342**, 1471–7.

Latronico, N., Bolton, C.F. (2011). Critical illness polyneuropathy and myopathy: a major cause of muscle weakness and paralysis. *Lancet Neurology*, **10**, 931–41.

Lawrence, M. (1995). The unconscious experience. *American Journal of Critical Care*, **4**, 227–32.

Lazarus, R.S., Folkman, S. (1984). *Stress, Appraisal, and Coping*. New York: Springer.

Le, A., Friese, R.S., Hsu, C.H., *et al.* (2012). Sleep disruptions and nocturnal nursing interactions in the intensive care unit. *Journal of Surgical Research*, **177**, 310–14.

Ligtenberg, J.J., Arnold, L.G., Stienstra, Y., *et al.* (2005). Quality of interhospital transport of critically ill patients: a prospective audit. *Critical Care*, **9**, R446–51.

McCrae, N. (2012). Whither nursing models? The value of nursing theory in the context of evidence-based practice and multidisciplinary health care. *Journal of Advanced Nursing*, **68**, 222–9.

McEwen, B.S. (2005). Stressed or stressed out: what is the difference? *Journal of Psychiatry & Neuroscience*, **30**, 315–18.

McKinley, S., Stein-Parbury, J., Chehelnabi, A., Lovas, J. (2004). Assessment of anxiety in intensive care patients by using the Faces Anxiety Scale. *American Journal of Critical Care*, **13**, 146–52.

Magarey, J.M., McCutcheon, H.H. (2005). 'Fishing with the dead'—recall of memories from the ICU. *Intensive & Critical Care Nursing*, **21**, 344–54.

Majumdar, S.S., Padiglione, A.A. (2012). Nosocomial infections in the intensive care unit. *Anaesthesia and Intensive Care*, **13**, 204–8.

Martin, S.J., Yost, R.J. (2011). Infectious diseases in the critically ill patients. *Journal of Pharmacy Practice*, **24**, 35–43.

Mazi, W., Senok, A.C., Al-Kahldy, S., *et al.* (2013). Implementation of the World Health Organization hand hygiene improvement strategy in critical care units. *Antimicrobial Resistance and Infection Control*, **2**, 15.

Meerlo, P., Sgoifo, A., Suchecki, D. (2008). Restricted and disrupted sleep: effects on autonomic function, neuroendocrine stress systems and stress responsivity. *Sleep Medicine Review*, **12**, 197–210.

Mehta, S., Burry, L., Cook, D., *et al.* (2012). Daily sedation interruption in mechanically ventilated critically ill patients cared for with a sedation protocol: a randomized controlled trial. *JAMA*, **308**, 1985–92.

Melzack, R. and Wall, P.D. (1965). Pain mechanisms: a new theory. *Science*, **150**, 971–9.

Muskett, H., Shahin, J., Eyres, G., *et al.* (2011). Risk factors for invasive fungal disease in critically ill adult patients: a systematic review. *Critical Care*, **15**, R287.

National Pressure Ulcer Advisory Panel & European Pressure Ulcer Advisory Panel (2009). *Pressure Ulcer Treatment*. Technical Report, National Pressure Ulcer Advisory Panel, Washington, DC.

Nelson, J.E., Mulkerin, C.M., Adams, L.L., *et al.* (2006). Improving comfort and communication in the ICU: a practical new tool for palliative care performance measurement and feedback. *Quality & Safety in Health Care*, **15**, 264–71.

Niël-Weise, B.S., Gastmeier, P., Kola, A., *et al.* (2011). An evidence-based recommendation on bed head elevation for mechanically ventilated patients. *Critical Care*, **15**, R111.

Nijs, N., Toppets, A., Defloor, T., *et al.* (2009). Incidence and risk factors for pressure ulcers in the intensive care unit. *Journal of Clinical Nursing*, **18**, 1258–66.

Niven, D.J., Bastos, J.F., Stelfox, H.T. (2014). Critical care transition programs and the risk of readmission or death after discharge from an ICU: a systematic review and meta-analysis. *Critical Care Medicine*, **42**, 179–87.

O'Grady, N.P., Alexander, M., Burns, L.A., *et al.* (2011). Guidelines for the prevention of intravascular catheter-related infections. *Clinical Infectious Diseases*, **52**, e162–93.

O'Grady, N.P., Murray, P.R., Ames, N. (2012). Preventing ventilator-associated pneumonia. Does the evidence support the practice? *JAMA*, **307**, 2534–9.

Park, G., Coursin, D., Ely, E.W., *et al.* (2001). Commentary. Balancing sedation and analgesia in the critically ill. *Critical Care Clinics*, **17**, 1015–27.

Park, G.R., McElligot, M., Torres, C. (2003). Outreach critical care—cash for no questions? *British Journal of Anaesthesia*, **90**, 700–1; author reply 701–2.

Parkin, B., Turner, A., Moore, E., *et al.* (1997). Bacterial keratitis in the critically ill. *British Journal of Ophthalmology*, **81**, 1060–3.

Patak, L., Gawlinski, A., Fung, N.I., *et al.* (2006). Communication boards in critical care: patients' views. *Applied Nursing Research*, **19**, 182–90.

Penoyer, D.A. (2010). Nurse staffing and patient outcomes in critical care: a concise review. *Critical Care Medicine*, **38**, 1521–8.

Penrod, J.D., Pronovost, P.J., Livote, E.E., *et al.* (2012). Meeting standards of high-quality intensive care unit palliative care: clinical performance and predictors. *Critical Care Medicine*, **40**, 1105–12.

Perpiñá-Galvañ, J., Richart-Martínez, M. (2009). Scales for evaluating self-perceived anxiety levels in patients admitted to intensive care units: a review. *American Journal of Critical Care*, **18**, 571–80.

Pickard, R., Lam, T., Maclennan G, *et al.* (2012). Types of urethral catheter for reducing symptomatic urinary tract infections in hospitalised adults requiring short-term catheterisation: multicentre randomised controlled trial and economic evaluation of antimicrobial- and antiseptic-impregnated urethral catheters (the CATHETER trial). *Health Technology Assessment*, **16**, 1–197.

Plummer, M.P., Blaser, A.R., Deane, A.M. (2014). Stress ulceration: prevalence, pathology and association with adverse outcomes. *Critical Care*, **18**, 213.

Prendergast, V., Jakobsson, U., Renvert, S., *et al.* (2012). Effects of a standard versus comprehensive oral care protocol among intubated neuroscience ICU patients: results of a randomized controlled trial. *Journal of Neuroscience Nursing*, **44**, 134–46.

Prendergast, V., Kleiman, C., King, M. (2013). The Bedside Oral Exam and the Barrow Oral Care Protocol: translating evidence-based oral care into practice. *Intensive & Critical Care Nursing*, **29**, 282–90.

Puntillo, K.A., Morris, A.B., Thompson, C.L., *et al.* (2004). Pain behaviors observed during six common procedures: results from Thunder Project II. *Critical Care Medicine*, **32**, 421–7.

Raghavendran, K., Nemzek, J., Napolitano L.M., *et al.* (2011). Aspiration-induced lung injury. *Critical Care Medicine*, **39**, 818–26.

Resar, R., Pronovost, P., Haraden, C., *et al.* (2005). Using a bundle approach to improve ventilator care processes and reduce ventilator-associated pneumonia. *Joint Commission Journal on Quality and Patient Safety*, **31**, 243–8.

Richards, K.C. (1998). Effect of a back massage and relaxation intervention on sleep in critically ill patients. *American Journal of Critical Care*, **17**, 288–99.

Rincon, H.G., Granados, M., Unutzer, J., *et al.* (2001). Prevalence, detection and treatment of anxiety, depression, and delirium in the adult critical care unit. *Psychosomatics*, **42**, 391–6.

Roberts, B.L., Rickard, C.M., Rajbhandari, D., *et al.* (2006). Patients' dreams in ICU: recall at two years post discharge and comparison to delirium status during ICU admission: a multicentre cohort study. *Intensive & Critical Care Nursing*, **22**, 264–73.

Roberts, B.L., Rickard, C.M., Rajbhandari, D., *et al.* (2007). Factual memories of ICU: recall at two years post-discharge and comparison with delirium status during ICU admission: a multicentre cohort study. *Journal of Clinical Nursing*, **16**, 1669–77.

Royal College of Nursing (2012). *Catheter Care* (2nd edn). Report, Royal College of Nursing, London.

Rosenberg, J.B., Eisen, L.A. (2008). Eye care in the intensive care unit: narrative review and meta-analysis. *Critical Care Medicine*, **36**, 3151–5.

Sakr, Y., Lobo, S.M., Moreno, R., *et al.* (2012). Patterns and early evolution of organ failure in the intensive care unit and their relation to outcome. *Critical Care*, **16**, R222.

Samuelson, K.A. (2011). Unpleasant and pleasant memories of intensive care in adult mechanically ventilated patients—findings from 250 interviews. *Intensive & Critical Care Nursing*, **27**, 76–84.

Samuelson, K., Lundberg, D., Fridlund, B. (2006). Memory in relation to depth of sedation in adult mechanically ventilated intensive care patients. *Intensive Care Medicine*, **32**, 660–7.

Sax, H., Allegranzi, B., Uçkay, I., *et al.* (2007). 'My five moments for hand hygiene': a user-centred design approach to understand, train, monitor and report hand hygiene. *Journal of Hospital Infection*, **67**, 9–21.

Schumm, K., Lam, T.B. (2008). Types of urethral catheters for management of short-term voiding problems in hospitalized adults: a short version Cochrane review. *Neurourology and Urodynamics*, **27**, 738–46.

Schweickert, W.D., Pohlman, M.C., Pohlman, A.S., *et al.* (2009). Early physical and occupational therapy in mechanically ventilated, critically ill patients: a randomised controlled trial. *Lancet*, **373**, 1874–82.

Scottish Intensive Care Society Audit Group (2013). *Audit of Critical Care in Scotland 2013: Reporting on 2012*. Report, NHS National Services Scotland, Edinburgh.

Selye, H. (1946). The general adaptation syndrome and the diseases of adaptation. *Journal of Clinical Endocrinology*, **6**, 117–230.

Selye, H. (1998). A syndrome produced by diverse nocuous agents. 1936. *Journal of Neuropsychiatry and Clinical Neurosciences*, **10**, 230–1.

Seron-Arbeloa, C., Zamora-Elson, M., Labarta-Monzon, L., *et al.* (2013). Enteral nutrition in critical care. *Journal of Clinical Medicine Research*, **5**, 1–11.

Sessler, C.N., Gosnell, M.S., Grap, M.J., *et al.* (2002). The Richmond Agitation–Sedation Scale: validity and reliability in adult intensive care unit patients. *American Journal of Respiratory and Critical Care Medicine*, **166**, 1338–44.

Shirey, M.R. (2008). Nursing practice models for acute and critical care: overview of care delivery models. *Critical Care Nursing Clinics of North America*, **20**, 365–73.

Shorter, M., Stayt, L.C. (2010). Critical care nurses' experiences of grief in an adult intensive care unit. *Journal of Advanced Nursing*, **66**, 159–67.

Shuman, E.K., Chenoweth, C.E. (2010). Recognition and prevention of healthcare-associated urinary tract infections in the intensive care unit. *Critical Care Medicine*, **38**(Suppl), S373–9.

Skrobik, Y., Chanques, G. (2013). The pain, agitation, and delirium practice guidelines for adult critically ill patients: a post-publication perspective. *Annals of Intensive Care*, **3**, 9.

Steinhauser, K.E., Christakis, N.A., Clipp, E.C., *et al.* (2000). Factors considered important at the end of life by patients, family, physicians, and other care providers. *JAMA*, **284**, 2476–82.

Sterling, P. (2004). Principles of allostasis: optimal design, predictive regulation, pathophysiology, and rational therapeutics. In *Allostasis, Homeostasis, and the Cost of Physiological Adaptation* (ed. P. Schulkin). Cambridge: Cambridge University Press.

Theaker, C., Mannan, M., Ives, N., *et al.* (2000). Risk factors for pressure sores in the critically ill. *Anaesthesia*, **55**, 221–4.

Thomas, L.A. (2003). Clinical management of stressors perceived by patients on mechanical ventilation. *AACN Clinical Issues*, **14**, 73–81.

Tracy, M.F., Chlan, L. (2011). Nonpharmacological interventions to manage common symptoms in patients receiving mechanical ventilation. *Critical Care Nurse*, **31**, 19–28.

Tschudin-Sutter, S., Pargger, H., Widmer, A.F. (2010). Hand hygiene in the intensive care unit. *Critical Care Medicine*, **38**(Suppl), S299–305.

University College London Hospitals NHS Foundation Trust (2013). UCLH vision, values and objectives. (www.uclh.nhs.uk/aboutus/wwd/Pages/Visionandobjectives.aspx (accessed 12 January 2013).

van Rompaey, B., Elseviers, M.M., Schuurmans, M.J., *et al.* (2009). Risk factors for delirium in intensive care patients: a prospective cohort study. *Critical Care*. 13(3): R77.

van Rompaey, B., Elseviers, M.M., van Drom, W., *et al.* (2012). The effect of earplugs during the night on the onset of delirium and sleep perception: a randomized controlled trial in intensive care patients. *Critical Care*, **16**, R73.

Varley, A.J., Williams, H., Fletcher, S. (2009). *Continuing Education in Anaesthesia, Critical Care, and Pain*, **9**, 114–18.

Vasilevskis, E.E., Han, J.H., Hughes, C.G., *et al.* (2012). Epidemiology and risk factors for delirium across hospital settings. *Best Practice & Research. Clinical Anaesthesiology*, **26**, 277–87.

Verhaeghe, S., Defloor, T., Van Zuuren, F., *et al.* (2005). The needs and experiences of family members of adult patients in an intensive care unit: a review of the literature. *Journal of Clinical Nursing*, **14**, 501–9.

Verran, B., Aisbitt, P. (1988). *Neurological and Neurosurgical Nursing*. London: Edward Arnold.

Vincent, J.L. (2005). Give your patient a fast hug (at least) once a day. *Critical Care Medicine*, **33**, 1225–9.

Vincent, J.L., Rello, J., Marshall, J., *et al.* (2009). International study of the prevalence and outcomes of infection in intensive care units. *JAMA*, **302**, 2323–9.

Wade, D.M., Howell, D.C., Weinman, J.A., *et al.* (2012). Investigating risk factors for psychological morbidity three months after intensive care: a prospective cohort study. *Critical Care*, **16**, R192.

Warfield, C., Manley, K. (1990). Developing a new philosophy in the NDU. *Nursing Standard*, **4**, 27–30.

Watt, B. (1996). *Patient: The True Story of a Rare Illness*. London: Viking.

Webster, J., Osborne, S., Rickard, C.M., *et al.* (2013). Clinically-indicated replacement versus routine replacement of peripheral venous catheters. *Cochrane Database of Systematic Reviews*, **4**, CD007798.

Welch, J.R. (2014). Critical care nursing. In *Oh's Intensive Care Manual* (7th edn) (eds A.D. Bersten, N. Soni). Oxford: Butterworth-Heinemann.

West, M.A., Guthrie, J.P., Dawson, J.F. (2006). Reducing patient mortality in hospitals: the role of human resource management. *Journal of Organizational Behavior*, **27**, 983–1002.

Wong, H.R. (2012). Clinical review: sepsis and septic shock—the potential of gene arrays. *Critical Care*, **16**, 204.

Xie, H., Kang, J., Mills, G.H. (2008). Clinical review: The impact of noise on patients' sleep and the effectiveness of noise reduction strategies in intensive care units. *Critical Care*, **13**, 208.

Zhang, Z., Pan, L., Ni, H. (2013). Impact of delirium on clinical outcome in critically ill patients: a meta-analysis. *General Hospital Psychiatry*, **35**, 105–11.

Zolfaghari, P.S., Wyncoll, D.L. (2011). The tracheal tube: gateway to ventilator-associated pneumonia. *Critical Care*, **15**, 310.

Further reading

Paw, H., Shulman, R. (2013). *Handbook of Drugs in Intensive Care* (5th edn). Cambridge: Cambridge University Press.

CHAPTER 4
Respiratory problems

Physiology and anatomy

The primary functions of the respiratory system are to supply oxygen to metabolically active tissues and to remove carbon dioxide, which is a waste product of metabolism. These processes are closely linked to transport of blood by the circulatory system:

$$O_2 + \text{Fuel} = \text{Energy} + CO_2 + H_2O$$

Respiration has four components:

(1) mechanical movement of gases into and out of the lungs
(2) exchange of these gases across a membrane
(3) carriage of gases to and from the tissues by the circulatory system
(4) metabolic processes within the cell to produce energy.

Movement of gases

Ventilation is the product of movement of the chest wall and diaphragm. A trans-airway pressure (P_{ta}) gradient is generated between mouth and alveoli that drives the movement of O_2 and CO_2. The gradient may be negative (as in normal breathing) or positive (in positive pressure mechanical ventilation). The transpulmonary pressure (P_{tp})—the difference between alveolar and pleural pressure—is a slight negative pressure (approximately –5 cmH_2O) which maintains lung expansion within the chest and prevents alveolar collapse (see Figure 4.1).

During normal spontaneous breathing, inspiration occurs when the diaphragm and intercostal muscles contract, pulling the lungs downwards and outwards. This creates a negative P_{ta} (approximately –4 cmH_2O) that sucks more air in. With normal lungs even a small change in pressure can move a large volume of air, and during deep inspiration it is possible for this negative pressure to reach as much as –170 cmH_2O (Harik-Khan *et al.* 1998). Expiration occurs when the inspiratory muscles relax and the elastic nature of the lung tissue causes a recoil to the neutral position. A slightly positive pressure is then briefly exerted on the lung and air is forced out.

Lung elasticity is influenced by the alveolar surface tension which tends to pull the alveoli closed, thus resisting expansion. This surface tension is decreased by surfactant, a lipoprotein secreted by the epithelial lining of the lung. Reduced production of surfactant may limit the ability of the alveoli to expand (see Box 4.1) Causes of pulmonary surfactant deficiency). Lung elasticity is also affected by the tendency of elastic fibres in the lung to contract.

When breathing becomes difficult or increased during exercise, other respiratory muscles may be used to increase ventilation. These 'accessory muscles of respiration' consist of neck, trapezius, pectoral, and external intercostal muscles in inspiration, and abdominal and internal intercostal muscles in expiration.

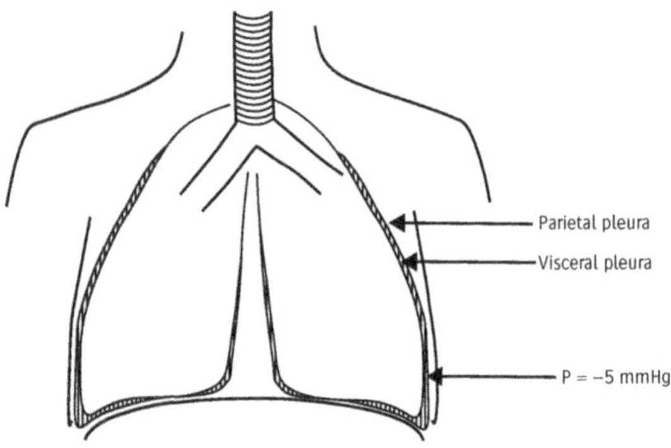

Figure 4.1 Maintenance of negative pleural pressure.

Box 4.1 Causes of pulmonary surfactant deficiency

General

- Systemic inflammation, sepsis
- Hypoxaemia and hyperoxia
- Acidosis
- Starvation

Specific

- Acute respiratory distress syndrome (ARDS), infant respiratory distress syndrome (IRDS)
- Atelectasis
- Pulmonary vascular congestion
- Pulmonary oedema
- Pulmonary embolus
- Excessive pulmonary lavage/hydration (e.g., humidification)
- Drowning
- Extracorporeal oxygenation

Work of breathing

The effort involved in moving air into and out of the lungs is known as the work of breathing. Normally, relatively little effort is required to breathe, but the work of breathing can greatly increase in severe respiratory and circulatory disease, and may eventually lead to exhaustion. Work of breathing is affected by:

- the resistance of airways to flow of air
- the elasticity of lung tissue
- any other obstruction to flow
- chest wall compliance.

These factors together determine the compliance of the respiratory system, expressed as the change in lung volume divided by the change in pressure required to produce that change in volume ($\Delta V/\Delta P$, ml/cmH_2O). Compliance is the inverse of stiffness. Thus, when a lung is compliant it will be less stiff and expand easily, and vice versa when non-compliant. The greatest compliance is seen when small changes in pressure induce the greatest change in volume. Poorly compliant stiff lungs require more effort for inspiration. On the other hand, highly compliant lungs make inspiration relatively easy, but expiration more difficult, for example when elastic tissue has been destroyed, as in emphysema.

Lung compliance can be classified into static and dynamic compliance.

1. **Static compliance** This refers to compliance measured under static conditions produced by brief occlusion (at least 2 seconds) of the airway at the end of inspiration to allow a plateau pressure to be reached. This allows an assessment of compliance without the pressure associated with flow resistance.

$$C_{st} = \frac{\Delta V}{\text{end-inspiratory occluded (plateau) pressure}}$$

where C_{st} is the static compliance of the respiratory system and ΔV is tidal volume. The normal range is 60–100 ml/cmH_2O.

2. **Dynamic compliance** This is the change in pressure from end-inspiration to end-expiration:

$$C_{dyn} = \frac{\Delta V}{\text{end-inspiratory pressure (immediate)} - \text{end-expiratory pressure}}$$

where C_{dyn} is the dynamic compliance of the respiratory system and ΔV is tidal volume.

In healthy lungs there is little difference between static and dynamic compliance at all respiratory rates. However, in patients with airway obstruction, dynamic compliance decreases rapidly as the respiratory rate rises while there is little change in the static compliance (see Table 4.1).

Table 4.1 Causes of altered lung compliance

Decreased by:	Increased by:
Hypervolaemia	Hypovolaemia
Increased pulmonary smooth muscle tone	Decreased pulmonary smooth muscle tone
Increased surface tension, e.g. with decreased surfactant	Decreased surface tension, e.g. with increased surfactant
Fibrosis, infiltration/oedema, atelectasis	Loss of alveolar and elastic tissue, e.g. with emphysema

Gas exchange

Gas exchange only takes place distally in the respiratory lobule. The remainder of the respiratory tract is not available for gas exchange and is known as dead space. There are three types of dead space.

1. **Anatomical dead space** This is where gas exchange cannot occur (i.e. nose, pharynx, trachea, and bronchi) and is approximately 150 ml in a normal-sized adult. Thus 150 ml of any tidal volume (usually 5–8 ml/kg for a normal spontaneous breath) does not contribute to either oxygenation of blood or removal of carbon dioxide.
2. **Alveolar dead space** Here, alveoli are ventilated but not perfused with pulmonary blood and so are unable to contribute to gas exchange.
3. **Physiological dead space** This is the sum of anatomical and alveolar dead space. It can be increased by old age, anaesthesia, mechanical ventilation, chronic lung disease, and pulmonary embolism. Hypoventilation increases the ratio of dead space to tidal volume although not the actual dead space volume (See Table 4.2).

In normal lungs, an enormous surface area (approximately 70 m^2) is available for gas exchange because of the convoluted surfaces of the alveoli that are in contact with a fine network of blood vessels throughout the pulmonary capillary membrane. The close contact between individual red blood cells and the respiratory membrane enables rapid and efficient diffusion of gases across the membrane (see Figure 4.2).

Gas diffusion

Diffusion is defined as the movement of molecules from an area of high concentration to an area of low concentration. The diffusion of gases across the respiratory membrane is affected by two laws describing the physical properties of gases: Dalton's law of partial pressures and Boyle's law.

Dalton's law of partial pressures

The first part of Dalton's law refers to the pressures exerted by gases:

> The pressure exerted by a mixture of gases is equal to the sum of the pressures each gas would exert if it alone occupied the space.

The partial pressure of a gas is the force it exerts when contained within a space, and is a measure of the amount of that gas. Air is made up of three main gases, nitrogen (N_2, 79% of air), oxygen (O_2, 20.9%), and carbon dioxide (CO_2, 0.03%). The partial pressure of oxygen (PO_2) or carbon dioxide (PCO_2) has a suffix depending on where

Table 4.2 Lung volume definitions

Term	Volume	Definition
Tidal volume (V_T)	5–8 ml/kg (~500 ml)	Volume of gas/air that will move in or out of lungs in a normal quiet breath
Minute ventilation (MV)	5–8 ml/kg × 12 breaths/min (~5–7 L/min)	Volume of gas/air that moves in and out of lungs over a minute
Vital capacity (VC)	3000–4800 ml	Maximum volume of gas that can be exhaled after a maximum inspiration
Anatomical dead space	2 ml/kg (~150 ml)	Volume of gas filling conducting airways (nose down to lower airways but not bronchioles)
Functional residual capacity (FRC)	1800–2400 ml	Volume of air remaining in the lungs after normal exhalation
Effective alveolar ventilation per unit time (V_A)		Expired minute volume (V_E)—physiological dead space (V_D)
Physiological dead space		Equals anatomical + alveolar dead space. As this varies depending on alveolar ventilation and perfusion, a ratio of dead space to tidal volume (V_D/V_T) is used instead (normally <0.3)

it is measured, e.g. P_AO_2 and P_ACO_2 in the alveoli, and P_aO_2 and P_aCO_2 in arterial blood.

The second part of Dalton's law refers to pressure exerted by saturated vapours:

The pressure exerted by a saturated vapour depends on the temperature and the particular liquid.

Air is normally humidified by the nose on inspiration and thus contains water vapour. This exerts a pressure that depends on body temperature, with higher temperatures causing more water to vaporize. As the total pressure of the gases within air is fairly constant at the same altitude, the presence of water vapour effectively decreases the quantities of other gases within the mixture entering the alveoli.

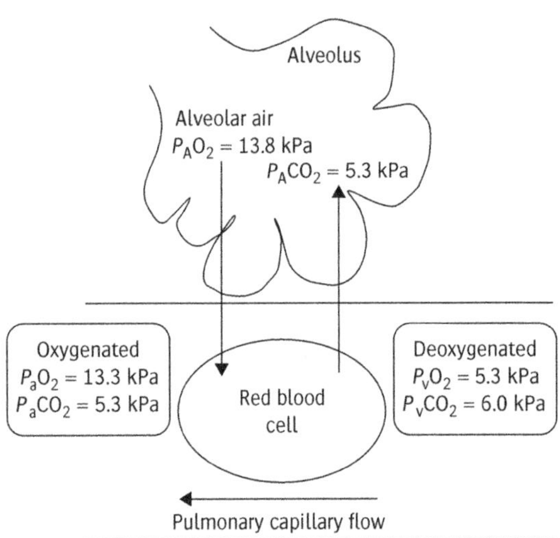

Figure 4.2 Gas exchange in the lungs.

Boyle's law

The partial pressure of any gas is proportional to its percentage by volume in the mixture.

Dry air is a mixture of N_2 (79%) + O_2 (20.9%) + CO_2 (0.03%). Air at sea level has an atmospheric pressure of 101 kPa (760 mmHg). Thus, according to Boyle's law, each gas exerts a partial pressure proportional to its percentage in air so, for example, O_2 exerts a partial pressure of 20.9 kPa (20.9% × 101 kPa), and CO_2 exerts a partial pressure of 0.03 kPa (0.03% × 101 kPa). With humidified air, the pressure exerted by water vapour is approximately 6.3 kPa at normal body temperature. There is a much higher CO_2 concentration in the lungs because they contain CO_2 diffused out of the pulmonary circulation, so the contents of alveolar gas will differ from those of inspired gas. The oxygen content of alveolar gas can be calculated using the alveolar gas equation (see Box 4.2).

In normal lungs the difference between alveolar and arterial PO_2 is about 2 kPa in youth and 3.3 kPa in old age. This A–a (alveolar–arterial) oxygen gradient

Box 4.2 The alveolar gas equation

$$\text{Alveolar } PO_2 = [\text{inspired } PO2 \times (\text{atmospheric pressure} - \text{water vapour pressure})] - (\text{arterial } PCO_2 / \text{respiratory quotient}).$$

The respiratory quotient is the ratio of carbon dioxide produced to oxygen consumed (usually ~0.8).

exists because there is a proportion of blood that passes through the lungs but is not oxygenated. It can be calculated using the alveolar gas equation and the arterial PO_2 measured on blood gas analysis. An increase in the A–a oxygen gradient is evidence of an abnormality in the ventilation/perfusion ratio.

The following factors affect diffusion across the pulmonary capillary membrane.

1. The difference between partial pressures of gases in the alveoli and the pulmonary capillary.
2. The area of the respiratory membrane. Any processes limiting the area available for gas exchange such as acute respiratory distress syndrome (ARDS) or emphysema can have a major effect on respiratory function.
3. The thickness of the respiratory membrane. Any factors increasing thickness (e.g. oedema) will impair pulmonary function.
4. The diffusion or solubility coefficient of the gas involved. Carbon dioxide is far more soluble than oxygen and thus diffuses faster and more efficiently.

The largest component of inspired air is nitrogen. Nitrogen is not soluble and does not pass into the capillaries. Therefore nitrogen in inspired air acts as a gas reservoir remaining in the alveoli, which maintains alveolar expansion and helps prevent collapse (atelectasis). This function is lost with a very high inspired concentration of oxygen as there will then be relatively little nitrogen.

Ventilation/perfusion match and mismatch

Another important determinant of gas exchange is the relationship between alveolar ventilation (V) and pulmonary capillary perfusion (Q). In the perfect situation, a well-ventilated alveolus would be adjacent to a correspondingly well-perfused capillary, giving the ideal V/Q ratio of 1:1 (usually expressed simply as 1). However, there is normally some mismatch between ventilation and perfusion in different parts of the lungs. This is partly due to the effects of gravity which increase the force required to move blood through vessels further above the heart, so that when the individual is upright, lower areas of the lung receive a better blood supply than upper areas (see Box 4.3). The body adapts by preferentially ventilating the better-perfused lower areas, but this response is lost when the patient is sedated and mechanically ventilated.

Box 4.3 Causes of ventilation/perfusion mismatch

- Pulmonary embolus
- Partial/complete obstruction of the pulmonary artery
- Extrinsic pressure on pulmonary vessels (pneumothorax, tumour)
- Destruction of pulmonary vessels
- Decreased cardiac output
- Obstruction of the pulmonary microcirculation (ARDS)

A three-compartment model illustrates V/Q relationships and changes in various disease states.

1. Physiological dead space (i.e. areas of wasted ventilation) generate a V/Q >1. Here, a V/Q mismatch occurs as poorly perfused areas of lung continue to be ventilated (e.g. when emboli obstruct pulmonary capillaries) and therefore the ratio of ventilation (V) to perfusion (Q) is increased.
2. Perfectly matched areas of ventilation and perfusion give a V/Q of 1.
3. Venous admixture (where non-oxygenated blood mixes with oxygenated blood after passage through the lungs) means that perfusion has been wasted (e.g. when there are diffusion defects or right-to-left shunts) giving a V/Q <1. Right-to-left shunts occur when there is continuing perfusion of poorly ventilated lung (when alveoli are collapsed, consolidated, or filled with fluid (oedema)), or when venous blood bypasses the lung completely (e.g. right-to-left ventricular septal defect) (see Box 4.4).

Two intrinsic responses allow some adjustments aimed at optimizing V/Q matching. The first involves the pulmonary capillary response to a low PO_2. If the alveolus is poorly ventilated, the P_AO_2 will be low, resulting in a correspondingly low P_aO_2 in adjacent pulmonary capillaries. This initiates 'hypoxic pulmonary vasoconstriction' which reduces pulmonary blood flow to the affected region and makes more blood available

Box 4.4 Situations causing right-to-left shunts

- Obstructive lung disease (emphysema, bronchitis, asthma)
- Restrictive lung disease (ARDS, pneumonia, fibrotic lung disease)
- Hypoventilation for any reason (e.g. excess sedation, respiratory muscle weakness)
- Right-to-left intracardiac shunt (e.g. ventricular or atrial septal defect)

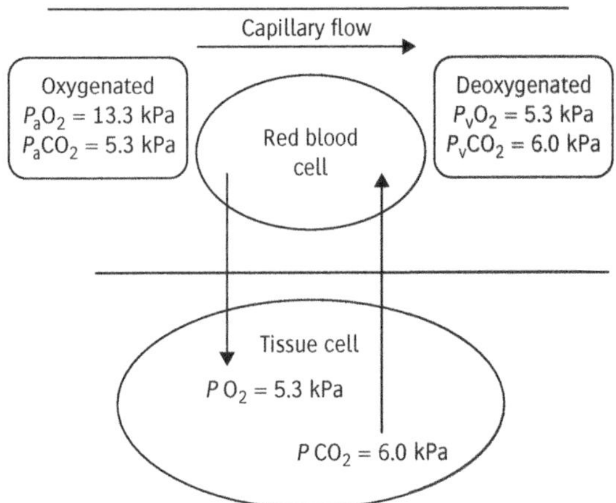

Figure 4.3 Gas exchange in the tissues.

to perfuse other, better ventilated alveoli. The second response involves localized bronchoconstriction when there are low levels of carbon dioxide caused by low blood flow in that area (e.g. due to pulmonary embolism). Here, the P_ACO_2 in adjacent alveoli will also be low, triggering constriction of local bronchioles and limiting ventilation of the underperfused area.

Carriage of gases

Oxygen is not a highly soluble gas, so the quantity of oxygen required by the human body could not be delivered if it was simply carried in solution. Therefore most oxygen is transported by haemoglobin. At a normal level of haemoglobin (15 g/dl), 20 ml O_2 is carried per 100 ml of blood, whereas only 0.3 ml O_2 is carried dissolved in plasma.

The chemical structure of haemoglobin allows a varying affinity to oxygen molecules depending on various factors including local PO_2, pH, and temperature. At a normal P_aO_2 (13.3 kPa), approximately 98% of the haemoglobin oxygen-binding capacity is utilized. This is the situation usually found in pulmonary capillaries. Oxygen-saturated haemoglobin is termed oxyhaemoglobin, while unsaturated haemoglobin is termed deoxyhaemoglobin (see Figure 4.3).

In the venous circulation, the oxyhaemoglobin saturation is reduced to 70–75% as by then oxygen has been released to the tissues. This still provides a large reservoir for conditions when oxygen demand suddenly increases, for example in exercise or in shock states where supply is reduced. In these circumstances, more oxygen can be released from haemoglobin in order to maintain aerobic metabolism; and in extreme situations venous oxyhaemoglobin saturation levels may drop to as low as 20–30%. Where O_2 supply fails to meet demand, tissues shift increasingly to anaerobic metabolism, resulting in lactate production and a metabolic acidosis.

Several important factors affect the release of oxygen from haemoglobin (oxyhaemoglobin dissociation). In some cases, the oxyhaemoglobin dissociation curve shifts to the right, i.e. oxygen is more readily released to the tissues at a given arterial PO_2. When the oxyhaemoglobin dissociation curve shifts to the left, oxygen is less readily released. These shifts have minimal effects on tissue oxygenation in the normal P_aO_2 range, but can be highly significant in patients with low P_aO_2.

Right shift of the oxyhaemoglobin dissociation curve

This is a compensatory mechanism to augment tissue oxygenation. Factors shifting the dissociation curve to the right include:

- decreased pH (acidosis)
- increased body temperature
- increased PCO_2
- increased 2,3-diphosphoglycerate (2,3-DPG), which is a substance contained within red blood cells formed during anaerobic glycolysis; levels are increased as a compensatory response to hypoxia, anaemia, and increased pH.

Left shift of the oxyhaemoglobin dissociation curve

Factors shifting the dissociation curve to the left include:

- increased pH
- decreased PCO_2
- decreased temperature
- decreased 2,3-DPG

- fetal haemoglobin (HbF)—HbF has a greater affinity for oxygen to enhance transfer of oxygen across the placenta
- carboxyhaemoglobin (COHb)—carbon monoxide has 250 times the affinity of oxygen for haemoglobin, so a small amount of carbon monoxide can bind to large amounts of haemoglobin, making it unavailable for oxygen transport.

Two further points are important in understanding the carriage of oxygen.

1. Once haemoglobin is fully saturated, no further increase in inspired O_2 can significantly increase the amount of oxygen carried by the blood unless the patient is placed in a hyperbaric oxygen chamber where the pressure is approximately double that of atmospheric pressure. Here, the amount of oxygen dissolved in plasma will increase significantly.
2. The P_aO_2 can decrease quite considerably before there is any major fall in oxyhaemoglobin saturation. Thus haemoglobin is still 90% saturated at around a PO_2 of 8 kPa.

Oxygen delivery to the tissues depends on haemoglobin concentration (Hb), oxygen saturation (S_aO_2) and cardiac output (see Chapter 5). Tissue oxygen delivery (DO_2) is given by

$$DO_2 = \text{cardiac output (CO)} \times \text{Hb} \times S_aO_2 \times 1.34 + (D_aO_2 \times 0.003)\,\text{ml/min}$$

where 1.34 ml O_2 is carried by each gram of haemoglobin and $P_aO_2 \times 0.003$ represents the dissolved plasma fraction (see Figure 4.4).

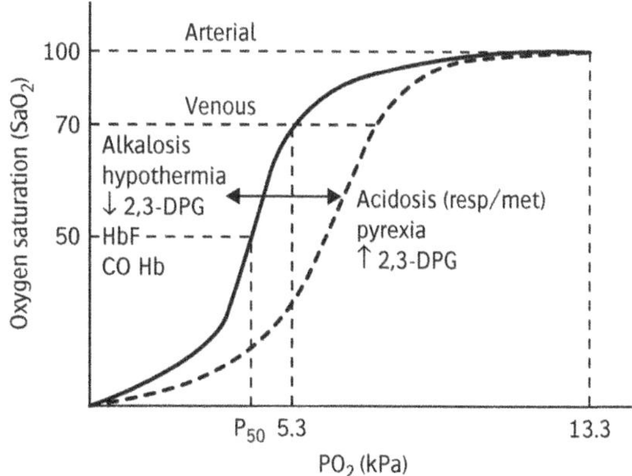

Figure 4.4 Oxyhaemoglobin dissociation curve (Bohr). HbF = fetal haemoglobin; COHb = carbon monoxide bound to haemoglobin (carboxyhaemoglobin); P_{50} = pressure at which haemoglobin is 50% saturated; 2,3-DPG = 2,3-diphosphoglycerate.

Carbon dioxide transport

Six mechanisms are involved in movement of carbon dioxide from the tissues to the alveoli (see Table 4.3). Unlike oxygen, the relationship between PCO_2 and the total amount of carbon dioxide in the blood is linear over the physiological range, so changes in PCO_2 have a more direct effect on the blood's carbon dioxide content. Carbon dioxide binding to haemoglobin is affected by the oxyhaemoglobin saturation. This is known as the Haldane effect, where deoxygenated blood increases the capacity for carbon dioxide transport and oxygenated blood enhances the unloading of carbon dioxide.

Cellular metabolic processes to produce energy

Oxygen diffuses through the capillary membrane and interstitial spaces into the cells where it then diffuses into specialized organelles (mitochondria). Here, in conjunction with a fuel source (predominantly glucose or fatty acids, but also amino acids and lactate), the oxygen is consumed and reduced to water. Carbon dioxide and heat are also generated as waste products.

This process enables an additional phosphate molecule to be added to adenosine diphosphate (ADP), forming adenosine triphosphate (ATP)—this is known as 'oxidative phosphorylation'. This phosphate bond acts as a high energy store. ATP is transported out of the

Table 4.3 Mechanisms of carbon dioxide transport

Plasma	Red blood cells	Percentage carried
As dissolved CO_2	As dissolved CO_2	~10%
Protein bound (carbamino compounds)	Carbaminohaemoglobin (combined with Hb)	1% protein bound, 20% carbaminoHb
As bicarbonate ((HCO_3^-)	As bicarbonate (HCO_3^-)	~70%

Table 4.4 Definitions of terms

Term	Definition	Example/formula
Acid	A substance containing weakly held hydrogen ions (H^+) which is easily split into hydrogen ions and the remaining substance.	Carbonic acid (H_2CO_3) → H^+ + HCO_3^-
Base	A substance which can combine with hydrogen ions (H^+). Extremely active metabolically and can have a major effect on cell function.	Bicarbonate (HCO_3^-) + H^+ → H_2CO_3
pH	The scale on which hydrogen ions are measured. It is the negative logarithm to the base 10 of the concentration of hydrogen ions.	$pH = -\log_{10} [H^+]$ Normal range 7.35–7.45
Acidosis	An abnormal process causing a relative increase in hydrogen ions and thus a decrease in pH. It can be due to an increase in acid or a decrease in base.	pH <7.35
Alkalosis	An abnormal process causing a relative decrease in hydrogen ions and thus an increase in pH. It can be due to a decrease in acid or an increase in base.	pH ≥7.45
Buffer	A substance with the ability to bind and release hydrogen ions, thus maintaining a relatively constant pH	Phosphoric acid and its salts, disodiumhydrogen phosphate, and monosodium dihydrogen phosphate

mitochondria and, on release of the phosphate bond, the energy is released enabling normal cell functions to occur, including protein synthesis, membrane pump activity to adjust intracellular electrolyte and water content, and repair processes.

Acid–base balance

The carbon dioxide produced as a waste product of cellular metabolism combines with water in solution to produce carbonic acid (H_2CO_3). H_2CO_3 can readily dissociate into hydrogen (H^+) ions and bicarbonate (HCO_3^-) ions which can affect the level of intracellular acidity (pH). As intracellular pH must be kept within relatively narrow limits for normal metabolic activity to occur, removal of carbon dioxide is essential (see Table 4.4). Mechanisms for maintaining acid–base balance can be divided into three distinct responses.

1. Buffering (immediate)— hydrogen ions are combined with other substances (such as bicarbonate) in less volatile chemical compounds.
2. The respiratory response (especially important in the first 2–3 hours)— CO_2 is eliminated on expiration, so less CO_2 is available to produce carbonic acid.
3. The renal response (over hours to days)— acid is eliminated in the urine. Urine pH is usually lower than that of pH, showing that the kidneys remove hydrogen ions from the blood.

Arterial blood gas analysis

This provides an indication of respiratory status and important data regarding the body's metabolic state. It gauges the ability of the body to maintain homeostasis (metabolic equilibrium). The variables measured are pH, PCO_2, and PO_2, while bicarbonate (HCO_3^-) and base excess are derived from formulae (see Box 4.5). Normal values for these variables are given in Table 4.5.

Physiological approach to acid–base balance

Several different theories have been developed to explain acid–base balance (Adrogué *et al.* 2009). The traditional

Box 4.5 Standard measures of bicarbonate and base excess

- Standard bicarbonate is defined as the concentration of bicarbonate in equilibrated plasma at 37°C and a P_aCO2 of 5.3 kPa.
- Standard base excess is defined as the milliequivalent (mEq or mmol) of strong acid necessary to titrate a blood sample at 37°C and a $PaCO_2$ of 5.3 kPa to a pH of 7.40.

Table 4.5 Normal values of arterial blood gases

Property	Value
pH	7.35–7.45
P_aCO_2	4.6–6.0 kPa
P_aO_2	10.0–13.3 kPa
HCO_3^-	22–26 mmol/L
Base excess	−2 to + 2
O_2 saturation	>95%

'physiological approach' still generally informs bedside interpretation. It focuses on the pH as a function of the relative levels of bicarbonate (reflecting metabolic processes) and PCO_2 (determined by respiration).

The lungs directly affect acid–base balance by increasing levels of CO_2 and the level of acidity (respiratory acidosis), or the converse (respiratory alkalosis). Metabolic factors also contribute to acid–base abnormalities. Metabolic acidosis occurs when levels of HCO_3^- and other buffer substances in the body fall, allowing levels of free hydrogen ions to increase (see Box 4.6). Metabolic alkalosis is characterized by raised levels of HCO_3^- and other buffers, with decreased levels of free hydrogen ions and a rise in pH (see Box 4.7).

The Henderson–Hasselbalch equation describes the relationship between the partial pressure of carbon dioxide (PCO_2), bicarbonate (HCO_3^-) and pH:

$$pH = 6.1 + \left(\log_{10} HCO_3^- / 0.03PCO_2\right).$$

Thus, if HCO_3^- falls or PCO_2 rises, the pH will fall. When bicarbonate is standardized to a normal PCO_2 and temperature, any abnormality must be due to a metabolic cause. Thus, standard bicarbonate is an indicator of metabolic abnormalities contributing to acidosis or alkalosis.

The base excess is a marker of the levels of bicarbonate and also other bases. When bicarbonate values fall below the normal range, the base excess becomes 'negative' (i.e. a 'base deficit'). Conversely, when bicarbonate levels rise, there is a positive base excess.

When interpreting any abnormality of pH, both PCO_2 and HCO_3^- must be considered, as well as the pH itself (see Table 4.6)

Compensated acidosis/alkalosis

When the body successfully responds to an acid–base imbalance, the pH is returned towards normal. This may

Box 4.6 Causes of respiratory acidosis (usually associated with hypoventilation)

- Obstructive lung disease
- Oversedation/other causes of depression of respiratory centre
- Neuromuscular disorders
- Hypoventilation during mechanical ventilation
- Pain, chest wall deformities, respiratory muscle fatigue, etc.

Box 4.7 Causes of respiratory alkalosis (usually associated with hyperventilation)

- Hypoxaemia
- Anxiety states
- Pulmonary embolus, fibrosis, etc.
- Pregnancy
- Hyperventilation during mechanical ventilation
- Brain injury
- High salicylate levels
- Fever
- Asthma
- Severe anaemia

Table 4.6 Alterations in different types of acidosis and alkalosis

	pH	P_aCO_2	Bicarbonate (HCO_3^-)
Acute respiratory acidosis	Low	High	Normal
Acute respiratory alkalosis	High	Low	Normal
Acute metabolic acidosis	Low	Normal or low	Low
Acute metabolic alkalosis	High	Normal	High

There may also be mixed or combined acidosis or alkalosis due to a combination of causes.

Table 4.7 Alterations in compensated acidosis and alkalosis

	pH	P_aCO_2	Bicarbonate (HCO_3^-)
Compensated respiratory acidosis	Near normal	High	High
Compensated respiratory alkalosis	Normal	Low	Low
Compensated metabolic acidosis	Near normal	Low	Low
Compensated metabolic alkalosis	Near normal	High	High

be by either respiratory and/or renal compensation. For example, a respiratory acidosis caused by hypoventilation in chronic pulmonary disease will be compensated by the kidneys producing and retaining bicarbonate, i.e. a metabolic compensation.

These compensatory mechanisms have only a limited range and compensation is usually only complete in chronic respiratory acidosis. In other cases, the pH does not completely return to normal (Table 4.7). If the primary abnormality continues, the patient may be unable to maintain a normal pH. Management of acid–base imbalance then usually depends on determining and treating the underlying cause.

Physiochemical approach to acid–base balance

The more recently developed 'physiochemical approach' to understanding acid–base balance suggests that, in addition to PCO_2, strong ions in solution within the body are key determinants of pH. Strong ions are those molecules which dissociate entirely in solution to their ionic form. In extracellular fluid (such as blood), these are mainly sodium (Na^+), potassium (K^+), and chloride (Cl^-). The difference between the sum of positive ions (cations), such as sodium and potassium, and the sum of negative ions (anions), such as chloride, is known as the 'strong ion difference' (SID). Laboratory studies demonstrate that pH is determined by (i) the strong ion difference, (ii) the total of weak acids in the plasma (mostly comprising serum proteins such as albumin and inorganic phosphate), and (iii) PCO_2. Changes in any of these components will alter pH. This approach considers more of the complexities of biological processes and may provide a more complete explanation of what is happening in some conditions. However, it requires many more variables to be measured and calculated, and the data produced can be difficult to interpret. The physiological approach is thus likely to remain the main model used in most critical care units for some while (Adrogué *et al.* 2009).

Neuronal control of respiration

The involuntary regulation of respiratory drive is controlled by a group of neurons in the brain medulla that form the respiratory centre (see Figure 4.5). The respiratory centre is moderated by the influence of the apneustic and pneumotaxic centres located in the pons. The apneustic centre is inhibited by the pneumotaxic centre and by stimuli from receptors in the lung (Hering–Breuer or stretch receptors).

Everyday control of respiration is further modified by several other factors, the most important of which are stimuli from chemoreceptors.

Central chemoreceptors

These are located bilaterally and ventrally in the medulla, and are in direct contact with cerebrospinal fluid (CSF). Chemoreceptors act directly on the respiratory centre to modulate respiratory effort. The most powerful stimulus to these receptors is an increase in hydrogen ion concentration in the CSF, which can be directly related to increased PCO_2 in the blood supply to the brain.

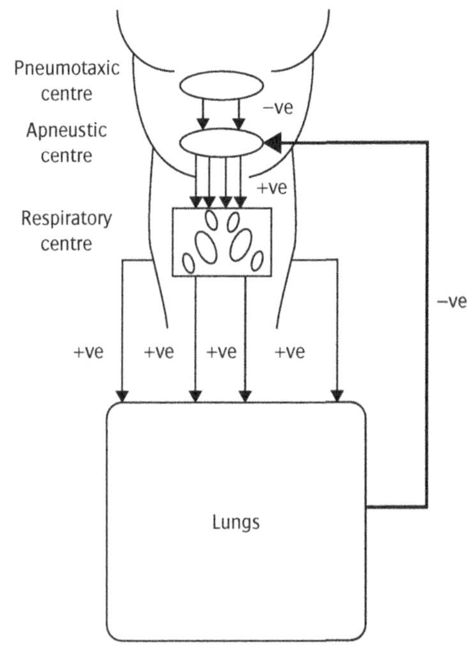

Figure 4.5 Neuronal control of respiration.

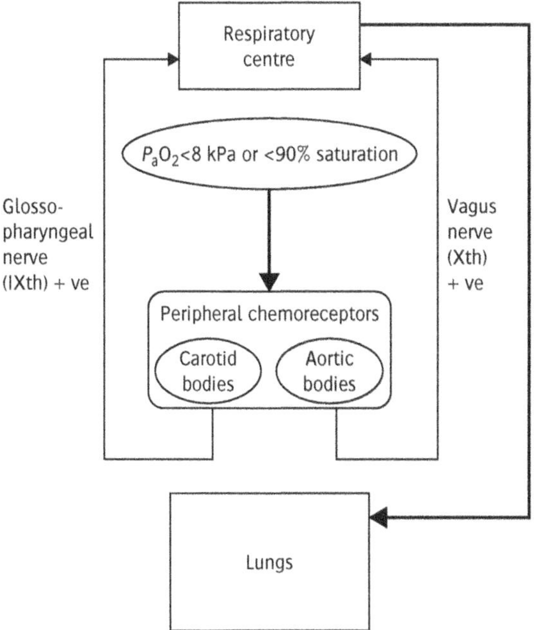

Figure 4.6 Mechanisms of peripheral chemoreceptor effects on respiration.

Peripheral chemoreceptors

These groups of oxygen-sensitive cells are located at the bifurcation of the internal and external carotid arteries and on the aortic arch. They stimulate the respiratory centre to increase respiratory effort when oxygen tension falls below 8 kPa. Peripheral chemoreceptors are sensitive to P_aO_2 rather than O_2 content, so conditions where the P_aO_2 is normal but O_2 content is low (e.g. in chronic anaemia, carbon monoxide poisoning, or methaemoglobinaemia) do not stimulate respiration (Figure 4.6).

Factors other than PaO_2 that affect the response of peripheral chemoreceptors include:

- increases in H^+ not due to raised PCO_2 (e.g. lactic acidosis)
- increases in temperature
- increased PCO_2 (a minor although faster response than that from central chemoreceptors)
- nicotine.

Peripheral chemoreceptors can also cause peripheral vasoconstriction, increased pulmonary vascular resistance, systolic arterial hypertension, tachycardia, and increased left ventricular perfusion.

Other mechanisms that influence respiration

- Hering–Breuer inflation reflex—this is generated by stretch receptors situated in the walls of the bronchi and bronchioles. When lungs overinflate, the receptors are stimulated to send impulses back to the respiratory centre terminating inspiration. This protects against pulmonary damage.
- Deflation reflex—the rate of breathing is increased when lungs are compressed or deflated. The precise mechanism is unknown.
- Irritant reflex—receptors located subepithelially in trachea, bronchi, and bronchioles cause an increase in ventilatory rate when lungs are compressed or exposed to noxious gases. They may also trigger a reflex cough and cause bronchoconstriction.
- Juxtapulmonary–capillary receptors (J-receptors)—these are located in the interstitial tissues between the pulmonary capillaries and alveoli and stimulate rapid shallow breathing when activated by pulmonary capillary congestion, capillary hypertension, oedema of the alveolar walls, humoral agents (e.g. 5-hydroxytryptamine (5-HT)) and lung deflation.
- Baroreceptors—these have a primarily cardiovascular function, but when stimulated by hypotension increase ventilatory rate as well as raising heart rate. When stimulated by hypertension they cause a decrease in ventilatory rate.
- Exercise—neural signals from the cerebral cortex to exercising muscles appear to have a collateral transmission to the respiratory centre, producing an increased rate and depth of breathing. Limb movement also transmits sensory signals up the spinal cord to the medulla.

Assessment of respiratory status

Remember that any primary lung dysfunction may also affect other systems, for example level of consciousness, cardiovascular status, and emotional state. The ability to perform personal needs and maintain vital defence mechanisms may also be reduced. The importance of preventative as well as therapeutic roles cannot be overemphasized; the nurse must maintain an overall view of the patient that does not neglect these other features while also managing the main causes of distress.

History

Initial assessment should first focus on the key priorities of ensuring a patent airway, adequate oxygenation, ventilation, and circulation, clarifying the level of consciousness, and performing a top-to-toe, front-and-back examination (i.e. a rapid assessment of Airway, Breathing, Circulation, Disability; with Exposure). Nonetheless, it is essential to obtain the patient's background and history as soon as possible. Patients in acute respiratory distress are often unable to provide detailed information, so all efforts should be made to obtain details from alternative sources such as relatives and friends, general practitioner records, and previous hospital notes, including the results of any previous investigations.

The nursing and medical histories should be done as a collaborative process to avoid unnecessary repetition. A great deal of data can be collected while attending to other urgent needs (see Box 4.8 and Table 4.8).

Physical assessment

Considerable information about the patient's condition can be gained from simply looking and listening.

Patient condition

Close observation of the general appearance, the effort of breathing/level of fatigue, and potential for maintaining respiration is essential. Useful indicators of failing respiratory function include the following.

1. Sweating (indicates use of considerable effort to maintain function and increased sympathetic drive).
2. Inability to speak in sentences or move limbs (indicates lack of breath and energy limitation due to poor respiratory function).
3. Restlessness, confusion, and altered level of consciousness (may indicate cerebral hypoxia or a high PCO_2, although other causes may also be responsible). If conscious level is decreased, the patient's ability to protect the airway should be assessed by checking the gag reflex.
4. Distress.
5. Posture.

Box 4.8 Useful information from history-taking

- Timespan of current problem plus any relevant past medical history, particularly the degree (if any) of chronic respiratory disability
- Previously tried manoeuvres found to be of benefit in reducing respiratory problems and breathlessness
- Current medications
- Type and time of occurrence of dyspnoea (e.g. on exertion only, position related, etc.)
- Sputum—colour, consistency, amount
- Pain (if any)—site, timing, modes of relief employed by patient
- Lifestyle/social factors—smoking, drug-taking, exposure to toxic substances, etc.
- Mood state and immediate anxieties

Table 4.8 Abnormal respiratory patterns

Name	Characteristics
Apnoea	Complete absence of spontaneous ventilation
Hypoventilation	Decreased alveolar ventilation with decreased rate and/or depth of breathing; results in an increased P_ACO_2 and, consequently, a rise in P_aCO_2
Hyperventilation	Increased alveolar ventilation with increased rate and/or depth of breathing; results in a decreased P_ACO_2 and, consequently, a fall in P_aCO_2
Hyperpnoea	Increased depth of breathing, with or without increased frequency
Tachypnoea	Increased rate of ventilation
Cheyne–Stokes	Periods of apnoea of 10–30 sec, followed by a progressively increasing rate and volume of breaths that reach a peak and then decline to another period of apnoea; this pattern of respiration is associated with cerebral dysfunction
Kussmaul breathing	Increased rate and depth of breathing commonly associated with diabetic ketoacidosis; it produces a decrease in P_ACO_2 and a low P_aCO_2
Biot's breathing	Short episodes of deep inspirations of the same volume and frequency followed by 10–30 sec of apnoea; this pattern is associated with meningitis

Eupnoea is the term for normal spontaneous ventilation.

Colour

The oral (buccal) mucosa as well as the peripheries should be viewed. The patient's colour can range from pink, and therefore probably relatively well oxygenated, to frankly cyanosed. Carbon monoxide poisoning may produce a characteristic 'cherry-red' colour due to carboxyhaemoglobin. Peripheral cyanosis is seen in conditions of poor circulation (vasoconstriction due to cold, poor cardiac output, arterial pathology, etc.) and does not necessarily indicate hypoxaemia. Central cyanosis, seen as blue lips and buccal mucosa, is indicative of a low P_aO_2. Central cyanosis is seen when >5 g/dl of haemoglobin is unsaturated, and therefore grossly anaemic patients may not exhibit cyanosis even if severely hypoxic.

Respiratory pattern

Assess the movement of the chest wall, considering the following.

1. Are both sides moving equally? Pneumothorax, mechanical dysfunction such as rib fractures and flail chest, pleural effusion, and major lobar collapse may cause diminished expansion of one side of the chest relative to the other.
2. Are the normal muscles of inspiration being used? Diaphragmatic splinting or paralysis, neuropathy, myopathy, Guillain–Barré syndrome, and myasthenia gravis can all affect the ability to use the diaphragm and intercostal muscles in the usual way.
3. Use of accessory muscles of inspiration to assist inspiration suggests that significant extra effort is required to create the negative pressure necessary for adequate inspiration. Inspiration may be more difficult owing to obstructive or restrictive disease, or because the demands of the body on the respiratory system are greatly increased. The accessory muscles of expiration may be being used to assist in expelling air when there is increased airway resistance (e.g. in asthma).
4. Respiratory rate should be counted and the depth observed together to give a clear picture of respiration. A high respiratory rate with shallow breaths may indicate pain preventing normal inspiration, whereas a high rate with normal-sized breaths may indicate hyperventilation. Hypoventilation may be due to central causes including head injury and stroke, or to iatrogenic or self-administered sedatives (e.g. benzodiazepines or opiates). It is not always possible to interpret these signs correctly without considering other data, so caution should be applied before attaching too great a significance to them (Table 4.8). For other respiratory patterns associated with specific neurological dysfunction see Chapter 8.

Palpation

The position of the trachea should be assessed for mediastinal shift by placing a finger either side of the trachea just above the sternal notch. Tracheal deviation is indicative of mediastinal shift caused either by large volumes of pleural air or fluid filling the pleural space and pushing the lung away from the chest wall (i.e. away from the problem side), or by lobar/lung collapse drawing the trachea towards the lung space (i.e. towards the problem side).

Tactile vocal fremitus refers to the vibrations felt when the patient speaks. Sound is usually transmitted well through solid structures and poorly through air; therefore conditions replacing air with more solid matter in the lungs (e.g. consolidation following pneumonia) may increase the transmission of sound. The fingertips or palm of the examiner's hand are placed on each side of the patient's chest. The patient is then asked to speak and a similar degree of vibration should be felt bilaterally (except over the heart). Inequality in transmission may be due to consolidation (increased transmission) or pneumothorax/pleural fluid (decreased transmission).

Percussion

This technique is relatively infrequently used by nurses and requires some practice to become skilled. The middle phalanx of the middle finger is pressed against the chest wall and struck with the tip of the other middle finger. The normal sound over the lungs is low pitched, long, and resonant (hollow). Increased density (e.g. from a pleural effusion) produces a stony dull sound, while decreased density (such as in pneumothorax or emphysema) causes hyper-resonant (loud, lower-pitched) or tympanitic (loud, long, high-pitched, drum-like) sounds.

Auscultation

Air entry to both lung fields

This is a basic procedure to assess air flow is occurring to all areas of the lung. Causes of reduced or non-existent air entry in the self-ventilating patient vary from lobar collapse and pleural effusion to pneumothorax and hypoventilation.

Normal breath sounds

These may be vesicular (soft, low-pitched, with no break between inspiration and expiration, inspiration usually longer than expiration, best heard in the lung periphery); bronchial (louder, high-pitched, with a pause between inspiration and expiration, and with inspiration equal to or shorter than expiration, heard over the trachea); or bronchovesicular (combination of the above sounds, heard over major airways in most other parts of the lung).

Bronchial sounds heard over areas of the lung other than the trachea suggest underlying consolidation or the presence of a pleural effusion just below. Here, the sound is due to the transmission of breath sounds from the main airway through the medium of consolidated or compressed lung rather than a direct flow of air. This phenomenon is known as 'bronchial breathing'. Absent or reduced/distant breath sounds may be heard over a pleural effusion or pneumothorax.

Abnormal breath sounds

1. Crackles (fine) are high-pitched rustles related to the reopening of small airways or the presence of intra-alveolar fluid. They can be heard in pulmonary oedema and pulmonary fibrosis at end-inspiration, and in pneumonia and bronchiectasis during both inspiration and expiration.
2. Crackles (coarse) are lower pitched, usually heard over larger airways, and are indicative of sputum or fluid in those areas.
3. Wheezes are generally heard on expiration as a result of expired air being forced through narrowed airways. Such conditions include asthma and other causes of bronchoconstriction (e.g. anaphylaxis, toxic gas inhalation). Wheeze may be heard in heart failure ('cardiac asthma'). Inspiratory wheeze (stridor) is associated with major airway obstruction such as a tumour or the presence of a foreign body. This is also heard in epiglottitis and laryngeal oedema (e.g. post-extubation). If wheezes are heard during both inspiration and expiration they are often caused by excessive airway secretions.
4. Pleural friction rubs are rough, grating, crackling sounds heard on inspiration and expiration over areas of pleural inflammation (pleurisy) where the normally smooth surfaces of parietal and visceral pleura are roughened and rub on each other.

Pulse oximetry

This non-invasive device utilizes a probe placed externally over a pulse (e.g. on a finger, toe, or earlobe). It provides almost immediate, continuous, and reasonably accurate readings of arterial oxygen saturation (S_pO_2) allowing early identification of hypoxaemia. The underlying principle relies on oxyhaemoglobin and deoxyhaemoglobin absorbing light at different wavelengths. The standard oximeter contains two light-emitting diodes (LEDs), one emitting red light at a frequency of 660 nm (corresponding to the peak level of light absorption for oxyhaemoglobin), and the other emitting infrared light at a frequency of 940 nm (corresponding to the peak level of light absorption for deoxyhaemoglobin). As light from the LEDs passes through tissue, most of it will be absorbed by connective tissue, skin, pigmentation, fat, bone veins, and venous blood. Light not absorbed by these tissues is sensed by a photoreceptor at the base of the probe (see Figure 4.7), with fluctuations in the signal then due to variations in arterial blood flow during the cardiac cycle. The ratio of the oxyhaemoglobin absorption signal to the sum of the combined oxyhaemoglobin and deoxyhaemoglobin signals provides a measure of arterial saturation:

$$SpO_2 = \frac{\text{oxyHb}}{\text{oxyHb} + \text{deoxyHb}} \left(\begin{array}{c} \times 100 \text{ to obtain the} \\ \text{percentage saturation} \end{array} \right).$$

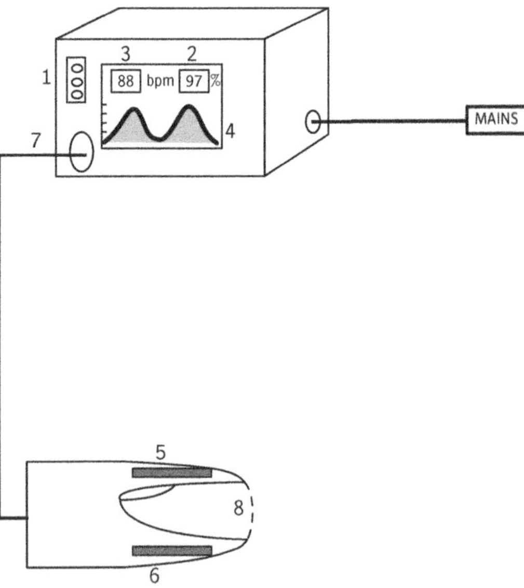

Figure 4.7 The pulse oximeter: 1, on–off, alarm settings; 2, S_aO_2 display; 3, heart rate display; 4, pulse waveform; 5, light-emitting diodes; 6, photodetector; 7, patient cable display; 8, patient's digit.

The accuracy of pulse oximetry is affected by several factors.

- An adequate peripheral circulation is needed such that the sensor can detect a sufficiently strong signal to give an accurate reading.
- Patient movement can cause artefact.
- Similarly, probe displacement with a partial loss of signal is a frequent occurrence that is sometimes erroneously interpreted as a fall in saturation. Attention to the quality of the displayed waveform is important; the probe position should always be checked if a sudden fall in saturation is seen. Transient falls in saturation may be observed following suction and repositioning of the patient, but if low saturations persist arterial blood gases should be obtained and analysed.
- Placement of the probe distal to a blood pressure cuff should be avoided as alterations in venous or arterial blood flow may affect the readings.
- Bright light from direct sunlight, surgical lamps, infrared warming lamps, etc. may interfere with signal processing. The probe may need to be covered with an opaque material in some cases.
- Caution should be applied where there is known or suspected abnormal haemoglobin (e.g. carboxyhaemoglobin, methaemoglobin, sickling cells) as these are not accurately differentiated by the standard oximeter. For example, smoke inhalation raises levels of carboxyhaemoglobin, i.e. haemoglobin with carbon monoxide rather than oxygen attached. Carboxyhaemoglobin has a similar pattern of light absorption to oxyhaemoglobin, which means that falsely high oxygen saturation levels may be given by the pulse oximeter. Methaemoglobin is found when the iron within the haemoglobin is in the ferric (Fe^{3+}) rather than the ferrous (Fe^{2+}) form and does not bind with oxygen. There is usually very little methaemoglobin present, but it can be significantly increased in a few rare inherited conditions and by various medications including nitrates, metoclopramide, primaquine, and lidocaine.
- Certain dyes and pigments, including methylthioninium chloride (methylene blue), indocyanine green, and blue, black, or green nail polish, can also cause inaccurate oximeter readings (McMorrow and Mythen 2006).
- As a standard pulse oximeter only utilizes two light wavelengths appropriate for oxyhaemoglobin and deoxyhaemoglobin, some abnormal forms of haemoglobin may confuse the situation. Some new models utilize light emitted at multiple wavelengths and can better differentiate the various forms of haemoglobin. However, these devices are expensive and not widely used as yet. An alternative is to periodically check pulse oximeter readings against those obtained from a co-oximeter (blood gas analyser) which uses multiple light wavelengths.

Nursing considerations:

- high and low alarm limits appropriate to the individual patient should be reviewed and set at least every shift
- the probe site should be rotated regularly as, depending on both the type of probe and patient factors, both pressure and heat injuries can be caused by the probe, sometimes in less than 3–4 hours (Wille *et al.* 2000)
- heated probes are not suitable for long-term monitoring in an ICU patient.

End-tidal carbon dioxide ($ETCO_2$) monitoring/capnography

Carbon dioxide concentration can be continually monitored in both inhaled and exhaled breaths in mechanically ventilated patients. The approach is based on the premise that, in lungs with a normal ventilation/perfusion relationship, the end-tidal concentration ($ETCO_2$) measured at the end of expiration can be used as an indicator of alveolar PCO_2 and this, in turn, reflects the adequacy of alveolar ventilation which correlates well with P_aCO_2. Guidelines recommend that capnography be used during endotracheal intubation and tracheostomy procedures to confirm tube placement in the trachea, and in some countries its use is mandated in any patient receiving mechanical ventilation (Thomas *et al.* 2011).

A sensor is placed between the endotracheal (or tracheostomy) tube and the ventilator circuit. An integral transducer detects the amount of infrared radiation absorbed by the expired air, with the $ETCO_2$ value being derived from the level of radiation specifically absorbed by CO_2 in the expired breath. The technique provides a continuous indication of CO_2 elimination without the need for arterial blood sampling, and so is particularly useful in patients without arterial access. The correlation may be less strong in cases of ventilation/perfusion mismatch or if there is significant air-trapping in the alveoli (e.g. in asthma).

Arterial blood gases

Measurement of the P_aO_2 and P_aCO_2 in arterial blood gives a clear indication of respiratory function. However, results must always be interpreted in the context of the inspired oxygen concentration and the patient's clinical condition. For example, a compromised tiring patient may be able maintain a near normal P_aCO_2 until almost the point of collapse. The functions of arterial blood gas measurement are:

- measurement of oxygenation
- estimation of the effectiveness of ventilation
- determination of acid–base balance (see earlier).

Tissue hypoxia

Tissue hypoxia is defined as an inadequate availability of oxygen for cellular metabolism. This can be due to one or more of hypoxaemia (hypoxic hypoxia), anaemia (anaemic hypoxia), circulatory impairment (circulatory hypoxia), or impaired cellular utilization of oxygen (cytotoxic dysoxia).

Hypoxaemia (hypoxic hypoxia) is addressed in more detail in the next section. In anaemic hypoxia the oxygen tension of arterial blood is normal but the oxygen-carrying capacity is inadequate. This may simply be due to low levels of haemoglobin or a deficiency in the ability of the haemoglobin to carry oxygen, for example in carbon monoxide poisoning when haemoglobin binds with carbon monoxide in preference to oxygen. In circulatory hypoxia the arterial blood that reaches the tissues may have a normal oxygen tension and content, but the volume of blood (and therefore the amount of oxygen) delivered is insufficient to meet tissue needs. This is commonly due to one of the following:

- stagnant hypoxia—slow peripheral capillary flow due to low cardiac output, vascular insufficiency, or neurochemical abnormalities
- arteriovenous shunt—where some tissues are bypassed by oxygenated arterial blood.

Cytopathic dysoxia is the impairment of the ability of cells to utilize oxygen. This occurs when there is inhibition of mitochondrial respiration. Examples include cyanide or carbon monoxide poisoning and prolonged severe sepsis.

Hypoxaemia

A low oxygen saturation in the blood is termed hypoxaemia. This is often arbitrarily defined as a saturation below 90–92% or P_aO_2 <8.0 kPa. Tissue hypoxia does not always result as the body compensates in both the short and long term to overcome the low P_aO_2, for example by an increase in cardiac output, increased oxygen extraction by the tissues, or, over time, by an increase in haemoglobin as seen, for instance, in chronic obstructive airways disease or living at altitude.

Hypocapnia

Hyocapnia is a low carbon dioxide tension in the blood (<4.6 kPa), usually due to hyperventilation.

Hypercapnia

Hypercapnia is a high carbon dioxide tension in the blood (>6.0 kPa), usually due to hypoventilation or an increase in dead space ventilation, but occasionally due to increased carbon dioxide production (e.g. with excessive carbohydrate intake) that is not adequately cleared by an increase in minute ventilation.

Methods of respiratory support

A wide range of respiratory support can be offered, from simple supplemental oxygen therapy to mechanical ventilation and the use of extracorporeal systems (see Table 4.9)

The aims of respiratory support are:

- to partially or completely return hypoxaemia and/or hypercapnia (and therefore respiratory acidosis) to acceptable levels
- to assist mechanical failure
- to relieve physiological stress and reduce physiological workload, especially the work of breathing and cardiac work.

Priorities in caring for patients requiring respiratory support

Safety

A method of back-up ventilation for the patient must always be immediately available. This is usually a manual bag–valve system incorporating a self-inflating resuscitator (sometimes known by the propriety name 'Ambu bag') that can be attached to a mask or via a catheter mount to the endotracheal or tracheostomy tube. This must be regularly checked as part of a standard safety routine by the nurse responsible for the patient. An appropriate size of oropharyngeal (Guedel)

Table 4.9 **Methods of oxygen delivery for respiratory support**

Mode of delivery	Oxygen percentage available	Associated problems	Safety priorities	Use
Nasal cannulae	Disposable delivery system (max. 44%): 2 L/min 23–28% 3 L/min 28–30% 4 L/min 32–36% 5 L/min 40% 6 L/min plus.	Limited % O_2 available Inaccurate delivery of oxygen, particularly with high minute volumes Requires patent nasal passages If patient mouth breathes amount of oxygen delivered will be altered Drying and uncomfortable for nasal passages	Regular monitoring of respiratory rate and pattern If patient unstable use pulse oximeter to monitor O_2 saturation Positioning of cannulae inside nares Check O_2 flow rate	Low levels of O_2 supplementation
Semi-rigid masks (e.g. Hudson, MC, etc.)	Disposable delivery system: 4 L/min ~35% 6 L/min ~50% 8 L/min ~55% 10 L/min ~60% 12 L/min ~65%	Inaccurate delivery of O_2 particularly with high respiratory rate and pattern Limits patient activities such as eating and drinking Drying of patient's mucosa and of secretions Rebreathing may occur with high minute volumes	Regular monitoring of minute volumes If patient unstable use pulse oximeter to monitor O_2 saturation Check positioning of mask and O_2 flow rate	Low to medium levels of O_2 supplementation
Venturi-type mask (high flow system) (e.g. Ventimasks, Inspiron, etc.)	Disposable delivery system with use of Venturi nozzle appropriate for desired percentage: 2 L/min, 24% 4 L/min 28% 8 L/min 35% 10 L/min 40% 15 L/min 60% If humidification used an extra attachment is required	Can still be drying for patient Patients requiring large inspiratory flow rates may not achieve required inspired O_2 saturation Limits patient activities such as eating and drinking	Regular monitoring of respiratory rate and pattern Check positioning of mask and O_2 flow rate If patient unstable use pulse oximeter to monitor O_2 saturation	Medium to high levels of O_2 supplementation
Humidified oxygen using nebulizer system (e.g. Aquapak)	Disposable delivery system Varying rates of flow to deliver 28–60% O_2.	Inaccurate delivery of O_2, particularly with use of high volumes Limits patient activities such as eating and drinking	Check positioning of mask, O_2 flow rate, and setting of O_2 percentage on nebulizer system Regular monitoring of respiratory rate and pattern If patient unstable, use pulse oximeter	Low to medium levels of O_2 supplementation
Non-rebreathe masks with reservoir bag	90–95% depending on respiratory rate and run at 15 L/min		Ensure reservoir bag is fully inflated before placing on patient Reservoir bag should be kept partially inflated at all times	Medium to high levels of O_2 supplementation Emergency situations, short-term use only

(continued)

Table 4.9 Continued

Mode of delivery	Oxygen percentage available	Associated problems	Safety priorities	Use
High flow nasal cannula (HFNC) oxygen	Disposable delivery system incorporating nasal cannulae for administration of 21% to<100% humidified O_2. driven by a high flow O_2 meter	Requires patent nasal passages Despite humidification, dryness, nasal discomfort, and epistaxis have been reported	Regular monitoring of respiratory rate and pattern Positioning of cannulae inside nares Check O_2 flow rate Pulse oximetry to monitor O_2 saturation	Medium to high levels of O_2 supplementation
Continuous positive airway pressure (CPAP)	40–100% with disposable tight- fitting CPAP mask (or helmet), tubing, 2.5–15 cmH_2O expiratory pressure valve, and high flow oxygen supply (via ventilator or wall oxygen supply)	Tight-fitting mask causes discomfort, pressure sores, etc. Leakage of high gas flows into eyes may cause corneal drying and abrasion Eating and drinking are very difficult Air swallowing may cause discomfort and increased risk of gastric regurgitation Patient may experience feelings of claustrophobia due to tight-fitting mask Increased noise associated with high flows may disturb patient In systems without a high flow generator, flow may be inadequate, causing increased inspiratory resistance	Regular monitoring of respiratory rate and pattern Pulse oximetry to monitor O_2 saturation Provision of psychological support and comfort to assist patient tolerance Use of nasogastric tube to decompress stomach if necessary	Medium to high levels of O_2 supplementation
Non-invasive bi-level positive airway pressure (BiPAP)	Tight-fitting mask and tubing connected to standard or custom ventilator Can provide up to 100% O_2 and up to 100% ventilation	Same problems as for CPAP	Monitoring of O_2 saturation	When patient is tiring or to support respiratory decompensation with rising P_aCO_2 May be used long term for patients with chronic COPD, chest wall deformity, neuromuscular disease, etc.

airway and facemask should also be available at the bedside.

The concentration of inspired oxygen (FiO_2) that the patient is receiving should be checked against that prescribed. This is done using an oxygen analyser that is either intrinsic to the ventilator or a separate device attached to the circuit. The method of oxygen delivery should be capable of delivering the FiO_2 required. Standard oxygen masks (e.g. Hudson masks) cannot deliver very precise levels of oxygen, and it is difficult to achieve FiO_2 values >0.4 using standard masks in patients with a high minute ventilation (see Table 4.9).

Equipment alarms are a reliable though sometimes oversensitive way of identifying sudden or life-threatening changes. However, they are only as useful as the alarm settings used. The vigilance of staff is key, so the bedside nurse must regularly review these settings and ensure that they are appropriate to the individual patient and their situation. The usual aim is to consider the patient's current physiological status as a baseline and to allow some fluctuation around that baseline without permitting any dangerous deviations.

Ventilator alarms

Alarm settings should be checked to ensure that they are switched on, are audible and visible, and are set to fit the patient's circumstances. A pragmatic approach is to set the alarm limits 25% above and below the desired level for each variable. Alternatively, the following are appropriate for most patients.

- Expired minute volume alarms should be set:
  - upper limit at 2l above current expired minute volume,
  - lower limit 2l below current expired minute volume.
- Airway pressure alarms should be set:
  - upper limit at 30–40 cm H_2O (at the most)
  - lower limit at 5 cm H_2O below current airway pressure reading.
- Pulse oximeter alarms are usually set at 90% oxygen saturation. However, this may change according to the patient's condition and underlying comorbidity (e.g. in COPD).
- Cardiac monitor alarms also provide a useful warning for respiratory problems and should be set appropriately (see Chapter 5 for guidance).

Suction equipment

This is essential for both emergency situations and routine use in intubated or tracheostomized patients. It should always be checked to ensure that it is capable of producing an appropriate level of suction, and that sufficient suction catheters of the correct size for the patient's endotracheal or tracheostomy tube and condition of secretions are available (see section on suction technique later in this chapter).

Problems associated with patients undergoing respiratory support

There are many potential problems associated with supporting a compromised respiratory system, and also with taking over the patient's respiratory function using some form of mechanical ventilation. All patients requiring respiratory support have some degree of respiratory failure (see Box 4.9), classically categorized as Type I or Type II:

- In Type I respiratory failure the main problem is the lung parenchyma: the patient is hypoxaemic (P_aO_2 <8 kPa/S_aO_2 <90%) but has normal (or even low) levels of carbon dioxide.
- Type II respiratory failure is 'pump failure' in which ventilation is inadequate and the patient is both hypoxaemic and hypercapnic (P_aCO_2 >6.0 kPa).

Non-invasive respiratory support may be considered in the circumstances detailed in Table 4.10. Non-invasive respiratory support involves use of oxygen therapy, continuous positive airway pressure (CPAP), intermittent positive pressure breathing (IPPB), and bilevel positive airway pressure (BiPAP). These systems deliver support through tight-fitting nasal or oral masks, full facemasks, or helmets (see Table 4.9).

Hypoxaemia

Management of hypoxaemia involves oxygen therapy (see Table 4.9). Patients with chronic carbon dioxide retention are much more dependent on a hypoxic respiratory drive. They may need carefully controlled oxygen therapy aimed at achieving their likely or known baseline oxygen saturation, which may be 88–92% or even lower. A proportion of such patients may suffer reduced respiratory drive and worsening hypercapnia if given excessive oxygen to increase their saturations above their baseline levels. Continuous observation of respiratory rate and regular monitoring of P_aCO_2 is needed to ensure that this does not occur. It should be remembered that worsening

Box 4.9 Definition of respiratory failure

Arterial blood gases

- P_aO_2 <8.0 kPa with patient breathing air and at rest
- P_aCO_2 >6.0kPa in the absence of primary metabolic acidosis
- ± pH <7.25 in the absence of primary metabolic acidosis

Patient

- Respiratory rate >40 or <6–8 breaths/min
- Deteriorating vital capacity (<15 ml/kg)

Table 4.10 Indications and contraindications for use of non-invasive ventilation (NIV)

Indications for NIV	Clinical condition	Contraindications	Preconditions
• Acute exacerbation of COPD • Type 2 respiratory failure secondary to chest wall deformity or neuromuscular disorder • Cardiogenic pulmonary oedema • As aid to weaning from invasive ventilation	• Sick but not moribund • Able to protect own airway • Haemodynamically stable	• Severe hypoxaemia. • Reduced consciousness (e.g. GCS <11) • Facial injury. • Vomiting • Fixed upper airway obstruction • Undrained pneumothorax • Excessive respiratory secretions	• Ensure a plan is in place to manage the patient if the trial of NIV fails. • Discuss/decide which environment is best for the patient (critical care unit or ward).

of the patient's underlying condition and/or increasing fatigue may also induce the same clinical pattern, so it should not be automatically assumed that excessive oxygen administration is the cause in every case.

- Chest physiotherapy will assist in removal of secretions. Deep breathing and coughing may also help reopen areas of collapsed lung.
- Positioning of the patient to optimize ventilation/perfusion matching is important too (see section on shunting). This usually involves sitting the patient upright, although if there is a one-sided (unilateral) chest problem, the patient should be placed on their side with the problem lung uppermost so that the good lung receives more perfusion.

Hypercapnia

Management of hypercapnia depends on the cause. Spontaneously breathing patients may require NIV, or intubation and mechanical ventilation if NIV is failing and/or they are not protecting their airway. Respiratory stimulants such as doxapram or reversal of excessive depressant medication may be needed (e.g. with naloxone for excessive opiate dosing). Mechanical problems such as sputum retention, pneumothorax, or a large pleural effusion may need to be addressed.

Maintenance of airway and sputum clearance

Effective humidification facilitates clearance of thick tenacious secretions and prevents drying of mucosa and cilia associated with inhalation of dry oxygen (see section on humidification). As ipratropium thickens secretions, its use should be carefully considered in the critical care patient as its modest bronchodilator effects may be outweighed by an increased risk of plugging in the airways.

Regular prompting of and/or assistance with deep breathing and coughing can reduce the incidence of atelectasis and help the patient clear secretions. Periodic deep breaths can be programmed into some mechanical ventilation regimens but, more often, manual hyperinflation is performed at intervals by giving one or more slow deep breaths using a Mapleson C/Waters circuit (2 L reservoir bag with an adjustable valve) aiming for a tidal volume 50% above the baseline. An inspiratory hold is briefly applied at the end of inspiration before rapid release of the bag in order to generate a relatively high expiratory flow. A similar function can be delivered by a non-invasive mechanical insufflator–exsufflator. These devices are used with a facemask, a mouthpiece, or attached to an endotracheal/tracheostomy tube. They also work by generating a positive airway pressure and then switching to a negative pressure which produces high expiratory flow and stimulates a cough.

Suctioning via the oro- or nasopharynx may assist in removal of sputum (see section on suction). Chest physiotherapy and postural drainage are also useful.

Fatigue related to work of breathing

It is important to limit any other stress or activity likely to produce fatigue and to provide periods specifically for complete rest without interference. Ensure that a day–night schedule is clear and differentiated and allows sleep.

Fear and anxiety

Severe respiratory failure and critical illness in general is extremely frightening. Management involves providing comfort and reassurance with a calm and confident approach to the patient. Include the family as much as possible in care and interactions. Allow time for expression of worries, and ensure that the patient is given full information expressed appropriately to ensure understanding. There is sometimes a place for anxiolytic medications such as benzodiazepines, but these should be used with considerable caution as there can be significant side effects.

Poor nutritional intake due to shortage of breath and loss of appetite

Provide frequent small nutritious meals if the patient is able to eat, with hot or cold drinks in between. Drinks may need to be fortified to supplement meals (e.g. with high calories). Encourage the family to become involved in meals and obtain details of the patient's likes and dislikes. Maintain a full record of nutritional intake and ensure that the medical staff are made aware of any significant deficits.

Impaired verbal communication due to shortage of breath and presence of mask

Provide alternative methods of communication such as an alphabet board or pen and paper. Use closed questions for specific information so that the patient can nod or shake their head to answer, and instruct the family in these methods. Anticipate the patient's information needs so that unnecessary questions can be avoided (see Chapter 3).

Drying of mouth and upper airways due to high flow of dry gases

Humidify the inspired gases (see section on humidification). Check skin turgor and the condition of the buccal mucosa. Provide mouthwashes and oral hygiene measures as necessary. Monitor fluid balance and avoid dehydration unless the medical condition dictates otherwise.

Endotracheal intubation and tracheostomy

Positive pressure respiratory support requires a closed delivery system with some form of seal of the patient's airway to achieve effective ventilation. Non-invasive ventilation uses a tight-fitting mask to form a seal while invasive mechanical ventilation uses either a cuffed endotracheal (ET) tube or a tracheostomy tube. As well as sealing the airway, the cuff provides some protection against aspiration of gastric secretions, food, blood, saliva, etc., although this is not completely guaranteed. See Box 4.10 for indications of endotracheal and tracheostomy tubes.

Endotracheal tubes are usually placed orally, although nasal placements are used in children and occasionally in adult ICU patients (see later). Tracheostomy tubes require percutaneous or surgical insertion below the cricoid and thyroid cartilages (usually around the second or third ring of the trachea) (see Box 4.11).

The presence of a tube in the trachea is associated with various potential problems and possible long-term complications (see Boxes 4.12 and 4.13). Some issues are immediately identifiable, but others may not become apparent until much later, perhaps not until the ET or tracheostomy tube has been removed (extubation/decannulation). These complications include development of tracheal ulceration and stenosis caused by excessive pressure exerted by the cuff in the airway. Cuffs are inflated with air to provide the necessary seal and are designed to be high in volume, while exerting a relatively low pressure so as to reduce the incidence of tracheal injury. Some tubes for specialist purposes use auto-expanding foam in a relatively bulky cuff that still

Box 4.10 Indications for endotracheal and tracheostomy tubes

- To obtain or maintain a clear airway
- To prevent aspiration of gastrointestinal contents
- To facilitate delivery of positive pressure ventilation
- To enable delivery of high concentrations of oxygen
- To facilitate removal of pulmonary secretions.

Box 4.11 Sites of insertion

- Oral endotracheal tube—mouth to trachea
- Nasal endotracheal tube—nose to trachea
- Tracheostomy—percutaneous or surgical insertion below the cricoid and thyroid cartilages (usually between the second and third, or third and fourth rings tracheal rings)
- Minitracheostomy or cricothyroidotomy—percutaneous or surgical insertion through the cricothyroid membrane

Box 4.12 Problems associated with endotracheal tube placement

- Tracheal stenosis, ulceration, necrosis
- Tracheomalacia (degeneration of the cartilaginous rings)
- Clearance of secretions
- Loss of normal humidifying and warming mechanisms
- Loss of physiological positive end expiratory pressure (PEEP) (i.e. resistance to expiration exerted by the pharynx and upper airways which limits alveolar collapse)
- Damage to vocal cords and trauma on insertion
- Increased risk of nosocomial (hospital-acquired) pneumonia
- Maxillary sinusitis (with nasal tubes)

Box 4.13 Problems associated with tracheostomy tube placement

- Tracheal stenosis, fibrosis, tracheomalacia
- Loss of normal humidifying and warming mechanisms
- Loss of physiological PEEP
- Increased risk of nosocomial pneumonia

gives a low pressure seal. It is very easy to over-inflate endotracheal and tracheostomy tube cuffs, so regular checks of cuff pressure must be performed. The aim is to have a cuff inflated so that there is no air leak during ventilation, but inflated no more than necessary to obtain the seal. Capillary occlusion pressure within the tracheal wall is approximately 30 mmHg, but may be lower; therefore it is important to limit cuff pressure to <30 mmHg to ensure adequate perfusion of tracheal mucosa. This can be monitored with cuff pressure manometers. These are usually hand-held devices, although some new tubes have intrinsic manometers. Cuff pressure should be checked at least four times daily and also when any air leaks or other problems are identified. Estimation of cuff pressure, either by squeezing the external pilot balloon or inflating the cuff until no further leak is heard, is inaccurate and likely to lead to excessive cuff pressures. For most patients, target cuff pressures of no more than 20–25 cmH_2O should be maintained (<18 mmHg) (Intensive Care Society 2008). Nonetheless, when pulmonary inflation pressures are high, cuff pressures may have to be increased over the recommended levels to prevent leaks.

Any access to the trachea bypassing intrinsic protective mechanisms increases the likelihood of ventilator-associated pneumonia (VAP). Indeed, intubation and mechanical ventilation have been associated with a 7- to 21-fold increase in the risk of developing VAP (Hunter 2006). Non-invasive ventilation constitutes a lower risk, yet this cannot always provide enough support in severe respiratory failure or where the airway is unprotected. Placement of an artificial airway is the most significant factor. Secretions tend to accumulate above the cuff in the subglottic space and are likely to become colonized and eventually aspirated because no cuff will completely seal the airway all the time. Drainage of subglottic secretions either continuously or intermittently, using specifically adapted ET and tracheostomy tubes, is advocated as a method of reducing the risk of ventilator-associated pneumonia. However, no large trials have been conducted and a meta-analysis of 13 studies concluded that while subglottic secretion drainage is likely to reduce the incidence of pneumonia, mortality was not affected (Muscedere *et al.* 2011). Another issue with ET tubes is that they may become coated both internally and externally with a biofilm, i.e. micro-organisms adhering to the surface of the plastic. This colonization can lead to subsequent infection.

Various other measures have been advocated for prevention of ventilator-associated pneumonia and other complications, with some incorporated into so-called 'bundles' of interventions (Resar *et al.* 2005) (see Box 4.14). It is important to note that many of these recommendations are based on weak evidence; indeed, there are studies suggesting that some of these interventions may actually increase the risk of pneumonia! For example, peptic ulcer prophylaxis will increase gastric pH, thus allowing bacterial overgrowth, so that the colonized secretions can migrate up the oesophagus and trickle around the cuff into the lung, with a reported increase in VAP rates (e.g. Miano *et al.* 2009). Likewise, in a recent randomized controlled trial, daily sedation holds had similar clinical outcomes to a titrated sedation protocol but involved a greater nurse workload (Mehta *et al.* 2012).

Endotracheal tubes

Endotracheal tubes designed for oral placement are most commonly used for adults as they are easier to insert and secure. Nasal tubes are only occasionally used; they may be needed for awake fibreoptic intubation where the upper airway is compromised (e.g. by

Box 4.14 Suggested measures for prevention of ventilation-associated pneumonia and related complications

- Endotracheal/tracheostomy tube cuff pressure maintained at 20–25 cmH_2O (Intensive Care Society 2008)
- Subglottic secretion drainage for patients expected to be ventilated for more than 3 days (Muscadere *et al.* 2008).
- Patient positioned semi-recumbent (elevated as near as possible to 45°)*
- daily 'sedation holds' and assessment of readiness to extubate*
- regular oral care*
- peptic ulcer prophylaxis*
- deep vein thrombosis prophylaxis*

A synthesis of several North American and European guidelines also suggests that practitioners should:

- ensure that there is adequate humidification while ensuring that water does not accumulate in the ventilator circuit—heat–moisture exchangers will often be adequate
- suction only when necessary
- use structured weaning protocols with non-invasive ventilation where possible
- avoid disconnections/too frequent changes of the ventilator or in-line suction catheter circuit
- monitor gastric residual volumes and minimize gastric distension as far as possible
- follow strict guidelines on antibiotic usage so as to avoid overuse
- avoid paralyzing agents as far as possible
- ensure scrupulous hand hygiene and prevention of cross-infection (Gentile and Siobal 2010)

* These five elements together make up the US Institute for Healthcare Improvement 'Ventilator Bundle' (http://www.ihi.org), also adopted by the UK NHS Patient Safety First programme (http://www.patientsafetyfirst.nhs.uk).

a pharyngeal abscess or swelling) and the clinician is concerned that an oral endotracheal tube may not be safely passed under sedation and paralysis. Nasal tubes may be more comfortable than oral tubes, avoid the hazard of being constricted by the patient's teeth, and make oral hygiene less difficult. However, nasal placement generally means the tube diameter needs to be smaller, and the angle at the nasopharynx can make it more difficult to pass a suction catheter. Placement is much more traumatic and bleeding is a common complication, especially in patients with a coexisting coagulopathy. Nasal tubes are also associated with an increased risk of maxillary sinusitis, which should be considered if a nasally intubated patient develops unexplained pyrexia.

Types of tube used for adults

Single-use cuffed endotracheal tubes, usually made from polyvinyl chloride (PVC), are most commonly employed (see Box 4.15). Some specialized tubes are used for particular circumstances.

- Double lumen ET tubes are used for asynchronous ventilation, e.g. when there is a need to just ventilate one lung (as in some types of upper gastrointestinal or thoracic surgery). One lumen opens into the trachea and the other into a bronchus (usually the left—this should be ascertained prior to insertion).
- Adjustable flange ET tubes can be used for patients with larger necks or when there are problems sealing the airway with standard length tubes.
- Reinforced ('armoured') tubes containing a spiral of wire embedded into the wall of the tube to give it

Box 4.15 Usual adult sizes of endotracheal tube

- Men: oral, 8–9 mm internal diameter (ID); nasal, 7–8 mm ID
- Women: oral, 7–8 mm ID; nasal, 6–7 mm ID

Tube sizes ranging from 6.0 mm to 11.0 mm ID are routinely available. The tube diameter (external) should be significantly less than the cricoid diameter to decrease the risk of damage.

Note. Tube sizes for children vary with age or body weight from 2.5 mm for newborns to 8.0 mm for 12- to 15-year-olds. Various formulae are available to estimate the correct diameter for age.

added strength—useful where there are concerns of external compression from, for example, a tumour.

Note: endotracheal tubes for children are usually uncuffed as children are more susceptible to stenotic problems related to cuff pressure, particularly in the cricoid region that is narrowed until puberty.

Length of endotracheal tubes

Oral ET tubes are typically positioned at approximately 23 cm at the incisors for men and 21 cm for women. However, the optimal position will depend on body size and neck length and requires confirmation by checking air entry to both lungs and, subsequently, by chest X-ray. The end of the tube should be roughly 3–5 cm above the carina; a tube sitting on the carina (or, alternatively, a cuff herniating through the vocal cords) is likely to be uncomfortable for the patient and may make ventilation difficult.

In the UK, ET tubes are generally cut prior to insertion to a length 2–3 cm longer than the values given above so that there is a short length of tube protruding from the mouth to allow secure tying of the tube. This should generally safeguard against the tube migrating further into the airway (endobronchial intubation), and perhaps reduce the risk of accidental extubation by the patient.

Intubation

Ideally, intubation should be an elective procedure performed in a considered timely way before the patient is in extremis. If possible, the patient should not have eaten for at least 4 hours to reduce the risk of aspiration of stomach contents. However, it is often necessary to intubate in crisis situations when patients present as emergencies or suffer rapid deterioration. A 'rapid sequence' intubation using total intravenous anaesthesia rather than inhalational anaesthesia is used in these emergency situations to reduce the risk of aspiration. This is also standard practice for critical care patients.

It is vital to have all essential equipment readily available in one place (see Box 4.16). Many critical care units have emergency intubation trolleys for these purposes. Whether the procedure is elective or an emergency, careful preparation and safety are paramount.

- Prepare and check the manual ventilation circuit (including suitably sized tight-fitting masks) and suction equipment to ensure that all components are in place and working.
- Prepare the mechanical ventilator and ventilator circuit, attach the ventilator to the gas source, and check it is functioning and, with a doctor, that the settings are appropriate for the patient. The inspired oxygen concentration should initially be set at a higher level than the anticipated requirements of the patient.
- Prepare/calibrate capnograph and sensor (if available).
- Have an ET tube cut to the right length ready for insertion and the cuff checked so that it inflates correctly and evenly and does not deflate spontaneously.
- Draw up the required sedatives (induction agent) and neuromuscular blocker (paralyzing agent) selected by the clinician.
- Bring emergency drugs to the bedside in case of peri- or cardiac arrest (it is often simplest to position a cardiac arrest trolley nearby) and ensure that the patient has reliable intravenous access.

Box 4.16 Equipment for intubation over and above standard safety equipment

- Laryngoscopes—one curved, one straight blade (check that the light is working) of appropriate size for the patient
- Selection of endotracheal tubes of varying internal diameter
- Lubrication (e.g. KY Jelly)
- Magill's forceps
- Introducers (bougies)
- 10 ml syringe
- Tape to secure tube
- Catheter mount
- Cuff pressure manometer
- Sedating and paralyzing agents
- A back-up manual ventilation bag and mask
- An intubating laryngoscope (may be requested for anticipated difficult intubations)
- End-tidal CO_2 monitoring
- Mechanical ventilator (set up and calibrated in advance)

Before intubation, the procedure should be explained to the patient if there is time. In particular, the temporary loss of speech due to presence of an ET tube should be emphasized to reduce anxiety.

- The patient is ideally positioned either supine with a pillow under the occiput or, if the patient is orthopnoeic, remaining upright but able to be laid flat as soon as the manoeuvre begins. The ideal position for intubation is with the neck slightly flexed and head extended.

- Continuous observation of the patient including ECG monitoring, pulse oximetry, and blood pressure monitoring is essential.

Before administering any drugs:

- Pre-oxygenate the patient with 100% O_2 via a facemask.
- Be ready to apply cricoid pressure if requested—putting backward pressure on the cricoid cartilage using the finger pads of the thumb, forefinger, and middle finger to compress the pharynx so as to prevent reflux of gastric contents.

Following ET tube insertion and cuff inflation:

- Check air entry by auscultation/with capnography (if available), and then attach to the ventilator. Measurement of expired CO_2 (end-tidal CO_2), preferably with a continuous waveform display, allows the ETT position to be checked. If the ETT is not in the trachea, a few ventilations will eliminate any residual CO_2 that may be present, so that the end-tidal CO_2 reading will be zero or nearly zero. In contrast, a correctly placed ETT accesses a steady source of CO_2 from the lungs so there should always be CO_2 evident on expiration.
- Secure the tube (see next section).
- Check cuff pressure with a manometer.
- Carry out a full set of respiratory observations, including pulse oximetry.
- Consider the need for a nasogastric tube.
- Ensure that a chest X-ray has been ordered to confirm satisfactory tube position (tip 2–5 cm above the carina) and absence of pneumothorax.
- Sample arterial blood to confirm satisfactory P_aO_2 and P_aCO_2 levels after 10–15 min equilibration (or sooner if indicated), and then adjust the ventilator settings as necessary.

Specific nursing care of the intubated patient

Securing the tube

Movement of the ET tube can result in displacement of the tube, loss of cuff seal, traumatic extubation, and even oesophageal intubation, as well as causing considerable discomfort to the patient. Migration of a tracheostomy tube into the pre-tracheal tissue is also possible. Therefore it is essential to secure the tube and regularly check for any loosening of the tapes or other fixing device used. Unplanned extubation has been reported in 3–16% of ventilated patients (Peñuelas *et al.* 2011). Such extubations are associated with lower levels of sedation and higher levels of consciousness, anxiety, agitation, use of physical restraints; and insufficient staff vigilance (which may be due to inadequate staffing) (Curry *et al.* 2008). Patients able to talk about their self-extubation afterwards usually said they did so because they found the tube uncomfortable (Yeh *et al.* 2004). See Box 4.17 for potential complications of intubation.

> **Box 4.17 Potential complications of intubation**
>
> - Inability to intubate
> - Aspiration of gastric contents
> - Bleeding from trauma to the airway
> - Endobronchial intubation (usually right main bronchus)
> - Oesophageal intubation
> - Vocal cord damage
> - Perforation (rare)
> - Hypotension (usually due to vasodilator effects of anaesthetic agents unmasking covert hypovolaemia; occasionally due to cardiodepressant effects of the same drugs)
> - Arrhythmias (usually bradycardia due to hypoxia or vagal stimulation—atropine may be required if the patient does not respond to correction of hypoxaemia)
> - Dislodged teeth

The traditional method of securing adult tubes uses cotton tapes looped around the ET tube or through slits in the flange of the tracheostomy tube. These are passed round the patient's head either above or below the ears and tied at one side. They should be tight enough to allow only one finger between the tape and the patient's neck (see Figure 4.8) Securing endotracheal tube tapes). Another option is purpose-made fixing devices, usually using soft fabric bands with Velcro® fasteners.

Pressure from the constricting tapes/knot or fixing device is a problem and can cause tissue ulceration and necrosis. Regular changing of tapes and any foam or other cover of the tapes is needed, while checking the lips and skin underneath (and nostrils with nasal tubes). The patient's ears and occiput can develop pressure sores from tapes or other fixing devices. Note that intracranial pressure can be increased by tight tapes occluding venous blood flow from the head. Two people are needed to change tapes or fixing device to safeguard against movement of the tube during the process.

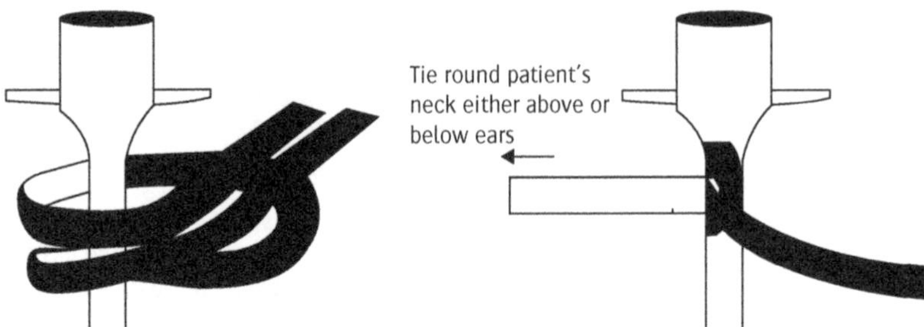

Figure 4.8 Securing endotracheal tube tapes. Tapes should always be tied around the plastic of the ET tube itself, not around the connector because it is possible for the connector to dislodge.

Prevention of upper airway damage

Pressure within the tube cuff should be checked routinely. Ideally, cuff pressure should be maintained at 20–25 cmH_2O, or at least as low as is compatible with a good seal. Low pressure, high volume cuffs should always be used. There is no evidence that periodic deflation of the cuff is of any benefit, and it may actually cause aspiration if large amounts of saliva/secretions have collected above the cuff.

Oral hygiene

Routine oral care may have to be increased in frequency, with extra care taken following intubation, particularly with an oral tube. The lips may become excoriated and dry, and should be protected with a moisturizing agent.

Extubation procedure (oral or nasal endotracheal tubes)

Preparation of the patient should include an explanation of the procedure to ensure cooperation during and after removal. Any nasogastric feeding should be stopped at least 4 hours beforehand (in case of vomiting/aspiration). Emergency equipment and monitoring, as for intubation, should be available (see Box 4.18). The patient should remain monitored/under close observation for the next few hours to ensure that they can maintain a safe airway and adequate respiratory function.

Box 4.18 Equipment for extubation

- Scissors
- Syringe
- Suction—tracheal and oral (Yankauer)
- Oxygen mask and tubing (or CPAP circuit)
- Disposable towel
- Mouthwash

The principles of extubation are as follows.

- Two healthcare practitioners are needed for safe extubation.
- The patient is usually most comfortable sitting up.
- The patient's airway and oropharynx should be as clear of secretions as possible prior to extubation.
- One nurse will cut the tapes/undo the fixing device and deflate the cuff, while the other will suction and withdraw the tube (i.e. suctioning to just below the tip of the tube and continuing while the tube is withdrawn.
- The patient may need prompting and/or assistance to cough up any further secretions, and then should have oral toilet or mouthwash to clear the mouth.
- The patient will almost always require oxygen via nasal cannulae, a mask, or CPAP depending on their condition.

Tracheostomy

Tracheostomy formation

Patients receiving invasive mechanical ventilation for more than 2–3 weeks usually have the oral endotracheal tube replaced with a tracheostomy tube. Tracheostomies are generally considered to be more comfortable for the patient, and will allow speech, eating, and drinking if well managed. Nonetheless, tracheostomy is an intervention that carries some risk and should not be undertaken lightly (see Box 4.19). It is either performed as a surgical procedure requiring a horizontal incision between the second and third tracheal rings or using a percutaneous technique (usually with a dilator system) to insert the tracheostomy tube. The percutaneous technique has fewer complications; a meta-analysis of studies involving 1212 patients concluded that the percutaneous approach resulted in significantly lower infection rates, less bleeding, and reduced mortality when

Box 4.19 Peri-operative complications of tracheostomy

- Haemorrhage
- Hypoxaemia
- Surgical emphysema
- Pneumothorax
- Air embolism
- Cricoid cartilage damage

compared with surgical tracheostomies performed in the operating theatre, (Delaney *et al.* 2006). In the UK most tracheostomies in critically ill patients are performed percutaneously in the ICU by intensivists rather than ENT surgeons (Intensive Care Society 2008).

After about 7 days, a tract forms along the path between the skin incision and the trachea. The tube can then be changed as required. Use of tracheostomy tubes with removable inner cannulae allows cleaning of the inner cannula to avoid encrustation and blockage with secretions. This is an important safety feature, especially in the longer-term ventilated patient.

Tracheostomy tubes

The type of tracheostomy tube used will vary according to the length of time the patient is likely to remain tracheostomized. The first tube placed will usually be a simple cuffed PVC tube without an inner cannula or fenestration. This can then be changed (usually after a period of at least 7 days) for a longer-term tube, such as one of the following.

- A long-term cuffed tracheostomy tube with a removable inner cannula that allows regular cleaning.
- A long-term cuffed tracheostomy tube with fenestrations (windows or holes in the tube) that allow redirection of exhaled breath through the vocal cords and therefore speech. This is usually only possible during spontaneous ventilation with cuff deflation. Fenestrated tubes come with both fenestrated and non-fenestrated inner cannulae, so the nurse must know which configuration is appropriate and in place at different times.
- A re-usable uncuffed silver tube (Negus tube) may be suitable for long-term tracheostomized self-ventilating patients. Use of such tubes is increasingly rare.

Routinely used tracheostomy tubes typically have an inner diameter (ID) of 5–10 mm, with an outer diameter (OD) up to 14 mm. It is important to check the dimensions of the tube used for an individual patient carefully as different manufacturers have different ways of denoting the inner and outer diameters; it is too simplistic just to say that a 'size 6' or a 'size 8' is being used. Tubes vary in length in proportion to the diameter, but it is also possible to obtain adjustable-flange tubes for patients with necks that are very short or long, or to avoid damaged areas of the trachea (e.g. in tracheomalacia).

Specific care of the patient with tracheostomy

Tracheostomy has been performed for literally thousands of years, and many of the associated practices have evolved without systematic study. Therefore much of tracheostomy care is essentially based on consensus expert opinion. The UK Intensive Care Society has produced a useful summary document to guide practice (Intensive Care Society 2008).

Safety priorities

Tracheal dilators and replacement tubes of the same size and one smaller size should be kept near the patient in case of accidental extubation. Routine and emergency equipment, including suction, manual ventilation circuit, airways, catheter mount, and mask, should be immediately available and checked routinely.

Care of the stoma

Following tracheostomy formation, a dry dressing such as a purpose-made polyurethane material is used. The stoma site should be inspected for infection or bleeding and cleaned using aseptic technique at least once daily. Normal saline solution should be sufficient in most cases.

If secretions from the tracheostomy are very copious, a hydrocolloid dressing may protect the skin better than a standard dressing, with secretions wiped away or suctioned as they appear.

If tracheostomy tubes with inner cannulae are used, they should be removed, checked, and cleaned as needed, usually four- to six-hourly, but more frequently if there are profuse/tenacious secretions. The cannula can be cleaned using mouthcare sponges, purpose-made brushes, or ribbon gauze soaked in normal saline solution.

Changing the tracheostomy tube

It is standard to wait at least 7 days or so after the initial insertion to allow the stoma to form before changing the tube. The frequency of tube changes thereafter is generally dictated by local policy, usually at least every 7–14 days

Box 4.20 Equipment for tracheostomy tube change

- Emergency equipment
- Tubes, one the same size, one smaller
- Tracheal dilators
- Lubricant jelly
- Bougie
- Sterile gloves
- Cleaning solution
- 10 ml syringe
- Tracheostomy dressing and new tapes

Box 4.21 Contraindications for use of a one-way speaking valve

- Unconscious and/or comatose patients
- Inflated tracheostomy tube cuff
- Foam-filled cuffed tracheostomy tube
- Severe airway obstruction
- Unmanageable thick secretions
- Severe risk of aspiration
- Severely reduced lung elasticity
- The device is not intended for use with endotracheal tubes or other artificial airways
- Sleeping patients

for a tracheostomy tube without a separate inner cannula to prevent encrustation and narrowing of the inner diameter which will increase the work of breathing. Tubes with an inner cannula are generally changed every month.

Tubes can be changed by an experienced nurse, but medical back-up should always be readily available in case of problems. Prior to assembling the equipment for the procedure, the patient should be prepared with an explanation of the requirement for a tube change and the steps involved. Two nurses are necessary for a safe procedure. It should be done aseptically. After preparation of the equipment (see Box 4.20), the new tracheostomy tube should be checked to ensure even inflation of the cuff and easy withdrawal of the introducer. The patient should be pre-oxygenated and have had the oropharynx and trachea suctioned. The stoma should be cleaned as normal and the tapes cut/fixing device unattached. When all is prepared, the existing tube cuff is deflated and the tube removed. The new tube is then inserted, the introducer withdrawn, the cuff inflated, the ventilator re-attached, and air entry checked. The tube can then be secured again.

Use of one-way 'speaking valves' with tracheostomies

One-way 'speaking valves' such as the propriety Passy–Muir valve® (invented by a patient called David Muir) can be used in both spontaneously breathing patients and ventilated patients with tracheostomy tubes (see Box 4.21 for instances when it is not appropriate to use these valves). There are specific models made to fit inside the ventilator circuit if needed. The valve allows gas flow into the lungs during inspiration (which may be from the ventilator) but closes as soon as gas flow ceases, redirecting exhalation past the deflated cuff and through the fenestrations if present (see Figure 4.9). Exhaled gas thus passes through the vocal cords allowing the patient to speak.

Removal of tracheostomy tube (decannulation)

A patient who has had a tracheostomy tube for some time should be fully assessed for any limiting factors associated with decannulation. Removal of the tracheostomy tube will result in an increase in dead space which can translate into an increase in the work of breathing. Patients with restrictive respiratory disease may not tolerate the increased demand so will require careful planning and a more gradual approach to decannulation, for example by the use of smaller-sized tracheostomy tubes over time rather than a straight removal. The ability to breathe around a capped-off tracheostomy tube (with the cuff deflated!) for over 4 hours without difficulty has been suggested as a positive predictor of the ability to spontaneously safeguard the airway after decannulation (Intensive Care Society 2008). Long-term critical care patients should be seen to have managed at least 24 hours with the cuff deflated and either a one-way speaking valve or a cap in place.

Assess the patient to ensure that:

- the original problem that necessitated tracheostomy has resolved
- there is no evidence of a functionally significant upper airway lesion (such as overgranulation or tracheal stenosis)
- there is no continuing requirement for respiratory support that cannot be met by non-invasive ventilation
- there is no other significant disease process or organ failure that could be worsened or interact with an increased work of breathing (e.g. a developing infection or circulatory failure)
- the patient cough allows easy expectoration of secretions

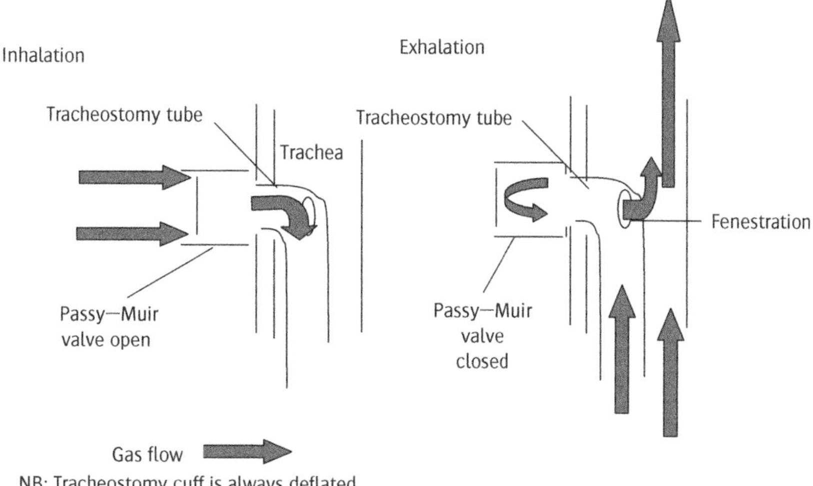

Figure 4.9 One-way speaking valve.

- pulmonary aspiration of oral secretions can be prevented.[1]

Decannulation procedure

Preparation is as for the extubation process described earlier, though a lightweight occlusive dressing should be added. No surgery or sutures are necessary as the stoma will generally close spontaneously over a few days.

The principles of tracheostomy tube removal are similar to those for extubation. In addition:

- stop any oral or nasogastric feeding at least 4 hours beforehand (in case of vomiting/aspiration)
- plan to decannulate earlier rather than later in the day when the patient is relatively rested and the full critical care team are available to manage any immediate complications that may arise
- clean the stoma site and seal the stoma with a sterile occlusive dressing after the tube has been removed, ensuring that no leak is present
- attach nasal cannulae or an oxygen mask as required.

Minitracheostomy

If there is a concern that the patient may not adequately clear secretions after decannulation, a small diameter (4.0 mm) cuffless minitracheostomy tube can be placed in the existing stoma, allowing tracheal suction to continue (a 10 FG suction catheter can be inserted through the tube). NB: minitracheostomy tube insertion is sometimes used as an emergency intervention for life-threatening upper airway obstruction, but it will not protect the airway as a cuffed tube would.

Ventilatory support (mechanical ventilation)

Mechanical ventilation is the form of respiratory support most associated with critical care. Therefore its functions are as previously stated: correction of hypoxaemia and/or hypercapnia, management of mechanical failure, relief of physiological stress, and reduction of physiological workload (see Box 4.22).

Ventilation is commonly used to manage the following.

- Acute respiratory failure:
  - in pneumonia, sepsis, the post-operative state (for patients with serious comorbidities/after high risk surgery), ARDS, cardiogenic pulmonary oedema
  - major trauma, pulmonary aspiration.

[1] Data from *Standards for the Care of Adult Patients with a Temporary Tracheostomy: Standards and Guidelines*, 2008, Intensive Care Society.

Box 4.22 Indications for ventilatory support

- Respiratory failure which is not corrected by other forms of respiratory support (e.g. status asthmaticus, ARDS, pneumonia, pulmonary oedema)
- Support of other failing organs, especially the heart, in order to reduce its workload
- Support of mechanical dysfunction (e.g. Guillain–Barré, flail chest, cervical spine fractures)
- Support of ventilatory function during use of high levels of sedation and anaesthesia necessary for other problems (e.g. status epilepticus, intra-operative anaesthesia)
- Therapeutic ventilation to reduce intracranial pressure (e.g. following head injury or extensive neurosurgery)

- Acute exacerbation of chronic obstructive pulmonary disease.
- Coma (e.g. due to brain injury, hepatic encephalopathy).
- Neuromuscular disease.

Ventilatory support includes methods of negative and positive pressure ventilation, high frequency ventilation, oscillation; and extracorporeal systems. Invasive and non-invasive approaches are available, although severe respiratory failure usually requires invasive ventilation. Most ventilators used in critical care are positive pressure ventilators; these are now discussed in detail. Other types of ventilation will be described briefly and referenced for further information.

Positive pressure ventilation

Elimination of carbon dioxide is a function of the volume of air moved in and then out of the lungs. Positive pressure ventilation entails air being driven into the airways under a positive pressure which inflates the lungs and moves the air from the upper respiratory tract through to the alveoli. The pressures required are much higher than those in normal breathing, and the effects of this abnormal process are often harmful. Furthermore, the gas mixture also has to be propelled through tubing (the ET/tracheostomy tube) with a smaller diameter than the patient's own trachea. This increases resistance to air flow and therefore increases the pressures required to deliver the same tidal volume breath.

The key point is that delivering adequate ventilatory volumes while also ensuring that airway pressures are not damagingly high requires careful adjustment of ventilator settings and close monitoring.

There are similar functions or controls on most ventilators, although there are many individually named features. The terminology used by manufacturers for different sorts of ventilation is not standardized; the same or similar terms are given to mechanisms that may be somewhat different, while different terms are sometimes used to describe identical or near identical methods (Mireles-Cabodevila *et al.* 2009) (see Table 4.11).

Table 4.11 Table of ventilatory modes

Mode	Description	Clinical Use
Controlled mechanical ventilation (CMV): (a) volume-controlled (b) pressure-controlled	(a) Pre-set tidal volume and frequency of breaths are delivered. (b) Breaths are delivered to a pre-set pressure with tidal volume varying with lung compliance	Patient requires complete mechanical ventilatory support
Assist/control (triggered)	Pre-set tidal volume breaths are delivered in response to a patient attempting a spontaneous breath. A back-up delivers a pre-set rate of breaths if the patient does not achieve the required rate	Patient is able to initiate breaths but requires ventilatory assistance to maintain oxygenation and CO_2 removal
Synchronized intermittent mandatory ventilation (SIMV)	Pre-set tidal volume breaths are delivered at a pre-set rate but spontaneous breaths can be taken in between. Ventilator breaths are synchronized with spontaneous breaths	Patient is being weaned from ventilation or for greater patient comfort/reduction of sedation requirements.
Pressure support (PSV) assist	Following triggering by the patient, a breath is delivered to a pre-set pressure level. The tidal volume delivered will thus depend on lung compliance.	Patient is being weaned from ventilation or for greater patient comfort/reduction of sedation requirements.

Mechanics of ventilation

The delivered tidal volume multiplied by the respiratory rate gives the minute volume that determines elimination of CO_2. Four variables are manipulated to produce mechanical ventilation breaths with various characteristics:

(1) volume
(2) pressure
(3) flow
(4) time.

These variables are used to manage different aspects of the ventilator breath (after Mireles-Cabodevila *et al.* 2009):

(1) the control component (e.g. the target volume or pressure)
(2) the trigger that initiates the breath (e.g. the set time between ventilator breaths, or the reduction in flow in the ventilator circuit generated by a patient's spontaneous respiratory effort)
(3) limiting factor(s), i.e. the maximum value of a given variable, such as inspiratory pressure
(4) the cycle component, i.e. the variable used to terminate inspiration (e.g. achievement of the target volume).

The interaction between these elements can be seen in the following two examples.

Volume-controlled ventilation delivers a target volume of air to the patient (i.e. the tidal volume) through the ventilator. Additional patient-triggered breaths may be possible. This means that the minimum desired ventilatory volume will be administered. A set flow rate is the limiting factor. Once the target volume has been achieved, volume cycling ends inspiration so that expiration occurs. The pressure generated by delivery of the target volume is determined by the time for inspiration, the flow rate, and the compliance/stiffness of the lung. Therefore it is possible to have some control of the pressure by adjustment of inspiratory time and flow rate. High airway pressures are associated with an increased incidence of lung injury, so manipulation is generally aimed at limiting those pressures.

Pressure-controlled ventilation generates inspiration to a target pressure rather than a target volume. It may be generated automatically by the ventilator or triggered by the patient. The size of the breath is limited by a set constant inspiratory pressure maintained during inspiration, during which the flow decelerates. Cycling to expiration occurs at the end of a set inspiratory time. Tight control of airway pressures is possible with this configuration, but the risk is that falls in lung compliance or the development of a large air leak may result in inadequate ventilation. Likewise, an improvement in ventilation (e.g. after removal of a sputum plug) may result in very large tidal volumes. The inspiratory pressure and expired tidal volume must be closely monitored, along with the patient's overall clinical status.

As well as considering volume and pressure, time and flow settings require thought. The timing of different parts of the respiratory cycle can be important, i.e. the times for inspiration, expiration, and sometimes also the plateau periods of the ventilator breath. Adjustment of these phases means that the tidal volume can be delivered over shorter or longer proportions of the total time for each breath. The ratio of time for inspiration to time for expiration (I:E ratio) is normally set at 1:2 but can be adjusted to allow a longer period for expiration in patients such as asthmatics with outflow obstruction (e.g. 1:3 or 1:4). Longer periods for inspiration (e.g. 1:1) may be used for patients with non-compliant lungs such as those with ARDS.

It is also possible to alter some aspects of the flow of gas in the ventilator circuit. For example, cycling between inspiration and expiration can be based on how flow begins to slow before a target airway pressure is reached, such that the switch to expiratory flow occurs once inspiratory flow falls to a certain point (see Table 4.12).

Enabling spontaneous ventilation: triggering

Maintaining at least some spontaneous breathing effort by the patient improves the likelihood of eventual discontinuation of mechanical ventilation. Therefore, whenever possible, this should be continued in whichever mode of ventilation is deemed most suitable. The posterior sections of the diaphragm move more actively with spontaneous breathing and this ensures better ventilation of dependent lung regions in the supine position (Putensen *et al.* 2006). Other advantages include retention of diaphragmatic muscle bulk and less need for sedation. Therefore a range of technologies have been employed so that modern ventilators can more easily detect spontaneous respiratory effort, and can almost instantly supply a flow of gas that provides an adequate breath in response to that trigger. Patient-triggered breaths are usually generated by reductions in pressure or flow in the ventilator circuit caused by spontaneous inspiration.

Detection of spontaneous effort—and therefore initiation of the response from the ventilator—can happen

Table 4.12 Table of ventilatory settings

Ventilator setting	Typical range of adult patient	Typical range of ventilation capability	Function	Alarm limits	Safety checks
Inspired oxygen (FiO_2/% O_2).	Variable according to patient need and PO_2: from 21% to 100%.	FiO_2 = 0.21–1.0. % O_2 = 21–100%.	Manipulation of inspired O_2 to produce optimal patient oxygenation.	Automatic alarm setting. If FiO_2 falls/rises from set value, alarm is triggered.	Check digital display of ventilator. Use separate oxygen analyser in ventilator circuit to confirm setting.
Respiratory rate (frequency/min or breaths/min).	Usually 10–15 breaths/min but rate altered to manipulate minute volume (MV) and PCO_2/PO_2.	From 0–50 breaths/min (rates above 50 usually for paediatric use).	Delivery of adequate ventilation. Used to manipulate PCO_2 and PO_2.	Associated with expired MV alarm as respiratory rate/min × tidal volume (V_T) = MV. MV alarms typically set at 2 L above (upper alarm) and 2 L below (lower alarm) set ventilator MV.	The patient's respiratory rate/min should be manually counted each hour. If patient is on IMV/spontaneous modes then ventilator display should be checked.
Tidal volume (V_T) (ml).	Aim is 6–8 ml/kg but may be altered outside this range to optimize PCO_2 and PO_2.	0–1500 ml.	Size of each breath can be altered to suit patient size and to ensure optimal alveolar ventilation without hyperinflation.	Associated with expired MV alarm as above.	Check ventilator display of expired MV or V_T if available. If in doubt, use separate spirometer to confirm.
Minute volume (V_E or MV).	6–8 ml/kg x 10–15 breaths/min = ~2.5–12 L/min.	0–75 L.	As above.	MV alarms typically set at 2 L above (upper alarm) and 2 L below (lower alarm) set ventilator MV.	Check ventilator display of expired MV. If in doubt, use separate spirometer on inspiratory and expiratory limbs.
Positive end expiratory pressure (PEEP) (cmH_2O).	+2 to +20 cmH_2O. Increasing levels of PEEP bring increasing risk of barotrauma and a depressant effect on cardiac output due to decreased venous return.	+2 to +20 cmH_2O.	Maintenance of alveolar expansion during expiration gives increased time for gas exchange and thus increased PO_2. Also aids recruitment of collapsed areas of lung.	None. However, increased PEEP brings increasing airway pressures, so upper and lower airway pressure alarm limits should be adjusted to allow for PEEP.	Observe airway pressure display on ventilator. Pressure at end of expiration should not be less than set PEEP level.

Pressure support/ assist.	+5 to +40 cmH_2O. Levels set according to patient need and the resulting V_T produced for each breath.	+5 to +40 cmH_2O.	Used to maintain patient's respiratory muscles and to wean patient by gradual reduction of the amount of assistance of spontaneous breaths. High levels can provide complete ventilatory support.	Contributes to airway pressure and MV.	Observe airway pressure and MV. Spontaneous breaths should show a positive pressure rise of the amount set as assist.
Flow rate (*V*) (L/min).	Variable within limits (default is typically 60 L/min) must be adjusted to ensure required V_T is reached if inspiratory time is reduced.	2–100 L/min.	(1) Adjusts to achieve V_T in inspiratory time with optimal airway pressure. (2) Can be used to limit peak airway pressure by manipulation in conjunction with I:E ratio. (3) Can manipulate I:E ratio in pressure control ventilation.	None, but contributes to achieving set VT and thus MV, so MV alarms as before.	Regular checks of ABGs if flow rate is altered, as inadequate VT will affect PO_2 and PCO_2. Observe expired MV. Particular care for COPD patients when weaning is needed as flow must be adequate for increased inspiratory effort.
Inspiratory: expiratory ratio (I:E ratio). Ratio of time for inspiration to time for expiration in each breath.	Variable from 1:1 to 1:4. Normal I:E ratio is 1:2. Inverse ratio ventilation refers to inspiratory times which are longer than expiratory times, i.e. 2:1 up to 4:1. Note: in acute asthma it is usually 1:3/1:4.	In some ventilators the range is continuous from 4:1 to 1:4. In others, ratios are limited (i.e. 1:1, 1:2, 1:3, etc).	(1) Allows manipulation of peak airway pressure by altering inspiratory time. (2) Allows time for complete expiration in severe asthmatics so avoiding risk of air-trapping (incomplete expiration resulting in build-up of air in lungs).	Contributes to airway pressure, so alarm limits set at 40 cmH_2O or, as instructed, (upper) and 5–10 cmH_2O below current airway pressure reading for lower alarm.	Observe peak airway pressure for increases. If air-trapping (incomplete expiration) is suspected, inform medical staff. Check pressure and flow waveforms on ventilator graphic display. If flow does not return to zero before the next breath begins, air-trapping is likely.
Trigger/sensitivity alters the amount of effort required by patient to trigger a positive pressure breath from the ventilator.	Negative pressure inspiratory effort of −0 to −10 cmH_2O or reduction in base flow of between 1 and 3 L/min.	Not always quantified on ventilator. May simply range from minimum to maximum sensitivity.	Alters the patient's work of breathing (specifically, the work of inspiration) and assists weaning by altering sensitivity to patient effort, so ventilatory support can be reduced as patient strength increases.	None.	Careful observation of patient during weaning to ensure coping with respiratory effort, and ABGs to check PO_2 and PCO_2.
Base flow (for flow trigger system).	Not applicable.	Normally between 3 and 5 L/min. May vary according to ventilator model.	Provides a constant flow through the circuit which is reduced when the patient takes a breath. This reduction triggers full flow to support the breath.	None.	Check base flow is on after use of nebulizer in the circuit.

more quickly with a new development called 'neurally adjusted ventilatory assist' (NAVA). NAVA uses electrodes on the end of a nasogastric tube to detect the electrical activity of the diaphragm when it is stimulated to contract by the phrenic nerves. This enables an earlier response from the ventilator than that produced by flow or pressure changes (which will occur afterwards). It is also possible for the ventilator to adjust to variations in the strength of electrical activity of the diaphragm on a breath-by-breath basis so that more or less assistance is given by the ventilator depending on patient need. These effects improve patient–ventilator synchronization and comfort (Verbrugghe and Jorens 2011), although clinical outcome improvements have yet to be demonstrated. Importantly, the technique will not work with patients with significant phrenic nerve or diaphragm dysfunction.

Non-invasive ventilation

Non-invasive ventilators are relatively simple positive pressure devices which provide a gas flow at two levels of pressure (inspiratory and expiratory) that can be adjusted separately. NIV can be delivered via a tight-fitting nasal mask, a full facemask, or a helmet so intubation and its associated risks can be avoided. The ventilator cycles between the two levels of pressure based on either sensing the reversal of gas flow or timing. They can typically deliver up to 40 cmH_2O pressure on inspiration and up to 20 cmH_2O on expiration, though such pressure settings are rarely used.

Physiological effects of positive pressure ventilation

The effects of positive pressure are apparent not only in terms of respiratory function but also with regard to other organs including the cardiovascular system and kidneys. An understanding of these processes is vital as they may have a profound effect on the patient (see Table 4.13)

Decreased cardiac output and venous return

- *Manifested by*: hypotension, tachycardia, hypovolaemia, decreased urine output, increasing metabolic acidosis.
- *Caused by*: increased intrathoracic pressure during inspiration that reduces venous return and increases right ventricular afterload. As a result, right ventricular and, consequently, left ventricular output is reduced. If positive end-expiratory pressure (PEEP) is also used, intrathoracic pressure will be positive even in expiration,. which may reduce venous return and therefore cardiac output even further (according to the set level of PEEP). If the patient has been significantly distressed prior to commencing mechanical ventilation, there may be a sudden reduction in peripheral vascular tone related to loss of circulating catecholamines once ventilation begins, especially when sedation is also administered.
- *Treated by*: fluid filling, for example by using 200 ml challenges over 10–15 min until the stroke volume (if measured) shows no further increase. Otherwise, fill until the CVP increases by >3 mmHg after a fluid challenge and remains increased (see Chapter 5). Inotropic support may be necessary if fluid loading is not considered clinically appropriate (see Chapter 5). Alteration of ventilator settings, such as inspiratory and expiratory times, tidal volume, and the level of PEEP may also be considered.

Decreased urine output

- *Manifested by*: oliguria.
- *Caused by*: reduction in cardiac output stimulating release of antidiuretic hormone together with an increased renin–angiotensin–aldosterone response leading to greater salt and water retention.
- *Treated by*: fluid filling as previously. Close monitoring of urine output is required.

Increased incidence of barotrauma (trauma due to pressure) related to higher positive airway pressures

- *Manifested by*: high airway pressures on inspiration.
- *Caused by*: the higher pressures required during positive pressure ventilation to force air into airways resistant to airflow. Damage to the lung occurs and this may be manifested clinically as a pneumothorax or a pneumomediastinum. Resistance to flow is related to the radius of the airway (to the fourth power). Changes in lung compliance will also affect the pressures involved. This is particularly relevant in the asthmatic patient, where bronchoconstriction produces greatly increased resistance to flow and greatly increased airway pressures.
- *Treated by*: manipulation of inspiratory and expiratory times for each breath and by flow rates of inspiratory gas. The aim is to keep tidal volumes and plateau airway pressures low whenever possible, particularly in severe lung disease such as ARDS (see Box 4.23).

Table 4.13 Problems associated with mechanical ventilation

Problem	Details/action
High airway pressure Causes: (a) Life-threatening (i.e. investigate and rule out/treat at once): • endotracheal tube (or ventilator tubing) obstruction • pneumothorax • severe bronchospasm. (b) Other: • build-up of secretions in airway • patient breathing out of synchronization with ventilator ('fighting') • patient coughing • increased peak airway pressure resulting from a tidal volume set too high for patient, or inspiratory time set too short, or addition of PEEP • displacement of ET tube either downwards, causing coughing from irritation of the carina or slipping down the right main bronchus, or upwards, causing cuff herniation through the larynx, resulting in patient discomfort and agitation	Manifested by: airway pressure alarm sounds, persistent rise in peak airway pressure, evidence of patient distress, haemodynamic instability. Interventions: 1. If patient severely compromised, remove from ventilator and manually ventilate using rebreathe bag and 100% oxygen. Assess lung compliance (the degree of resistance to inspiration) and symmetry of inflation while bagging. Call for senior and medical help. 2. Perform suction to clear any secretions and to determine whether tube is patent. If secretions are very thick, review humidification and instil 2–3 ml normal saline down ET tube prior to suctioning. Repeat as necessary. 3. If cause is complete ET tube obstruction that cannot be cleared with suctioning, emergency reintubation will be necessary. If no one is immediately available to reintubate, it is possible to manually ventilate the patient following extubation using a Guedel airway and tight-fitting facemask. It is important to have the patient's neck resting on one pillow and to lift the jaw forwards to maintain a patent airway. If trained and proficient in its use, a laryngeal mask airway is an alternative to either reintubation or facemask bagging. 4. Auscultate lungs for signs of wheezing, reduction in air entry, and altered breath sounds. 5. If the cause is a pneumothorax and there is cardiovascular compromise immediate insertion of a chest drain or large needle will be necessary (by medical staff) to allow relief of tension (for details see chest drains) 6. If the patient is stable, attempt to ascertain the cause of the increased airway pressure. 7. Reassure and attempt to alleviate any cause of distress if the patient is restless and distressed by ventilation ('fighting'). This is suggested by tachypnoea, breathing out of synchronization with the ventilator, and continually coughing or gagging. Check insertion depth of ET tube to see whether it has migrated upwards or downwards 8. Check blood gases if restlessness and distress continue and/or peripheral oxygen saturation remains low. Increase FiO_2 and consult with medical staff 9. If the patient is restless and unable to settle on the ventilator but otherwise cardiovascularly stable with appropriate blood gases, review sedation and inform senior or medical staff if an increase in sedation ± muscle relaxant is indicated. 10. Review ventilator settings and discuss with senior or medical staff if settings seem inappropriate or addition of PEEP appears to have caused a problem.

(continued)

Table 4.13 Continued

Problem	Details/action
Low airway pressure Causes (a) Life-threatening: ● disconnection or major leak from the ventilator, burst cuff on endotracheal/ tracheostomy tube. (b) Other: ● leak in the ventilator circuits, loss of seal on cuff, bronchopleural fistula (with massive air leak through chest drain), ventilator dysfunction.	Manifested by: Sounds of air leak, decreased expired minute volume (MV), low airway pressure reading. Interventions: 1. Check patient is attached to the ventilator. 2. Check connections on ventilator tubing for leaks, tears, or cracks. 3. Check cuff pressure to ensure a seal is present. Use cuff pressure manometer to check the cuff pressure is <30 mmHg. If the leak continues inflate cuff further as necessary, and inform medical staff. 4. Check ventilator functioning. 5. Check ventilator is delivering its set tidal volume. 6. Check levels set for pressure alarm limits are appropriate. 7. If low airway pressure continues and tidal volume is not being delivered, the ET tube or the ventilator may need changing. Manually ventilate the patient and inform senior nursing or medical staff.
Low minute volume Causes: (a) Life-threatening: ● disconnection from the ventilator ● inappropriate ventilator settings (i.e. flow rate may be too low to allow set volume in time allocated by set respiratory rate) ● hole in ventilator tubing. (b) Other: ● leak caused by tubing connections working loose ● loss of seal on cuff ● presence of bronchopleural fistula with chest drain in situ.	Manifested by: Low MV alarm sounding, MV read-out shows less than set MV, audible cuff leak, patient may appear distressed and haemodynamically compromised, oxygen saturation may drop, and patient may appear cyanosed. Interventions: 1. Unless cause of low MV is immediately apparent, manually ventilate patient. 2. Check ventilator tubing from machine to patient, testing connections and looking for holes. 3. Review ventilator settings to ensure MV is capable of being delivered and that ventilator is not malfunctioning. 4. Auscultate trachea to detect any leak around the cuff. Refill cuff as before. 5. Monitor air leak through chest drain if present. If increased, inform medical staff. Ventilation may have to be increased or altered to allow for leak.
High minute volume Causes: (a) Life-threatening: ● possible ventilator malfunction (b) Other: ● patient making respiratory efforts which are excessive ● inappropriate ventilator settings	Manifested by: Sounding of high MV alarms, patient making respiratory effort. Interventions: 1. Ascertain any causes of tachypnoea such as pain, hypoxaemia, hypercapnia. 2. Review ventilator settings with senior and/or medical staff.

Hypoxaemia Causes: (a) Life-threatening: • pneumothorax, pulmonary embolus, sputum plug, or other body obstructing major airway, severe haemodynamic compromise, severe bronchospasm, severe pulmonary oedema, ventilator malfunction. (b) Other: • Build-up of thick secretions, increase in severity of disease, atelectasis, bronchospasm, repositioning of patient causing increase in shunt, leak in ventilator tubing, patient fighting ventilator, pulmonary oedema.	Manifested by: Peripheral O_2 saturation <90%, arterial blood gases show fall in P_aO_2 to <8–10 kPa, patient is restless (unless heavily sedated ± paralysed), tachycardic, possibly hypotensive, and cyanosed. Interventions: 1. If hypoxaemia is severe and/or causing haemodynamic compromise ventilate patient on 100% oxygen. Call for help 2. Check ventilator is delivering set ventilation and that alarm limits are appropriate 3. Check arterial blood gases and ensure that pulse oximeter is picking up a good signal 4. Auscultate chest for air entry and abnormal breath sounds, depending on findings, suction and/or chest physiotherapy may be necessary. Observe symmetry of lung movement and consider pneumothorax 5. Ascertain cause of hypoxaemia—reposition patient if recently placed on side, in consultation with medical staff consider need for chest X-ray, review haemodynamic causes such as decreased cardiac output. Review need for further sedation 6. In consultation with medical staff, ventilator settings such as FiO_2, tidal volume, I:E ratio, etc. may be altered
Hypercapnia Causes: Life-threatening: • no urgently life-threatening causes but long-term uncorrected hypercapnia may cause severe metabolic problems. Other: • inadequate MV either from patient if in weaning modes or ventilator settings • compensation for metabolic alkalosis, carbohydrate overload, or increased CO_2 related to increased metabolic rate (see Chapter 10) • air-trapping (intrinsic or auto-PEEP).	Manifested by: P_aCO_2 >6.0 kPa, patient appears restless and agitated with tachypnoea if on weaning modes, or may show signs of increased respiratory effort if on controlled ventilation. *Note*: Chronic CO_2 retainers (e.g. COPD) may tolerate high levels of P_aCO_2. In patients with severe pulmonary disease, such as ARDS where there is risk of further lung damage with the high airway pressures necessary to reduce P_aCO_2, it may be preferable to tolerate high leve1s of CO_2 provided that acidosis is adequately compensated ('permissive hypercapnia'). Interventions: 1. Ensure the patient is receiving the set MV or, if weaning, is achieving the MV required 2. Check air entry and perform suction to discount any sputum plugging or obstruction 3. Review ventilator settings with medical staff and alter MV if necessary. A decrease in ventilation may be necessary if the patient is air-trapping.
Auto-PEEP (intrinsic PEEP air-trapping) Causes: • increased resistance to airflow and increased work of breathing • incomplete/impeded exhalation either as a result of high MV (>10 L/min) or in respiratory or cardiac disease, particularly chronic airway limitation.	Manifested by: Failure of alveolar pressure to return to zero at end-exhalation Interventions: 1. Ensure low compressible volume ventilator tubing is used. 2. Review ventilator settings with medical staff and decrease MV by decreasing respiratory rate or alter inspiratory flow rate to decrease inspiratory time and increase expiratory time. 3. Reduce metabolic workload to reduce respiratory demand.

Box 4.23 Typical targets of positive pressure ventilation

- Correction of hypercapnia is done by increasing minute volume (tidal volume and respiratory rate), usually aiming for a P_aCO_2 near the patient's normal level (generally 4.4–5.7 kPa). Note that occasionally air-trapping may occur with too great a minute ventilation and an inability to sufficiently clear the volume of inspired gas. In such situations, a reduction in minute ventilation may paradoxically improve P_aCO_2 levels.
- Correction of hypoxaemia is achieved by manipulating FiO_2 and PEEP, usually aiming for an S_pO_2 of 94–98%, or 90±2% in patients with chronic CO_2 retention. These targets may be relaxed over time in patients with severe respiratory failure as they will 'acclimatize' to the lower levels of oxygen.
- Prevention of adverse effects of ventilation, particularly injury due to over-distension of the lungs by excessive volumes and/or pressures. This is especially important with lungs that are already damaged (e.g. in ARDS). Harm can be minimized by:
  - ensuring that tidal volumes are ≤6 ml/kg body weight
  - limiting plateau pressure to ≤30 cmH_2O (Acute Respiratory Distress Syndrome Network 2000; Petrucci and De Feo 2013).
- If it is impossible to maintain P_aCO_2 ≤6.0 kPa without high tidal volumes or plateau pressures, it is preferable to allow an increased P_aCO_2. This is known as permissive hypercapnia. This will cause the blood pH to fall, at least in the short term. While some authorities do not allow the pH to fall below 7.20–7.25, others are less concerned. Indeed, some animal data have shown a protective effect from respiratory acidosis.

Sputum clearance and airway management

The presence of an endotracheal or tracheostomy tube means that normal humidification and warming of inspired air by the upper airway tract—in particular, by the nasal passages—are bypassed. The delivery of dry cold gas, often at a high flow rate, has several deleterious effects on the trachea and bronchi:

- increased viscosity of mucus which may dry and encrust the airways causing inflammation and ulceration;
- depressed ciliary function
- atelectasis from obstruction of small airways by thickened mucus.

The overall effect is to grossly impair movement or clearance of secretions. This may result in obstruction of major segments of lung or blockage of the tube itself.

Two other factors contribute to the problem:

- decreased ability of the intubated patient to cough, either due to the presence of the tube itself or to suppression of the cough reflex by analgesia or sedation
- loss of the natural periodic sigh, i.e. the larger than normal breath taken at intervals by the spontaneously breathing individual to expand their lung bases and alveoli that may not fully expand during regular breathing.

If the patient is dehydrated, the moisture content of mucus will be further reduced and extra humidification will be required. Accumulation of secretions causes airway blockage, leading to atelectasis and then shunt due to the reduced availability of air for gas exchange. The degree to which this will cause problems is related to the underlying disease process. For example, patients with pneumonia who produce large amounts of purulent secretions or those with cystic fibrosis or bronchiectasis will require more intervention.

Methods of managing sputum clearance

Humidification

Ideally, the chosen method of humidification should:

- allow inspired gas to be warmed to near body temperature so as to carry a high water content; an inspired gas temperature 34–37°C provides a water content of 33–44 mgH_2O/L and a relative humidity of 100% (Restrepo and Walsh 2012)
- be simple, easy to use, and adaptable for a variety of methods of respiratory support/ventilation
- avoid increases in airway resistance or altered compliance
- not increase the risk of infection.

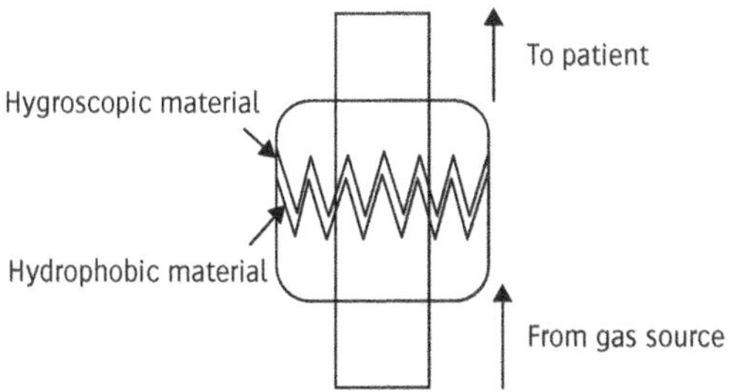

Figure 4.10 Heat–moisture exchanger.

Several methods of humidification are available.

1. **Heat–moisture exchangers (HMEs)** These filters are hygroscopic on the patient side and hydrophobic on the gas source side (Figure 4.10). The hygroscopic material picks up moisture and heat from the patient's exhaled breath which is then transferred to the inhaled gas as the patient breathes in again, providing a form of passive humidification.
   - Advantages: decreased infection risk (most HMEs are bacteriostatic), low cost, light, disposable.
   - Disadvantages: the level of humidification available is fixed and may be insufficient for high gas flow rates or very thick secretions. HMEs may increase resistance to air flow in the circuit and also add to dead space. This may be problematic, particularly in patients ventilated with low tidal volumes.
2. **Nebulizers** These devices deliver aerosolized water particles. There are two main types. Pneumatic or jet nebulizers use a high velocity gas jet which takes water from a reservoir and passes it through a baffle to create fine particles. Ultrasonic devices generate high frequency sound waves and mechanical vibration over a reservoir to produce a fine mist. Droplets produced are deposited in the upper airway, bronchi, and alveoli, depending on their size. Only the smallest particles (<3 μm) are likely to reach the alveoli, so there will also be deposition in the bronchioles, bronchi, and upper airways—and in the tracheal tube and ventilator circuit (Galluccio and Bersten, 2014).
   - Advantages:
     (a) the amount of humidification can be increased and decreased according to patient need
     (b) the quantity of water delivered is not limited by temperature and, with ultrasonic nebulizers, supersaturation is possible
     (c) delivery of topical medication is also possible, although drug delivery is not completely predictable.
   - Disadvantages:
     (a) risk of infection from bacterial contamination of the water is higher, so sterile water should always be used.
     (b) over-hydration is possible, particularly with ultrasonic nebulizers where supersaturation may occur
     (c) there may be increased airway resistance with nebulizers located in the circuit.
3. **Hot-water bath humidifiers** Gas is driven over, or through, a heated water bath. Humidity can only be achieved at temperatures between 45 and 60°C. As the humidified gas passes through the tubing to the patient it cools and condenses, producing a fully saturated gas at about 37°C.
   - Advantages: effective and efficient humidification.
   - Disadvantages:
     (a) Infection is a hazard. Water temperatures of 45°C provide an effective growth medium for contaminating bacteria. Sealed sterile water units are now more commonly employed. Temperatures must be maintained near the 60°C level to limit the growth of contaminants.
     (b) Efficiency is not constant and may be altered by fluctuating gas flow, water temperature, and the area of the vaporizing surface.
     (c) There is a risk of scalding the airway. Thermostatic control and temperature sensors situated at the patient end of the circuit are essential.
4. **Cold water humidifiers** Gas from an oxygen flowmeter passes via a Venturi system allowing manipulation of oxygen concentration through a water reservoir. Most types are disposable and provide oxygen concentrations from 28% to 60%, although these are not reliable at high minute volumes. The oxygen is only partially humidified, depending on gas flow rates, and therefore is incompletely saturated.
5. **Instillation of normal saline** It has been common practice to administer boluses of normal saline into the trachea on the basis that this may loosen and clear secretions and can stimulate a cough. However, the technique has fallen out of favour with both the UK Intensive Care Society (2008) and the American Association for Respiratory Care (2010) who stated that it should not be done routinely. Of note, evidence for both benefit and harm is mixed, although most of the studies are considered to be poor quality (Paratz and Stockton, 2009). There are reports of

desaturation and also of increased sputum yield with saline instillation. A recent better quality randomized clinical trial found that patients receiving saline instillation before tracheal suctioning had less microbiologically proven pneumonia, although this made no difference to length of stay or mortality (Caruso *et al.* 2009).

Suctioning and bronchial hygiene

Removal of secretions using a suction catheter placed in the trachea is essential for maintaining airway patency. It should be performed when there is evidence of secretions in the large airways manifested as crackles or wheezes.

An important precaution when suctioning patients with borderline hypoxaemia is the use of pre-oxygenation with 100% oxygen, ideally through the ventilator rather than by manual means (Demir and Dramali 2005; American Association for Respiratory Care 2010). Use of a closed suction system is recommended to maintain ventilation, minimize lung de-recruitment, and reduce the risk of desaturation (American Association for Respiratory Care 2010; Maggiore *et al.* 2003).

Reported deleterious effects of suctioning include:

- increased respiratory rate and decreased tidal volume (Seymour *et al.* 2009)
- decreased P_aO_2 (Dyhr *et al.* 2003)
- decreased mixed venous oxygen saturation due to falls in cardiac output and arterial oxygen saturation (Clark *et al.* 1990)
- microatelectasis
- cardiac dysrhythmias associated with vagal stimulation and hypoxaemia
- haemodynamic instability
- increased intracranial pressure
- laryngospasm (in non-intubated patients)
- bronchoconstriction
- tissue damage, haemorrhage

Evidence for tissue damage and mucosal trauma is from research which is over 30 years old. It is likely that improvements in catheter construction and attention to limiting negative pressure levels have reduced the risk of such injury. Nonetheless, a study of nurses' and physiotherapists' technique has found that suction is regularly applied over 2.5 times an agreed safe level, even when manometer readings of the pressures are available (Donald *et al.* 2000).

Closed suction systems that allow suction without disconnecting the patient from the ventilator have become the accepted standard in critical care, especially for patients with high oxygen requirements or PEEP, or who are at risk of lung de-recruitment (American Association for Respiratory Care 2010). The closed suction system consists of a suction catheter protected by a flexible plastic sleeve attached to a T-shaped catheter mount. An instillation port is available for either injecting saline into the endotracheal lumen or flushing the system with saline (see Figure 4.11).

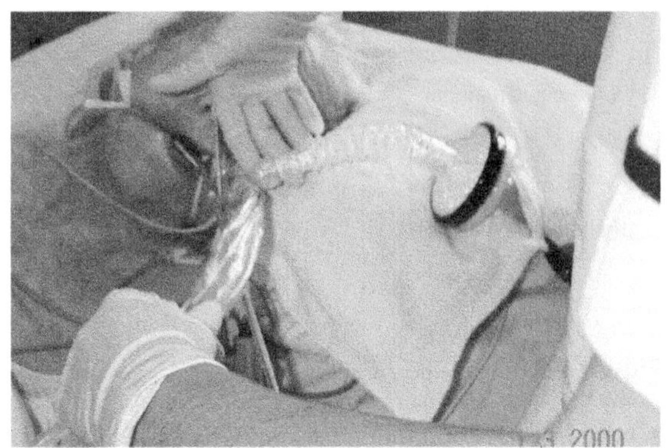

Figure 4.11 A closed suction system.

The main advantage of closed suction systems are:

- no requirement to break the ventilator circuit in order to suction (which could result in loss of PEEP)
- fewer episodes of lung de-recruitment so better preservation of lung volumes (Maggiore *et al.* 2003)
- possible reduced incidence of eye infection due to splash contamination (Parkin *et al.* 1997) and reduced risk of cross-infection in general: another study showed visible droplets scattered up to 168 cm away from the patient following suction with open systems (Ng *et al.* 1999).

There have also been reports of lower levels of desaturation and ventilator-associated pneumonia (VAP) when closed systems are used. However, a recent systematic review concluded that, overall, there was no significant difference between open and closed suctioning with regard to oxygenation and VAP rates (Overend *et al.* 2009).

Manufacturers have recommended changing the closed suction system every 24–48 hours to prevent build-up of bacterial colonization. However, Stoller *et al.* (2003) and others have shown that there is no increase in the incidence of VAP when suction systems are changed weekly or only when obviously soiled.

The key principles for suctioning are as follows.

1. The experience is very unpleasant for the patient. It has been described as feeling like choking or loss of breath; and so should be performed as briefly

and effectively as possible to maximize efficacy and minimize trauma. Therefore suctioning should not be done routinely but only when there are signs that secretions are present in the upper airways.

2. Unless it is certain that suction can be performed without breaking a closed circuit, goggles and mask or a full-face visor should be worn to protect the nurse against splashing of secretions.
3. Pre-oxygenation with 100% oxygen for >30 sec should be used in patients at risk of desaturation.
4. Suction levels should be set as low as will still be effective, ideally <20 kPa (150 mmHg/200 cmH_2O), to minimize the risk of trauma and desaturation.
5. The technique should be aseptic:
   - with handwashing (or use of alcohol gel) prior to the procedure
   - use of new clean (but non-sterile) gloves.
6. When using an open suction system:
   - a new disposable glove should be worn on the dominant hand (suction catheter handling hand) with each catheter used
   - catheters should be sterile, inserted once, withdrawn, and then discarded.
7. When using a closed suction system, the catheter and sleeve should be examined regularly to ensure that the catheter is patent and the sleeve intact.
8. Catheters should have an end-of-catheter lumen and more than one side lumen to minimize trauma. A single side lumen is more likely to cause tracheal trauma.
7. Ideally, the correct size of suction catheter should not exceed half the internal diameter of the endotracheal tube.
8. In most cases, the catheter generally only needs to be inserted to the end of the ET or tracheostomy tube (van de Leur *et al.* 2003).
9. Suction should be applied only as the catheter is withdrawn.
10. The whole procedure of insertion and withdrawal should not take more than 30 sec (the suction itself should be <15 sec) in order to reduce the risk of complications.
11. When suction is complete, the closed suction system catheter should always be withdrawn so that the black marker line is visible in the sleeve. If the catheter remains in the ET tube or the catheter mount, it will occlude the lumen and increase airway resistance. The closed suction system catheter should always be washed through with normal saline.
12. Observation of ECG and S_pO_2 should be continuous during the procedure.[2]

Chest physiotherapy

Techniques such as vibration, gravity-assisted positioning, percussion, and hyperinflation can all improve clearance of secretions. These methods should be taught by a specialist physiotherapist and practised under guidance.

1. **Vibration** Vibratory force is applied through the chest wall during the expiratory phase of the respiratory cycle with two hands firmly placed on the chest, shaking at a frequency of about 200/min—often in conjunction with ventilator or manual hyperinflation. This increases expiratory flow so that secretions move into larger proximal airways where they are more easily suctioned or coughed out. It is most effective when coordinated with the patient's intrinsic or controlled respiratory cycle (Shannon *et al.* 2010).
2. **Gravity-assisted positioning (GAP) or postural drainage** Changing the patient position enables gravitational drainage of secretions in the bronchial tree. It is most often used in conjunction with other techniques such as manual hyperinflation and chest wall vibration. Remember that there is better perfusion of dependent lung areas so shunt/venous admixture may increase if the dependent lung has very poor air entry.
3. **Percussion** This technique is infrequently used in critically ill patients because of the risk of dysrhythmias and haemodynamic instability. Loosening and movement of secretions is achieved by percussing a cupped hand over the patients chest wall. When percussion is performed, it is usually done in association with GAP.
4. **Hyperinflation** This is the deliberate administration of one or more breaths that are 50% greater than the tidal volume being routinely delivered. The purpose of hyperinflation is to re-expand collapsed alveoli, and mobilize and remove excessive bronchial secretions. It can be achieved using a manual technique or through most ventilators.
   - A Mapleson C/Water's circuit or self-inflating resuscitator (e.g. 'Ambu bag') is generally used. A study

[2] Data from American Association for Respiratory Care, Endotracheal suctioning of mechanically ventilated patients with artificial airways, 2010, *Respiratory Care*, Volume 55, pp. 758–64, 2010 Daedalus Enterprises Inc.

of manual hyperinflation in 100 stable ventilated patients found that static compliance, PaO_2:FiO_2 ratio and A–a gradient were all significantly improved for a period after the treatment (Patman *et al.* 2000). Physiotherapists often introduce a plateau phase for a few seconds after inflation, followed by a rapid exhalation to simulate a patient's normal cough and move secretions proximally. It is difficult to be precise about the volumes given in practice—even with significant experience—and with high flow oxygen attached to the circuit, very large tidal volumes can be unintentionally achieved (Singer *et al.* 1994). Ideally, a manometer (pressure gauge) should be sited in the circuit to limit the pressure generated to <40 cmH_2O.

- Ventilator hyperinflation is the delivery of an augmented breath via a ventilator. It is used less often than manual hyperinflation but has similar efficacy (Dennis *et al.* 2012).
- Intermittent positive pressure breathing (e.g. using a Bird respirator) uses positive pressure during inspiration to augment spontaneous breaths, returning to atmospheric pressure during expiration. It requires expert manipulation of the settings to achieve effective results (Sorenson and Shelledy 2003).
- Mechanical insufflation–exsufflation (MI-E) (e.g. with the Philips CoughAssist Device) again uses positive pressure to augment lung inflation, which is then followed by a rapid switch to a negative pressure. This change in pressure mimics the change in flow that would normally occur during a cough, and hence assists in secretion clearance. It has most often been used in patients with neuromuscular disease.
- In non-ventilated cooperative patients, the active cycle of breathing technique (ACBT) consisting of breathing control (relaxed breathing), thoracic expansion exercises (deep breathing), and forced expiration ('huffing') can mobilize and help clear bronchial secretions. ACBT is most frequently used in patients with bronchiectasis and cystic fibrosis, but is also a useful adjunct in critical care patients with a high secretion load.

Patient needs

All of the techniques for clearing sputum can cause some discomfort and distress. Analgesia should be timed where possible to cover any planned physiotherapy. The patient should be given a full explanation of the necessity and nature of any procedure. Patient cooperation should always be sought. See Box 4.24 for a summary of requirements for sputum clearance.

> **Box 4.24 Requirements for sputum clearance**
>
> 1. Adequate humidification.
> 2. Suctioning and bronchial hygiene.
> 3. Chest physiotherapy.
> 4. Systemic hydration.
>
> Note: The underlying disease process will affect the intensity of each intervention.

Communication difficulties associated with intubation

These problems affect the patient, family, and the staff who care for them. It is a priority to explain why communication is difficult, and to give reassurance that the inability to talk is a temporary situation which will resolve once the tube is removed. Alternative means of communication must be sought and established so that the patient, family, and carers become familiar with the methods that work best for the individual.

It is essential that the patient and family feel well informed and that they have every opportunity to ask questions and clarify issues. However, the presence of an ET or tracheostomy tube often reduces communication to closed questions requiring only 'yes' or 'no' answers. This is obviously very limiting and should only be used until the patient can adopt alternative methods (see Chapter 3 for more details).

Methods of non-verbal communication

The patient's family often needs encouragement and help to continue talking to their relative even when there is little or no response, particularly with regard to expressing their personal thoughts and feelings.

Speech and language therapists (SALTs) are invaluable in providing assistance and technical aids. A SALT should be contacted early, especially for patients likely to have a lengthy stay. They are also able to assist with swallowing and other upper airway problems associated with tracheal intubation.

The family should be asked to identify topics of interest to the patient. Provision of suitable newspapers, a radio, MP3 players, television, etc. will all assist the patient to feel more normal.

Box 4.25 Factors contributing to psychological problems

- Discomfort
- Fear
- Loss of control
- Disorientation
- Disease pathology

Psychological problems associated with intubation and ventilation

Most critically ill patients have greatly increased levels of anxiety and general stress, compounded by their inability to express these feelings. These issues are discussed in Chapter 3. It is essential that the nurse works to recognize the often subtle signs of anxiety and stress and responds to them appropriately (see Box 4.25).

Nutritional problems associated with intubation and ventilation

This is discussed in detail in Chapter 9. A full standard oral diet is impossible for the patient with an ET tube, although patients with tracheostomies may manage if a normal swallow function has returned and the cuff can be safely deflated. Some patients can manage to eat semi-solid or puréed foods or drink water with the cuff inflated, but this approach should be used with caution, at least to begin with. Whether this causes harm to the swallowing apparatus is not known. Other forms of nutritional support, including enteral and parenteral feeding, must be utilized as needed. The effects of malnutrition on the critically ill patient are severe, and efforts should be made to establish appropriate levels of intake.

Particular problems can be encountered in the patient who is weaning from ventilation.

1. Overfeeding of carbohydrate will cause the body to lay down fat stores. Burning carbohydrate produces considerably more CO_2 than that produced by the breakdown of fat for energy needs, and the patient may need to increase their minute volume to remove excessive CO_2. This will increase physiological workload and may prove too much for weakened respiratory muscles. In these circumstances, provision of half the non-protein calories as fat should be considered.
2. Depletion of important minerals and trace elements such as zinc and magnesium may have a deleterious effect on respiratory muscle function. Supplementation may aid recovery of muscle mass, especially if the supply of these nutrients has been inadequate in the long term, but the evidence base is scanty. Likewise, correction of serum phosphate is frequently performed but has no good supportive evidence base.
3. Patients exhibiting an inflammatory or septic response (i.e. fever, high levels of urinary nitrogen excretion, high metabolic rate) may fail to utilize nutrition to regenerate their depleted muscle tissue, making weaning a protracted process.
4. Malnourished patients have an increased risk of developing pneumonia and other complications due to associated dysfunctions of the immune system and the possible reduction of surfactant production found in fatty acid deficiency.
5. Malnutrition is associated with a reduced diaphragmatic mass, reduced maximal voluntary ventilation, and reduced respiratory muscle strength. These deficits will detract from the patient's ability to wean from the ventilator.
6. Non-ventilated patients may also have problems maintaining adequate nutritional intake when they have oxygen masks in situ or feel breathless when attempting to eat.

Strategies for assisting the breathless patient to eat include:

- using nasal cannulae for oxygen administration during meals
- nutritional supplements such as high calorie (fat/carbohydrate) drinks
- small, frequent, nutritious, and tempting (!) food portions
- an upright and comfortable position in which to eat
- thoughtful timing of meals (e.g. not just after physiotherapy).

Increased infection risk associated with intubation and ventilation

A 'foreign body' in the airway increases the likelihood of infection in several ways.

1. The tube bypasses normal physical and physiological mechanisms of resistance such as cilia and the mucous membrane of the upper airways.

2. The trauma associated with the presence of the tube and suctioning provides an opportunity for bacterial colonization. In addition, the cuff of the endotracheal tube is not a perfect seal and secretions from upper airways and gastric regurgitation may trickle into the lungs.
3. Interventions such as suctioning require scrupulous attention to aseptic principles in order to avoid direct delivery of any bacterial contamination to the bronchi and respiratory lobules.
4. Critically ill patients are already at increased risk from infection due to high levels of skin-barrier-penetrating instrumentation (cannulae, catheters, drains, etc) and underlying immunosuppression, either from underlying disease processes or from treatments such as corticosteroids.

Alternative modes of ventilation and respiratory support

Improving ventilation

Maintaining some spontaneous respiratory effort improves the likelihood of eventual discontinuation of mechanical ventilation so, whenever possible, this should be continued in whichever mode of ventilation is used. The posterior sections of the diaphragm move more actively with spontaneous breathing and this ensures better ventilation of dependent lung regions in the supine position (Putensen *et al.* 2006). Other advantages include retention of diaphragmatic muscle bulk and less need for sedation.

Inverse ratio ventilation

This technique consists of reversing the normal inspiratory–expiratory ratio and controlling inspiratory gas flow by limiting the airway pressure, slowing or decelerating the rate of inspiratory flow, or adding an additional end-inspiratory pause.

Two methods are generally used to administer inverse ratio ventilation.

1. The ventilator is time-cycled with a pre-set inspiratory pressure limit and a long inspiratory phase. This is pressure-controlled inverse ratio ventilation (PC-IRV).
2. The ventilator is volume-cycled with an end-inspiratory pause and a slow or decelerating inspiratory flow rate. This is volume-controlled inverse ratio ventilation (VC-IRV).

Inspiration may commence before expiratory flow has finished and this will generate a degree of auto-PEEP. While oxygenation may be improved, this may lead to excessive air-trapping and a rise in P_aCO_2.

Advantages of VC-IRV:

- delivery of a guaranteed tidal volume
- precise manipulation of the inspiratory flow pattern
- decreased peak inspiratory flow rates with a similar or lower shear force.

Disadvantages of VC-IRV include:

- changes in peak alveolar pressures which may be excessive if peak inflation pressures are not carefully monitored.

Advantages of PC-IRV include:

- possibly better gas distribution than constant flow VC-IRV due to the decelerating flow pattern
- avoidance of pressures above those set on the ventilator

Disadvantages of PC-IRV include:

- variation in delivered tidal volume with alterations in respiratory system compliance and resistance
- opposing pressure exerted by any level of auto-PEEP may reduce the volume delivered
- greater shear forces may be generated compared with VC-IRV by the fast flow at the beginning of inspiration, and this may contribute to tissue injury

Limitations of inverse ratio ventilation

1. The breathing pattern imposed (I:E ratio ≥1:1) is difficult for a patient to tolerate unless well sedated ± paralysed.
2. Air-trapping can occur in alveoli with high expiratory resistance, leading to hyperinflation and possibly an increased incidence of barotrauma.
3. In PC-IRV, the longer inspiratory time allows equilibration between alveolar and airway pressure causing an increase in peak alveolar pressure compared with VC-IRV where the peak airway pressure always exceeds alveolar pressure.
4. Rises in mean airway pressure and auto-PEEP may affect venous return, increasing right ventricular afterload and decreasing cardiac output.

Other measures for supporting respiration

Other options may need to be considered with ARDS or other severe lung pathology where conventional ventilation is unable to provide adequate oxygenation and/or sufficient CO_2 elimination.

Supporting adequate oxygenation

Nitric oxide gas inhalation

Nitric oxide is a pulmonary vasodilator which crosses the alveolar membrane when inhaled. It then acts locally on the pulmonary circulation, dilating the vasculature and increasing blood flow. This improves ventilation/perfusion (V/Q) matching, and thus gas exchange, as blood flow is only increased in ventilated areas. As soon as it enters the blood, nitric oxide is bound to haemoglobin and has no further significant systemic effects.

Nitric oxide gas is added to the gas delivery of the ventilator or in the inspiratory limb. Volumes are measured in parts per million (ppm) by a monitor and optimal delivery levels identified by titrating the nitric oxide against either P_aO_2 or S_pO_2. Optimal levels should be regularly re-evaluated but are usually in the 5–20 ppm range. Withdrawal of nitric oxide should be done gradually as there may be rebound pulmonary hypertension and hypoxaemia.

Although significant increases in oxygenation are seen with inhaled nitric oxide, at least in the short term, these are not definitively associated with an improvement in overall mortality (Afshari *et al.* 2011). An increased risk of renal impairment has been observed (Afshari *et al.* 2011).

Safety aspects:

- Nitric oxide combines with oxygen to produce a small amount of the toxic substance nitrogen dioxide (NO_2). Levels of NO_2 >0.005 ppm are rarely seen, but levels >5 ppm are considered dangerous.
- Nitrogen dioxide can further combine with water to produce nitric acid, so catheter mounts and ventilator circuits should be used with HME filters and prevented from accumulating high levels of condensation or water pooling.
- Some patients may also develop significant (>5% total haemoglobin) methaemoglobinaemia (i.e. the ferric (Fe^{3+}) form of Hb rather than the usual ferrous (Fe^{2+}) form) when NO combines with haemoglobin. As oxygen carriage is affected by methaemoglobin, levels should be monitored by regular blood gas analysis.

Prone positioning

The severely injured lung is likely to have dysfunctional regions ranging from areas with irreversible damage and alveolar collapse to some potentially reversible areas of infiltration and consolidation. This variability means that potentially functional areas of ventilation tend to be poorly matched with perfusion. This may be compounded by placement of the patient in the standard supine position as this is apt to promote ventilation of the anterior portions of the lung. Placement in the prone position improves oxygenation in a significant proportion of patients (termed 'responders'), although the mechanism is not completely understood. A recent multicentre study showed mortality benefit from early prone positioning for at least 16 hours per day in severe ARDS (Guérin *et al.* 2013). However, not all patients can be turned prone and the risk–benefit of any manoeuvre must be evaluated (see Box 4.26). There are risks of displacement of the ET/trachesotomy tube and other devices, pressure damage, and haemodynamic instability (see also Box 4.27). Safe prone positioning requires at least four personnel, with one person responsible purely for turning the patient's head and safeguarding the ET tube.

Box 4.26 Relative contraindications to prone positioning

- Spinal instability
- Increased intracranial pressure
- Abdominal compartment syndrome
- Shock
- Multiple trauma
- Massive resuscitation or haemodynamic instability
- Pregnancy
- Abdominal surgery
- Extreme obesity

Box 4.27 Problems associated with the prone position

- Facial and conjunctival oedema
- Pressure ulcers on knees, shoulders, iliac crests, and face
- Limited access to endotracheal and nasogastric tubes
- No immediate access for resuscitation in the event of cardiac arrest
- Shoulder problems

Some units use special beds that allow alteration of the support pressures to reduce support under the abdomen and increase support at the head, chest, and pelvis during prone positioning. This allows the abdomen to expand during inspiration. If a special bed is not used, pillows should be placed under the pelvis and chest and a specific head support or two pillows used. Positioning of the arms is important, and a variety of arrangements have been recommended. The 'swimmer's position' has one arm above the head and one by the patient's side. Alternatively, both arms can be placed above the head. Some units use special boards to allow the arms to be extended to the side.

Reducing hypercapnia

High frequency ventilation

High frequency ventilation (HFV) incorporates techniques using rapid ventilation frequencies (up to 2000 breaths/min) with very small tidal volumes (<5 ml/kg). These methods were developed in part from the observation that panting dogs ventilate effectively even though the tidal volumes involved are less than the volumes of anatomical dead space. Two types of HFV currently used are high frequency oscillation and high frequency jet ventilation.

Delivery requires specialized ventilators, as conventional machines provide insufficient tidal volumes at high frequencies due to compression of gas within the ventilator itself.

High-frequency oscillation

A rapidly oscillating gas flow is created by a device that acts like a woofer on a loudspeaker, producing a high frequency rapid change in direction of gas flow. The oscillator is set using the delta pressure (ΔP), i.e. the measure of the pressure swing between inspiration and expiration, the frequency (in Hertz), and the mean airway pressure. Oxygenation is thought to be improved by increases in transpulmonary pressure and recruitment of collapsed alveoli. Mean airway pressures are increased, but peak pressures are less than in conventional ventilation. However, there may be haemodynamic instability and patients usually need to be heavily sedated ± paralysed. Unfortunately, two recent multi-centre studies from the UK (Young *et al.* 2013) and Canada (Ferguson *et al.* 2013) showed no benefit and even harm in terms of survival.

High frequency jet ventilation (HFJV)

High pressure air and oxygen are blended and supplied to a non-compliant injection (jet) system. The normal pressure of this gas (known as the driving pressure) is around 2.5 atmospheres. This can be adjusted to alter the rate of flow from the maximum down to zero. Added (warmed and humidified) gas is entrained from an additional circuit via a T-piece attached to the ET tube. The entrainment circuit should provide a flow of at least 30 L/min. Efficient humidification (usually via a hotplate vaporizer humidifier) is necessary because of the high flows of otherwise dry gas. The usual frequency set is between 100 and 200 breaths/min delivering tidal volumes of 2–5 ml/kg.

In an entrainment system, the tidal volume delivered by the ventilator increases with driving pressure and decreases with respiratory frequency. It remains the same with alterations in I:E ratio. The system requires either a special jet endotracheal tube or a cannula via an adapter fixed to a standard ET tube.

Jet ventilation may have advantages for some specific groups of patients such as those with bronchopleural fistula because peak airway pressures will be less than with conventional ventilation, but there is as yet no evidence that there is any improvement in survival or length of stay. It requires considerable skill to maintain a patient successfully on HFJV and therefore it is only used in a small minority of critical care units.

Extracorporeal respiratory support

Extracorporeal membrane oxygenation (ECMO) uses technology developed for cardiopulmonary bypass in cardiac surgery. Modern systems are venous–venous extracorporeal circuits with a blood pump circulating blood at <5 L/min past a membrane with a high surface area interfacing with an oxygen–air mix. A heat exchanger in the system can be used to regulate blood temperature. Exposure of venous blood to the membrane allows oxygenation and removal of carbon dioxide along the concentration gradients across the membrane. It is usually necessary to supplement these processes with some low level mechanical ventilation.

The CESAR trial compared patients with high lung injury scores or severe respiratory acidosis (causing pH <7.20) that were randomized to either stay in the admitting critical care unit and receive conventional ventilation or be transferred to a specialist centre where they could receive optimized conventional ventilation or ECMO (Peek *et al.* 2009). While patients treated at the ECMO centre had a significantly lower overall mortality, 25% received optimized conventional ventilation only. The ECMO-treated patients actually showed no mortality benefit. This suggests that outcomes are enhanced in specialized respiratory centres, perhaps regardless of whether or not they offer ECMO or not. Five such centres have been established in the UK. Importantly, ECMO is associated with significant morbidity including vascular occlusion by the cannulae, haemorrhage (including stroke) from the high dose anticoagulation required, and neurocognitive problems in survivors (Hodgson *et al.* 2012). Thus its use should be carefully considered.

Extracorporeal carbon dioxide removal ($ECCO_2R$) aims only to remove CO_2 by the extracorporeal circuit. This is possible with much lower flow rates than those required for ECMO (>1 L/min); CO_2 can be removed through a low blood flow–high gas flow circuit because it has a much higher solubility coefficient than oxygen. Some oxygen can still be delivered across the extracorporeal membrane depending on the patient's need. The rationale is that $ECCO_2R$ and ECMO minimize further damage and facilitate healing of injured lungs because overall ventilation volumes and pressures can be reduced. An early trial of $ECCO_2R$ ensured that atelectasis was avoided with simultaneous low frequency positive pressure ventilation at a rate of 3–5 breaths/min with limited peak airway pressures (35–45 cmH_2O) and a constant level of PEEP (15–25 cmH_2O) (Gattinoni *et al.* 1986). $ECCO_2R$ has been shown to effectively clear CO_2 and to improve some aspects of the pulmonary disease process, but this has yet to be seen to make a difference to mortality (Stewart *et al.* 2011). A currently available commercial device—the Novalung Interventional Lung Assist device—has not been formally trialled, so the impact on outcome is unknown. This device used to rely on the patient's blood pressure to drive blood flow through the extracorporeal circuit via an arteriovenous circuit; however, the manufacturer has recently launched a venovenous pumped device.

Weaning from mechanical ventilation

Weaning is the reduction of mechanical ventilatory support until effective self-ventilation and extubation can be achieved. This is a straightforward and reasonably rapid process for most patients. However, in some cases weaning is difficult and may be prolonged—and occasionally impossible (Boles *et al.* 2007). Patients in the prolonged weaning group (>1 week) are few in number but have long stays in critical care, disproportionately high costs, and increased mortality (Peñuelas *et al.* 2011). They include patients with complications after major surgery and those with such conditions as chronic airflow limitation, poor left ventricular function, polyneuropathy/myopathy (a common consequence of critical illness), or respiratory paralysis (e.g. myasthenia gravis).

Short-term weaning

- Planning of weaning should begin as soon as the reasons for beginning and continuing mechanical ventilation have ceased to be clinically significant. It is not always clear when this point has been reached but the possibility should be considered sooner rather than later. Assessment of readiness to wean should be part of the daily patient review, looking especially at cerebral, respiratory, and haemodynamic functions, including the ability to voluntarily make respiratory effort and cough. Vital sign observations in the normal range, an FiO2 <0.4, minimal ventilatory support, and little or no requirement for inotropes or vasopressors are useful indicators (Boles *et al.* 2007), but the weaning process can be commenced well before these criteria are met in anticipation of progressive improvement over the next hours or days. Avoiding heavy sedation and/or a daily period of reduced or no sedation gives the patient a better chance of demonstrating readiness to wean—and of being able to communicate and actively engage in the weaning process.
- Daily assessment of physiological readiness is recommended (Boles *et al.* 2007), for example by using the rapid shallow breathing index (RSBI) described by Yang and Tobin (1991). This screening tool assesses the ability to generate deep breaths without becoming tachypnoeic. The patient should be observed breathing using a T-piece or CPAP circuit (which could be via the ventilator). After 1 min, the respiratory rate is divided by the average tidal volume (in litres) of breaths for that minute (see Box 4.28). A high f/VT ratio identifies patients unlikely to pass a spontaneous breathing trial, whereas values <105 identify patients with the potential to complete a spontaneous

Box 4.28 Screening the patient using the RSBI

The patient breathes at a respiratory rate of 20 breaths/min, producing an expired minute volume of 8 L over 1 min:

respiratory rate (f) = 20 breaths/min
minute volume (V_E) = 8 L
average tidal volume (V_T) = V_E/f = 8/20 = 400 ml (or 0.4 L)
RSBI = f/V_T = 20/0.4 = 50

Yang and Tobin (1991)

breathing trial (although not all of these will go on to wean straight away).

- A spontaneous breathing trial can then be performed, either via a T-piece circuit or by staying on the ventilator with no more CPAP or pressure support than is needed to overcome the resistance of the circuit, i.e. <7–10 cmH_2O pressure support and <5 cmH_2O PEEP (see Brochard and Thille 2009). The spontaneous breathing trial should be undertaken for at least 30 min, and for up to 2 hours for patients considered more at risk of failing to manage off the ventilator. Ideally, the trial should be performed when the patient is most likely to be reasonably rested, usually earlier rather than later in the day. The patient should be given a full explanation of what is to happen with an opportunity to ask any questions. They should be made comfortable in a sitting position to allow expansion of lung bases, and assessed to see if suctioning is required.
- Close observation and monitoring of the patient's appearance, respiratory rate, S_pO_2, ECG, pulse, and blood pressure should continue throughout the trial period, with an arterial blood gas analysed after about 20 min. If there are no adverse signs after 30 min, extubation may be possible. However, if after 30 min the patient has not tolerated the spontaneous breathing trial, ventilatory support should be restarted as it was before the trial took place. Occasionally the stress of a spontaneous breathing trial causes some deterioration, so the level of support may need to be increased for a period. If the patient's breathing seems adequate but sputum clearance is a problem, the patient may manage with a minitracheostomy which can be sited before extubation.

Failure of a spontaneous breathing trial can be identified by (adapted from Boles *et al.* 2007):

- agitation, anxiety, or profuse sweating for >5 min
- respiratory rate >35 breaths/min for >5 min
- oxygen saturation <90% for >5 min
- heart rate increased or decreased by >20% for >5 min.
- systolic BP >180 or <90 mmHg continuously for >1 min.

Any failure to wean should be systematically evaluated, and possible causes of reduced respiratory muscle capacity or increased respiratory load identified so that these can be treated (if possible): see Table 4.14 and Figure 4.12. An **A**irway/lung, **B**rain, **C**ardiac, **D**iaphragm, **E**ndocrine schema sets out some of the routine assessments and therapies that can be used, as well as more advanced investigations and treatments for specific issues, for example nerve conduction studies to assess neuropathy or levosimendan (or other agents) to treat left ventricular failure compromising weaning (Heunks and van der Hoeven 2010).

Table 4.14 Causes of ventilator dependency

Cause	Description
Neurological system	Reduced central drive (respiratory centre/brainstem injury, drug effects) Cervical spinal cord injury Peripheral nerve disease/damage
Respiratory system	Mechanical load: issues with respiratory system mechanics, e.g. reduced compliance (acute/chronic lung disease, pulmonary oedema), or imposed load Inadequate ventilatory muscle function: insufficient inherent strength/endurance; poor metabolic state/nutrition/oxygen delivery or extraction, muscle atrophy Gas exchange problems: cardiovascular pathology, ventilation/perfusion mismatching
Cardiovascular system	Cardiac intolerance of ventilatory muscle work, peripheral oxygen demands
Psychological factors	Impaired cognitive function (e.g. delirium), mood (e.g. depression), anxiety; motivation/engagement

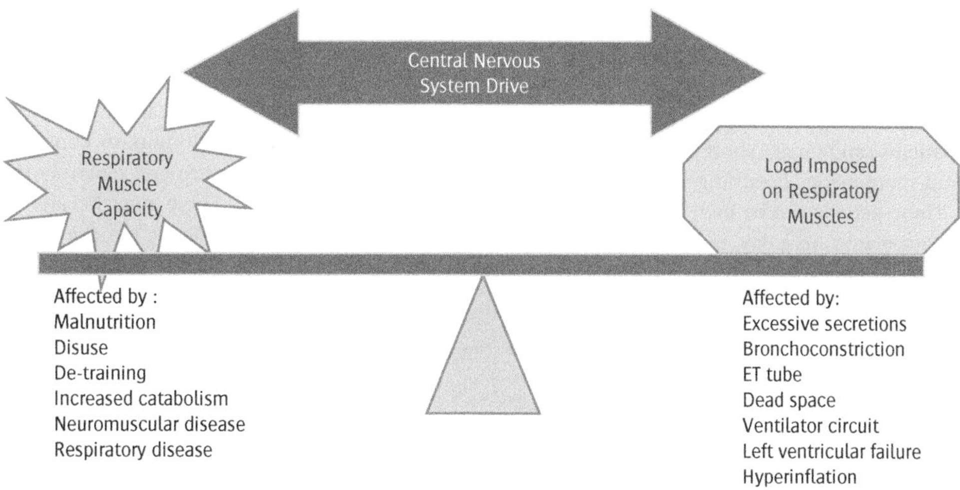

Figure 4.12 The balance required for weaning.

Long-term weaning

There is good evidence that facilitating at least some spontaneous breathing as early as possible in a period of mechanical ventilation is beneficial as it reduces the rate of muscle atrophy found in mandatory modes (Brochard and Thille 2009). Nonetheless, the precise mode of ventilatory support used during weaning is less important than the development and delivery of a consistent package of care tailored to the individual patient. A structured planned multidisciplinary approach is needed, with regular review by the physiotherapist, speech and language therapist, and dietician. Other professionals should be brought in for specific problems, for example the pain control specialist, the pharmacist for drug advice, or an occupational therapist regarding specialist equipment. Input from a psychologist is often very important, as a positive attitude should be fostered and maintained.

The principles of effective long-term weaning are as follows.

1. For patients failing to wean early, all essential physical functions should be optimized as much as possible, with attention paid to psychological aspects such as understanding, mood, and motivation as well.
2. Weaning is frequently a trial and error process, sometimes with limited progress followed by setbacks. No single weaning method has produced consistently superior results as each patient is different.
3. A clear weaning plan should be written, setting out step-by-step reductions in ventilatory support over increasingly longer periods over several days. Pressure support ventilation is most often used, with assist–control ventilation advocated as an alternative (Boles *et al.* 2007). The weaning process may take some weeks but often needs review and adjustment every few days, so a complete whole-patient assessment is required at least once or twice weekly. Rest periods should be scheduled and night-time sleep optimized; if any sedation is needed for this, it should be given early in the night so that it does not compromise weaning during the day.
4. Consistent measures of respiratory function should be agreed so that all staff know what is considered acceptable for a particular patient, for example a respiratory rate <30–35 breaths/min, tidal volumes >4–5 ml/kg, and blood gas values in the normal range or, at least, not significantly worsening. How the patient looks and feels is also important to monitor and respond to.
5. A complete up-to-date record of the plan, ventilator settings at different times of the day, all weaning attempts, and achievements should be kept and referred to so that a logical, consistent, and structured approach can be continued. It may be useful for the patient to have an easy-to-read progress chart showing what improvement is being made.
6. In the longer-term weaning patient, pressure support is typically reduced by 1–4 cmH_2O per day. It is often beneficial to return to higher levels at night to allow a stress-free period during sleep. Once pressure support is <10–12 cmH_2O, patients with

tracheostomies (the majority of those receiving prolonged ventilation) may have brief cuff deflations to enable speech.

7. Having weaned to a pressure support level of 5 cmH_2O, most patients can manage short periods of cuff deflation and spontaneous breathing via a tracheostomy mask. These periods can be increased each day (e.g. two 1-hour periods in a day, two 2-hour periods the next day, two 3-hour periods the day after, then two 4-hour periods, one 6-hour period, and so on. This regime may be accelerated or slowed down depending on the strength of the patient.
8. The level of ventilator support should be gradually reduced until the patient can breathe without support (other than that required to overcome ventilator resistance) for at least 24 hours.
9. Extubation or decannulation can then be considered provided that the patient is considered fit enough to maintain a patent and safe airway without artificial aids (see sections on 'Extubation procedure' and 'Removal of tracheostomy tube').

Rehabilitation

Some patients need time to rebuild global muscle strength in order to wean successfully. In these cases, it is often best to not reduce ventilatory support for several days, or even weeks. It may even be necessary to increase the level of support during rehabilitation, to reduce their work of breathing. A structured programme of rehabilitation can be used to mitigate the short-, medium-, and long-term consequences of critical illness and its treatment—such as the effects of protracted bed rest. There may be anxiety about mobilizing critically ill patients, but there is emerging evidence that judicious early mobilization is feasible, safe, and can improve functional outcomes (Pohlman *et al.* 2010). Hanekom *et al.* (2011) published useful criteria to help decide which patients can safely engage in physical activity, although such decisions should also be agreed by the multidisciplinary team. Typically, there is a progression from sitting upright in bed to sitting over the edge of the bed, standing, bed to chair transfer, marching on the spot, and then walking. Functional goals should be set in conjunction with the patient and/or their carers with due regard to what the patient could do before being critically ill. Specialist equipment such as hoists, chairs, standing frames, and tilt tables can be used to facilitate these activities (Needham *et al.* 2009).

If ventilatory dependence continues for more than 3 months, referral to a specialist weaning centre should be considered. Factors contributing to weaning failure are shown in Figure 4.13.

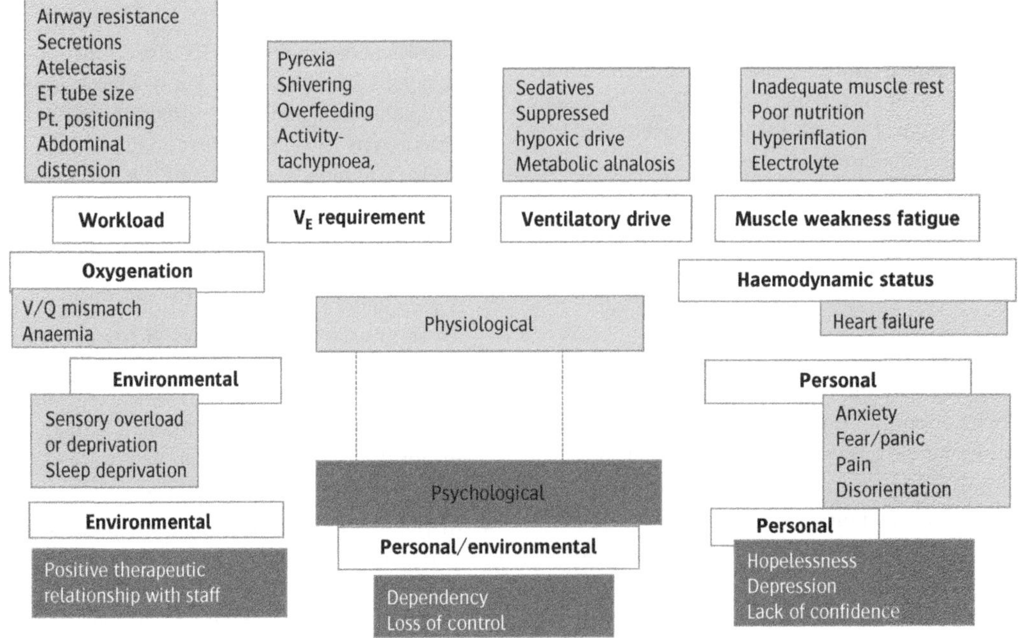

Figure 4.13 Factors contributing to weaning failure.

Specific respiratory problems

Pneumothorax

Pneumothorax is the presence of air between the visceral and parietal pleura, caused by traumatic or iatrogenic injury, or a spontaneous rupture resulting in a hole between the alveolar or bronchial wall and the pleura which allows air to escape into the pleural space. The subsequent loss of lung area for gas exchange can lead to significant respiratory compromise, especially in patients whose lung function is already limited.

Tension pneumothorax

A tension pneumothorax develops when an opening in the alveolar wall functions as a one-way valve through which air enters the pleural space on inspiration but cannot return to the lung on expiration. There is rapid accumulation of air in the pleural space which increases in volume and pressure until the lung on that side collapses. This displaces mediastinal structures away from the affected lung, and can significantly compromise venous return and ventricular contraction. The effects of this are immediate and life-threatening.

The clinical consequences of tension pneumothorax are as follows.

- Tachycardia and an initial rise followed by a fall in blood pressure as cardiac output decreases due to increased intrathoracic pressure, impeding venous return and compressing the heart.
- Cyanosis, respiratory distress, and agitation. Oxygen saturation will quickly fall.
- If the patient is ventilated, airway pressures sharply rise. Expired minute volume may reduce.
- If not immediately treated, cardiovascular collapse and cardiac arrest will follow.

On examination, the patient will have unilateral chest movement. Air entry and breath sounds are greatly diminished on the affected side. There will be a displaced apex beat and hyper-resonance on percussion. The trachea may be shifted from the midline away from the affected side.

Bronchopleural fistula

A fistula connecting lung and pleural space will produce the same effect as a pneumothorax, although it is less likely to close spontaneously. It may require surgical intervention.

Interventions

1. Tension pneumothorax is a medical emergency. Immediate help must be obtained. Relief of the tension by insertion of a large gauge needle or intravenous cannula in the second intercostal space in the mid-clavicular line is performed as a first-line treatment (or, less commonly, a chest drain is quickly inserted if it is ready to hand). Patients on positive pressure ventilation will not suck in air through a needle/cannula unless they are making spontaneous breathing efforts. Once placed, a chest drain can be attached to underwater seal drainage (see next section).
2. Pneumothorax: If a pneumothorax is not life-threatening, there is time for the diagnosis and exact position of the problem to be confirmed by chest X-ray, and a drain inserted, if required, in an appropriate location under aseptic conditions. Asymptomatic pneumothoraces <30% of the hemithorax in size can be left undrained but should be closely monitored. Various body fluids (e.g. pleural effusion, blood) can also occupy the pleural space. Treatment options include needle aspiration, insertion of a pigtail catheter, or a chest drain.

Insertion and care of underwater seal chest drain

Chest drains are inserted into the pleural space (Havelock *et al.* 2010) to allow one-way drainage of:

- air
- pleural effusion
- blood
- chyle (digested fat drained by the lymphatic system)
- empyema (pus in the pleural cavity).

Chest drains range in size from 8 to 32 FG. They are inserted percutaneously through an intercostal space in the chest wall and into the pleural space. The size of the tube depends on what is to be drained, with larger sizes required for drainage of blood. An aseptic procedure to penetrate the chest wall and insert the drain is required. The recommended site of insertion is in the mid or posterior axillary line, usually in the fourth or fifth intercostal space. The second intercostal space in the mid-clavicular line can be used for an anterior pneumothorax. Ultrasound imaging should be used to enable safe and accurate placement.

Insertion

1. The procedure should be explained to the patient. Whenever possible, consent should be obtained.
2. If reasonably awake, the patient is generally placed in an upright or semi-upright reclining position, leaning over pillows placed on a bed-table in front of them, or lying on the opposite side.
3. The underwater seal bottle is primed with a specified amount of sterile water sufficient to cover the drainage tube. This prevents backflow of air or fluid into the pleural space. Underwater seal bottles have a recommended water level clearly marked, so any fluid drained thereafter can be easily measured. There should not be excessive fluid in the bottle as the high pressure this exerts may prevent drainage of air and resolution of the pneumothorax.
4. As with any insertion procedure, the site should be cleaned and covered with sterile drapes. The area is infiltrated with local anaesthetic.
5. The chest drain is then placed, using the Seldinger guidewire technique or direct placement. In the Seldinger approach, a hollow needle is inserted into the pleural space, a guidewire is passed through the needle, the needle is withdrawn, and then dilators are passed over the guidewire to create a tract for the tube itself to be sited and then connected to the drainage system. A blunt dissection technique can be used as an alternative method, particularly for larger size drains.
6. The drain is positioned in the upper chest for pneumothoraces and in dependent areas for drainage of fluid. When the drain is correctly positioned, air or fluid will drain out and there will be movement of the fluid level in the drainage tube with respiration.
7. The chest drain is generally sutured in place. A purse string suture may be sewn round the entry site to prevent any air leaks when the drain is removed, although this is not always necessary. A sterile dressing is used to cover the insertion site, together with adhesive tape to secure the tubing at the insertion site and further down the chest wall.
8. The drainage bottle should always be positioned below the level of the patient's chest to avoid backflow of water into the lung.
9. A chest X-ray should be taken to check the position of the drain and lung re-inflation.
10. Suction (usually –10 to –20 cmH_2O) may be added if the lung fails to re-inflate despite a well-placed drain.
11. The drainage bottle is generally placed below the level of the heart to assist drainage of fluid. During transfer (e.g. to the CT scanner) it can safely rest on the patient's bed provided that positive pressure ventilation is being administered as this will prevent backflow of fluid back into the patient's chest.

Problems associated with insertion and drainage

1. Inadvertent puncture of the lung or other structures is possible during chest drain insertion. This may cause a bronchopleural fistula, identified by a flow of air bubbles into the chest drain bottle either continuously or during expiration. If blood drainage exceeds 1000 ml or continues at >200 ml/h for 4 hours, there may have been trauma to a local blood vessel. A doctor should then be informed, coagulation studies performed and corrected if abnormal, and referral to a thoracic surgeon considered. Deep tension sutures may occasionally stop bleeding.
2. Blockage of the drainage system may result in a build-up in pressure within the pleural space, or even a tension pneumothorax. Therefore chest drains should never be clamped without careful thought and close observation. Clamping for more than a few seconds is not recommended for any patient apart from those post-pneumonectomy. Loss of the respiratory swing of the meniscus in the drain tubing may indicate obstruction, especially if accompanied by signs of distress and lack of drainage. However, these signs can also occur as the pneumothorax or haemothorax resolves, so the patient's overall condition should be assessed. Drainage of a haemopneumothorax may require gentle milking of the drainage tubing or irrigation of the drain with sterile normal saline solution to prevent obstruction from a clot. These manoeuvres should be performed with caution, as high pressures which may cause discomfort and/or injury can be generated in the system.
3. Leaks can occur at the insertion site, the connection between drain and tubing, or the connection between tubing and bottle. Check the drain, tubing, and drain bottle for signs of leakage at regular intervals. Continuous bubbling not related to respiration or fluid escaping at the connections are signs of leakage. Make all connections secure, and if there are still signs of leakage examine the site itself to ensure that the drain has not slipped out.
4. Continuous bubbling of air which still continues despite all care being taken may indicate a bronchopleural fistula. Inform a doctor. Suction may be added to the drainage system, although very often this does

not stop bubbling until the patient is removed from positive pressure ventilation.

Prevention of infection

1. The dressing should be checked daily and changed if obviously wet or soiled, using standard aseptic technique.
2. Hands should be washed and gloves worn for handling the drain or redressing the site.

Removal of chest drains

1. Re-expansion of the lung should be checked on X-ray following prior discontinuation of any suction. There should be no air leak or any significant drainage.
2. There is no need to clamp drains prior to removal.
3. A full explanation must be given and patient cooperation obtained if possible. Chest drain removal can be uncomfortable, so analgesia should be considered and, if required, be given in time to have a good effect.
4. Aseptic technique is essential.
5. If a purse string suture has been used, two people are generally needed to remove the drain. The securing suture is removed and the ends of the purse string freed. The drain is then withdrawn at end-inspiration to prevent air being drawn into the pleural space on removal of the drain. If present, purse strings are pulled tight and secured.
6. An occlusive dressing is then applied to the drain site.

Acute respiratory distress syndrome (ARDS)

ARDS is a form of severe respiratory failure caused by a variety of direct and indirect pulmonary injuries that produce similar pathophysiological changes. It is the pulmonary manifestation of multiple-organ dysfunction syndrome, and reflects similar disease processes in other body systems (see Chapter 10). The lung may be affected to a greater or lesser degree. The pathophysiology and management of patients with ARDS is set out in Chapter 10.

ARDS is characterized by an acute deterioration, with:

- diffuse acute pulmonary infiltrates on X-ray which are not just due to heart failure or fluid overload
- decreased pulmonary compliance
- increased alveolar–arterial oxygen difference and hypoxaemia
- a precipitating factor (see Box 4.29).

Box 4.29 **Disorders associated with ARDS**

- Infection: pneumonia, sepsis
- Trauma
- Aspiration: gastric acid, hydrocarbons, near drowning
- Inhalation: smoke, corrosive gases
- Haematological: massive blood transfusion, post-cardiopulmonary bypass
- Metabolic: pancreatitis, acute liver failure
- Drug overdose: heroin, barbiturates
- Miscellaneous: eclampsia, amniotic fluid embolism, etc.

Asthma

Asthma is an acute reversible airway restriction caused by bronchospasm in response to a range of stimuli including allergens, infections, and exercise. The disease is characterized by bronchial smooth muscle contraction, inflammation of small airways, mucosal oedema, and excessive mucus production.

Management

Reduction of bronchospasm and inflammation

1. Bronchodilation with a β_2-adrenergic agonist, usually salbutamol, inhaled from an oxygen-driven nebulizer.
2. Anticholinergic drugs (e.g. ipratropium bromide) are given to relax smooth muscle and enhance the effect of the β_2 agonist. However, its efficacy in acute exacerbations is limited and its anticholinergic effect will increase sputum thickness, thus potentially contributing to difficulties in removing thick sputum plugs which are a hallmark of the condition.
3. Intravenous magnesium sulphate and/or infusions of aminophylline or salbutamol may be given if there is no response to inhaled medications. These agents all relax bronchial smooth muscle.
4. Steroids such as hydrocortisone or prednisolone reduce hypersensitivity, although an effect is not usually seen for some hours. Hydrocortisone can be given intravenously three or four times a day if there are concerns regarding absorption.
5. Antibiotics should be commenced if bacterial infection is deemed likely from the history and investigations. However, many asthma patients do not need antibiotics.

Support of respiratory function

1. Oxygen therapy: high concentrations as necessary to maintain S_pO_2 at 94–98%.
2. Humidification and intravenous fluid to achieve adequate hydration so as to avoid/reduce mucus plugging and facilitate clearance.
3. Physiotherapy (and bronchoscopy) as required.
4. Ventilation (usually invasive) if:
   - P_aCO_2 is rising
   - patient is obtunded
   - patient is fatigued
   - P_aO_2 is falling
   - patient is not responding to treatment.

Sedatives, especially in large doses, should not generally be given unless the patient is about to be ventilated as they can reduce respiratory drive and cause hypoventilation, resulting in worsening respiratory failure. However, judicious use may be very helpful in calming an agitated patient, but this should be done under close supervision.

Avoidance of iatrogenic complications

1. Air-trapping—manifested by a rising end-expiratory pressure (intrinsic PEEP or auto-PEEP), an expiratory wheeze continuing right up to the beginning of the next breath, and sometimes increased chest girth. Review of flow and volume graphic waveforms on the ventilator allows identification of air-trapping as the flow will not be seen to return to zero before the next breath is taken. To treat air-trapping, a long expiratory time should be considered, for example a prolonged I:E ratio (1:3 or more) and/or a slow respiratory rate to allow complete expiration to occur. Occasionally, in very severe asthmatics, disconnection from the ventilator and manual chest decompression are required.
2. Barotrauma is a significant risk when positive pressure is applied to very bronchoconstricted lungs with low compliance. Peak airway pressures should be kept below 35 cmH_2O. This can generally be achieved with low respiratory rates (6–10 breaths/min), small tidal volumes (e.g. 6 ml/kg), and/or long expiratory times. All these measures can result in hypoventilation and thus hypercapnia. Some clinicians are concerned if the hypercapnia causes a decrease in pH to <7.20, but there is no supporting evidence base that values below this level are harmful. Elongating expiratory times means that inspiratory times may be shortened, so it is sometimes useful to increase the inspiratory flow rate or reduce the respiratory rate in order to allow an adequately sized breath to still be taken (Stather and Stewart, 2005).
3. Sedation and muscle relaxants may be needed to enable effective ventilation, but drugs with the potential to stimulate histamine release (e.g. 'natural' opiates or derivatives) should be avoided. Ketamine has bronchodilator properties and may be useful in asthma. In more severe cases, sevoflurane or other inhalational anaesthetics can be used, although care should be taken for adequate scavenging or room air flow to avoid environmental pollution and staff risks.

Chronic obstructive pulmonary disease (COPD)

COPD is a product of chronic bronchitis, bronchiectasis, emphysema, and asthma. Most sufferers have a mixture of chronic bronchitis and emphysema. Acute exacerbations usually occur as a result of infection, but may also be related to atmospheric pollution or surgery (with use of inhalational anaesthetics). Inappropriate use of sedatives or high concentration oxygen therapy can precipitate acute decompensation.

Management

Much of the treatment is similar to that of asthma. Nebulized medications may need to be driven by air rather than oxygen (see next section). Infection is the precipitating cause of exacerbation in many cases, so antibiotics should be given if infection is suspected.

Support of respiratory function

1. Oxygen therapy: caution is required with oxygen therapy in COPD as a subset of such patients become dependent on hypoxic stimulation of respiratory drive due to chronic carbon dioxide retention causing loss of their hypercapnic drive. In these cases, higher concentrations of oxygen (>28%) should be administered via an accurate delivery system, such as a Venturi mask, and titrated to a specific target S_pO_2 that should be set relative to the patient's normal range; this is usually lower than that of patients without chronic lung disease. A target S_pO_2 of 90–92% is generally appropriate in the first instance. Serial arterial blood gases should be monitored for evidence of increasing CO_2. Remember that increasing hypercapnia may be related to patient fatigue rather than excessive oxygen.
2. Judicious use of non-invasive ventilation such as BiPAP is often a better and more effective option than invasive ventilation for patients with COPD

(Keenan and Mehta, 2009). NIV should be considered for patients with acute exacerbations of COPD where P_aCO_2 is >6.0 kPa and pH is <7.35 for over an hour despite standard medical treatments having been given (British Thoracic Society *et al.* 2008).

3. Removal of chest secretions: deep breathing, effective humidification of inspired gas, management of anxiety, and encouragement with expectoration will assist the spontaneously breathing patient. Aids such as a nasopharyngeal airway or minitracheostomy may enable manual clearance of sputum. If ventilation is required, direct bronchoscopic clearance of thick secretions may be useful. Sleep should be encouraged and facilitated to prevent the patient becoming fatigued and/or agitated.
4. A respiratory stimulant such as doxapram can be used to treat patients with reduced consciousness and increasing hypercarbia, but is only recommended if non-invasive ventilation is unavailable or considered inappropriate (National Institute for Health and Care Excellence 2010).
5. Invasive mechanical ventilation: the decision to intubate and ventilate patients with COPD should be carefully considered. Weaning from ventilation is often difficult and, for those who survive, subsequent quality of life can be very poor. Nonetheless, if there is a reversible precipitating factor such as recent surgery or a treatable infection, ventilation may provide support until recovery has taken place. However, if respiratory failure is the result of a continuing deterioration of the disease itself, ventilation simply prolongs life without prospect of improvement. Weaning may prove impossible and quality of life may be worsened. There is a need for advance discussions between the multidisciplinary team and the patient and their relatives to decide whether ventilation is appropriate in these cases. If it is used, ventilation should aim to maintain the patient's normal P_aCO_2 (which will usually be above the normal range), but this may not be possible if lung function has decompensated badly. Weaning tends to be a lengthy process because of poor respiratory reserve, comorbidities, and nutritional state. Pressure support can be gradually decreased and patient effort built up over days or weeks.
6. Nutrition: patients with COPD are usually chronically malnourished due to impairment of appetite, dyspnoea during meals, and chronic ill health. Early nutritional support is generally advisable, but these patients should not be required to cope with any excess CO_2 production related to carbohydrate overload. Care should be taken to ensure that equal amounts of fat and carbohydrate contribute to calorie intake.

Pulmonary embolus (PE)

Pulmonary embolus is the occlusion of a pulmonary artery by a thrombus and may be single or multiple. Emboli are most commonly thrown off from a deep vein thrombosis (DVT) within the pelvic or leg veins, or from a mural thrombus within the right heart. The severity of the effect is related to the size of the embolus and the ability of the patient to compensate adequately for the strain on the right ventricle.

Symptoms

These range from tachypnoea, tachycardia, dyspnoea, and pleuritic or substernal chest pain through to hypotension, shock, and cardiac arrest.

Diagnosis is made initially by clinical suspicion (history, clinical features), abnormal tests including a raised central venous pressure, an abnormal chest X-ray (e.g. reduced blood flow (oligaemia) to an area of lung or evidence of pulmonary infarction (classically a wedge-shaped peripheral shadow)), and ECG changes indicative of right heart strain (e.g. right axis deviation, S1, Q3, T3 configuration, partial right bundle branch block), and hypoxaemia). A computed tomography–pulmonary angiography (CT–PA) scan provides definitive evidence. A ventilation-perfusion scan may also be useful, but definitive diagnosis is often difficult. Echocardiography should be performed to assess right ventricular function as this is a major determinant of a poor prognosis.

Management

- Anticoagulation, initially with heparin (subcutaneous low molecular weight (LMW) unless the patient is in renal failure when unfractionated heparin should be infused intravenously). LMW heparins have the advantage that they do not require coagulation monitoring. Oral warfarin is usually commenced after 1–2 days and the heparin continued until 1–2 days after the patient has been fully anticoagulated with warfarin. New oral antithrombin inhibitors have been developed that are at least as safe as warfarin and do not require regular coagulation monitoring.
- Thrombolytic therapy should be used when there is haemodynamic compromise. Evidence for benefit from thrombolytic therapy when there is right ventricular dysfunction but without haemodynamic compromise is lacking, as the risk of severe bleeding offsets earlier dispersal of the embolus.

- Respiratory support (oxygen, CPAP, mechanical ventilation). There is a risk of cardiovascular collapse during intubation because of loss of sympathetic reflexes, vasodilatation, and reduced ventricular filling.
- Pulmonary embolectomy (radiological or surgical) may need to be performed in acute severe life-threatening situations.
- Prevention using elastic anti-embolism stockings, intermittent pneumatic compression devices, exercises, and mobilization. An inferior vena cava filter can be placed radiologically if anticoagulation is contraindicated.
- If cardiovascular embarrassment is evident, the patient must be initially fluid loaded to ensure optimal right ventricular filling. Inotropes may subsequently be required. For further management see Chapter 5.

Pneumonia

Pneumonia is an inflammatory process caused by bacterial, viral, fungal, tuberculous, protozoan, or rickettsial causes. Chemical (e.g. gastric aspiration) or gas inhalation may result in a pneumonitis. Pneumonia is usually characterized by dyspnoea, sometimes pleuritic pain, pyrexia, and purulent respiratory secretions; although one or more of these features may be absent on admission. Opacities on the chest X-ray may be seen, for example with lobar involvement in pneumococcal pneumonia, or generalized 'ground-glass' shadowing and pulmonary infiltrates with *Pneumocystis* pneumonia. Treatment depends on the aetiology and infecting agent, but all patients require similar support and management. Hospital-associated pneumonia (HAP) is defined as pneumonia occurring after the first 48 hours of hospital admission, while ventilator-associated pneumonia (VAP) is defined as a pneumonia occurring after 48 hours in intubated patients. Aspiration of micro-organisms is the main route for pneumonia in intubated patients as the endotracheal tube holds the vocal cords open and so facilitates aspiration. An inflated cuff reduces the risk of aspiration, but does not completely eliminate it.

Management

- Antibiotic therapy
- Oxygen therapy, CPAP, and mechanical ventilation as needed to maintain adequate gas exchange
- Chest physiotherapy and bronchial hygiene to clear secretions
- Postural drainage and position changes
- Adequate nutrition
- Prevention of further infection

References and bibliography

Abroug, F., Ouanes-Besbes, L., Dachraoui, F., *et al* (2011). An updated study-level meta-analysis of randomised controlled trials on proning in ARDS and acute lung injury. *Critical Care*, **15**, R6.

Acute Respiratory Distress Syndrome Network (2000). Ventilation with lower tidal volumes as compared with traditional tidal volumes for acute lung injury and the acute respiratory distress syndrome. *New England Journal of Medicine*, **342**, 1301–8.

Adrogué, H.J., Gennari, F.J., Galla, J.H., *et al.* (2009). Assessing acid–base disorders. *Kidney International*, **76**, 1239–47.

Afshari, A., Brok, J., Møller, A.M., *et al.* (2011). Inhaled nitric oxide for acute respiratory distress syndrome and acute lung injury in adults and children: a systematic review with meta-analysis and trial sequential analysis. *Anesthesia and* Analgesia, **112**, 1411–21.

American Association for Respiratory Care (2010). Endotracheal suctioning of mechanically ventilated patients with artificial airways 2010. *Respiratory Care*, **55**, 758–64.

Bersten, A.D. (2009). Humidification and inhalation therapy. In *Oh's Intensive Care Manual* (6th edn) (eds A.D. Bersten and N. Soni). Philadelphia, PA: Butterworth-Heinemann.

Boles, J.M., Bion, J., Connors, A., *et al.* (2007). Weaning from mechanical ventilation. *European Respiratory Journal*, **29**, 1033–56.

British Thoracic Society, Royal College of Physicians of London, Intensive Care Society (2008). *The Use of Non-Invasive Ventilation in the Management of Patients with Chronic Obstructive Pulmonary Disease Admitted to Hospital with Acute Type II Respiratory Failure (with Particular Reference to Bilevel Positive Pressure Ventilation).* http://www.brit-thoracic.org.uk/Portals/0/Clinical%20 Information/NIV/Guidelines/NIVinCOPDFullguidelineFINAL.pdf (accessed 1 May 2012).

Brochard, L. and Thille, A.W. (2009). What is the proper approach to liberating the weak from mechanical ventilation? *Critical Care Medicine*, **37**(Suppl), S410–15.

Caruso, P., Denari, S., Ruiz, S.A., *et al.* (2009). Saline instillation before tracheal suctioning decreases the incidence of ventilator-associated pneumonia. *Critical Care Medicine*, **37**, 32–8.

Clark, A.P., Winslow, E.H., Tyler, D.O., *et al.* (1990). Effects of endotracheal suctioning on mixed venous oxygen saturation and heart rate in critically ill adults. *Heart and Lung*, **19**, 552–7.

Curry, K., Cobb, S., Kutash, M., Diggs, C. (2008). Characteristics associated with unplanned extubations in a surgical intensive care unit. *American Journal of Critical Care*, **17**, 45–51.

Delaney, A., Bagshaw, S.M., Nalos, M. (2006). Percutaneous dilatational tracheostomy versus surgical tracheostomy in critically ill patients: a systematic review and meta-analysis. *Critical Care*, **10**, R55.

Demir, F., Dramali, A. (2005). Requirement for 100% oxygen before and after closed suction. *Journal of Advanced Nursing*, **51**, 245–51.

Dennis, D., Jacob, W., Budgeon, C. (2012). Ventilator versus manual hyperinflation in clearing sputum in ventilated intensive care unit patients. *Anaesthesia and Intensive Care*, **40**, 142–9.

Donahoe, M. (2011). Acute respiratory distress syndrome: a clinical review. *Pulmonary Circulation*, **1**, 192–211.

Donald, K.J., Robertson, V.J., Tsebelis, K. (2000). Setting safe and effective suction pressure: the effect of using a manometer in the suction circuit. *Intensive Care Medicine*, **26**, 15–19.

Dushianthan, A., Goss, V., Cusack, R., *et al.* (2014). Altered molecular specificity of surfactant phosphatidycholine synthesis in patients with acute respiratory distress syndrome. *Respiratory Research*, **15**, 128.

Dyhr, T., Bonde, J., Larsson, A. (2003). Lung recruitment manoeuvres are effective in regaining lung volume and oxygenation after open endotracheal suctioning in acute respiratory distress syndrome. *Critical Care*, **7**, 55–62.

Esteban, A., Anzueto, A., Alía, I., *et al.* (2000). How is mechanical ventilation employed in the intensive care unit? An international utilization review. *American Journal of Respiratory and Critical Care Medicine*, **161**, 1450–8.

Ferguson, N.D, Cook, D.J., Guyatt, G.H., *et al.* (2013). High-frequency oscillation in early acute respiratory distress syndrome. *New England Journal of Medicine*, **368**, 795–805.

Galluccio, S.T. and Bersten, A.D. (2014). Humidification and inhalation therapy. In *Oh's Intensive Care Manual* (7th edn) (eds A.D. Bersten and N, Soni). Butterworth-Heinemann, London

Gattinoni, L., Pesenti, A., Mascheroni, D., *et al.* (1986). Low-frequency positive-pressure ventilation with extracorporeal CO_2 removal in severe acute respiratory failure. *JAMA*, **256**, 881–6.

Gentile, M.A., Siobal, M.S. (2010). Are specialized endotracheal tubes and heat-and-moisture exchangers cost-effective in preventing ventilator associated pneumonia? *Respiratory Care*, **55**, 184–96.

Guérin, C., Reignier, J., Richard, J.C, *et al.* (2013). Prone positioning in severe acute respiratory distress syndrome. *New England Journal of Medicine*, **368**, 2159–68.

Hanekom, S., Gosselink, R., Dean, E., *et al.* (2011). The development of a clinical management algorithm for early physical activity and mobilization of critically ill patients: synthesis of evidence and expert opinion and its translation into practice. *Clinical Rehabilitation*, **25**, 771–87.

Harik-Khan, R.I., Wise, R.A., Fozard, J.L. (1998). Determinants of maximal inspiratory pressure. The Baltimore Longitudinal Study of Aging. *American Journal of Respiratory and Critical Care Medicine*, **158**, 1459–64.

Havelock, T., Teoh, R., Laws, D., *et al.* (2010). Pleural procedures and thoracic ultrasound: British Thoracic Society Pleural Disease Guideline 2010. *Thorax*, **65**(Suppl 2), ii61–76.

Heunks, L.M., van der Hoeven, J.G. (2010). Clinical review. The ABC of weaning failure—a structured approach. *Critical Care*, **14**, 245.

Hodgson, C.L., Hayes, K., Everard, T., *et al.* (2012). Long-term quality of life in patients with acute respiratory distress syndrome requiring extracorporeal membrane oxygenation for refractory hypoxaemia. *Critical Care*, **16**, R202.

Hunter, J.D. (2006). Ventilator associated pneumonia. *Postgraduate Medical Journal*, **82**, 172–8.

Intensive Care Society (2008). *Standards for the Care of Adult Patients with a Temporary Tracheostomy*. Report, Intensive Care Society, London.

Keenan, S.P., Mehta, S. (2009). Noninvasive ventilation for patients presenting with acute respiratory failure: the randomized controlled trials. *Respiratory Care*, **54**, 116–26.

Lellouche, F., Mancebo, J., Jolliet, P., *et al.* (2006). A multicenter randomized trial of computer-driven protocolized weaning from mechanical ventilation. *American Journal of Respiratory and Critical Care Medicine*, **174**, 894–900.

McMorrow, R.C., Mythen, M.G. (2006). Pulse oximetry. *Current Opinion in Critical Care*, **12**, 269–71.

Maggiore, S.M., Lellouche, F., Pigeot, J., *et al.* (2003). Prevention of endotracheal suctioning-induced alveolar derecruitment in acute lung injury. *American Journal of Respiratory and Critical Care Medicine*, **67**, 1215–24.

Marcy, T.W., Marini, J.J. (1991). Inverse ratio ventilation in ARDS: rationale and implementation. *Chest*, **100**, 494–504.

Mehta, S., Burry, L., Cook, D., *et al.* (2012). Daily sedation interruption in mechanically ventilated critically ill patients cared for with a sedation protocol: a randomized controlled trial. *JAMA*, **308**, 1985–92.

Miano, T.A., Reichert MG, Houle TT, *et al.* (2009). Nosocomial pneumonia risk and stress ulcer prophylaxis: a comparison of pantoprazole vs ranitidine in cardiothoracic surgery patients. Chest. 136(2):440–7.

Mireles-Cabodevila, E., Diaz-Guzman, E., Heresi, G.A., *et al.* (2009). Alternative modes of mechanical ventilation: a review for the hospitalist. *Cleveland Clinic Journal of Medicine*, **76**, 417–30.

Muscedere, J., Rewa, O., McKechnie, K., *et al.* (2011). Subglottic secretion drainage for the prevention of ventilator-associated pneumonia: a systematic review and meta-analysis. *Critical Care Medicine*, **39**, 1985–91.

NICE (National Institute for Health and Clinical Excellence) (2010). *Chronic Obstructive Pulmonary Disease: Management of Chronic Obstructive Pulmonary Disease in Adults in Primary and Secondary Care*. NICE Clinical Guideline http://www.nice.org.uk/nicemedia/live/13029/49425/49425.pdf (accessed 1 May 2012).

Needham, D.M., Truong, A.D., Fan, E. (2009). Technology to enhance physical rehabilitation of critically ill patients. *Critical Care Medicine*, **37**(Suppl), S436–41.

Ng, K.S., Kumarasinghe, G., Inglis, T.J. (1999). Dissemination of respiratory secretions during tracheal tube suctioning in an intensive care unit. *Annals of the Academy of Medicine, Singapore*, **28**, 178–82.

Overend, T.J., Anderson, C.M., Brooks, D., *et al.* (2009). Updating the evidence-base for suctioning adult patients: a systematic review. *Canadian Respiratory Journal*, **16**, e6–17.

Paratz, J.D., Stockton, K.A. (2009). Efficacy and safety of normal saline instillation: a systematic review. *Physiotherapy*, **95**, 241–50.

Parkin, B., Turner, A., Moore, E., *et al.* (1997). Bacterial keratitis in the critically ill. *British Journal of Ophthalmology*, **81**, 1060–3.

Patman, S., Jenkins, S., Stiller, K. (2000). Manual hyperinflation: effects on respiratory parameters. *Physiotherapy Research International*, **5**, 157–71.

Peek, G.J., Mugford, M., Tiruvoipati, R., *et al.* (2009). Efficacy and economic assessment of conventional ventilatory support versus extracorporeal membrane oxygenation for severe adult respiratory failure (CESAR): a multicentre randomised controlled trial. *Lancet*, **374**, 1351–63.

Peñuelas, O., Frutos-Vivar, F., Fernández, C., *et al.* (2011). Characteristics and outcomes of ventilated patients according to time to liberation from mechanical ventilation. *American Journal of Respiratory and Critical Care Medicine*, **184**, 430–7.

Petrucci, N., De Feo, C. (2013). Lung protective ventilation strategy for the acute respiratory distress syndrome. *Cochrane Database of Systematic Reviews*, **28**(2), CD003844.

Pohlman, M.C., Schweickert, W.D., Pohlman, A.S.,.*et al.* (2010). Feasibility of physical and occupational therapy beginning from initiation of mechanical ventilation. *Critical Care Medicine*, **38**, 2089–94.

Putensen, C., Muders, T., Varelmann, D., *et al.* (2006). The impact of spontaneous breathing during mechanical ventilation. *Current Opinion in Critical Care*, **12**, 13–18.

Resar, R., Pronovost, P., Haraden, C., *et al.* (2005). Using a bundle approach to improve ventilator care processes and reduce ventilator-associated pneumonia. *Joint Commission Journal on Quality and Patient Safety*, **31**, 243–8.

Restrepo, R.D., Walsh, B.K. (2012). Humidification during invasive and noninvasive mechanical ventilation. *Respiratory Care*, **57**, 782–8.

Seymour, C.W., Cross, B.J., Cooke, C.R., *et al.* (2009). Physiologic impact of closed-system endotracheal suctioning in spontaneously breathing patients receiving mechanical ventilation. *Respiratory Care*, **54**, 367–74.

Shannon, H., Stiger, R., Gregson, R.K., *et al.* (2010). Effect of chest wall vibration timing on peak expiratory flow and inspiratory pressure in a mechanically ventilated lung model. *Physiotherapy*, **96**, 344–9.

Singer, M., Vermaat, J., Hall, G., *et al.* (1994). Hemodynamic effects of manual hyperinflation in critically ill mechanically ventilated patients. *Chest*, **106**, 1182–7.

Sorenson, H.M., Shelledy, D.C. (2003). AARC clinical practice guideline. Intermittent positive pressure breathing—2003 revision and update. *Respiratory Care*, **48**, 540–6.

Stather, D.R., Stewart, T.E. (2005). Clinical review: mechanical ventilation in severe asthma. *Critical Care*, **9**, 581–7.

Stewart, N.I., Jagelman, T.A., Webster, N.R. (2011). Emerging modes of ventilation in the intensive care unit. *British Journal of Anaesthesia*, **107**, 74–82.

Stoller, J.K., Orens, D.K., Fatica, C., *et al.* (2003). Weekly versus daily changes of in-line suction catheters: impact on rates of ventilator-associated pneumonia and associated costs.*Respiratory Care*, **48**, 494–9.

Sud, S., Sud, M., Friedrich, J.O., *et al.* (2010). High frequency oscillation in patients with acute lung injury and acute respiratory distress syndrome (ARDS): systematic review and meta-analysis. *BMJ*, **340**, c2327.

Taccone, P., Pesenti, A., Latini, R., *et al.* (2009). Prone positioning in patients with moderate and severe acute respiratory distress syndrome: a randomized controlled trial. *JAMA*, **302**, 1977–84.

Thomas, A.N., Harvey, D.J.R., Hurst, T. (2011). *Standards for Capnography in Critical Care (revised)*. Report, Intensive Care Society, London.

van de Leur, J.P., Zwaveling, J.H., Loef, B.G., *et al.* (2003). Endotracheal suctioning versus minimally invasive airway suctioning in intubated patients: a prospective randomised controlled trial. *Intensive Care Medicine*, **29**, 426–32.

Verbrugghe, W., Jorens, P.G. (2011). Neurally adjusted ventilatory assist: a ventilation tool or a ventilation toy? *Respiratory Care*, **56**, 327–35.

Wille, J., Braams, R., van Haren, W.H., *et al.* (2000). Pulse oximeter-induced digital injury: frequency rate and possible causative factors. *Critical Care Medicine*, **28**, 3555–7.

Yang, K.L., Tobin, M.J. (1991). A prospective study of indexes predicting the outcome of trials of weaning from mechanical ventilation. *New England Journal of Medicine*, **324**, 1445–50.

Yeh, S.H., Lee, L.N., Ho, T.H., *et al.* (2004). Implications of nursing care in the occurrence and consequences of unplanned extubation in adult intensive care units. *International Journal of Nursing Studies*, **41**, 255–62.

Young, D., Lamb, S.E., Shah, S., *et al.* (2013). High-frequency oscillation for acute respiratory distress syndrome. *New England Journal of Medicine*, **368**, 806–13.

Further reading

Asthma

British Thoracic Society/Scottish Intercollegiate Guidelines Network (2012). *British Guideline on the Management of Asthma*. Report, British Thoracic Society, London. http://www.brit-thoracic.org.uk/Portals/0/Guidelines/AsthmaGuidelines/sign101%20Jan%202012.pdf (accessed 1 May 2012).

Pulmonary embolism

Pastores, S.M. (2009). Management of venous thromboembolism in the intensive care unit. *Journal of Critical Care*, **24**, 185–91.

Pneumonia

Lim, W.S., Baudouin, S.V., George, R.C., *et al.* (2009). BTS guidelines for the management of community acquired pneumonia in adults: update 2009. *Thorax*, **64**(Suppl 3), iii-1–55.

Woodhead, M., Welch, C.A., Harrison, D.A., *et al.* (2006). Community-acquired pneumonia on the intensive care unit: secondary analysis of 17,869 cases in the ICNARC Case Mix Programme Database. *Critical Care*, **10**(Suppl 2), S1.

CHAPTER 5
Cardiovascular problems

Anatomy and physiology

The principal functions of the cardiovascular system are (see also Figure 5.1):

1. Carriage of oxygen to the tissues from the lungs.
2. Carriage of carbon dioxide from the tissues to the lungs.
3. Carriage of nutrients from the digestive tract to the tissues.
4. Carriage of metabolic waste from the tissues to the kidneys.
5. Carriage of hormones from endocrine glands and other sources to site of action.
6. Transport and radiation of excess heat.

The cardiovascular system includes:

1. The systemic circulation, consisting of aorta, arteries, capillaries, and veins, which is supplied by the left ventricle (LV).
2. The pulmonary circulation, consisting of the pulmonary artery, capillaries, and veins, which is supplied by the right ventricle (RV).

Flow of blood through the heart

Venous blood returns to the right atrium via the inferior and superior venae cavae. The atria act as a top-up system which forces extra blood into the respective ventricles immediately prior to ventricular contraction (Figure 5.2).

The pressure created by commencement of ventricular contraction closes the valves between the atria and ventricles. Continuing ventricular contraction then forces blood out from the right ventricle into the pulmonary artery, and from the left ventricle into the aorta. Owing to the disparity of pressures between pulmonary and systemic circulations, the left ventricle is considerably thicker and more muscular. It also has a globular shape as opposed to the half-moon shape of the right ventricle.

Pressure changes during a cardiac cycle

Ventricular pressure changes

In the left ventricle:

- a peak pressure of ~120 mmHg (rising with age) is generated during systole
- during diastole, pressure falls to a thoracic cavity pressure of ~0 mmHg
- left ventricular pressure changes are therefore 120/0 mmHg.

In the right ventricle:

- systolic pressure is ~25 mmHg. The same volume of blood is ejected as the left ventricle but at a lower pressure
- during diastole, pressure falls to the thoracic cavity pressure of ~0 mmHg
- right ventricular pressure changes are therefore 25/0 mmHg.

Aortic pressure changes

- The peak pressure is the same as the left ventricular systolic pressure, namely ~120 mmHg.
- During diastole, aortic pressure is maintained by elastic recoil of the arterial walls and falls to ~80 mmHg.
- Aortic pressure changes are therefore ~120/80 mmHg.

Anatomy and physiology

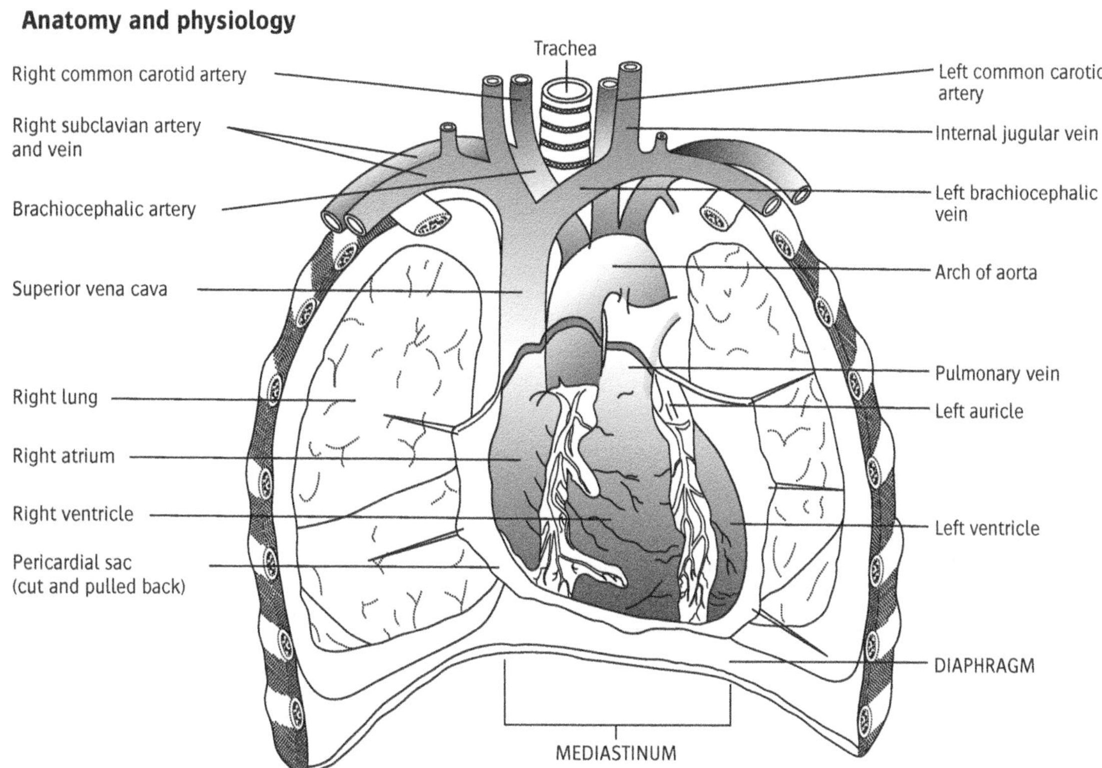

Figure 5.1 General view of the heart in the anatomically correct position.

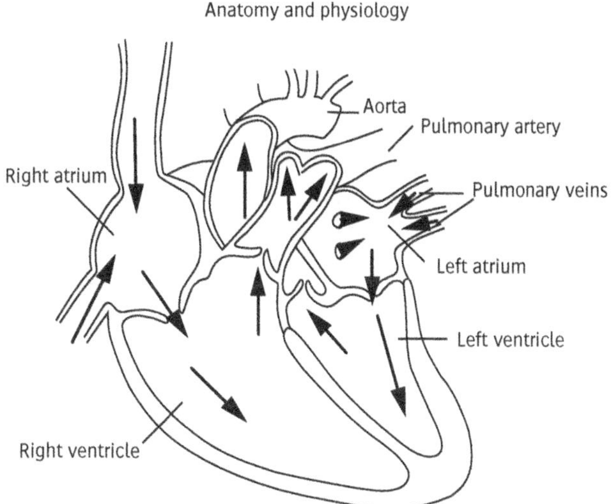

Figure 5.2 Diagram of a cross-section of the heart showing direction of flow.

Pulmonary artery pressure changes

- Maximum pressure is the same as right ventricular pressure, namely ~25 mmHg.
- During diastole, pulmonary artery pressure falls to ~8 mmHg.
- Pulmonary artery pressure changes are therefore 25/8 mmHg.

Atrial pressure changes

These are more complex due to bulging of the tricuspid and mitral valves during ventricular systole, and downward movement of the atrioventricular ring following opening of the pulmonary and aortic valves. Upward return of the atrioventricular ring and filling from the venae cavae and pulmonary veins will increase atrial pressures until the mitral and tricuspid valves open again and atrial contraction occurs.

Excitation, contraction, and conduction

Features of cardiac muscle

Syncytium

Cardiac muscle is similar to skeletal muscle apart from the syncitium, a lattice-like interconnection of fibres between muscle cells. This forms a complex network that allows almost simultaneous spread of excitation and contraction. The atria form one syncytium that is divided from the ventricular syncytium by fibrous tissue. This division allow separate atrial and ventricular contractions.

Automatic rhythmicity

Some areas of muscle fibre have the ability to depolarize rhythmically without external stimulation. This occurs because the fibre membrane is permeable to sodium, allowing continual leak of sodium ions into the cell. This increases the electrical charge until it hits a 'threshold' level, triggering an action potential. After the action potential occurs the membrane is temporarily less permeable to sodium but more permeable to potassium ions. Potassium thus leaks out, creating a negative charge across the membrane.

The speed of rhythmic depolarization is determined by the length of time taken to increase the membrane potential to the 'threshold' level once more. Sinoatrial node fibres have the fastest inherent rhythmicity and thus usually act as the heart's pacemaker.

Membrane potential

All cells have an electrical potential across the cell membrane, which is negative inside the cell in resting conditions. The potential is due to differences between ion composition in intra- and extracellular fluids. This is maintained by the Na^+/K^+ pump, which transports Na^+ ions to the outside of the cell while transporting potassium ions inside. The membrane is highly permeable to K^+ ions but much less permeable to Na^+. K^+ ions tend to leak out, leaving large negatively charged ions inside the cell that produce the relative negative charge.

Prolonged muscle contraction

The action potential includes a plateau phase that lasts for ~0.3 sec before returning to baseline owing to the slow repolarization of cardiac muscle.

Increased speed of contraction and repolarization with increased cardiac rate

This is partly due to a shortened period of systolic ejection, but mostly to a shortened diastolic period. Thus, in prolonged tachycardia, the time for muscle rest and coronary blood flow is greatly reduced. The absolute refractory period is protected to prevent tetanic or chaotic excitation (Table 5.1).

Depolarization

A stimulus alters the permeability of the polarized cell membrane by inactivating the Na^+/K^+ pump and allowing Na^+ ions to diffuse rapidly into the cell via 'fast sodium channels'. This results in a reversal of the electrical charge. When polarity reduces from a resting potential of –80 mV to –35 mV, calcium channels are opened, causing an immediate influx of Ca^{2+} ions. Combined with the continuing sodium ion influx, polarity across the membrane is increased to + 30 mV. The cells on either side are then stimulated and membrane permeability altered, thus depolarization becomes self-propagating. This is known as an action potential and calcium release is triggered to allow muscular contraction (see below). If the critical level of depolarization is not reached, depolarization will remain local to the cell and calcium release will not be activated.

Table 5.1 Duration in seconds of contraction and replorization

Event	Duration at rate of 75 bpm	Duration at rate of 200 bpm
Cardiac cycle	0.80	0.30
Systole	0.27	0.16
Action potential	0.25	0.15
Absolute refractory period	0.20	0.13
Relative refractory period	0.05	0.02
Diastole	0.53	0.14

Repolarization

The first phase of repolarization is closure of the fast sodium channels. K^+ moves out of the cell while Ca^{2+} and Na^+ ions influx via slow channels. This is the plateau phase of repolarization (phase 2), which is represented on the electrocardiogram (ECG) as the ST segment. During phase 3, the slow channels close and influx of Ca^{2+} and Na^+ ions is halted. There is increased permeability to K^+ ions with further movement of K^+ out of the cell until the negative polarity of the cell's resting state is restored. This appears as the T wave on the ECG. Finally, phase 4 of repolarization reactivates the Na^+/K^+ pump, allowing the ratio of Na^+ to K^+ ions inside the cell to be regained.

The refractory period

Cardiac muscle cells will not respond to further stimulation between phases 0 and 3 of the action potential. This is the 'refractory period'. The *absolute* refractory period covers phases 0 to 2 of depolarization and repolarization. No stimulus can elicit a response during this period. On the ECG, this is denoted by the period from the beginning of the QRS complex to just after the beginning of the T wave. The *relative* refractory period covers phase 3 of repolarization when membrane potential is more negative than –50 mV. A relatively strong stimulus will trigger a response but conduction is slower than when fibres are fully repolarized. This period is represented by most of the T wave. The occurrence of an ectopic stimulus during the relative refractory period can initiate life-threatening dysrhythmias. This is known as an 'R on T' ectopic.

Mechanical response to depolarization

In response to an action potential, Ca^{2+} ions are released from the sarcoplasmic reticulum within the cell (Figure 5.3). Further Ca^{2+} influx can also occur through opening of Ca^{2+} channels in the cell membrane.

Free Ca^{2+} ions activate contraction ('systole') by combining with the protein troponin that is situated on actin filaments. Calcium-bound troponin reorients the filament, uncovering binding sites on the actin which can then interact and form cross-bridges with the myosin filaments. Release of energy from ATP allows the two filaments to move past each other, shortening the distance between two Z bands. This shortening is the basis of myocardial contraction. Calcium is taken up again by the sarcoplasmic reticulum and contraction ceases as the binding sites are once again covered. The sarcomere lengthens and relaxation occurs (see Figure 5.3).

Conduction

For virtually simultaneous contraction to take place throughout the individual chambers of the heart, there must be a very fast conduction pathway. Electrical stimulation can be conducted from cell to cell, but this is too slow to provide optimal contraction. All specialized cells within the conduction pathway possess automaticity but the discharge rate varies. The fastest discharge rate (60–100 beats per minute (bpm) at rest), and thus the normal pacemaker of the heart, is the sinoatrial (SA) node.

The action potential moves through the atria via a number of tracts; thus the action potential from different atrial areas will arrive at the atrioventricular (AV)

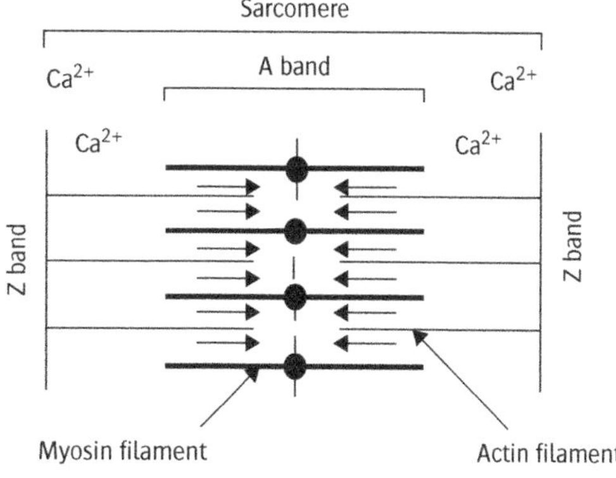

Figure 5.3 Diagram of sarcomeres (arrow shows direction of contraction.

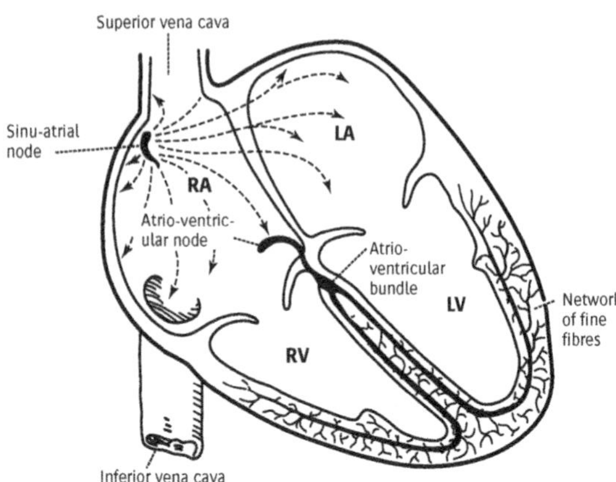

Figure 5.4 The conduction system of the heart.

This figure was published in *Foundations of Anatomy and Physiology*, 3rd Edition, Ross, J.S., Wilson, K.J.W., p. 144, Copyright Elsevier (1973).

node at different times. As the AV node is normally the only electrical pathway between atria and ventricles, the action potential is delayed here to allow all action potentials to be conducted to the ventricles at the same time. The normal AV nodal delay is approximately 0.1 sec. The AV node is continuous with the bundle of His and excitation spreads rapidly down this bundle, then into right and left bundle branches, the Purkinje fibres, and the rest of the ventricles.

Depolarization starts on the left of the ventricular septum and passes to the right across the mid-portion. It then moves down to the apex and out to the ventricular walls (Figure 5.4). The electrical events of the cardiac cycle are seen on the ECG. This records fluctuations in electrical potential from the heart. These fluctuations (currents) are conducted by body fluids containing large quantities of electrolytes which conduct current and are measured on the body surface (Figure 5.5).

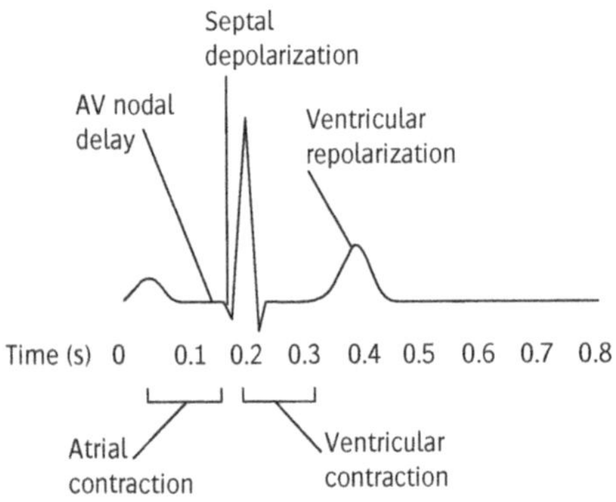

Figure 5.5 Electrical and mechanical events during the cardiac cycle

Automatic discharge rate of cardiac tissues

- Sinoatrial (SA) node: 60–100 bpm.
- Atrioventricular (AV) node: 40–60 bpm.
- Ventricular tissue: 20–40 bpm.

External regulation of the heart rate

The heart rate is influenced by two major external controls:

- the autonomic nervous system
- circulating catecholamines.

Autonomic influence

SA and AV nodes are both innervated by parasympathetic and sympathetic fibres. Parasympathetic stimulation via the vagus nerve causes release of acetylcholine near the nodal cells, causing:

- decreased heart rate by delayed depolarization
- decreased force of contraction
- delayed conduction of impulses through the AV node.

Sympathetic stimulation releases norepinephrine (noradrenaline) near the nodal cells. This stimulates specific receptor sites (β_1-adrenergic receptors) causing:

- a faster heart rate, mediated by an increase in the rate of nodal depolarization
- increased strength of cardiac contraction
- increased rapidity of cardiac impulse conduction.

Influence of catecholamines

The release of epinephrine (adrenaline) and norepinephrine into the bloodstream by the adrenal medulla will also have a direct effect on the heart in the same way as sympathetic nervous stimulation.

Heart rate and blood pressure

Two reflexes adjust heart rate to blood pressure (BP) via the cardioregulatory centre in the medulla.

The aortic reflex

Aortic and carotid sinus baroreceptors respond to alterations in systemic BP and sensory impulses sent to the cardioregulatory centre to produce the responses shown in Table 5.2.

Table 5.2 The aortic reflex

Alteration in BP	Cardioregulatory centre response	Physiological response
Raised BP	Increase in vagal stimulation or a decrease in sympathetic stimulation	Lower heart rate causing a decrease in cardiac output and BP
Lowered BP	Increase in sympathetic stimulation or a decrease in vagal stimulation	Increased heart rate and force of contraction causing a rise in cardiac output and BP

The Bainbridge reflex

Receptors in the venae cavae stimulated by an alteration in venous return send sensory impulses to the cardioregulatory centre (Table 5.3).

Haemodynamics

Under physiological conditions the normal heart should generally be able to meet the metabolic demands placed upon it. However, a diseased heart or alterations in the peripheral circulation may affect cardiac performance. Determinants of cardiac performance can be divided into:

- cardiac output
- preload
- heart rate
- afterload
- stroke volume
- contractility.

Table 5.3 The Bainbridge effect

Alteration in venous return	Cardioregulatory response	Physiological response
Increased venous return	Increase in sympathetic stimulation and a decrease in parasympathetic stimulation	Increased heart rate
Decreased venous return	Increase in parasympathetic stimulation and a decrease in sympathetic stimulation	Decreased heart rate

When assessing haemodynamic status, interrelationships between these factors should be taken into account.

Cardiac output

Cardiac output (CO) is the amount of blood ejected from the left ventricle in one minute. It is determined by stroke volume and heart rate, and therefore manipulation of either can alter CO:

$$\mathrm{CO} = \text{heart rate} \times \text{stroke volume}.$$

The usual range is 4–7 L/min. CO can be adjusted to body size by dividing it by body surface area (BSA). This is termed the cardiac index (CI):

$$\mathrm{CI}(\mathrm{l/min/m^2}) = \frac{\mathrm{CO(l/min)}}{\mathrm{BSA(m^2)}}.$$

The normal range for CI is 2.5–4.0 L/min/m^2. Body surface area is determined using a nomogram derived from height and weight. Cardiac output normally decreases by about 1% per annum after the age of 25 years.

Heart rate

Elevated heart rates can compromise cardiac output by:

- increasing the amount of oxygen consumed by the myocardium
- reducing diastolic time, resulting in less time for coronary artery perfusion
- shortening the ventricular filling phase of the cardiac cycle, decreasing the volume pumped with the next contraction.

Slow heart rates may also be detrimental. Although a longer filling time may initially increase cardiac output, if the heart is diseased the myocardium may be so depressed that the muscle cannot contract long enough to eject this volume. A healthy heart should be able to tolerate a range of heart rates from 30 to 170 bpm for relatively prolonged periods; however, if cardiac function is compromised, this range may be considerably narrower.

Other factors affecting heart rate include temperature, psychological state (stress), thyroid function, and arrhythmias.

Stroke volume

Stroke volume (SV) is the amount of blood ejected by the left ventricle during a single contraction. It is the difference between end-diastolic volume (EDV), the amount of blood left in the ventricle at end-diastole, and end-systolic volume (ESV), the blood volume left in the ventricle at end-systole. The normal range of stroke volume is 60–100 ml.

The volume of blood ejected by each ventricular contraction (stroke volume) depends on:

- myocardial muscle contractility
- preload (the volume of blood filling the ventricle)
- afterload (the resistance to blood flow from the ventricle)
- heart rate (tachycardia reduces the time for diastolic filling).

Ejection fraction

The ejection fraction (EF) is the stroke volume expressed as a percentage of end-diastolic volume. This is most commonly measured by echocardiography. For example, a stroke volume of 70 ml and an end-diastolic volume of 120 ml produces an EF of 70/120 × 100 = 58%.

Healthy individuals usually have an ejection fraction of 50–70%. Damage to the myocardium may impair its ability to pump blood, therefore reducing the EF. In severe heart failure the EF may be <20%. However, it is possible to have heart failure with a normal EF. In diastolic dysfunction caused by hypertrophy, ventricular filling is impaired. Thus the stroke volume and EDV are both reduced, but EF does not change significantly. For this reason, a low EF is generally associated with systolic rather than diastolic dysfunction.

Preload

This refers to the degree of stretch of the muscle fibres at the end of diastole. The greater the volume of blood in the ventricle, the more the degree of muscle fibre stretch. This self-regulatory system allows the force of contraction to equal the volume of blood that needs to be ejected. Starling's law of the heart states that the force of myocardial contraction is determined by the length of the muscle cell fibres (Figure 5.6).

The volume of blood in the ventricle at diastole is dictated by the venous return (the volume of blood returning to the heart) and the contractile ability of the ventricle. There is an optimal range of stretch beyond which the force of contraction is reduced rather than increased. Beyond a certain distance there are probably too few actin–myosin binding sites overlapping to provide adequate contraction.

The factors affecting ventricular preload are shown in Table 5.4. Specific causes of a decreased left ventricular preload but normal right ventricular filling include pulmonary embolus and mitral stenosis. Since preload is difficult to measure at the bedside, the pressures required to fill the ventricles are used as indirect guides to ventricular end-diastolic volume, i.e. the RV end-diastolic (filling) pressure (= central venous pressure) for the right ventricle, and the LV end-diastolic (filling) pressure (= pulmonary artery wedge pressure) for the left ventricle.

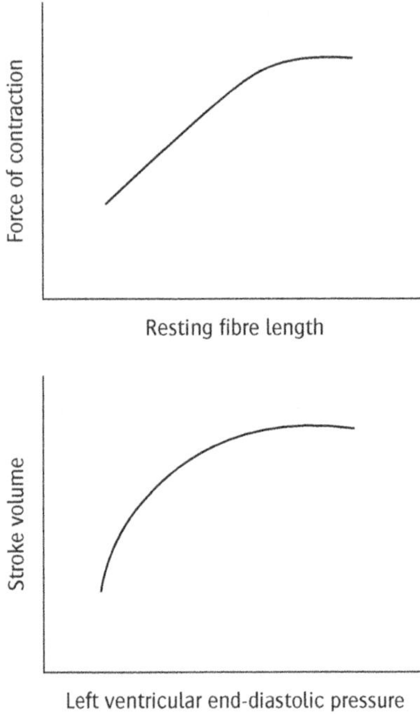

Figure 5.6 Starling's law.

Table 5.4 Factors influencing ventricular preload

Decreased preload	Volume loss—haemorrhage, vomiting, polyuria Vasodilatation—pyrexia, drugs (e.g. nitrates), septicaemia, neurogenic shock, anaphylactic shock Tachycardia (potentially insufficient diastolic filling time) Impeded venous return (e.g. high intrathoracic pressure, pericardial tamponade, pulmonary embolus)
Increased preload	Volume gain—renal failure, excess blood products, excess IV fluids Vasoconstriction—hypothermia, drugs (e.g. epinephrine, norepinephrine), heart failure, pain, anxiety Bradycardia

Afterload

Afterload is the resistance to the outflow of blood that must be overcome by the ventricles during systole. The most important factor determining afterload is the vascular resistance. The pulmonary vascular resistance (PVR) dictates RV afterload and the systemic vascular resistance (SVR) dictates LV afterload.

The bedside measurement of 'afterload' is derived from the cardiac output (CO) and mean arterial pressure (MAP):

$$SVR = \frac{MAP - RAP}{CO} \times 80 \times dyn.sc.cm^{-5}$$

and

$$PVR = \frac{(MPAP - RAP)}{CO} \times 80 \times dyn.sc.cm^{-5}$$

where MPAP is mean pulmonary artery pressure, PAWP is pulmonary artery wedge pressure, and RAP is right atrial pressure. 80 is a conversion factor to present the units of resistance as dyn sec cm^{-5} (1 dyn = 10^{-5} N). The normal ranges are 800–1200 for SVR and 50–200 for PVR.

Afterload has an inverse effect on ventricular function. As resistance to ejection increases, so does ventricular workload. A dysfunctional ventricle may not be able to maintain stroke volume against a high resistance; thus cardiac output frequently falls in the face of increasing peripheral vasoconstriction. The opposite is seen with vasodilatation; the heart has less resistance to pump against and cardiac output usually increases as a consequence.

A satisfactory BP that allows an adequate perfusion pressure of the vital organs must be achieved without compromising blood flow (and thus organ perfusion). Factors affecting afterload are shown in Table 5.5. Specific causes of increased right ventricular afterload include pulmonary valve disease, pulmonary embolus, and pulmonary hypertension. Specific causes of increased LV afterload include aortic valve stenosis and systemic hypertension.

Contractility

Contractility refers to the ability to shorten myocardial muscle fibres without altering their length or preload. The force of contraction of cardiomyocytes alters in response to neural stimuli and plasma catecholamine levels. Norepinephrine is liberated at sympathetic neuromuscular junctions and binds to $ß_1$-adrenergic myocardial membrane receptors. The mechanism is mediated by cyclic AMP and protein kinase A, producing an increase in intracellular levels of calcium and ATP, and thereby facilitating excitation–contraction coupling. Factors affecting contractility are shown in Table 5.6.

Table 5.5 Factors affecting afterload

Increased afterload	Vasoconstricting drugs (e.g. epinephrine, norepinephrine)
	Anxiety
	Hypovolaemia
	Hypothermia
	Cardiogenic shock
	Hypertension
Decreased afterload	Vasodilatating drugs (e.g. nitrates, hydralazine, nitroprusside)
	Anaphylactic shock
	Sepsis
	Hyperthermia
	Neurogenic shock

Blood flow

The heart generates the pressure which forces blood into the circulation. The actual rate of blood flow depends on the difference between pressure produced by the heart and that at the end of the vessel, i.e. the difference between mean arterial and central venous pressure. If pressure in the arterioles is high due to vasoconstriction, there will be a lower blood flow for the same pressure induced by ventricular contraction. Other factors affecting flow include vessel diameter, blood viscosity, and vessel length. These form the resistance to blood flow.

Poiseuille's law states that the ability of blood to flow through any given vessel is:

- proportional to the pressure difference between the two ends of the vessel, and to the fourth power of the vessel diameter,

Table 5.6 Factors affecting contractility

Increased contractility	Positive inotropic drugs Endogenous catecholamines
	Aerobic metabolism
	Hypervolaemia
	Hyperthyroidism
Decreased contractility	Negative inotropic drugs Functional loss of myocardium Anaerobic metabolism (intracellular acidosis)
	Hypocalcaemia
	Hypomagnesaemia
	Hypovolaemia
	Hypoxia

- inversely proportional to the vessel length and blood viscosity.

That is:

$$\text{Blood flow} = \frac{\text{pressure} \times (\text{diameter})^4}{\text{length} \times \text{viscosity}}$$

Regulation of blood flow

The main regulators of blood flow in the different tissue beds are the arterioles. These vessels produce the greatest decrease in diameter and thus the highest resistance to flow. Their tiny size, and the fact that resistance is inversely proportional to the fourth power of their diameter, means that any alteration in diameter will result in a major change in blood flow. This alteration in diameter is mediated by the strong muscular wall, which can alter diameter by up to a factor of 5.

The smooth muscle within the vessel wall responds to two regulatory stimuli:

- the local requirements of tissues when nutrient supply falls below need or exceeds demand, i.e. autoregulation
- autonomic signals, particularly sympathetic stimulation.

Autoregulation of blood flow

In most tissues the most powerful stimulus for regulating blood flow is the need for oxygen. Exceptions are the kidney, as the concentration of electrolytes and metabolic waste plays a major role in renal blood flow regulation, and the brain, where CO_2 levels will also control cerebral blood flow. The alteration of flow to match oxygen requirements allows an automatic and immediate response to increases in cell activity. If tissue PO_2 falls then arteriolar dilatation occurs, producing an increase in blood flow; conversely, if tissue PO_2 rises then arteriolar constriction occurs and blood flow is reduced. The system allows oxygen delivery to be adjusted according to cellular activity, and blood flow to be redirected to areas of need.

Autonomic control of blood flow

Arteries, veins, and, in particular, arterioles are supplied by sympathetic nerves that moderate the state of vasoconstriction by transmitting a continuous stream of impulses to maintain vasomotor tone. Vasoconstriction is produced by increased sympathetic impulse activity and vasodilatation by reduced sympathetic impulses. Autonomic control allows an appropriate distribution of blood flow to major regions of the body.

Factors altering autonomic control of blood flow include:

- body temperature
- exercise
- changes in blood volume.

Blood pressure

Arterial pressure is the product of cardiac output and vascular resistance. Thus, either a change in cardiac output or a change in vascular resistance will alter the BP.

Normal regulation of blood pressure

The mechanisms involved are:

- neural control of vasoconstriction and contractility
- capillary fluid shift mechanisms, which alter blood volume
- renal excretory and hormonal mechanisms, which alter blood volume and vasoconstriction.

Neural control

The vasomotor centre in the brainstem controls vasomotor tone and heart rate via the sympathetic and parasympathetic nervous systems. Vasomotor tone (Box 5.1) is primarily controlled by sympathetic nervous outflow. Heart rate and contractility (Box 5.2) are controlled by the balance of sympathetic and parasympathetic stimulation and inhibition. The vagus nerve is the primary parasympathetic pathway; stimulation will reduce heart rate and decrease contractility. Sympathetic stimulation increases heart rate and the force of contractility.

The *baroreceptor system* consists of receptors sensitive to the degree of stretch exerted by pressure in the arteries. These receptors are situated in the aortic arch and carotid sinuses. They transmit impulses that increase in rate as the BP rises. These impulses inhibit sympathetic outflow from the vasomotor centre, so heart rate, contractility and vasomotor tone are reduced. If the BP falls, the baroreceptors are stimulated less and so impulses decrease. Thus the

Box 5.1 Vasomotor tone

- Increased sympathetic activity = vasoconstriction
  The decrease in arteriolar diameter and the venous reservoir will initially increase venous return and BP
- Decreased sympathetic activity = vasodilatation
  Increases in arteriolar diameter and the venous reservoir decrease venous return and BP

Box 5.2 Heart rate and contractility

- Increased sympathetic stimulation = increased heart rate + increased force of contraction
- Decreased sympathetic stimulation = decreased heart rate + decreased force of contraction
- Increased parasympathetic stimulation = decreased heart rate + decreased force of contraction

vasomotor centre loses its inhibition and increases sympathetic signals to the heart and vessels.

Capillary fluid shift mechanism

This is a longer-term mechanism for blood pressure regulation. It is particularly important when blood volume is either too low or too high. Increased circulating blood volume will raise systemic pressure and hydrostatic pressure within the capillaries. This will increase the shift of fluid across capillary membranes into the interstitial space. A decrease in circulating blood volume will lower capillary hydrostatic pressure and allow oncotic pressure exerted by plasma proteins to pull fluid by osmosis from the interstitial space into the capillaries. This response takes between 10 min and several hours to readjust the arterial pressure back towards normal.

Renal excretory and hormonal mechanisms

The kidneys play an important role in the long-term control of BP and circulatory volume. Formation of urine by the kidneys is regulated by pressure in the renal arteries. A fall in BP will produce a fall in renal artery blood flow, which will decrease or stop the formation of urine. Alternatively, a rise in blood pressure will produce an increased urine output.

A secondary hormonal mechanism, the renin–angiotensin system (described in Chapter 7), responds to falls in BP that reduce renal perfusion. Angiotensin II, a hormone produced by this mechanism, is a potent vasoconstrictor that increases BP. It also stimulates the adrenal cortex to secrete aldosterone which acts on the distal tubules and collecting ducts of the kidney to increase reabsorption of sodium and water. This results in an increase in circulating volume, which will also increase BP.

The vasomotor centre can be stimulated by higher cerebral centres. The limbic system and hypothalamus mediate emotionally induced alterations in BP such as vasovagal collapse brought on by bad news. The midbrain mediates the initial hypertension associated with severe pain and the later fall in BP following prolonged severe pain.

An elevated intracranial pressure can produce reflex increases in arterial blood pressure due to medullary hypercapnia or hypoxia. The increase in arterial pressure increases medullary perfusion, thus potentially reducing hypercapnia and hypoxia by increasing minute ventilation.

Diagnostic and investigative procedures

The electrocardiogram (ECG)

All critically ill patients require continuous ECG monitoring. The aims of cardiac monitoring are:

- early detection of changes in heart rate and rhythm
- assessment of the effectiveness of treatment strategies.

Basic principles of ECG monitoring

- Electrodes are placed on the chest wall to detect electrical activity initiated by the heart. Activity that is moving towards an electrode produces an upward (positive) deflection on the recording, while that moving away produces a downward (negative) deflection. The baseline (isoelectric line) is where positive and negative deflections begin and end.
- The electrodes are connected by a cable to a monitor that displays a continuous waveform reflecting each phase of the heart's electrical activity.
- The impulses produced by cardiac activity are amplified 1000-fold to be seen on the monitor.
- The ECG waveform can be adjusted to optimize size, brightness, and position. A choice of leads is possible but lead II is usually selected as the direction of electrical current passing through the ventricles is directed towards this lead, resulting in a large positive waveform that can be easily interpreted.

Placement of ECG electrodes

The electrodes are small disposable adhesive pads that are pre-gelled (to facilitate conduction) and readily attached to the chest wall by simply peeling off the backing paper and pressing firmly to the skin. The skin must be clean and dry, and it may be necessary to shave chest hair to facilitate contact. It is imperative to have good contact between skin and electrode or the ECG waveform will be distorted and artefacts will appear.

The electrodes can remain in situ for several days, as the gel does not usually dry out. However, skin irritation by the adhesive or the conducting jelly can occur. The electrode positions should be rotated regularly to avoid soreness, and the skin checked for sensitivity.

Thin wires snap or clamp onto the electrodes and are connected to designated leads on the patient cable. These are coloured and usually designated RA (right arm), LA (left arm), and RL (right leg or earth), and should be connected to the corresponding electrode. Three- or five-electrode systems are usually used (see Figure 5.7). Five electrodes are commonly used in the critical care setting because multiple leads offer a more comprehensive electrical picture of the heart and increase the liklihood that ischaemic episodes are detected. When five leads are used the two additional leads are designated left leg and chest (or V1–6). The colours of the leads are not universal and two different systems exist (used in North America or Europe), but other regions may be mixed (see later).

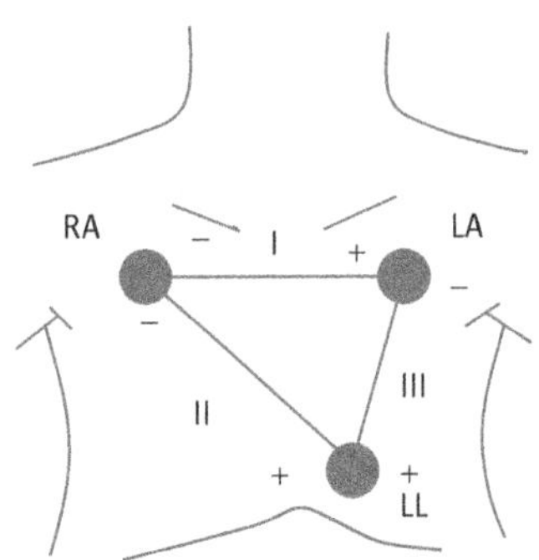

(a) The standard position of electrodes for 3 lead monitoring

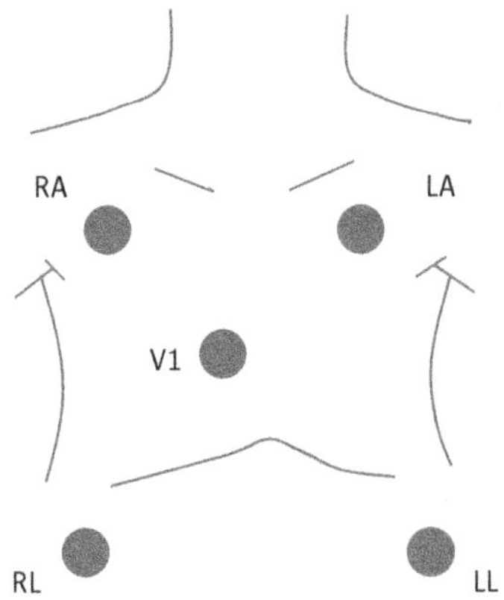

(b) The standard position of electrodes for 5 lead monitoring

Figure 5.7 Placement of ECG electrodes

The 3-lead monitoring system

The right arm (RA) lead is connected to an electrode placed just below the clavicle on the right shoulder, The left arm (LA) lead is connected to an electrode below the left clavicle, and the left leg (LL) lead is connected to an electrode positioned near the apex of the heart. This provides three views of the heart; each lead views the heart from the perspective of the positive electrode towards the negative electrode. Each lead is bipolar and contain boths positive and negative electrodes. RA is always negative, LL is always positive, and LA changes polarity depending upon which lead is selected (positive in lead I, and negative in lead II). Lead I provides a lateral view of the heart, including the left ventricle and atrium, and leads II and III view the inferior surface including the right and left ventricles.

The 5-lead monitoring system

The right arm (RA) and left arm (LA) electrodes are positioned just below the clavicle as in the 3-lead monitoring system The right leg (RL) and left leg (LL) electrodes are placed just below the last ribs, and V1 (chest lead) is placed in the fourth intercostal space to the right of the sternum. V1 is a positive electrode that views the heart directly below it. V1 and V6 are the best leads for differentiating wide QRS rhythms (e.g. identifying SVT from VT with aberrant conduction), and V1 can be moved (e.g. to the V5 position) to view the lateral left ventricle and atrium.

Adjusting the monitor

The displayed waveform must be clear and distinct. Fine adjustments to brightness and size can be made on the monitor. The amplitude of the R wave is of particular importance as the monitor calculates heart rate by recognizing and counting this wave. If the height of the wave cannot be increased sufficiently to record an accurate heart rate, the position of the electrodes, or the lead displayed, may need to be changed to obtain a greater electrical potential.

High and low rate alarm limits should be set according to the patient's clinical condition. Frequent false alarms undermine the rationale for alarm setting and may cause the patient undue anxiety.

Most ratemeters count the number of ventricular beats (R waves) per minute and display this as the heart rate. Most meters will count all large upward deflections as they cannot distinguish ventricular beats from muscle potentials caused by skeletal muscle contractions. Thus patient movement or muscle tremors may cause falsely elevated heart rate readings. These can also be seen if the R and T wave are the same size and the monitor is recognizing both as R waves. To rectify this, the waveform amplitude should be increased until the R wave is higher than the T wave, or the electrode positions or ECG lead displayed should be changed.

Falsely low heart rates occur if the R wave is of insufficient size to be detected (the amplitude should be increased until the wave is recognized), or if there is a disturbance in signal transmission from skin to monitor. This may be due to a defective electrode, separation of electrode from skin, or disconnection of one of the patient leads.

Electrical interference from other bedside devices can occur. This will appear as a series of fine rapid spikes (artefact) which distort the ECG baseline. This may be due to incorrect earthing of a device which should be identified and checked. Artefact may also be caused by patient shivering (particularly if the electrodes are positioned over skeletal muscle) or loose cable connections.

A wandering baseline can occur when the isoelectric line regularly moves up and down rather than in a straight line. This is invariably due to movement of the chest wall during respiration. The only solution is to alter the electrode positions by placing them at the lowest ribs and apex of the chest (Table 5.7).

Arrhythmias and conduction disturbances

Disorders of cardiac rhythm are commonplace in the ICU patient. ECG monitoring allows prompt recognition and immediate intervention. All ECG rhythms should be examined in the context of the patient's clinical condition and intervention decided on this, rather than the rhythm itself.

ECG definitions

There are a number of definitions that provide a background for understanding the ECG.

- *Sinus rhythm*: rhythm originating in the sinoatrial (SA) node of >60 bpm and <100 bpm.
- *Sinus tachycardia*: rhythm originating in the SA node >100 bpm.
- *Sinus bradycardia*: rhythm originating in the SA node <60 bpm.

These rhythms usually reflect either a normal heart or a normal physiological response to an external factor such as exercise.

- *Isoelectric line*: the baseline of the ECG tracing (i.e. no electrical activity is occurring).
- *Positive deflection*: upward movement of the ECG tracing from the baseline.
- *Negative deflection*: downward movement of the ECG tracing from the baseline.
- The *P wave* corresponds to atrial depolarization and is seen in normal sinus rhythm. P waves are best seen in leads II, III, VI, and V2. No P waves are seen in atrial fibrillation, while a peaked wave is classically seen with chronic pulmonary hypertension and an M-shaped wave with mitral valve disease.
- The *PR interval* should be in the range 0.12–0.2 sec. A longer interval (>0.2 sec) is seen with first-degree heart block while a shorter interval (<0.12 sec) is seen with rapid atrioventricular (AV) conduction (e.g. Wolff–Parkinson–White (WPW) syndrome).
- The *QRS complex* (Figure 5.8) corresponds to ventricular depolarization; the width should be <0.12 sec. A greater width is seen with delayed conduction through the ventricular conducting system

Table 5.7 Summary of problems associated with ECG monitoring

Problem	Cause	Action
Falsely high rate	Patient movement, fitting, tremors	Ensure electrodes are not placed over skeletal muscle
	T wave same height as R wave	Increase amplitude, change position of electrodes
Falsely low rate	Lead disconnection	Check leads
	Separation of electrode from skin	Check/replace electrodes
	Insufficient height of R wave	Increase amplitude, change position of electrodes
Artefact	Shivering, tremors	Ensure patient is warm
	Electrical equipment	Check other electrical equipment in use at the bedside (e.g. electric razors, fans)
Wandering baseline	Respiration causing chest wall movement	Adjust position
		Reposition electrodes to lowest ribs to minimize effect

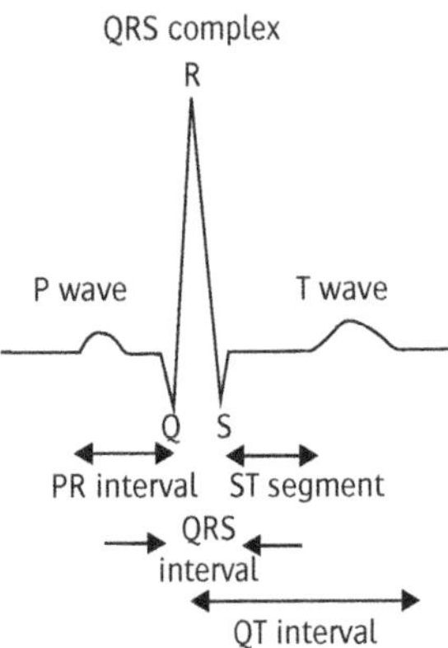

Figure 5.8 The QRS complex.

(e.g. bundle branch block). The QRS height can assess left or right ventricular hypertrophy. A pathological Q wave is seen in myocardial infarction (MI) and should be >25% of the height of the following R wave and >0.04 sec in width.

- The *Q–T interval* varies with heart rate and is approximately 0.35–0.43 sec long when the heart rate is 60 bpm. It is prolonged in hypocalcaemia and shortened by hypercalcaemia.
- The *ST segment* is elevated (in convex shape) from the baseline (isoelectric line) in myocardial infarction and depressed during myocardial ischaemia (see later). Concave ST segment elevation is seen in pericarditis.
- The *T wave* corresponds to ventricular repolarization and should normally be 'positive' (i.e. pointing upwards) in leads I, II, V4, V5, and V6. An inverted T wave may be seen in myocardial ischaemia and infarction, and in types of bundle branch block. It is peaked during hyperkalaemia and flattened by hypokalaemia.

Timing of the ECG

The paper used to record the ECG trace is made up of small and large squares. Each small square measures 1 mm and each large square 5 mm. The paper runs at a standard speed of 25 mm/sec; thus each small square takes 0.04 sec to pass the recording pen and each large square takes 0.2 sec. This allows the timing and rate of the ECG trace to be calculated.

Systematic analysis of the ECG rhythm strip

When first attempting to identify arrhythmias, use a step-by-step sequence to ensure that all aspects of the rhythm are analysed and thus avoid missing important information. Ideally, a recorded strip (traditionally lead II, but any monitoring lead can be used) should be taken to systematically analyse the rhythm. One suggested sequence is as follows.

1. Determine the rate.
2. Determine the regularity of the rhythm.
3. Identify the P wave and its shape.
4. Identify the QRS complex.
5. Determine the relationship between P waves and QRS complexes (i.e. is there one P wave to every QRS?).
6. Calculate the P–R interval.
7. Examine the shape and width of the QRS complex.

Classification of arrhythmias

Arrhythmias can be classified as disorders of impulse formation or impulse conduction.

1. Disorders of impulse formation—may be due to dysfunction of the pacemaker rate of the sinoatrial node allowing escape rhythms from other pacemakers. In conjunction, excessively rapid impulse generation may produce atrial, junctional, and ventricular tachycardias via re-entry pathways (see Table 5.8).
2. Disorders of impulse conduction—refers to situations where conduction is slowed, blocked, or uses an alternative pathway (see Table 5.9).

Precipitating causes of arrhythmias

As well as focal arrhythmias associated with cardiac disease itself, alterations of underlying physiology and biochemistry may also precipitate arrhythmias. The

Table 5.8 Disorders of impulse formation

Site	Disorder (rhythm)
Supraventricular	Sinus arrhythmia Sinus bradycardia Sinus tachycardia Atrial ectopic beats Atrial flutter Atrial fibrillation Sick sinus syndrome
Junctional (nodal)	AV nodal (junctional) premature beats AV nodal (junctional) tachycardia
Ventricular	Venticular ectopic beats Ventricular tachycardia Ventricular fibrillation Torsades de pointes

Table 5.9 Disorders of impulse conduction

Slowed or blocked conduction	First-degree atrioventricular block Second-degree atrioventricular block Third-degree atrioventricular block Bundle branch block
Alternative pathways	Wolff–Parkinson–White (WPW) syndrome Lown–Ganong–Levine syndrome

patient's condition should always be reviewed for precipitating treatable causes, such as the following.

1. Myocardial ischaemia due to poor coronary artery perfusion, or related to low cardiac output states, hypoxaemia, or sepsis.
2. Autonomic control may be affected by central neurological damage.
3. Alterations in electrolyte and acid–base balance (e.g. hypo- and hyperkalaemia, -calcaemia, -magnesaemia, and -phosphataemia, and metabolic and respiratory acidosis) (see Table 5.10).
4. Endocrine influence, particularly thyroid.
5. Effects of drugs.

Disorders of impulse formation

1. Sinus arrhythmia (Figure 5.9):

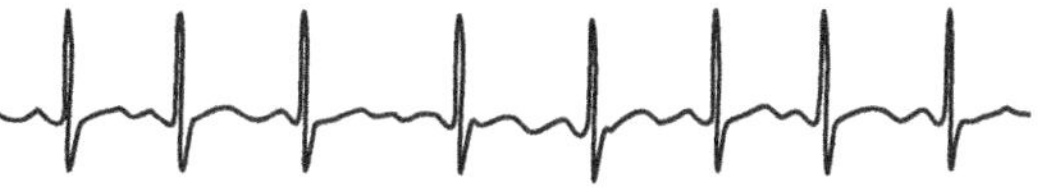

Figure 5.9 Sinus arrhythmia.

Spacing between normal P and QRS complexes varies regularly, usually with respiration; in young patients this is due to an increased venous return on inspiration.

Aetiology: Physiological in most young patients but occasionally associated with inferior MI.

Treatment: None.

2. Sinus tachycardia (Figure 5.10):

P waves and QRS complexes are normal but the rate is increased to >100 bpm.

Aetiology: Physiological in exercise and emotional slates. Pathologically, it is associated with underlying fever, fluid volume deficit, heart failure, anaemia, thyrotoxicosis, stimulants such as amphetamines, and drugs such as atropine and epinephrine.

Treatment: Directed at finding and treating the underlying cause.

3. Sinus bradycardia (Figure 5.11):

Normal P and QRS complexes but the rate is <60 bpm.

Aetiology: Physiological in athletes and fit people but associated pathologically with myocardial infarction, sick sinus syndrome, myxoedema, raised intracranial pressure, and drugs such as β-blockers, digoxin, verapamil, and cholinergic drugs.

Treatment: Usually only needed if BP is compromised or where cardiac failure prevents the patient from compensating for the slow rate with increased myocardial contraction. Atropine 0.3 mg, followed by supplemental doses as necessary, may be used to block vagal tone and increase the rate. Occasionally, in sick sinus syndrome, transvenous pacing may be necessary.

4. Atrial ectopic (premature) beats (Figure 5.12):

A stimulus for a beat occurs earlier than expected, arising not in the sinoatrial node but in another part of the atrium. The distance between the

Table 5.10 Arrhythmias caused by metabolic changes

Metabolic change	ECG change
Hyperkalaemia	Tall ('tented') T waves ± wide QRS complexes ± absent P waves
Hypokalaemia	Flattened T waves U waves (seen after T wave)
Hypercalcaemia	Short Q–T interval
Hypocalcaemia	Prologed Q–T interval
Hypothermia	J wave (small wave appearing immediately after QRS complex) Bradycardia
Digoxin effect	ST depression Inverted T wave ('reverse tick'), not a sign of toxicity Any arrhythmia may occur with toxicity

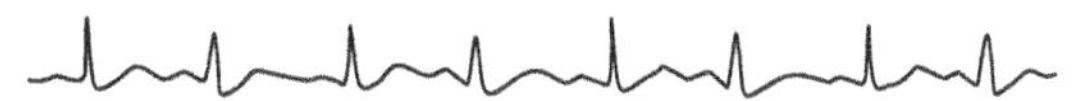

Figure 5.10 Sinus tachycardia

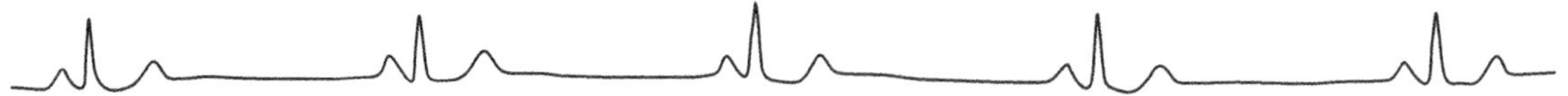

Figure 5.11 Sinus bradycardia.

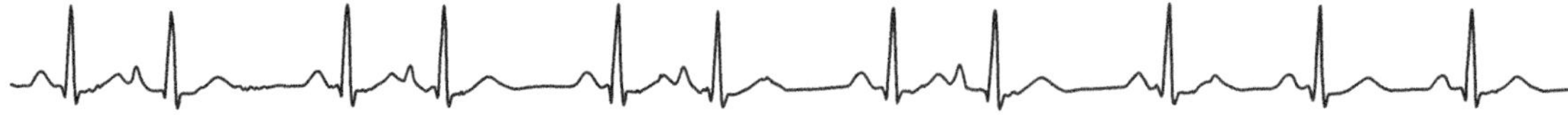

Figure 5.12 Atrial ectopic beats

previous beat and the ectopic beat is much shorter than normal and may be followed by a longer than normal interval before the next beat occurs ('compensatory pause').

Aetiology: These beats are often present in the normal heart but may be induced by stimulants such as caffeine, nicotine, and stress. They may occur pathologically as a result of infections, ischaemia, electrolyte imbalance, underlying heart disease, or drug toxicity such as excess theophylline and digoxin.

Treatment: Only indicated in the healthy person if the ectopic beats are symptomatic or precipitate atrial tachycardia. Avoidance of recognized provoking factors is usually sufficient. Digoxin or β-blockers may be used if symptomatic.

5. Supraventricular tachycardia (SVT) (Figure 5.13):

A rapid, regular rhythm, with a rate of 140–220 bpm, usually of sudden onset. P waves may be present but abnormal or obscured by the rapid rate QRS complex. There may be difficulty in distinguishing SVT with aberrant ventricular conduction from a ventricular tachycardia. Carotid sinus massage (see later) or IV adenosine (initially 3 mg rapid bolus followed by 6mg bolus and then 12 mg bolus if no effect in 1–2 min) can slow the rate sufficiently to allow diagnosis of the tachycardia.

Aetiology: SVT can occur in patients with healthy hearts or those with heart disease and conduction abnormalities such as Wolff–Parkinson–White syndrome. It is distinguished from sinus tachycardia by its sudden onset or cessation.

Treatment: Supraventricular tachycardia is usually successfully treated with IV β-blockers, amiodarone, or verapamil. Patients in heart failure should receive verapamil or β-blockers with caution. Giving verapamil to those receiving β-blockers may induce severe hypotension and bradycardia. Other options for SVT include cardioversion or, occasionally, overdrive pacing.

6. Atrial flutter (Figure 5.14):

This ectopic atrial rhythm produces characteristic 'sawtooth' or 'picket fence' P waves. The atrial rate is usually 250–300 bpm with a variable ventricular rate depending on the degree of AV nodal block. If one QRS occurs to every two P waves, the ventricular rate is 125–150 bpm. If one QRS occurs to every three P waves, the ventricular rate is 75–100 bpm. The QRS complex is normal unless there is aberrant conduction.

Aetiology: There is usually underlying heart disease (e.g. myocardial ischaemia).

Treatment: If there is haemodynamic compromise or a very fast ventricular rate then synchronized DC cardioversion should be considered. If the rate is acceptable and the patient is stable, IV amiodarone, verapamil, or digoxin can be given.

7. Atrial fibrillation (AF) (Figure 5.15):

This irregular QRS pattern has no discernible P waves but a QRS width that is usually normal. The atria fibrillate at a rate of 400–600 bpm. The ventricular rate is usually >100 bpm.

Aetiology: Chronic AF can occur from chronic heart disease, while paroxysmal AF occurs from a variety

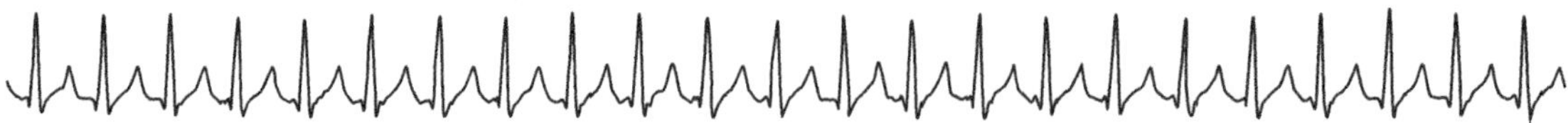

Figure 5.13 Supraventricular tachycardia

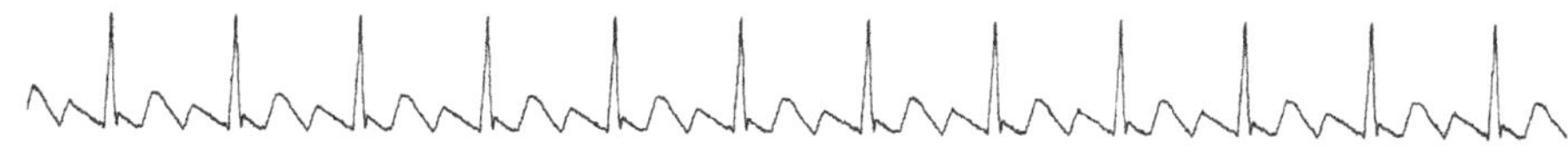

Figure 5.14 Atrial flutter.

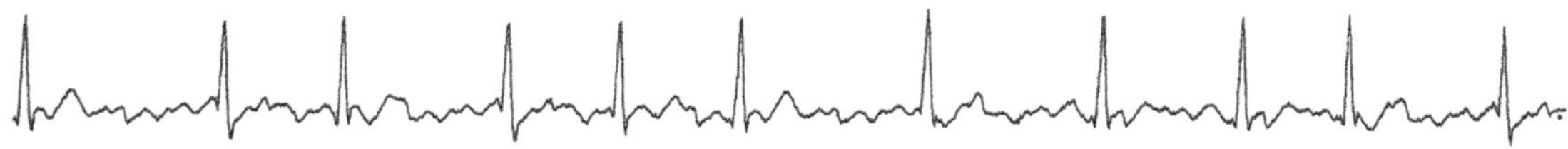

Figure 5.15 Atrial fibrillation

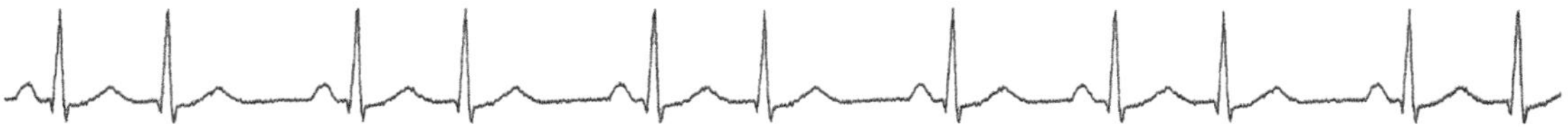

Figure 5.16 AV junctional (nodal) premature beats (ectopics).

of acute disorders as well as WPW syndrome. Digoxin toxicity may cause AF and should be suspected if the ventricular rate is slow, or there is evidence of AV block, with associated ventricular ectopics.

Treatment: In chronic AF, the aim is to control the ventricular rate. Digoxin is often used. In paroxysmal AF, the aim is to restore sinus rhythm following treatment of the primary cause. If there is haemodynamic compromise, cardioversion may be required, but if the AF has lasted more than a few days the patient should be first adequately anticoagulated to reduce the risk of emboli. Amiodarone IV can be used to restore sinus rhythm. Digoxin IV will slow the rate but will not convert the rhythm to sinus rhythm.

8. AV junctional (nodal) premature beats (ectopics) (Figure 5.16):

A premature stimulus arises from the AV node which is conducted simultaneously through the ventricle and retrogradely through the atria. The QRS complex is usually normal.

Aetiology: AV junctional ectopics may occur in healthy people but are most commonly associated with heart disease. They can also be a sign of digoxin toxicity.

Treatment: Management is similar to atrial ectopics.

9. Junctional (nodal) tachycardia (Figure 5.17):

This rapid regular rhythm originating in the AV node has no upright P waves, but inverted P waves may be seen. QRS waves are normal unless there is aberrant conduction. Rate is up to 140 bpm. Differentiation between atrial and junctional tachycardia may be difficult at fast rates.

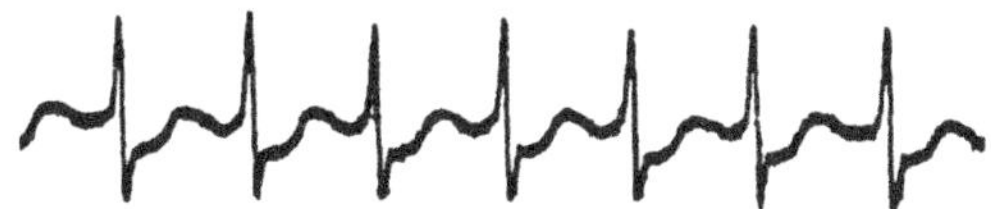

Figure 5.17 Junctional (nodal) tachycardia

Aetiology: This is classified and treated as an SVT. A non-paroxysmal or accelerated junctional rhythm may be caused by digoxin toxicity, myocardial infarction, or myocarditis.

Treatment: As for SVT, if paroxysmal. Discontinuing digoxin treats an accelerated junctional rhythm caused by digoxin toxicity. Correction of any underlying physiological disturbance may be sufficient to terminate the arrhythmia.

10. Junctional (nodal rhythm) (Figure 5.18):

Failure of the SA node to generate impulses will result in the AV node taking over as pacemaker. There are no discernible P waves. The QRS is normal unless there is aberrant conduction. The intrinsic rate is slower (40–70 bpm) and the rhythm is regular.

Aetiology: A junctional rhythm can occur in a normal person. It is usually associated with myocardial infarction or increased vagal tone and occasionally seen with digoxin toxicity.

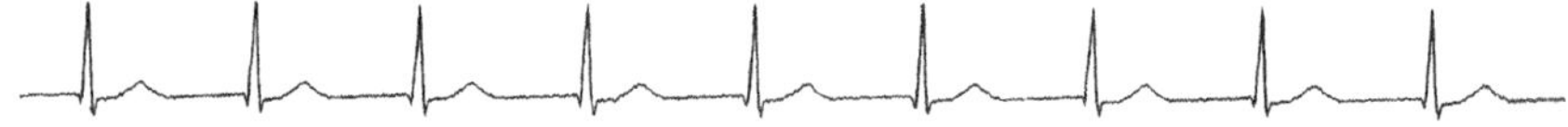

Figure 5.18 Junctional (nodal) tachycardia

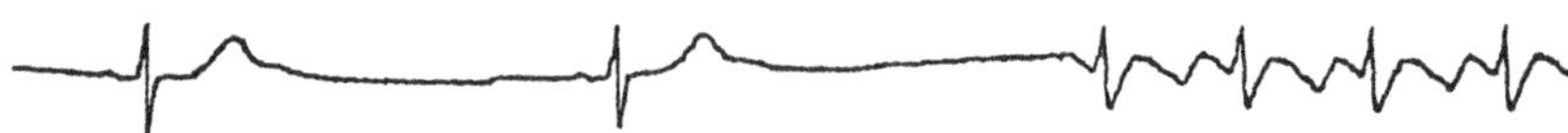

Figure 5.19 Sick sinus syndrome

Treatment: Discontinue digoxin if toxicity is suspected. Treatment is usually only necessary if there are symptoms or haemodynamic compromise. Atropine can be given if excessive vagal tone is suspected. Pacing is rarely needed.

11. Sick sinus syndrome (Figure 5.19):

A variety of disruptions to rhythm occur including sinus bradycardia, sinus arrest, wandering pacemaker (where the origin of the impulse occurs in different parts of the atria), and atrial ectopic beats. These may be accompanied by episodes of rapid atrial arrhythmias, such as AF, atrial flutter, and SVT.

Aetiology: Intrinsic disease of the sinoatrial node and conducting system causes palpitations and fainting episodes (Stokes–Adams attacks). These may be idiopathic in the elderly but can be associated with infarction affecting the atria, rheumatic heart disease, and pericarditis.

Treatment: Permanent pacing is often required, with pharmacological control of tachyarrhythmias if necessary (e.g. with β-blockers).

12. Ventricular premature contractions (ectopics) (Figure 5.20):

A stimulus arises earlier than expected from the Purkinje fibre network in the ventricles. No P wave is present prior to the beat, although an inverted P wave from retrograde conduction may be seen afterwards. The QRS is widened and bizarre in shape with a notch and increased amplitude. A compensatory pause may follow the beat. Bigeminy occurs when each normal beat is accompanied by an ectopic beat. Trigeminy occurs when every second normal beat is followed by an ectopic beat. Multifocal ectopic beats appear as different shaped QRS complexes and arise from different areas within the ventricle.

Aetiology: A common arrhythmia that can occur at any age. It is common in myocardial disease or as a result of increased myocardial irritability (e.g. hypoxia, hypokalaemia, and digoxin toxicity). Ectopic beats are associated with heart disease in the over forties if they are frequent, occur in runs, and are multifocal.

Treatment: Occasional ventricular premature contractions require no treatment. If multifocal, occur in runs, are frequent (>5/min), or occur very close to the apex of the T wave of the previous beat, they may require treatment if the patient is symptomatic. Correction of underlying disorders such as hypokalaemia, digoxin toxicity, and hypoxia is essential.

13. Ventricular tachycardia (Figure 5.21):

A ventricular ectopic focus stimulates a series of rapid and regular beats with no P waves and a bizarrely shaped and widened QRS complex. The rate is 100–220 bpm.

Aetiology: Occurs commonly following myocardial infarction or from digoxin toxicity. The stimulus arises in the Purkinje fibres and may continue

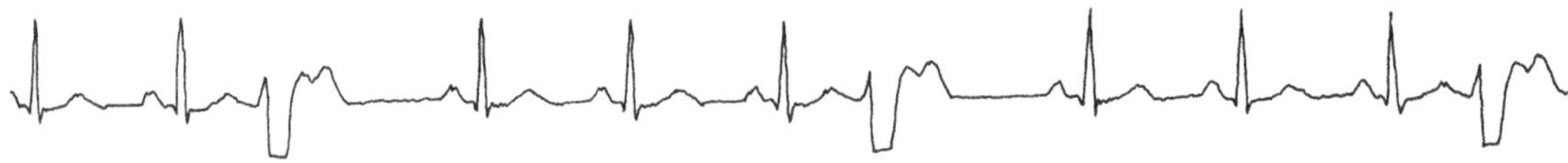

Figure 5.20 Ventricular premature contractions (ectopics).

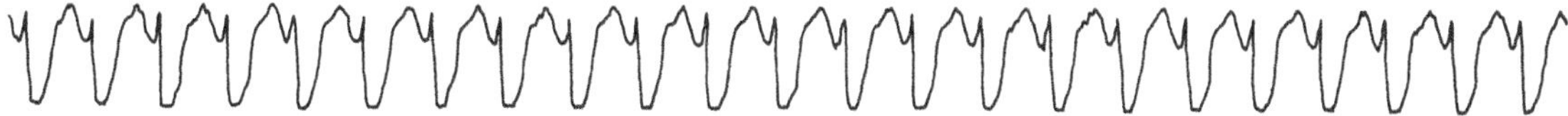

Figure 5.21 Ventricular tachycardia.

as a re-entry mechanism (see later). The fast rate and loss of coordinated atrial contraction into the ventricles produces a severe drop in cardiac output which may require cardiopulmonary resuscitation (CPR).

Treatment: Defibrillation is the treatment of choice if there is haemodynamic deterioration. If the patient is stable, β-blockers or amiodarone IV can be given. Intravenous magnesium may also be helpful. Potassium and magnesium levels should be checked, and other underlying physiological and biochemical disorders corrected.

14. Torsades de pointes (Figure 5.22):

This specific variety of ventricular tachycardia means 'twisting of the points'. The QRS complex is ventricular in origin and broadened, but the axis changes from positive to negative and back again. It is a transitional rhythm between ventricular tachycardia and fibrillation, and is associated with a prolonged Q–T interval.

Aetiology: Development is more likely with a prolonged Q–T interval (>0.44 sec). Precipitating conditions include hypokalaemia, hypocalcaemia, and hypomagnesaemia, or anti-arrhythmic agents, such as disopyramide, which increase the Q–T interval. Prolonged Q–T with subsequent torsades has reported with tricyclic antidepressants and phenothiazines (e.g. haloperidol), as well as with insecticide poisoning.

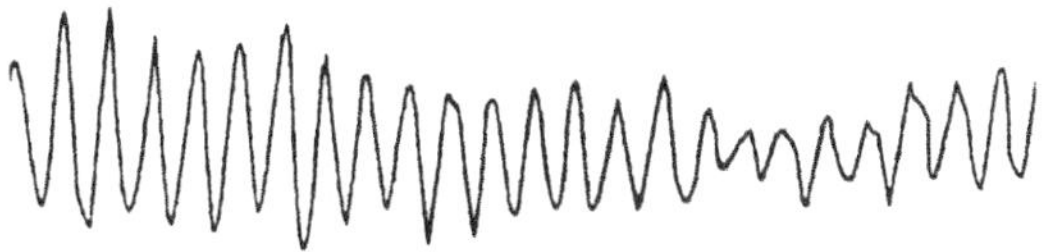

Figure 5.22 Torasdes de pointes.

Treatment: The rhythm should be recognized and treated accordingly, as conventional treatment for VT will cause the condition to worsen. Correction of any underlying electrolyte imbalance and discontinuation of any pharmacological cause is crucial. IV magnesium is now considered the treatment of choice.

15. Ventricular fibrillation (Figure 5.23):

This is rapid, chaotic, and ineffectual contraction of the ventricle, always accompanied by complete loss of cardiac output. Unless CPR is carried out immediately the patient will die.

Aetiology: Associated with ischaemic heart disease, hypoxia, metabolic disturbances, following electrocution, and drug toxicity (e.g. digoxin, tricyclic antidepressant overdose).

Treatment: Immediate defibrillation is the only treatment for VF. Following successful defibrillation the patient may, if needed, be treated with an anti-arrhythmic drug such as a β-blocker or amiodarone to prevent recurrence.

Disorders of impulse conduction

16. First-degree heart block (Figure 5.24):

Delay in impulse conduction occurs at the AV node. The PR interval is >0.20 sec.

Aetiology: First-degree block can occur in normal or diseased hearts. It may be a precursor to second- or third-degree block.

Treatment: First-degree block does not require treatment and is only significant if it precedes second- or third-degree block.

17. Second-degree heart block:

There are two types: Mobitz type I (Wenkebach) and Mobitz type II.

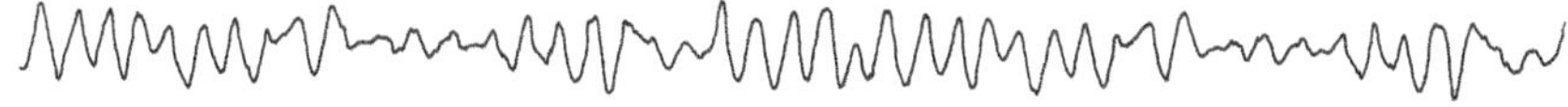

Figure 5.23 Ventricular fibrillation

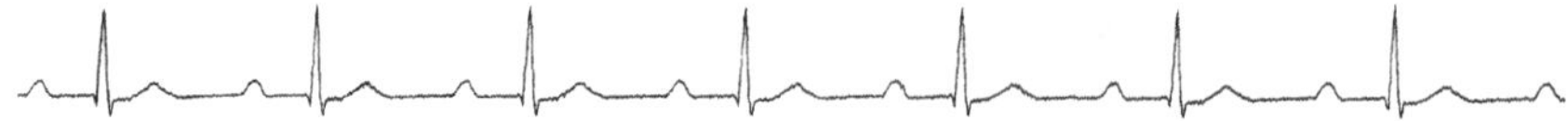

Figure 5.24 First-degree heart block

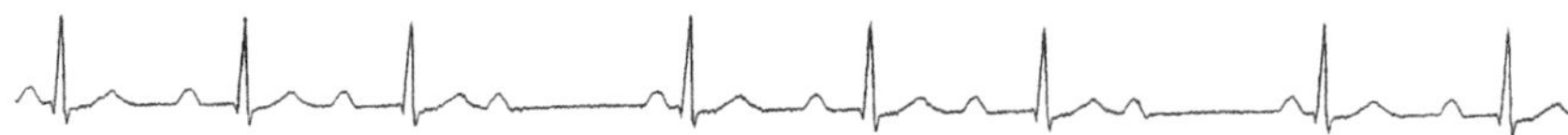

Figure 5.25 Mobitz type I

In Mobitz type I (Wenkebach) (Figure 5.25) a delay at the AV node gradually increases through a series of beats until conduction of the impulse does not occur. The whole process is then repeated. The QRS complex is normal.

Aetiology: Mobitz type I is usually associated with acute reversible conditions and is relatively benign.

Treatment: Only necessary if there is haemodynamic compromise associated with the block.

In Mobitz type II (Figure 5.26), a varying ratio of P waves to QRS complexes is conducted through the AV node (e.g. 2:1, 3:1, etc.). The PR interval in conducted beats remains constant.

Aetiology: Mobitz type II block indicates more severe impairment of AV conduction and is associated with myocardial infarction. It may precede complete heart block.

Treatment: Monitoring is essential but treatment depends on the cardiac output. If this is compromised or the ventricular rate is very slow, treatment is indicated. Atropine or isoprenaline IV may be given. Alternatively, transvenous pacing may be required.

18. Third-degree (complete) heart block (Figure 5.27):

There is a complete block of conduction between atria and ventricles at the AV node. The atrial rate continues at a normal or slightly faster rate but the QRS rate will be slower. There is no relationship between the P wave and the QRS complex. If the QRS originates in the AV node the rate will be 50–60 bpm and the QRS width will be normal. If the QRS originates in the ventricles the rate will be 30–40 bpm with a widened QRS.

Aetiology: Most commonly due to acute myocardial infarction and idiopathic degeneration of the conducting system with age. It can occur following cardiac surgery, particularly after mitral or aortic valve surgery.

Treatment: In anterior myocardial infarction, treatment is urgent as occurrence of complete heart block is associated with more extensive infarction. In other patients, treatment will depend on symptoms and haemodynamic compromise. The definitive treatment is transvenous pacing, although external cardiac pacing can be used for short periods to maintain cardiac output. If this is not available IV atropine or an isoprenaline infusion can be tried.

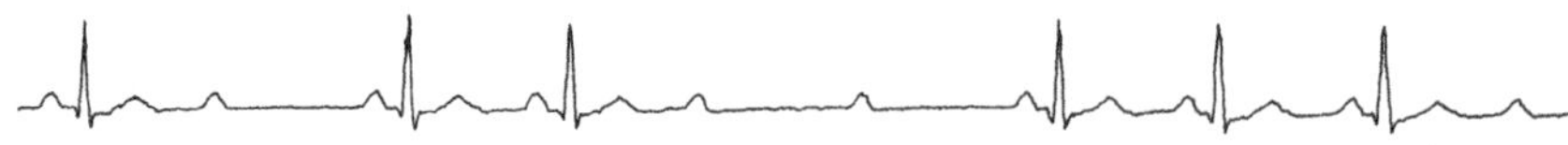

Figure 5.26 Mobitz type II

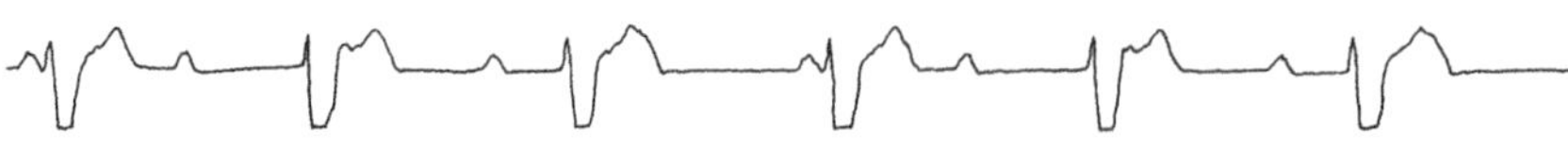

Figure 5.27 Third-degree heart block.

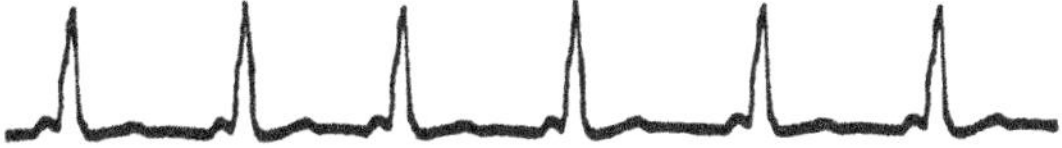

Figure 5.28 Wolff–Parkinson–White syndrome.

19. Wolff–Parkinson–White (WPW) syndrome (Figure 5.28):

This consists of episodes of paroxysmal tachyarrhythmia characterized by a shortened PR interval and widened QRS complex. In the non-tachyarrhythmic state the QRS complex has a notch known as the delta wave which indicates early ventricular stimulation via the accessory conduction pathway that bypasses the AV node. The PR interval is shortened due to rapid conduction through the accessory pathway which, unlike the AV node, does not slow conduction.

Aetiology: Strands of myocardial tissue act as a bridge of conducting tissue across the non-conducting AV ring. This conduction pathway is known as the bundle of Kent. The accessory pathway can support arrhythmias, most commonly AF and paroxysmal SVT.

Treatment: If haemodynamically unstable in AF or paroxysmal SVT, cardioversion should be performed. Amiodarone IV is the drug treatment of choice. Digoxin should be avoided as it lengthens AV nodal block and may increase conduction via the aberrant pathway.

Mechanisms of tachyarrhythmias

Re-entry tachycardias: there are several available routes for impulse conduction. Re-entry is thought to occur under the following circumstances.

- Ischaemia, high potassium levels, and blockage of the Purkinje system produce an area of depressed conduction so stimuli are conducted in only one direction in one of the available routes.
- Conduction is slow so that the normally functioning route is repolarized and available for a second depolarization.

Therefore a stimulus is conducted down the normal conduction route but blocked through the depressed area in that direction. The impulse is then slowly propagated retrogradely through the depressed area in the opposite direction and then restimulates the normal route, which has by now repolarized. Re-entry tachycardias can occur in any area of the conduction system and are probably the cause of various supraventricular and ventricular tachycardias.

Monitoring the Q–T interval

The normal value depends on the heart rate. As it increases, the Q–T interval shortens and vice versa. The formula for correcting the Q–T interval for heart rate (QT_c) is:

$$QT_c = QT/\sqrt{}(R-R\ \text{interval})$$

where QT is the interval from the beginning of the QRS complex to the end of the T wave, and the R–R interval is the time between two successive R waves.

The QT_c is prolonged if it is >0.44 sec. A prolonged QT_c interval is associated with hypokalaemia, hypocalcaemia, hypomagnesaemia, and tricyclic drugs. It can lead to torsades de pointes.

The 12-lead ECG

This is performed in order to:

- make a clinical diagnosis
- monitor changes over time.

The frequency of recording a 12-lead ECG depends on the patient's clinical condition and diagnosis. In the absence of cardiac problems this may be daily or less frequently, while those who have undergone cardiac surgery or have cardiac dysfunction (e.g. myocardial infarction, unstable angina) may require more frequent recordings.

The 12-lead ECG records the flow of current in several planes to obtain a more comprehensive view of the heart's electrical activity than is given by a 3-lead ECG. This is achieved by placing one electrode on each limb and six electrodes on the chest wall. The electrode placed on the right leg acts as an earth and is not an electrical lead.

The electrodes should be placed over positions of least muscle mass to avoid interference from skeletal muscle (i.e. the inside of the wrist and the inner aspect of the ankle). Ideally, electrodes should be in the same position for each serial ECG.

The standard leads (limb leads)

Three major planes of electrical activity can be viewed using the limb leads, termed I, II, and III, which record differences in electrical forces between each of the limb electrodes (Table 5.11).

Table 5.11 The 12-lead ECG

Lead	Electrode 1	Electrode 2
I	RA	LA
II	RA	LL
III	LA	LL
VR	RA	LA and LL
VL	LA	RA and LL
VF	LL	RA and LA

RA, right arm; LA, left arm; LL, left leg.

These views form a hypothetical triangle with the heart at the centre. Electrical current flows between negative and positive poles. When current flows towards a positive pole the ECG shows an upward (positive) deflection, and when it flows away from a positive pole the deflection is downwards (negative).

The complete 12-lead EGG consists of:

- three limb leads—I, II, and III
- three augmented (modified) limb leads termed aVL (augmented view left), aVR (augmented view right), and aVF (augmented view foot or left leg)
- six chest leads—V1, V2, V3, V4, V5, and V6.

Electrodes recording the limb and augmented limb leads

These show the direction of viewing the heart (from electrode 1 to electrode 2); thus each lead will have characteristic upward and downward deflections.

The chest leads

The positions of the chest leads are:

- V1—fourth intercostal space to the right of the sternum
- V2—fourth intercostal space to the left of the sternum
- V3—midway between V2 and V4
- V4—fifth intercostal space mid-clavicular line
- V5—anterior axillary line at same level as V4
- V6—mid-axillary line at same level as V4.

All 12 leads show different electrocardiographic patterns due to the different positions of the electrodes. The direction of deflection depends on the view of the heart in that particular electrical lead. Some waves may change polarity (a normally negative deflection becomes positive) due to pathology. Figure 5.29 shows a normal 12-lead EGG.

The ECG should be analysed for rate, rhythm, axis, P wave, PR interval, QRS complex, QT interval, ST segment, and T wave to enable the diagnosis of:

- abnormal rhythms and conduction
- changes secondary to ischaemic heart disease
- changes secondary to pericardial disease
- changes secondary to metabolic and other diseases
- ventricular hypertrophy.

Axis

This is the sum of ventricular electrical forces during depolarization. Figure 5.30 shows the orientation of the limb leads. The normal heart axis between –30° and + 90° (i.e. towards the left as the left ventricular mass is greater than the right). If the axis lies outside –30° this

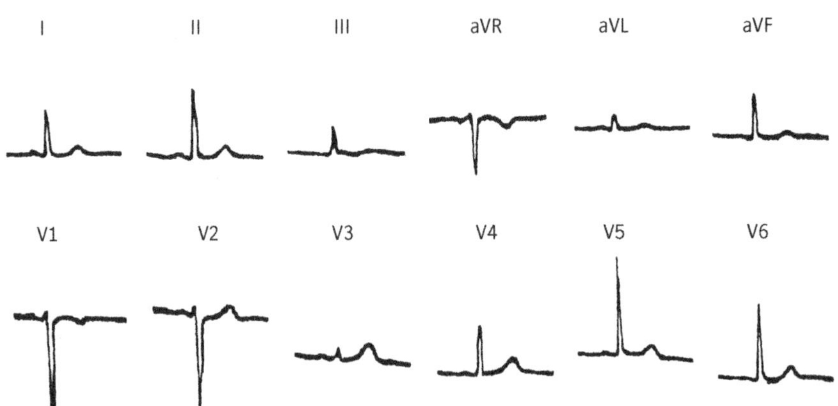

Figure 5.29 Waveform of the 12-lead ECG in a patient with normal heart function

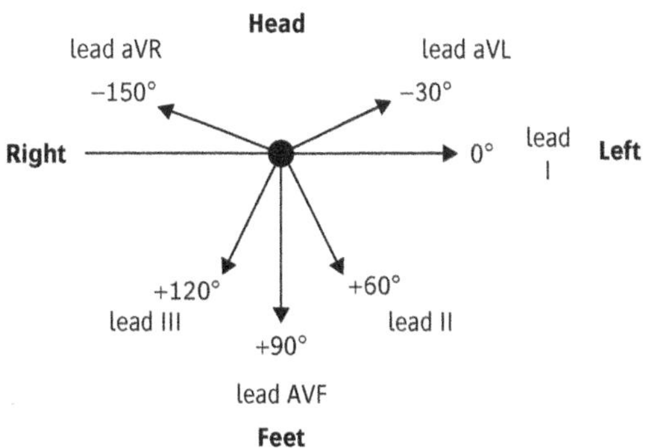

Figure 5.30 Orientation of the limb leads.

is termed left axis deviation, and if greater than +90° it is termed right axis deviation. The axis is calculated by determining the vector of forces between lead I (0°) and lead aVF (+90°) (see Figure 5.31).

Analysis of 12-lead EGG

A variety of disease processes can be assessed from 12-lead EGG analysis.

Changes secondary to ischaemic heart disease: The area of the heart affected by injury, ischaemia, or infarction can be determined by observing which leads show abnormal changes (Table 5.12):

- Changes in the anteroseptal area are indicated by leads V1–V4.
- Changes in the anterolateral area are indicated by leads I, aVL, V5,and V6.

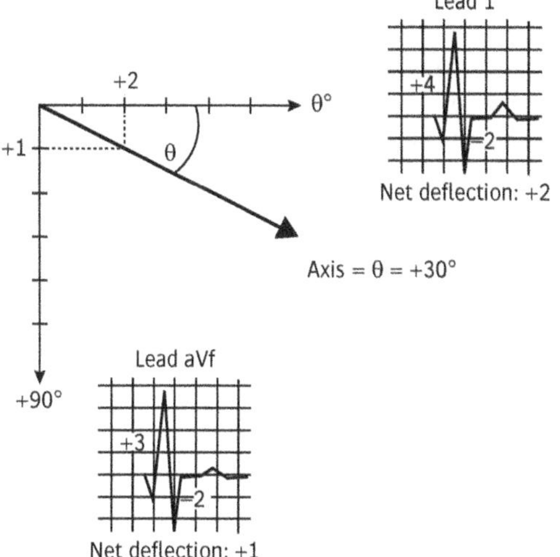

Figure 5.31 Calculation of the axis.

Table 5.12 Changes secondary to ischaemic heart disease

ECG change	Cause
ST segment depression	Myocardial injury/ischaemia
ST segment elevation (convex)	Myocardial injury/ischaemia
Pathological Q wave	Myocardial infarction
T wave inversion	Myocardial injury/ ischaemia/infarction

- Changes in the inferior area are indicated by leads II, III, and aVF.
- Changes in the posterior area are indicated by a mirror-image (i.e. upside-down changes) seen in leads Vl and V2.

Changes secondary to pericardial disease

Concave ST segment elevation and tachycardia may be seen in acute pericarditis, while low voltages (and, occasionally, alternating QRS complexes) may be seen with a large pericardial effusion.

Changes due to ventricular and atrial hypertrophy

Large QRS complexes are suggestive of hypertrophy. This may be normal in adults <35 years old. Left ventricular hypertrophy is present when the sum of the R wave in V5 or V6 plus the S wave in Vl exceeds 35 mm. In right ventricular hypertrophy a 'dominant' R wave is seen in lead Vl (i.e. a large R wave relative to the S wave), but with a normal width QRS complex.

A 'strain pattern' is seen when ST depression and T wave inversion coexist in the appropriate leads and is suggestive of ischaemia in the hypertrophied ventricle.

Changes due to other diseases

ECG changes of pulmonary embolism are those of acute right heart strain and may include:

- sinus tachycardia
- right axis deviation
- 'Sl–Q3–T3'—deep S wave in lead I, pathological Q wave and inverted T wave in lead III
- right ventricular strain
- partial right bundle branch block (i.e. M-shaped QRS complex but width <0.12 s)
- peaked P waves
- atrial fibrillation.

Invasive monitoring

Although invasive monitoring is commonplace on the ICU, the potential value of such techniques must be carefully considered prior to catheter insertion. They can be potentially hazardous due to complications arising either from the insertion. or by remaining in situ. However, they can also provide invaluable information for monitoring disease processes and adjusting therapeutic strategies.

The nurse must be fully aware of the techniques and their potential hazards and complications in order to minimize risk. Each device carries its associated complications, but the very fact of its being invasive means infection is a potential problem. Local policies and practices should be followed for changes of dressings, cannulae, and tubing (including transducers). Routine infection control measures should be instituted. These include:

- effective hand-washing
- the use of a strict aseptic technique when inserting or re-dressing cannulae
- clear semipermeable dressings over cannula sites to allow regular inspection
- minimal disturbance of the dressing; re-dress as necessary rather than routinely
- minimal use of three-way taps to limit potential entry for infection
- labelling lines and transducers with the date and time they were last changed.

Invasive lines should be well secured to prevent accidental removal by the patient or during rolling and turning. Some devices, such as pulmonary artery catheters (with associated cardiac output leads), are quite heavy and the weight will need to be supported by securing the catheter to the pillow or bedding.

Pressure monitoring

Bedside monitors display invasive pressures continuously. These pressures can include systemic arterial, pulmonary artery, and central venous pressures.

Transducers are needed to measure the pressure recorded within the heart or blood vessel and transmitting it to the monitor. Transducers come in varying shapes and forms depending on the manufacturer and the type of monitor used. They are now generally pre-assembled with all the patient tubing attached and are very easy to set up (see Figure 5.32).

In general, transducers are small fluid-filled devices. Tubing from the patient cannula is connected to one side of the transducer. On the other side a giving set is connected to a bag of 0.9% saline solution and kept under continuous pressure (usually 300 mmHg for arterial lines but less for venous lines) to prevent backflow of blood from the patient into the circuit. Adjacent to the transducer is a flushing device which ensures continuous delivery of fluid (3 ml/h) through the patient's cannula and allows the tubing to be manually flushed at any time (such as after taking blood samples). The flushing device keeps the cannula patent.

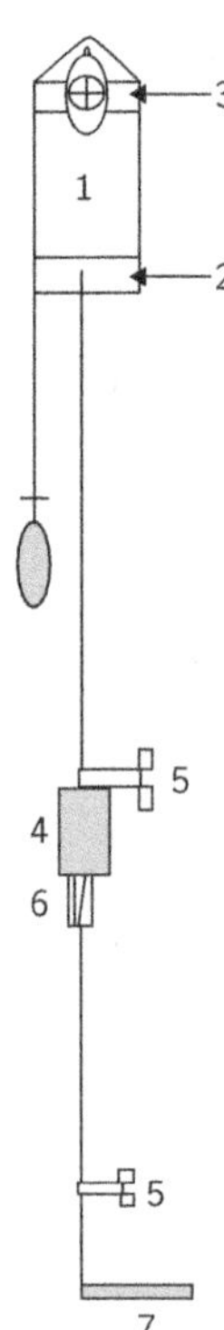

Figure 5.32 Transduced pressure monitoring system: 1, infusion fluid; 2, pressure bag; 3, pressure gauge; 4, transducer; 5, three-way tap; 6, flush device; 7, patient cannula.

Pressure is transmitted from the cannula through the fluid-filled pressure tubing to the transducer. From here it is relayed via an electrical cable to the monitor, where it is usually displayed as both a waveform trace and as a digital readout providing systolic, diastolic, and mean pressure measurements.

There are several points to remember to ensure accurate pressure readings.

- The transducer must always be level with the zero reference point. This is usually the right atrium (mid-axilla). If the patient is moved, the transducer must be realigned.

- The transducer must be calibrated to atmospheric pressure ('zeroed') before use, intermittently while in use (e.g. at the beginning of each shift), and whenever the patient's tubing or transducer is changed or disconnected. This procedure will vary according to the type of monitor being used, but basically entails turning the three-way tap in the circuit 'off' to the patient, thus exposing the transducer to atmospheric pressure (air), and pressing a zero button on the monitor. When the monitor shows a zero reading the three-way tap can be turned back 'on' to the patient and placed at the zero reference point. The transducer will now read an arterial or venous pressure calibrated to atmospheric pressure.
- Only dedicated manometer tubing should be used throughout the system. This is rigid tubing with a low compliance and small diameter. Soft flexible tubing should not be used, as the pressure changes will not be accurately conducted.
- Excessively long tubing or air bubbles in the tubing or transducer may cause a 'dampened' trace with consequent inaccurate readings. Overdamping results in falsely low systolic and falsely high diastolic pressure readings. The presence of three-way taps in the circuit will also 'dampen' the trace, Tubing that is too short will result in an under-damped trace with a systolic overshoot, as may hypertension, vasoconstriction, aortic regurgitation, and hyperdynamic states such as sepsis. An under-damped system will record falsely high systolic pressures and falsely low diastolic pressures.

Blood pressure (BP) measurement

Oscillometry

An automated machine uses a cuff to compress the limb and measures BP by sensing the arterial pulsations (oscillations) as a function of cuff pressure. The sensor on the cuff is placed in the correct position (an arrow on the cuff indicates its placement over an artery) and the cuff is automatically inflated. As the cuff deflates, the arterial pressure becomes equal to the cuff occluding pressure and blood begins to flow through the artery. The oscillations in the artery wall are small, but as the cuff deflates further flow is increased and the amplitude of the oscillations reaches a maximum. As the cuff completely deflates the oscillations lessen. This is due to a reducing resistance to flow as the cuff occluding pressure is now less than the diastolic pressure. The rapid increases and decreases in oscillations correspond to the systolic and diastolic pressures.

To ensure accurate BP recording the correct size of cuff is important. If the cuff is too narrow or applied too loosely the BP will be falsely high, and if it is too wide it will under-read. The bladder width should ideally be 40–50% of upper arm circumference. The bladder length should encircle 80% of the arm. The cuff should be at the level of the heart to maintain a true zero level.

Oscillometry is less useful when used on severely hypotensive patients as the oscillation amplitude may be too small to be accurate.

Intra-arterial cannulation

This allows continuous monitoring of BP and frequent blood sampling without disturbing the patient and avoiding repeated vessel puncture.

The radial, femoral, or dorsalis pedis arteries are the most commonly used. The radial artery is preferred as the hand usually has a good collateral circulation, the artery is near to the skin surface, and the cannula site is easily observed. However, in patients with Raynaud's disease or an inadequate ulnar circulation, hand ischaemia and skin necrosis can occur. The Allen test (occlusion of radial and ulnar arteries to blanch the hand, followed by release of the pressure on the radial artery to check the quality of the collateral circulation provided by the ulnar artery) has been shown to give unreliable results. If in doubt, perform Doppler ultrasound to determine arterial patency.

The femoral artery is frequently cannulated in severely hypotensive patients as the femoral pulse is often the most easily palpable and its superficial location makes it easy to access. However, if blood flow to the limb is compromised, the patient is exposed to a potentially large area of ischaemia. Regular assessment of pedal pulses and skin temperature should be carried out. Since the groin cannot be continually exposed and therefore observed, unseen haemorrhage at this site can have dire consequences. It is imperative that lower alarm limits are set on the monitor and a clear waveform is visible so that any accidental disconnection is discovered immediately. This is not the preferred cannulation site for diabetic patients (who may have poor wound healing and microcirculation problems) or patients with occlusive vascular disease. The risk of infection is also greater.

The dorsalis pedis artery can be used but is small and often difficult to cannulate. It also makes patient mobilization more difficult, and it can be difficult to obtain a good waveform. It should be avoided if possible in patients with peripheral vascular disease or diabetes. Thrombosis can occur, and the toes should be observed for ischaemia. Because of the greater distance from the heart and the smaller vessel lumen, the BP recorded from the dorsalis pedis (and also the radial artery) will be higher than that in the femoral artery, and may not necessarily reflect perfusion pressure in other regions.

Ideally, the brachial artery should not be used except for short-term placement when no other cannulation sites are available/accessible. As it is an end artery, vessel damage/thrombosis at this point may result in loss of blood supply to the forearm. Haematoma formation at the cannula site can result in median nerve compression. Nerve damage and reduced joint mobility can occur, as well as the potential risk of embolization. This site is also uncomfortable for the patient as mobility is reduced.

In summary, whichever artery is chosen:

- there should be a good collateral blood supply to the limb
- it must be easily observable with access for nursing care
- it should not be located in an area prone to contamination or where a wound exists
- it should not be sited in limbs that have vascular prostheses.

The arterial waveform

This reflects the pressure generated in the arterial tree following contraction of the left ventricle after electrical activation. Hence, when the arterial waveform is evaluated in conjunction with the ECG, the electrical activity BP may be associated with a high flow vasodilated state, as seen in sepsis (see Figure 5.33):

1. **Anacrotic notch** This is only seen in central aortic pressure monitoring or in some pathological conditions. During the second phase of ventricular systole there is a pre-systolic rise in pressure (the 'anacrotic notch') which occurs before the opening of the aortic valve.

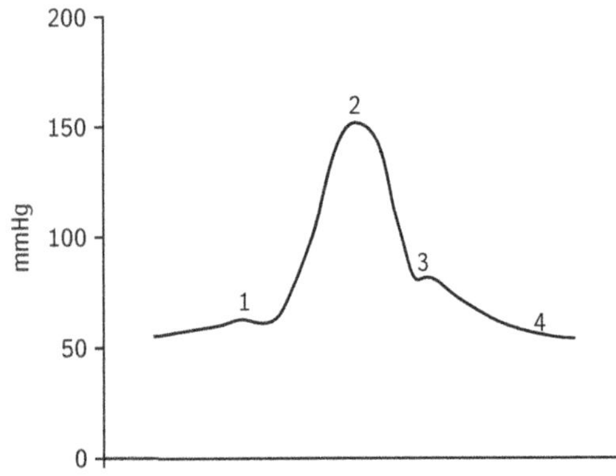

Figure 5.33 The arterial waveform: 1, anacrotic notch; 2, peak systolic pressure; 3, dicrotic notch; 4, diastolic pressure.

2. **Peak systolic pressure** This is the maximum LV systolic pressure. The sharp upward rise in pressure is generated by the outflow of blood from the ventricle into the arterial system.
3. **Dicrotic notch** This reflects aortic valve closure caused by a rise in aortic pressure. When this pressure exceeds that in the LV, the blood attempts to flow backwards, causing the valve to close. On the waveform trace the dicrotic notch marks the end of systole and the onset of diastole. The dicrotic notch is elevated in patients with decreased cardiac output and increased peripheral vascular resistance.
4. **Diastolic pressure** This is related to the degree of vasoconstriction in the arterial system and the diastolic time during the cardiac cycle. During diastole there must be sufficient time for blood to drain into the smaller arteriolar branches. If there is a short diastole, as in a fast heart rate, there is insufficient time for this to occur; consequently, diastolic pressure may be higher.

Pulse pressure (PP)

This is the difference between systolic and diastolic pressure. Factors that affect PP include changes in stroke volume (affecting systolic pressure) or changes in vascular compliance (affecting diastolic pressure).

Mean arterial pressure (MAP)

Most monitors compute MAP from the arterial waveform as the average pressure in the arterial system during one complete cycle of systole and diastole. At normal heart rates, systole usually requires one-third of the cardiac cycle time and diastole two-thirds; this is reflected in the equation for calculating MAP:

$$MAP = DBP + \frac{SBP - DBP}{3}$$

where SBP is systolic pressure and DBP is diastolic pressure.

Observation of the arterial waveform can provide useful clinical information.

1. **Atrial fibrillation** The characteristic rate and rhythm irregularity is reflected on the pressure monitor by variable amplitudes of the arterial waveform. This equates to the variable stroke volumes produced as a result of altered diastolic filling times. A 12-lead ECG is needed to make a firm diagnosis as multiple supraventricular ectopics can mimic the irregular rhythm.
2. **Pulsus alternans** There is a regular alternating of peak systolic pressure amplitude with the patient in

sinus rhythm. This is classically seen in patients with left ventricular failure.

3. **Aortic stenosis** This produces a narrow pulse pressure since the systolic pressure is lower and the slowed ventricular ejection through the stenotic valve causes a delayed systolic peak. The dicrotic notch is not well defined as the valve leaflets close abnormally at the onset of diastole.
4. **Aortic regurgitation** This causes a wide pulse pressure and (usually) a higher peak systolic pressure because the left ventricle receives more blood as it backflows through the incompetent valve during diastole.

Normal respiration can cause changes in amplitude of systolic pressure due to altered intrathoracic pressure. During inspiration in the spontaneously breathing person, intrathoracic pressure is lower (i.e. more negative), thereby causing a pooling of blood in the pulmonary vasculature. Thus less blood reaches the left side of the heart with peak systolic pressures being 3–10 mmHg lower. At expiration, blood that had pooled in the pulmonary bed is shunted to the left side of the heart, increasing LV filling volumes and causing a higher peak systolic pressure. The opposite is seen with mechanical positive pressure ventilation.

'Pulsus paradoxus' is the term used when the difference in peak systolic pressure is >10 mmHg between inspiration and expiration. This is simply an accentuation of normal. An exaggerated swing in systolic pressure over the respiratory cycle is seen on the monitor. Causes include pericardial disease (e.g. pericardial tamponade) which impedes ventricular filling, exaggerated inspiration by the patient, or pathological conditions causing gross changes in intrathoracic pressure during respiration (e.g. asthma). The commonest cause of an exaggerated 'respiratory swing' in the ICU patient is hypovolaemia, particularly when there are concurrently high airway pressures. Pulse pressure variation and stroke volume variation are described in more detail later.

Specific nursing care

Safety

Accidental disconnection can result in considerable blood loss unless detected immediately. For this reason the cannula site should always be visible (unless the femoral artery is used). Alarm limits (particularly the lower limit) must be set on the monitor; this will allow disconnection to be recognized immediately. This is essential if the femoral artery is used, as the site will not be continuously visible.

All connections within the circuit should be Luer locked and firmly connected. A loose connection can cause loss of pressure within the circuit, backflow of blood from the patient, and blood loss at the connection site.

Inadvertent administration of drugs can have dire consequences and arterial lines must be labelled clearly to avoid confusion with venous lines.

Limb perfusion

Perfusion distal to the cannula site must be observed regularly. Occlusion of the artery by a thrombus or adjacent haematoma can severely reduce blood flow to the area supplied by that vessel. *If the limb becomes cold, white, or painful, inform senior medical staff immediately.* The cannula should be removed and circulation assessed manually by capillary refill or the use of Doppler to identify pulsatile flow. If collateral circulation is good, the limb may be saved, but there is a danger, particularly if the brachial artery has been used, that circulation may not be restored. Vascular and/or radiological intervention may be needed.

Arterial spasm can also result in blanching and pain in the limb. This can be caused by very cold and frequent administrations of flush solution or accidental injection of a drug into the cannula. The cannula should be removed. The other limb can be warmed to encourage reflex vasodilatation, but the affected limb should not be warmed directly as this increases its metabolic rate. In the absence of a restored circulation, it may hasten and worsen the ischaemia. For accidental intra-arterial drug administration the cannula should be flushed vigorously using the flushing device. Another treatment option for persisting arterial spasm is to inject papaverine intra-arterially (see also Box 5.3).

Complications of intra-arterial cannulation

Specific complications have already been mentioned. In addition to thrombus formation, embolization, infection, and exsanguination due to disconnection, the following are also recognized complications:

- accidental intra-arterial injection of drugs
- air embolus (from air within the flush system)
- arteriovenous fistula
- pain
- aneurysm or false aneurysm formation
- local haematomas
- necrosis of skin and digits.

Removal of the cannula

When the catheter is removed, digital pressure should be applied for as long as necessary to achieve haemostasis. Assess the peripheral circulation, as thrombosis can occur after removal.

Box 5.3 Summary of problems associated with arterial cannulae

Over-damped trace

This causes a widened slurred waveform, and underestimates the systolic BP and overestimates the diastolic BP.

Causes

- Air bubbles in the circuit.
- Compliant tubing.
- Catheter kinks.
- Blood clot or fibrin in the catheter.
- Poor position of the limb causing the tip of the catheter to lie against the vessel wall.
- No fluid or low pressure in the infusion bag.

Action

- Inflate pressure bag to 300 mmHg, and check that there is sufficient infusion fluid.
- Withdraw blood and then flush the catheter.
- A 'square wave' test can be performed by opening the continuous flush valve for a few seconds and then releasing it. A square wave should be seen on the monitor, which will return to the baseline waveform within a few oscillations.
- Ensure that there are no air bubbles in the tubing by disconnecting the tubing from the catheter and flushing through to expel air before reconnecting.
- If necessary change the transducer.
- Remove any excess taps from the circuit.

Under-damped trace

This causes a narrow peaked waveform and overestimates the systolic BP and underestimates the diastolic BP.

Causes

- Long stiff tubing, increased vascular resistance.

Action

- Remove long lengths of tubing—the optimal length is 1.2 m.

No arterial waveform

This causes a straight line on the monitor.

Causes

- The taps to the patient or transducer are turned off.
- The catheter is disconnected from the tubing at the catheter connection, the three-way taps, or the transducer.
- The catheter tip is against the wall of the vessel.
- Asystole.

Action

- Ensure that all the taps to the transducer and patient are turned on.
- Check the catheter site and reconnect immediately if disconnected.
- Manipulate the catheter/limb to achieve a waveform.
- Check the ECG monitor and institute CPR immediately if there is no cardiac output.

Backflow of blood from the catheter towards the transducer

Causes

- The pressure bag is inflated at below the patient's BP.
- Loose tap connection or disconnection within the circuit.

Action

- Inflate pressure bag to 300mmHg.
- Check all connections are secure.

Central venous pressure (CVP) or right atrial pressure (RAP) measurement

To monitor CVP, a catheter is usually inserted via the internal jugular or subclavian veins. Long lines inserted via the femoral or brachial veins can also be used. The tip of the catheter does not need to lie inside the right atrium but should be within one of the larger veins leading to the heart inside the thoracic cavity. The CVP at this point equals the RAP which, in turn, equals the RV end-diastolic (filling) pressure. The pressure within the right atrium does not necessarily reflect either intravascular volume status or left heart pressures. Therefore it has limitations in the acute stages of critical illness. However, the access into a large vein also enables the infusion of hypertonic solutions, solutions that are irritant to peripheral veins, and drugs that require a rapid effect.

Single-, double-, triple-, and quadruple-lumen catheters are available. Multiple-lumen catheters are particularly useful as they allow dedicated lumens for drug infusions, especially vasoactive drugs, separate infusions of fluids that should not be mixed with others (such as total parenteral nutrition, sodium bicarbonate), and the bolus administration of drugs without inadvertent flushing of other drug infusions.

The catheter is inserted under sterile conditions, usually by the Seldinger technique. An introducer (a large bore needle or cannula) is inserted into the vessel, a flexible wire is fed into the vein via the introducer, and the introducer is then withdrawn completely. The catheter is then inserted over the wire to a satisfactory depth (usually 15–20 cm for jugular or subclavian lines) and the wire is removed.

The catheter position is usually confirmed by X-ray before drugs or infusion fluids are given. The tip position should be ascertained, and complications such as pneumothorax excluded. Ultrasound guidance is increasingly being recommended as standard practice, and should be particularly considered in anatomically difficult patients (e.g. those with a short fat neck) or after previous failed attempts. There must be an easy withdrawal of blood from all catheter lumens.

When the correct position is confirmed, a transducer system or giving set can be attached and drugs or infusions administered as necessary.

Potential complications associated with the insertion of a CVP catheter

1. **Arrhythmias** These may occur during insertion, especially when the introducer guidewire makes contact with the tricuspid valve or the catheter is inserted too far. If this occurs, the wire or catheter should be withdrawn several centimetres. Rarely, drugs or cardioversion are needed.
2. **Pneumo/haemothorax** This results from accidental pleural puncture during the procedure. Haemodynamic and respiratory status must be monitored closely during and after insertion. The post-insertion chest X-ray should be carefully examined. Not only may the patient be compromised if a pneumothorax is present, but if fluids and drugs are infused into the pleural space a potentially disastrous situation can result. A consequent pleural effusion may cause respiratory deterioration while drugs and fluids may be ineffective as they have not entered the systemic circulation. The catheter must be removed immediately; pleural aspiration/drainage may be required while supportive respiratory care is given.
3. **Haematoma caused by trauma to the vein and/or surrounding tissue** Observe the site for bleeding, bruising, and swelling. An artery may be accidentally punctured by the introducer while attempting insertion. If this is known to have occurred, particular attention must be focused on the site to identify bleeding or swelling. Prolonged direct pressure may be necessary to stop bleeding, although this cannot be achieved if the subclavian artery has been punctured. Occasionally, clotting products and even thoracotomy are necessary to control excess bleeding.
4. **Catheter in incorrect position** Occasionally, the catheter may follow a path away from the heart towards the head or down the arm. This will not give an accurate reading of CVP, and rapid fluid infusions may cause discomfort. The catheter should be repositioned.
5. **Air embolus** This may occur if the catheter is not properly connected to the appropriate tubing, or if one of the portals or three-way taps is left 'open to air' and the patient is making spontaneous breathing efforts (negative intrathoracic pressure sucking the air in). The catheter and tubing must be primed with fluid prior to insertion.

Measuring the CVP

This can be done using a transducer system (see Figure 5.32) or manually using a manometer. The latter method is now uncommon within the ICU setting as it is less accurate. Manual measurement allows only intermittent recordings to be made and requires a fluid-filled manometer tube to be connected to the catheter. The manometer is aligned so that the point on the scale of the manometer levelled with the right atrium of the

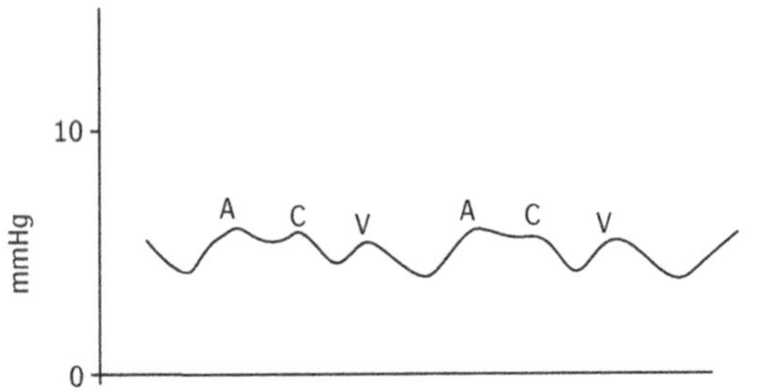

Figure 5.34 The right atrial waveform (A, C, and V waves).

patient is regarded as zero. The manometer is filled with fluid from a bag of normal saline or 5% glucose to a level well above the expected CVP. The manometer tap is then turned so that it is open to the patient. The fluid level falls until it rests at a level that represents the CVP. The reading is made from an adjoining scale. The fluid level in the manometer should gently rise and fall with respiration.

A transduced catheter will give a continuous display of CVP on a monitor. The waveform should show small undulations reflecting changes in pressure within the right atrium/large thoracic vein during the cardiac cycle (see Figure 5.34). Excessive undulations are seen with tricuspid regurgitation or if the tip is within the right ventricle.

The normal range for CVP is 3–6 mmHg in a healthy person. Any increase in intrathoracic pressure, such as positive pressure ventilation or positive end-expiratory pressure, will increase the CVP measured relative to atmospheric pressure. The juxtacardiac pressure (i.e. CVP minus intrathoracic pressure) may be considerably lower. Thus hypovolaemia can be camouflaged by a seemingly normal or high CVP, especially in the presence of concurrently high intrathoracic pressures, or when there is intense vasoconstriction which will also affect the venous system.

The right atrial pressure waveform has three characteristic positive deflections corresponding to the electrical events of the ECG.

1. **A wave**: reflects right atrial contraction and follows the P wave on the ECG. The descent after this represents atrial relaxation. An elevated A wave may be associated with right ventricular failure or tricuspid stenosis.
2. **C wave**: represents tricuspid valve closure and follows the QRS on the EGG tracing. The distance A–C should be the same as the P–R interval.

Table 5.13 Conditions affecting the CVP

Increased values	Decreased values
Right ventricular failure Pericardial tamponade Fluid overload Pulmonary hypertension Triscuspid regurgitation Pulmonary stenosis Peripheral vasoconstriction (e.g. cold, excess norepinephrine) Superior vena caval obstruction	Hypovolaemia Peripheral vasodilatation (e.g. sepsis, regional analgesia, sympathetic dysfunction)

3. **V wave**: represents the pressure generated to the right atrium by the contracting right ventricle despite the tricuspid valve being shut. It corresponds to the latter half of the T wave on the ECG. An elevated V wave is associated with tricuspid regurgitation.

Table 5.13 summarizes conditions that affect the CVP.

Removal of the CVP catheter

To reduce the risk of an air embolism the patient should lie flat or, if their condition allows, with the head tipped down when the catheter is withdrawn. If the patient is breathing spontaneously ask them to take a deep breath in and hold it. Gently withdraw the catheter while applying direct pressure with sterile gauze. Tell the patient to breathe normally after the catheter is removed. In the ventilated patient remove the catheter at end-inspiration. After removal apply direct manual pressure and when bleeding has stopped apply a transparent occlusive dressing over the site.

Pulmonary artery catheterization

In many critically ill patients, particularly those with pulmonary disease or isolated right or left heart dysfunction, the measurement of right atrial pressure gives no true indication of the function of the left side of the heart. If determinants of cardiac function (see later in this chapter) can be known and manipulated, better targeted treatment strategies can be instituted. This can be achieved invasively using a pulmonary artery catheter.

The pulmonary artery catheter

This catheter measures (or derives) a range of intracardiac and pulmonary artery pressures, vascular resistances, and cardiac output.

The standard pulmonary artery catheter consists of three or four lumens, is 110 cm long, and is marked in

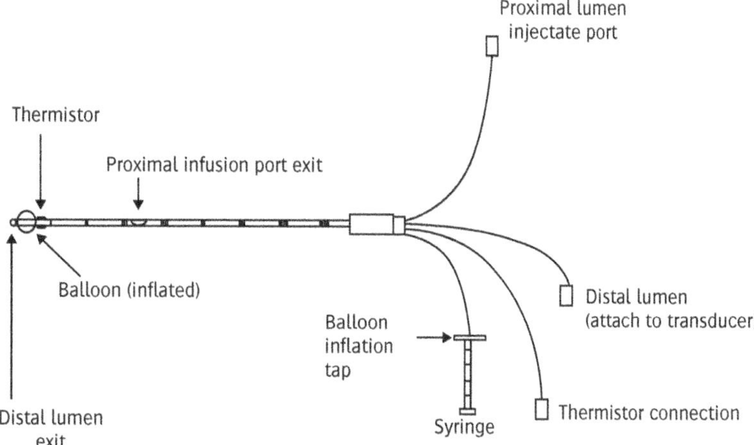

Figure 5.35 The standard pulmonary artery catheter.

10 cm increments to aid placement (see Figure 5.35). Various modifications include:

- extra lumens for drug/fluid administration
- thermistor and computer connector for cardiac output measurement
- continuous mixed venous oxygen saturation
- a pacing wire or external electrodes for temporary pacing
- measurement of right ventricular volume and ejection fractions

1. **The proximal lumen** opens 30 cm from the catheter tip. Thus when the tip is in the pulmonary artery in an adult, the opening of the proximal lumen lies within the right atrium. It is used to inject fluid for thermodilution cardiac output measurements, to monitor right atrial pressure, and for drug/fluid infusions.
2. **The distal lumen** runs the entire length of the catheter, opening at the catheter tip in the pulmonary artery. It is connected to a transducer which continually monitors pulmonary artery pressure and permits measurement of the wedge pressure. During catheter insertion it can measure all right intracardiac pressures as it is advanced through the heart. Blood samples can be withdrawn from this lumen to obtain blood. Blood withdrawn from the PA or RV outflow tract is known as 'mixed venous' blood (i.e. where blood from the inferior vena cava (IVC) and superior vena cava (SVC) are well mixed).
3. **The thermistor connection** connects the thermistor to the monitor cable to enable core and injectate fluid temperatures to be detected.
4. **The thermistor** lies 4 cm from the catheter tip and measures core blood temperature. Two insulated wires run the length of the catheter to end at the thermistor connection.
5. **The balloon inflation lumen** is used to inflate and deflate the balloon near the catheter tip to assist insertion ('flotation'), and also for recording the pulmonary artery wedge pressure. A 1.5 ml capacity syringe is attached at this point and a tap allows the lumen to be turned off to the syringe when not in use. Adult catheters accommodate the full 1.5 ml of air in the balloon, and this should be inflated only while the wedge pressures are being measured and then deflated immediately. Otherwise the pulmonary artery branch that the catheter sits in may be occluded for too long, and this may cause a pulmonary infarct. Over-inflation by injection of extra volumes may result in balloon rupture.

Insertion 1 the catheter

The most common insertion sites are the internal jugular and subclavian veins. The external jugular, antecubital, and femoral veins can also be used, but it is considerably more difficult to 'float' the catheter into a correct position from these sites.

Before insertion, all lumens of the catheter are flushed with normal saline solution, and the integrity of the balloon is checked by inflating it with 1.5 ml of air. The balloon should be seen to inflate evenly and symmetrically. A sterile sleeve adapter is placed over the catheter before insertion and this allows later manipulation while keeping the enclosed catheter portion sterile.

The catheter is inserted under strict aseptic conditions. Using the Seldinger technique, a larger size introducer cannula is first inserted into the vessel and the pulmonary artery catheter is then passed through a self-sealing valve at the top of the introducer into the vessel itself.

The distal lumen of the catheter is connected to the transducer and, by observing the monitor during placement, the location of the catheter tip can be determined by changes in waveform and pressure.

The catheter is advanced, with the balloon deflated, until it is beyond the end of the introducer cannula; it can then be inflated. If the internal jugular or subclavian veins are used, the catheter tip should enter the right atrium at 15–20 cm (femoral vein distance is 30 cm). The characteristic right atrial (RA) waveform will be seen at this point (see Figure 5.36).

The catheter is advanced until a right ventricular (RV) waveform is displayed on the monitor, and the ventricular systolic and diastolic pressures are noted. This should be achieved within 10–15 cm of entering the right atrium. Failing this, the balloon should be deflated, the catheter withdrawn, and the procedure repeated until the RV waveform is seen. If the RV is not entered, the catheter may advance down the inferior vena cava or into the coronary sinus (which may give the impression of a 'wedged' trace achieved well before the expected 50 cm insertion distance).

The catheter is further advanced, through the pulmonary valve, into the pulmonary artery where a change in waveform occurs (a rise in diastolic pressure). This point will be approximately 40–45 cm from the insertion site if the internal jugular vein is used.

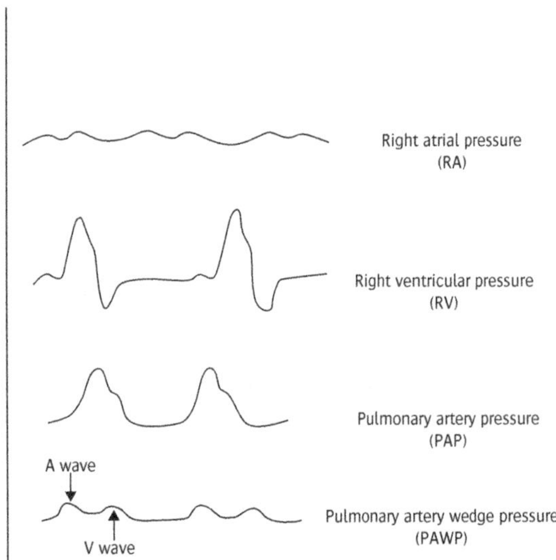

Figure 5.36 Pressure waveform characteristics during insertion of the pulmonary artery catheter.

The catheter is then advanced a further 5–10 cm until it is in a 'wedge' or occluded position. If the catheter is not wedged at this insertion depth, there may be some coiling in the right ventricle. The balloon should not be left inflated for more than 15 sec and a distinct pulmonary artery waveform should always be seen on the monitor.

Waveform characteristics

1. **Right ventricular pressure** The waveform shows tall upright peaks corresponding to ventricular systole. The baseline corresponds to ventricular diastolic pressure which is similar to RA pressure because of the low resistance across the tricuspid valve. Arrhythmias can occur as the catheter is passed through the RV due to irritation of the ventricle by the catheter tip or by its passage through the tricuspid valve. If ventricular ectopics occur, one can continue with the procedure, but if ventricular tachycardia occurs the catheter should be withdrawn from the ventricle. This normally self-corrects, though an anti-arrhythmic drug may be necessary if it recurs on reinsertion.
2. **Pulmonary artery pressure** Rapid ejection of blood from the RV into the PA represents the pulmonary artery systolic pressure (PASP). Since the pulmonary valve is open at this point, PASP equals the RV systolic pressure. At the end of systole the PA pressure falls and the pulmonary valve closes, creating a dicrotic notch on the waveform. The PA diastolic pressure is usually 5–10 mmHg higher than the right ventricular diastolic pressure.
3. **Pulmonary artery wedge pressure (PAWP)** When the balloon is inflated in a branch of the pulmonary artery, it occludes flow completely. Thus all influences on pressure measured at the catheter tip resulting from flow from the right side of the heart are removed. The pressure at the catheter tip therefore reflects only the pressure ahead of it. Assuming an open circuit through the pulmonary vasculature and into the left heart, the LV end-diastolic pressure equals the left atrial pressure, the pulmonary venous pressure, and the pulmonary capillary pressure. The pulmonary artery wedge (or occlusion) pressure is thus a good reflection of the LV end-diastolic pressure, except in certain circumstances. The PAWP waveform is characteristic of the pressure changes within the left atrium. Small A and V waves can be distinguished which represent left atrial and left ventricular systole. The pressure in the left atrium is usually slightly higher than in the right atrium and slightly less (1–3 mmHg) than the PA diastolic

pressure. PAWP is measured at the end of the A wave (i.e. at the end of ventricular diastole, and at the end of expiration). At this point, the intrathoracic pressure is closest to barometric pressure against which the pressure transducer is zeroed.

Measuring the PAWP

- *Slowly* inflate the balloon until the characteristic flattened waveform is seen on the monitor. The balloon is now occluding blood flow and is said to be 'wedged' (Figure 5.37).
- Stop inflating as soon as this waveform is seen.
- Freeze the monitor screen if the monitor has this facility. If not, read the wedge pressure from the monitor display; if the patient is mechanically ventilated, the lowest value should be taken as this corresponds to the PAWP at the end of expiration.
- Deflate the balloon rapidly. The balloon should not be left inflated for more than 15 sec.
- If a screen freeze facility is available, ascertain the wedge pressure by moving the cursor control on the monitor to the correct position on the waveform (see Figure 5.37).

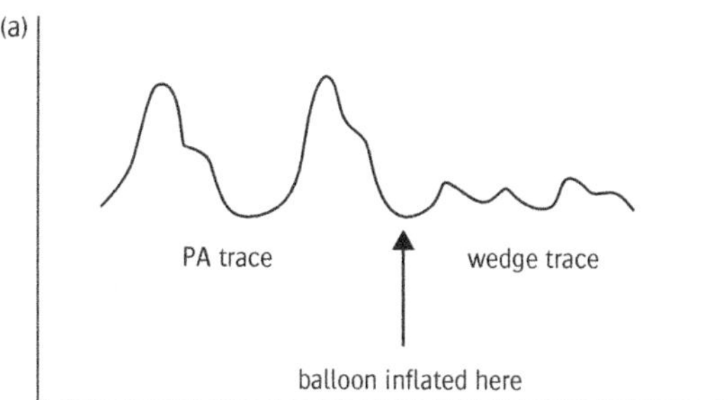

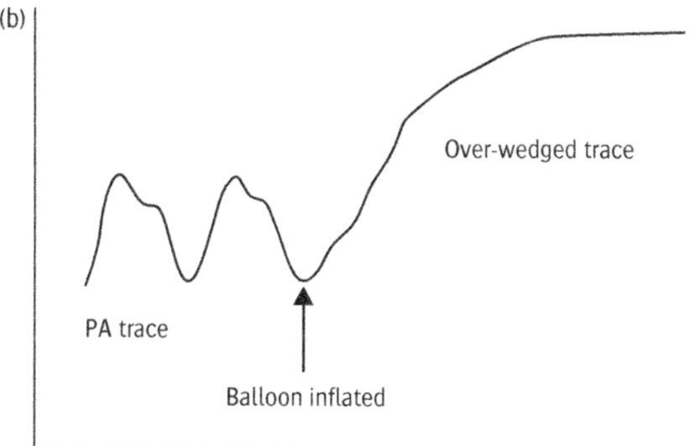

Figure 5.37 The pulmonary artery wedge trace: (a) waveform showing a wedge trace; (b) waveform showing an over-wedged trace caused by over-inflation of the balloon.

- Unfreeze the screen to restore the continuous pulmonary artery waveform.
- Ensure that a normal pulmonary artery waveform is present.

Special points:

- Do not use >1.5 ml of air in the balloon as there is a risk of rupture of the balloon or the blood vessel. If <1.2 ml of air is required to obtain the wedged waveform, the catheter tip is too far advanced. As this also carries an increased risk of pulmonary artery rupture, the balloon should be deflated and the catheter withdrawn slightly.
- The catheter is 'over-wedged' if the trace rises sharply while the balloon is being inflated. This is due to tramsmission of the high pressure within the over-inflated balloon to the transducer (see Figure 5.37). If this occurs when the balloon is inflated with <1.2 ml air, the catheter tip is situated in a small vessel; the balloon should be deflated *immediately* and the catheter withdrawn to a more proximal position.
- Inflation time must be kept to a minimum and the balloon should not remain inflated for more than 15 sec (approximately two to three cycles of respiration).
- Never flush the catheter when the balloon is inflated.
- Never inject fluid into the inflation port.

The correct wedge pressure can readily be achieved in a patient who is mechanically ventilated, but it is more difficult to gain accurate readings in patients who are breathing spontaneously (with or without ventilatory assistance), particularly if deep breaths are being taken as this may result in large 'respiratory swings' on the monitor.

During spontaneous respiration the PA and PAWP both fall during inspiration (i.e. as the intrathoracic pressure becomes more negative) and rise with expiration. All pressures are recorded at the end of expiration (i.e. closest to atmospheric pressure); therefore this is just before the pressures start to fall on the waveform trace. The opposite occurs in ventilated patients because positive pressure ventilation causes intrathoracic pressure to increase with inspiration, increasing PA and PAWP. During exhalation the pressures fall. Thus, in a ventilated patient, readings are made just before the trace on the waveform begins to rise (see Figure 5.38).

There are certain conditions where PAWP does not accurately reflect LVEDP. The PAWP is greater than left ventricular end-diastolic pressure (LVEDP) in:

- greatly raised intrathoracic pressure
- pulmonary venous obstruction
- mitral stenosis
- left atrial myxoma.

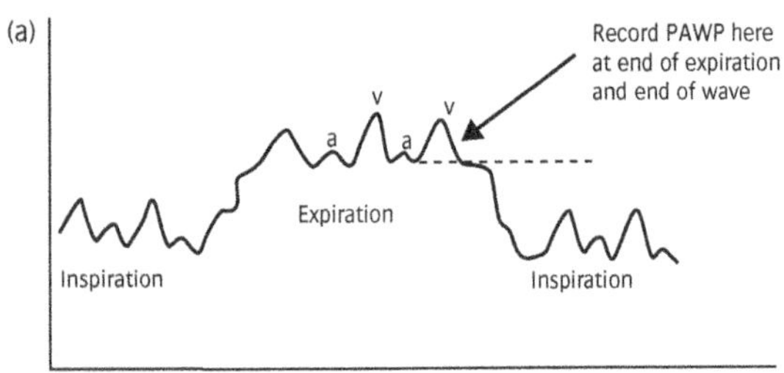

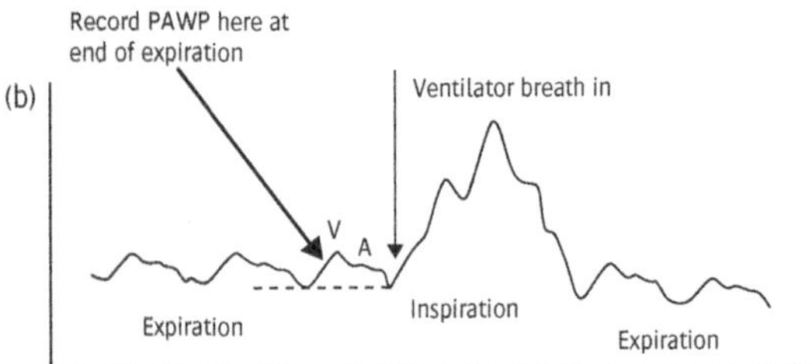

Figure 5.38 Where to measure the PAWP: (a) in a patient breathing spontaneously; (b) in a mechanically ventilated patient.

Catheter position in the pulmonary artery

The catheter tip should be located in a main branch of the pulmonary artery. Changes in tip position can cause potential harm. The catheter may migrate into a more distal branch of the pulmonary artery when the balloon is deflated, causing it to be partially or completely wedged. This can be identified by the characteristic wedged tracing on the waveform. The catheter must not remain in this position because of the potential risk of pulmonary artery occlusion or rupture and must be repositioned, usually by withdrawing it by 1–2 cm.

Occasionally, the catheter tip may slip back into the RV, giving a ventricular waveform tracing. The tip may cause irritability to the RV and predispose to arrhythmias (ventricular fibrillation, tachycardia, or ectopics). If this occurs, the balloon should be inflated and re-floated into the pulmonary artery.

The position of the catheter tip in the lung is important for accurate PAWP recordings. The lungs have three physiological ('West') zones of blood flow depending on the interaction of alveolar, pulmonary, arterial, and venous pressures (West *et al.* 1964). To reflect left atrial pressure the tip should lie in zone III where flow is continuous. If it is sited in zones I or II, alveolar pressures are reflected and may give a spuriously high reading of LVEDP. These zones are not fixed anatomically and will change gravitationally with body position. Hypovolaemia and positive end-expiratory pressure (PEEP) will increase the proportions of zones I and II. Thus the zone in which the catheter tip is located may change with body position, hypovolaemia, or PEEP. Paradoxically, therefore, the wedge pressure may rise with hypovolaemia. The correct position can be identified on a lateral chest X-ray where the catheter tip should be below the level of the left atrium. An alternative means of confirming a satisfactory zone III position is to increase the level of PEEP temporarily (e.g. by 5 cmH_2O) and check that the wedge pressure does not increase by at least half the increase in PEEP (e.g. 2–3 mmHg).

- **Zone I** The alveolar pressure is greater than the pulmonary arterial and venous pressures. Therefore there is no blood flow from the pulmonary capillary beds.
- **Zone II** The alveolar pressure exceeds the pulmonary venous pressure but the arterial pressure is high enough to allow some blood flow. PAWP recordings will be less accurate than if the tip is in zone III. PEEP may increase alveolar pressure, causing zone II to be similar to zone I.
- **Zone III** The pulmonary venous pressure exceeds the alveolar pressure and all pulmonary capillaries are open.

Specific complications of pulmonary artery catheterization

- Pulmonary artery rupture, or perforation due to the catheter tip, or over-inflation of the balloon. This is particularly important in patients with pulmonary hypertension and the elderly as they have less distensible arteries.
- Rupture of the right atrium.
- Air embolism due to rupture of the balloon.
- Ventricular arrhythmias: these can occur on insertion or removal of the catheter, or if the tip migrates back into the right ventricle.
- Pulmonary infarction: this results from loss of blood supply to a branch of the pulmonary artery due to the catheter spontaneously wedging if the catheter migrates forwards, or if the balloon remains inflated for long periods.
- Valvular damage: this can occur if the balloon is inflated while the catheter is withdrawn.
- Right-sided valvular vegetations: the proportion leading to clinically significant endocarditis or valve dysfunction is uncertain.
- Insertion problems such as arterial puncture, pneumothorax, etc.
- Knotting of the catheter during insertion.

See Table 5.14 for a summary of problems associated with pulmonary artery catheterization.

Table 5.14 Summary of problems associated with pulmonary artery catheterization

Problem	Potential cause	Action
Unable to wedge when balloon is inflated.	Catheter tip not in correct position. Balloon rupture. Pulmonary hypertension.	Inform medical staff. Catheter needs to be advanced. Remove catheter. May not be able to wedge. Use other readings (e.g. pulmonary artery diastolic pressure).
Over-wedged trace when balloon inflated.	Incorrect position of catheter. Tip is advanced too far and lies in a smaller vessel.	Inform medical staff. Catheter needs to be pulled back into larger vessel.
Blood in syringe when air removed from balloon.	Rupture of balloon.	Inform medical staff. Turn off stopcock to syringe. Catheter should be removed.
Spontaneous wedge (wedge trace seen when balloon not inflated).	Catheter has migrated into a small vessel.	Inform medical staff. Catheter must be withdrawn urgently until PA waveform is seen, otherwise there is a risk of pulmonary infarction.
RV waveform instead of PA trace	Catheter has slipped back into right ventricle.	Inform medical staff. Potential for ventricular arrhythmias. Catheter must be repositioned in the PA.
'Damped' pressure trace.	Loose connections. Catheter tip against vessel wall. Low pressure in bag. Excessive length of tubing from transducer. Air bubbles or blood in transducer. Fibrin deposition at tip.	Inform medical staff. Check connections are secure. Reposition catheter. Check pressure bag inflated to 300mmHg. Remove excess tubing. Check transducer; change if necessary. Flush catheter or replace (use a 2 ml syringe to aspirate or for a high pressure flush).

Removal of the pulmonary artery catheter

The PA catheter alone can be removed, leaving the introducer sheath in situ; therefore ascertain if only the catheter or both are to be removed. Infusions via the PA catheter should be transferred to the side arm of the introducer or other catheters, and any cardiac output equipment should be disconnected. Emergency equipment for defibrillation should be at hand, as there is a potential risk of ventricular arrhythmias as the catheter passes through the ventricle. The procedure is carried out aseptically.

- Assemble equipment.
- Explain procedure to patient.
- Place patient in supine position to reduce the risk of air embolism.
- Ensure that the balloon is deflated and a PA waveform is shown on the monitor.
- Unclip the sleeve adapter from the introducer sheath.
- Remove the dressing and cut any sutures.
- Remove during expiration in the spontaneously breathing patient, or time removal to the inspiratory cycle of the ventilator. This reduces the risk of air embolism.
- While observing the ECG monitor, gently withdraw the catheter. As the catheter tip passes from PA to RA the characteristic change in waveforms is seen. Particular observation of the ECG is necessary as the tip passes through the RV. If ventricular arrhythmias occur, continue withdrawing the catheter as these will often terminate once the catheter is removed.

If there is any difficulty in withdrawing the catheter, discontinue the procedure immediately. Do not use force as resistance may be due to knotting or kinking of the catheter, or it may be caught on a valve or other structure. Seek medical help. If the catheter is in the RV and unable to be withdrawn, and ventricular arrhythmias are occurring, consider inflating the balloon and advancing the catheter forward to try and stop the arrhythmias.

- When the PA catheter has been completely removed a haemostatic valve closes over the entrance in the introducer sheath. This should prevent entry of air and exit of blood, but occasionally it can be damaged by passage of the catheter. Therefore a sterile occlusive obturator cap should be placed in the introducer lumen.
- If the introducer is also to be removed, it is easier to remove the PA catheter first and then the introducer. The procedure is the same as for the removal of a central venous catheter (described earlier). Ensure haemostasis by manual pressure. Cover with an occlusive dressing.

Cardiac output measurement

The Fick method

This measurement is based upon the principle described by Adolph Fick which states that the amount of substance taken up by an organ is equal to its blood flow and the arterial–venous difference in concentration of the substance. In clinical practice, the Fick method generally uses the lungs as the organ and oxygen as the substrate. Cardiac output (CO) can be calculated as

$$CO = \frac{\text{oxygen consumption (ml/min)}}{\text{A} - \text{V oxygen difference}}.$$

This is cumbersome and generally unsuitable for use in critically ill patients as it demands a steady physiological state. Potential errors are created by any leaks in the ventilator circuit and humidification, and the flow-by facility on some ventilators needs to be accounted for. The error in CO measurement is estimated to be approximately 10%. This may be higher with active inflammatory processes in the lung as the technique does not measure the increase in local oxygen consumption secondary to the inflammation.

Oesophageal Doppler ultrasound

Oesophageal Doppler monitoring is a relatively non-invasive technique for continuously measuring a variety of haemodynamic parameters. Compared with pulmonary artery catheterization it is simple to insert, cost-effective, and safe.

The technique involves passing an ultrasonic flow probe down the oesophagus, attaching it to a monitor, and obtaining a waveform display that accurately reflects blood flow in the descending thoracic aorta. Using a nomogram of the patient's age, height, and weight, a good approximation of total cardiac output is obtained.

The machine consists of a probe containing two transducers mounted at its tip, a connecting cable, and a monitor giving a visual display of the blood flow velocity profiles. One of the probe transducers continuously emits ultrasound waves at a frequency optimal for the depth of penetration and sensitivity required for measuring blood flow in the descending thoracic aorta (4 MHz). The other transducer detects the reflected Doppler shifted signals.

Waveform characteristics

A stylized normal blood velocity profile as displayed on the monitor is shown in Figure 5.39. The x-axis denotes time and the y-axis the blood flow velocity. The basic signal resembles a row of triangles sitting on the time line. The triangle itself represents the blood flow velocity profile as a bolus of blood is pumped through the aorta. The base of the triangle represents the duration of blood flow through the aorta during systole—the 'flow time'. Blood moving away from the transducer is plotted above the time axis while blood flowing towards the transducer is plotted below.

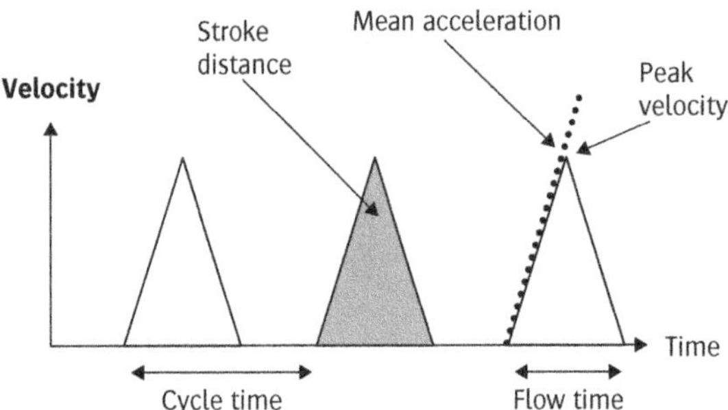

Figure 5.39 Normal blood velocity profile of oesophageal Doppler.

Regurgitant flow in the descending aorta, as seen in moderate to severe aortic regurgitation, produces a reverse flow signal throughout all of diastole. A short period of reverse flow in early diastole is a normal phenomenon in young people, feeding the coronary arteries.

- The **cycle time** is the time from the beginning of one systole to the beginning of the next. Expressed in milliseconds, it is analogous to the R–R interval on the ECG. The flow time (systole) and the filling time (diastole) are affected by heart rate. The flow time can be corrected to a heart rate of 60 bpm by the following equation:

$$\text{Corrected flow time} = \frac{\text{flow time}}{\sqrt{\text{cycle time}}}.$$

The normal corrected flow time is 330–350 msec.

- **Stroke distance** is the area within the triangle and is defined as the distance a column of blood travels down the descending aorta with each left ventricular stroke. The stroke volume of blood passing down the descending thoracic aorta is the stroke distance multiplied by the cross-sectional area of the aorta at the observation point.
- **Peak velocity** is the maximum speed at which blood is moving during systole, and is represented by the peak of the waveform This provides an indication of left ventricular contractility. although it is age-dependent as the peak velocity declines with age.
- **Mean acceleration** is the maximum acceleration at which blood is moving during systole. It is calculated as peak velocity divided by the time to reach peak velocity

from the beginning of systole. This too provides an indication of left ventricular contractility, although it is also age-dependent as acceleration declines with age.

Potential errors in the estimation of cardiac output using oesophageal Doppler

The device makes certain assumptions when calculating cardiac output including the following.

- The probe is facing the descending aorta at an angle of 45°.
- The stroke volume is computed using a nomogram utilizing age, height, and weight. Although formulated by measurements from many patients, it remains an average value. The accuracy has not been confirmed in bariatric patients.
- The proportion (approximately 70%) of blood passing through the observation point in the descending aorta (approximately 30% goes to coronary circulation, carotid, and upper limbs) is not significantly changed by alterations in cardiac output or blood pressure. Cross-clamping of the aorta during vascular surgery is an example of how this proportion is altered.

Contraindications for use

The oesophageal Doppler measurement of cardiac output will not be accurate in the following circumstances:

- during aortic vascular surgery when the aorta is cross-clamped
- when an intra-aortic balloon is in situ (causes local turbulence)
- with aortic coarctation
- with a working epidural catheter in place as this dilates the lower blood circulation, affecting the proportionality between upper and lower body.

However, trends can still be followed.

Electrocautery during surgery interferes with the Doppler signal; however, this is not a contraindication to its use.

Cautions/relative contraindications to its use include:

- patients who have oesophageal pathology (e.g. oesophageal varices)
- patients who have undergone recent surgery to the mouth, oesophagus, or stomach
- patients who have severe bleeding disorders.

Probe placement

At a depth of approximately 35–40 cm from the teeth in the normal-sized adult, the descending aorta lies parallel and very close to the oesophagus in the region of the T5–T6 vertebrae. The appropriate depth will change in tall or short people; this should be considered when the probe is inserted, otherwise it may be inadvertently focused on other vessels (e.g. pulmonary artery or coeliac axis) which may look similar to the aortic waveform.

At the correct depth, the probe detects blood flow from one of three structures—the heart, azygos vein, or descending thoracic aorta—depending on the orientation of the probe tip. The signals from each are distinct and can be easily recognized with experience.

Once in situ the probe can be rotated or moved slightly up or down until a clear aortic waveform appears on the monitor. The 'ideal' waveform should have a black central portion and a sharp outline in red, orange, yellow, and white. The colours correspond to the proportion of blood cells moving at a given speed at that point in time. White indicates the speed at which most of the blood cells are moving. Red shows the velocity at which few cells are moving and black indicates no movement at all.

Insertion of the probe

- Position the patient appropriately.
- Explain the procedure and ensure the patient is adequately sedated.
- Lubricate the probe tip with lubricating jelly.
- Gently insert the probe orally into the oesophagus.

Never force the probe. If firm resistance is encountered stop the procedure and seek medical advice. Occasionally, the probe needs to be inserted under direct vision using a laryngoscope, as there may be difficulty in bypassing the region adjacent to the endotracheal tube.

- Continue gently inserting the probe until the patient's teeth are midway between the two furthest external depth markers (indicating 35–40 cm from the tip).
- Connect the probe to the monitor.
- Rotate or move the probe up and down until a correct descending aortic waveform display is seen and the audio signal indicates the highest pitch. It may need to be inserted further in a tall person or pulled out 5 cm or so in a short person.
- The probe can be secured with paper tape to the endotracheal tube or catheter mount to prevent movement.

The probes are disposable and there is no recommended upper time limit for how long they may be left in situ. Care should be taken to avoid pressure effects of the probe on the lips and mouth.

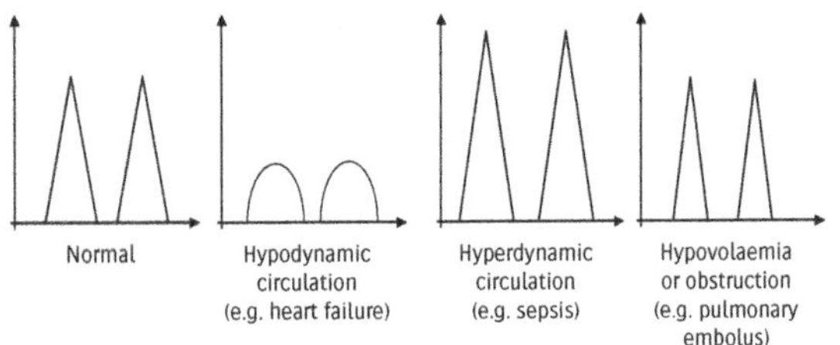

Figure 5.40 Stylized normal and pathological waveforms.

Interpretation of the waveform

Certain pathological conditions show characteristic changes in the waveform shape and can give immediate information concerning haemodynamic status (Figure 5.40). Studies have shown a close relationship between myocardial contractility and peak velocity, and an inverse relationship between increased systemic vacular resistance (SVR) and the corrected flow time.

1. ***Corrected flow time (FTc)***. The normal range is 330–350 ms. A lower value suggests vasoconstriction and a high SVR. This is usually due to hypovolaemia, but can also be due to cold, excessive vasopressor drugs, or obstruction (e.g. due to tamponade). A value higher than normal suggests vasodilatation. During hypovolaemia, unless severe, the peak velocity is usually maintained within age-related values and produces a narrow peaked waveform. However, in the presence of left ventricular dysfunction, the peak velocity is normally reduced, producing a short, rounded waveform.
2. **Peak velocity (PV)** The normal range seen within the descending thoracic aorta decreases with age. Normal values are:
   - at 20 years old, 90–120 cm/sec
   - at 50 years old, 60–90 cm/sec
   - at 70 years old, 50–80 cm/sec.

   Values falling below this range suggest a hypodynamic circulation such as cardiogenic shock, while values above suggest a hyperdynamic circulation (e.g. sepsis or pregnancy).
3. **Clinical profiles**
   - Sepsis. In a patient with sepsis (usually has a hyperdynamic circulation), an increase in peak velocity and corrected flow time is usually seen (provided that they are fluid resuscitated and do not have marked myocardial depression).
   - Cardiac failure. A patient in cardiac failure (a hypodynamic circulation) would show a flattened waveform with a decrease in peak velocity and a fall in corrected flow time because of compensatory vasoconstriction.
   - Hypovolaemia. A patient with hypovolaemia or flow obstruction (e.g. due to pulmonary embolus) would show a normal or slightly low peak velocity and a short corrected flow time.

Clinical utility of waveform analysis

Alterations in preload, afterload, and inotropic status produce consistent changes in FT_c and PV (Figure 5.41). Preload changes predominantly affect FTc, inotropic changes affect PV, while changes in afterload affect both FTc and PV.

Oesophageal Doppler can also be used for non-invasive optimization of left ventricular filling as immediate changes can be seen in the size of the waveform.

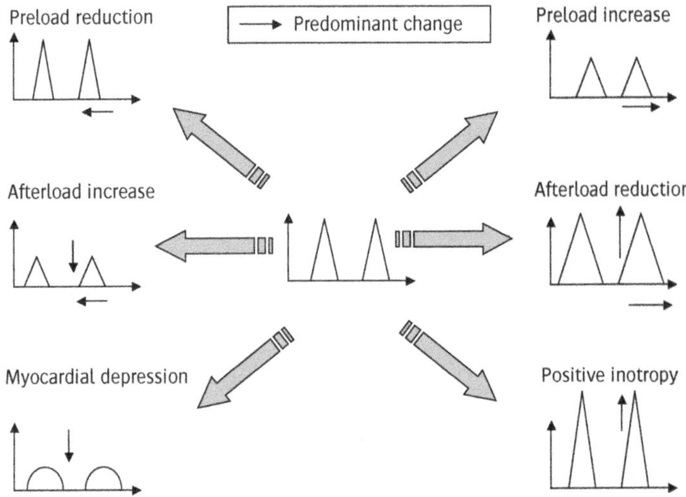

Figure 5.41 Waveform responses to clinical interventions.

Preload can be increased by fluid challenge or decreased by diuretics or nitrates. Afterload can also be decreased by administering short-acting nitrates.

Inotropes, vasodilators, vasopressors, fluid, and ventilator settings can be thus titrated to optimize cardiac output. Inotropes and vasopressors may produce an excessively narrow waveform indicating excessive constriction. This can be corrected by adequate administration of fluid or co-administration of a vasodilator.

Thermal and dye dilution methods

Thermodilution

Various techniques offer thermal or dye dilution techniques as a means of measuring cardiac output. These are inaccurate in patients with intracardiac shunts, aortic aneurysm, aortic stenosis, mitral or tricuspid insufficiency, pneumonectomy, large pulmonary emboli, and the use of an extracorporeal circulation.

Pulmonary artery catheter—intermittent thermodilution This method involves injection of an exact amount of 5 or 10 ml 5% glucose (preferably ice-cold for greater accuracy, although room temperature fluid can be used) into the right atrium via the proximal lumen of a PA catheter.

The injection must be rapid (within 3–4 sec). As the cold solution mixes with the blood, a thermistor at the tip of the PA catheter senses the change in blood temperature and a temperature–time curve can be plotted. An integral computer computes the output from the modified Stewart-Hamilton equation that takes into consideration the injectate volume, blood and injectate temperatures, and the specific heat and gravity of the blood and injectate. As the fluid is injected the temperature curve is displayed on the cardiac output monitor. This represents the change from a warmer to a cooler and back to a warmer temperature, with the area under the curve being inversely proportional to the cardiac output.

A closed injectate set is available whereby syringes of injectate can be drawn without disconnecting the circuit. Alternatively, prefilled syringes can be prepared and used at room or iced temperature.

A computer constant must be fed into the monitor before cardiac output measurements are made. This constant depends on the make and model of catheter, the volume of injectate fluid used, and the temperature of the injectate.

Once selected, the temperature of the injectate must be within a defined range for each set of measurements that are taken. The computer constants are found accompanying the catheter.

A minimum of three injectates should be performed with an average of three values falling within 10% of each other taken as the cardiac output value. A large respiratory swing (e.g. due to hypovolaemia or high airway pressures) may cause a variability of up to 50% in stroke volume. Therefore injectates should be evenly spaced across the respiratory cycle.

Because of inherent variability in injection technique and changes in stroke volume across the respiratory cycle, the variability of the thermodilution technique (one 'standard deviation') is approximately 7%. Thus a change in cardiac output >14% (2 standard deviations) is needed to be 95% confident that this is a true change rather than technique variability.

For problems encountered when determining cardiac output with thermodilution see Table 5.15.

Pulmonary artery catheter—continuous cardiac output ontinuous cardiac monitoring can be obtained using a modified pulmonary artery catheter and a cardiac output computer. The catheter has a special 10 cm long thermal filament which lies between the RA and RV when correctly positioned. The energy signal is emitted from this filament which emits pulses of heat. The algorithm in the computer identifies when the change in pulmonary artery temperature matches the input signal. Cross-correlation of the input and output signals produces a thermodilution washout curve. The modified Stewart–Hamilton equation is applied to determine cardiac output. This process occurs every 30–60 sec and the values are averaged to produce a continuously displayed parameter. However, data are collected over 2–7 min and therefore are not 'continuous' as rapid changes are detected as artefact and thus excluded by the software.

Peripheral thermodilution measurement

This system (PiCCO™) requires a specialized peripheral arterial thermodilution catheter and large-bore peripheral or central venous access connected to a monitor. Results and reliability differ depending on the location of the cannulae, with more central sites (the femoral artery being preferred) providing greater accuracy than the brachial or radial arteries. A bolus of fluid is injected rapidly through the venous catheter and the temperature change is detected in a thermistor located within the arterial catheter.

The mean of three thermodilution injectates falling within 10% of each other is taken as the cardiac output value.

As is the case with all arterial catheters, it is important to regularly assess for adequate perfusion downstream of the puncture site by clinical inspection, surface temperature

Table 5.15 Summary of problems associated with measuring cardiac output with a thermodilution pulmonary artery catheter

Problem	Potential cause	Action
Difficulty injecting solution through proximal lumen	Proximal lumen occluded/kinked. Catheter tip against wall of vessel.	Unkink/replace catheter. Reposition catheter.
Blood temperature not displayed	Faulty thermistor. Fibrin growth on thermistor.	Replace catheter.
Injectate temperature not displayed	Faulty injectate temperature probe.	Replace probe.
Wide discrepancies in serial CO recordings	Inaccurate amounts of injectate drawn up. Poor technique (uneven injection). Arrhythmias (atrial fibrillation, ventricular ectopics). Valvular disease (tricuspid insufficiency) causing turbulent flow. Patient movement during recordings. Malfunction of CO computer.	Ensure exact injectate volume drawn up. Inject evenly within 4 sec. Observe ECG, avoid injection during arrhythmias. Use alternative method for obtaining CO. Limit patient movement during recordings. Replace computer.
Inappropriately high values for CO	Incorrect injectate volume (usually too low or leaking connection). Injectate temperature too low. Incorrect computer constant. Poor injection technique.	Check correct volume to be used (5 or 10 ml). Check injectate temperature. Check computer constant. Inject evenly within 4 sec.
Inappropriately low values for CO	Incorrect injectate volume (usually too much). Injectate temperature too high. Start button pressed after beginning of injection. Incorrect computer constant. Delivery of injectate longer than 4 sec. Concomitant infusions at high flow rates (>150ml/h) through distal lumen.	Ensure correct injectate value. Check injectate temperature. Do not hold barrel of syringe when injecting. Press start button at the same time or just before beginning the injection. Check computer constant. Ensure injection is within 4 sec. If possible turn off concomitant infusions during measurements.

measurement, and/or applying a pulse oximetry sensor to a downstream digit. The PiCCO system uses a larger bore arterial catheter compared with those used for BP monitoring alone, so the risk of vessel obstruction is higher, leading to potential limb ischaemia and necrosis.

A number of additional derived parameters are obtained with this device (see Table 5.16 for normal ranges), including the following.

- Global end-diastolic volume (GEDV)—the volume of blood contained within the four chambers of the heart. This is used as a marker of cardiac preload.
- Intrathoracic blood volume (ITBV)—the volume of the four chambers of the heart plus blood volume within the pulmonary vessels. This is also used as a marker of preload.
- Extravascular lung water (EVLW)—the amount of water content in the lungs. It is used as a bedside quantification of the degree of pulmonary oedema.

Dye dilution method

This method involves injection of a dye or chemical into the blood (usually through a central venous catheter) and measuring the subsequent dilution after a designated time. The traditional dye used was indocyanine green; its subsequent dilution was measured by a densitometer downstream of where it was injected. Serial measurements are taken over a period of time and a dye dilution curve is produced. From this, cardiac output can be calculated. However, this dye is not generally used nowadays.

Table 5.16 Normal ranges of thermodilution parameters

Index range unit	Thermodilution parameters
Cardiac index	3.0–5.5 L/min/m^2
Global end-diastolic volume index (GEDVI)	680–800 ml/m^2
Intrathoracic blood volume index (ITBI)	850–1000 ml/m^2
Extravascular lung water index (ELWI)	3.0–7.0 ml/kg
Pulmonary vascular permeability index (PVPI)	1.0–3.0
Cardiac function index (CFI)	4.5–6.5 L/min
Global ejection fraction (GEF)	25–35%

Lithium dilution cardiac output (LiDCO™)

This method utilizes the dye dilution method with an indicator solution of lithium chloride (LiCl). The technique requires only an arterial line and a central venous catheter and therefore is less invasive than pulmonary artery catheterization.

The lithium chloride is injected as a bolus via the central venous catheter, and an arterial plasma concentration curve is measured by means of a sensor. The sensor is disposable and consists of a polycarbonate flow-through cell housing a lithium-selective electrode. When making a measurement, blood is sampled through this cell with a peristaltic pump, which limits the flow to 4 ml/min. The voltage across the lithium-selective membrane is related to the plasma lithium concentration by the Nernst equation. A correction is applied for plasma sodium concentration because of the relatively low selectivity of the membrane for Li^+ over Na^+. The voltage is measured using an isolated amplifier and, then digitized online, analysed, and stored. The cardiac output is calculated as follows:

$$\text{Cardiac output} = \frac{\text{LiCl dose} \times 60}{\text{Area} \times (1 - \text{PCV})} 1/\text{min}$$

where the LiCl dose is in mmol, area is the integral of the primary curve, and PCV is packed cell volume.

The dose of lithium used is 1/300th of the therapeutic dose and should not cause any adverse effects. The manufacturer recommendeds that measurements are limited to 10 per day and should not be used in patients on lithium therapy. To improve accuracy, three injectates should be performed and the measurements averaged.

The device cannot be used in patients who are being given non-depolarizing neuromuscular blocking agents such as atracurium and rocuronium, as these adversely affect the sensor.

Pressure waveform (pulse contour) analysis (PiCCO™, LiDCO Rapid™, Flotrac™)

The area under the systolic portion of the arterial pressure waveform and the shape of the pressure wave (including the position of the dicrotic notch) are utilized to provide continuous monitoring of cardiac output. However, this relationship is heavily influenced by the resistive and elastic characteristics of the arterial system. Numerous formulae have been developed to estimate stroke volume from these variables, with some taking aortic elastance and resistance into account. However, these formulae differ considerably when tested against each other.

Devices utilizing pulse contour analysis can be 'standalone' (e.g FloTrac™, LiDCO Rapid™) with proprietary algorithms providing an estimation of absolute stroke volume. Alternatively, they can be calibrated against intermittent measurements of cardiac output made with transpulmonary thermal or lithium dilution (LiDCO Plus™, PiCCO™), as described in the previous section.

Although tracking will be reasonably accurate in a stable patient, any significant change in the circulation will affect the compliance (stiffness) of the arterial system and alter the relationship between pressure and flow, making the measurement unreliable. This can occur, for example, with hypovolaemia, institution or alteration of the dose of a vasopressor, or pain/agitation causing an increase in blood pressure. The manufacturer of the PiCCO™ device recommends that the device should be re-calibrated at least eight-hourly, but this may be needed much more frequently (up to several times per hour) if the patient's haemodynamic condition is unstable, if there is a significant change in blood pressure, or if one measurement does not closely correspond to others.

Accuracy is also affected significantly if the arterial pressure waveform is either under- or over-damped, or if the line is physically kinked. Thus it is imperative to ensure and maintain an optimal pressure waveform to remove this source of inaccuracy.

Stroke volume and pulse pressure variation

Stroke volume variation (SVV) represents the variation of stroke volume (SV) over the ventilatory cycle and

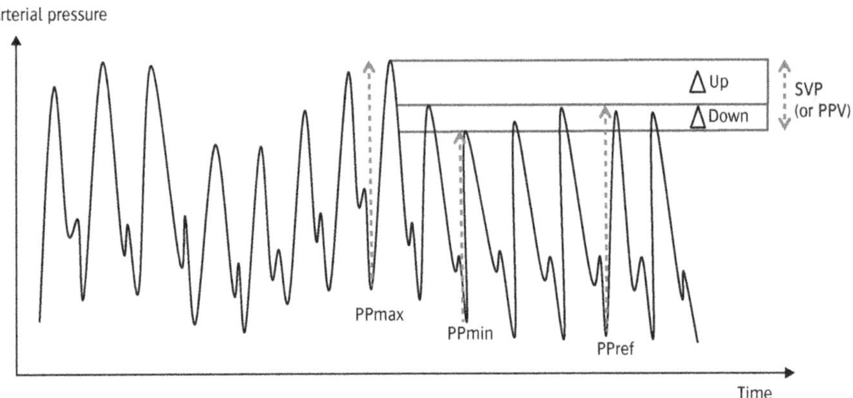

Figure 5.42 Arterial pressure variation during positive pressure ventilation without spontaneous effort. Key: Pref, reference pulse pressure (PP); Ppmax, maximal PP; Pmin, minimal PP; SPV, systolic pulse variation; PPV, pulse pressure variation; Up, increasing part of SPV from reference PP; D, decreasing part of SPV from reference PP.

reflects the sensitivity of the heart to the cyclic changes in cardiac preload induced by mechanical ventilation.

Pulse pressure variation (PPV) can be used to assess preload dependency and may increase in right ventricular dysfunction (see Fig 5.42)

During inspiration in positive pressure ventilation, pulse pressure (PP) first slightly increases and then after a few heartbeats it decreases. As venous return decreases, right ventricular preload decreases and results in a decrease in right ventricular ejection. This then leads to a decrease in left ventricular preload and left ventricular systolic volume of ejection.

Factors that may affect pulse pressure variation include:

- volume status
- arterial compliance
- heart rate
- spontaneous respiration
- tidal volume
- chest compliance
- lung compliance
- right ventricular failure.

Studies have suggested that values of PPV and SVV >10–15% can predict whether stroke volume will increase with volume expansion. Importantly, this does not necessarily mean that the patient needs fluid to improve perfusion, as perfusion may be adequate, but that their circulation is likely to respond positively to fluid with an increase in stroke volume.

Assessment of fluid responsiveness by SVV and PPV is only applicable in patients who are fully mechanically ventilated with tidal volumes ≥8 ml/kg, and who have a regular heart rhythm. Reliability deteriorates in patients making spontaneous breathing efforts, whose tidal volumes are low, or who have arrhythmias or multiple ectopics. As described earlier, it is also imperative to ensure a good quality arterial pressure (or stroke volume) waveform trace.

Other diagnostic techniques

Echocardiography

Ultrasound waves emitted in pulses by a probe directed at the heart are reflected back to the probe off the different surfaces and interfaces within the heart. A composite picture of these 'echoes' is built up and rebuilt multiple times per second producing a structural representation of the heart in motion in, either one dimension (M mode echo) or two (2D echo). As these can be viewed in real time, movement of the atrial and ventricular walls and opening and closing of the valve leaflets through the cardiac cycle can be imaged.

More sophisticated echocardiography machines have a Doppler ultrasound facility to measure the degree and direction of blood flow within the heart. This is particularly useful for assessing and quantifying valvular regurgitation and stenosis and septal defects non-invasively. Cardiac output can also be measured by Doppler echocardiography, measuring blood flow velocity through either the mitral or aortic valves or the ascending aorta by Doppler, and using the echocardiographic image to measure the valvular or aortic diameter.

The probe can be placed on the skin surface (transthoracic) in various locations such as the parasternal, apical (over the apex of the heart), or epigastric regions. The patient can either be resting supine or rolled onto their left-hand side. These changes in posture and probe site help to facilitate the view of a particular region of the heart. Signal acquisition is improved by smearing a conducting gel over the probe tip.

As ultrasound travels poorly through air, patients with hyperinflated lungs (e.g. emphysema) or after sternal opening (e.g. post-cardiac surgery) may be difficult to image. Likewise, patients with a thick chest wall may prove awkward to image. Use of trans-oesophageal echocardiography overcomes these problems as high-quality signals are obtained from behind the heart with minimal artefact. It can be performed in conscious sedated patients, but is also being used successfully in mechanically ventilated patients in the operating theatre and ICU environments. However, these probes are very expensive and require considerable expertise to use.

Uses of echocardiography

1. **Pericardial disease** A pericardial effusion or haemopericardium can be identified and drained, if needed. Constrictive pericarditis can also be diagnosed (e.g. as seen in tuberculosis).
2. **Myocardial disease:**
   - *Wall motion abnormalities*—lack of movement (akinesia) of a region of ventricle during systole indicates infarction or ischaemia, though the latter is often temporary. Reduced (hypokinetic) or abnormal (dyskinetic) movement of a ventricular segment may be seen with ischaemia. Paradoxical movement of a region (i.e. in the wrong direction during systole) indicates a ventricular aneurysm.
   - *Wall thickness*—hypertrophy can be diagnosed.
3. **Chamber size** The size of the four heart chambers can be estimated and dilatation or underfilling diagnosed. This can be used for assessment of the effect of drugs and other therapies such as PEEP. The left and right ventricular ejection fraction, i.e.(end diastolic volume—end systolic volume)/(end diastolic volume)can be used as a guide to contractility.
4. **Valvular defects** Valvular stenosis and regurgitation can be diagnosed by characteristic movement of the valves and by the appearance of abnormal flow jets using colour-flow Doppler. The latter technique can also be used to quantify the pressure gradient across stenotic or regurgitant valves.
5. **Septal and congenital defects** Atrial and ventricular septal defects, either congenital or acquired (e.g. post-infarction), can be readily imaged. The colour-flow facility, and/or injection of microbubbles or radiocontrast, enables the operator to determine whether a left-to-right or a right-to-left shunt exists, and its significance.
6. **Cardiac output estimation**
7. **Thrombi, vegetations, pulmonary emboli, and neoplasms** Although a negative result does not exclude the presence of intramural thrombi or valvular vegetations, echo is a very useful diagnostic technique, especially for larger lesions. The trans-oesophageal approach is superior in view of the better picture quality obtained and the superior ability to look at the posterior parts of the heart. Atrial myxomas can be readily imaged by this technique. A large pulmonary embolus cannot be directly imaged, but its presence is suggested by marked right ventricular strain and left ventricular under-filling.
8. **Aortic aneurysm** The trans-oesophageal approach is well suited for imaging the aortic root, aortic arch, and descending thoracic aorta for the presence of an aneurysm.

Nuclear scans

Radionuclide ventriculography involves the injection of ^{99}Tc-labelled blood (or albumin). A gamma camera placed over the heart counts the amount of radioactivity emitted by the technetium in the heart chambers at different points in the cardiac cycle. This is achieved by connection ('gating') to an electrocardiogram and is known colloquially as a MUGA scan (multiple gated analysis scan). The difference in counts at the end of diastole and systole can be used to determine the ejection fraction of both left and right ventricles. Regional wall motion abnormalities can also be detected.

Regional myocardial perfusion can be assessed by injection of thallium-201, which is taken up into the muscle. Non-perfused areas of muscle produce a defect on the subsequent scan. This can be permanent after an infarction, or transient in the case of ischaemia which can be produced by exercise, or infusion of dipyridamole or dobutamine.

Technetium pyrophosphate is also not taken up by normal myocardium and can be used as a diagnostic tool for myocardial infarction when either the ECG or cardiac enzyme results are inconclusive, not available, or non-interpretable.

Angiography

Cardiac catheterization involves insertion of a catheter either through a vein into the right heart or via an artery (usually brachial or femoral) into the left heart under fluoroscopy (X-ray imaging). The latter is usually performed in a specialized laboratory and enables a number of investigations and procedures.

1. Visualization of the coronary arteries by placement of the catheter into the individual coronary artery orifices followed by injection of a radio-opaque dye. The patency of the vessels (including previous bypass grafts) and the degree of collateral flow can be determined.
2. Assessment of the degree of stenosis or regurgitation of a damaged valve with quantification of the pressure gradient across the valve.
3. Angioplasty ± stent insertion, or valvuloplasty (i.e. dilatation of an artery or a stenosed valve), can be performed by inflation of a balloon sited near the tip of the catheter.
4. Diagnosis of a dissecting aortic aneurysm.
5. Diagnosis and assessment of intracardiac pressures, ejection fraction, congenital heart disease, shunts, etc., as well as the ability to perform an endomyocardial biopsy (e.g. cardiomyopathy, histological evidence of rejection of transplanted heart).
6. Sampling of blood for measure of oxygen saturation within the different heart chambers (used in diagnosis and quantification of intracardiac shunts).

As with any invasive procedure, cardiac catheterization carries a risk of complications, including arrhythmias, thromboembolism, vessel dissection, and infection.

Computed tomography (CT) and magnetic resonance imaging (MRI) scans

With improvements in CT and MRI scan technology with faster acquisition rates, CT (or MR) contrast angiography, where timed contrast is injected during a scan, can also be employed. While not yet as discriminatory as standard angiography, with a less distinct outline of the arteries, it is far less invasive and thus safer, and can also provide information on ventricular size and performance, with visualization of infarcted areas of myocardium and the amount of arterial calcification. An advantage of invasive angiography is that the cardiologist/radiologist can perform balloon angioplasty or stent insertion immediately, but the less invasive techniques can be used in low to moderate risk patients for excluding severe pathology.

Assessment of the patient with a cardiac disorder

This is achieved using information derived from a variety of sources, including:

- history
- pain assessment
- ECG
- non-invasive and invasive monitoring
- serum biochemical and haematological tests
- physical assessment (see Box 5.4)
- chest X-ray
- other diagnostic tests, e.g. echocardiography, angiography (see previous section).

History

Details should include type of pain, length of history, precipitating factors, relieving factors, social history (smoking, alcohol, drugs, etc.), and any relevant family history.

Pain assessment

The assessment of pain can be an important diagnostic tool and may help differentiate pain of cardiac origin

Box 5.4 Physical assessment of the patient

- Skin—colour (pale, cyanosed, mottled), cold, clammy, hot, oedema
- Respiration—rate, depth, tachypnoeic, dyspnoeic, using accessory muscles, orthopnoeic (breathless lying flat)
- Pulse—thready, full volume, bounding, tachycardia, irregular
- Pain—site, duration, severity, associated with movement, respiration or at rest
- Other—oliguria, nausea, vomiting, cough (possible pulmonary oedema), anxious, restless

from that of respiratory, oesophageal, or musculoskeletal disorders.

Characteristic descriptions of chest pain

Stable angina

Typically constricting retrosternal pain, radiating to the arms (usually the left), neck, or jaw. It often occurs in response to stimuli that increase the oxygen demand of the heart (e.g. physical exertion or emotion) and is relieved by resting.

Unstable angina

As in stable angina, but the periods of pain are prolonged, may occur at rest, and have no precipitating factors.

Myocardial infarction

Typically severe crushing retrosternal pain which may extend to the arms, neck, jaw, or back and often lasts >30 min. It is frequently accompanied by nausea, vomiting, and sweating. The onset of pain is not always associated with exertion and is not relieved by rest. However, some patients may have little or no pain, especially the elderly and diabetics.

Pericarditis

The pain is usually sharp and retrosternal and may be more apparent on inspiration. It is often worse when lying flat, but is relieved when sitting up and leaning forward.

Pleuritic pain

This is usually a sharp localized pain, worse on inspiration and coughing.

Pulmonary embolism

The pain is usually pleuritic in nature and may be associated with haemoptysis and breathlessness.

Oesophageal pain

Oesophageal pain is usually associated with, or eased by, food and is typically worse when lying flat. It may also be relieved by nitrates or antacids. Oesophageal rupture is usually preceded by vomiting.

Aortic dissection

The patient experiences a 'tearing' pain (as opposed to the crushing pain of myocardial infarction). This pain is typically felt in the back.

Musculoskeletal pain

Pain due to spinal or muscular disorders can usually be identified by the effect of movement and position. Unlike the other conditions, the chest wall is tender to touch at the specific location.

ECG: 12-lead and continuous monitoring

The 12-lead ECG must be viewed in conjunction with the patient's history, physical examination, and blood tests. An ECG showing unequivocal changes can be extremely valuable, particularly in confirming a diagnosis of myocardial infarction.

Non-invasive and invasive monitoring

The extent of monitoring will depend on the patient's condition. Increasingly complex regimens (e.g. for the treatment of cardiogenic shock) will require an increased complexity of monitoring.

Treatment strategies should be guided by data gained from invasive monitoring and used in conjunction with the assessment of physical signs (e.g. cool peripheries, pallor, confusion), biochemical tests, chest X-ray, ECG and echocardiography, and urine output.

Serum biochemical and haematological tests

Routine blood tests will include:

- biomarkers of cardiac injury (e.g troponin) and failure (brain-type natriuretic peptide (BNP))
- urea and electrolytes
- full blood count, liver function tests
- glucose
- clotting studies (usually only if anticoagulant therapy has been administered)
- cholesterol and triglyceride levels
- drug levels (e.g. if on digoxin or warfarin).

Other biochemical and haematological tests (as indicated), e.g.

- arterial blood gas analysis if acidosis or hypoxaemia are suspected,

Chest X-ray

Usually taken on admission and thereafter according to the patient's condition or after central-line insertions. It provides valuable information on heart size and shape, the presence of pulmonary oedema, and aortic dissection.

Priorities of care

The main function of the cardiovascular system is to maintain tissue perfusion. It must deliver an adequate supply of oxygen and nutrients, and remove carbon dioxide and other waste substances. The priority is to support the ability of the cardiovascular system to carry out these functions.

Adequate monitoring is essential to allow assessment of cardiac function and detection of arrhythmias. This should include a minimum of ECG monitoring and arterial blood pressure monitoring (preferably continuous). Central venous pressure, pulmonary artery pressure, and central or mixed venous oxygen saturation monitoring may also be indicated. Urine output will provide a guide to renal perfusion, while lactate and arterial base deficit are guides to the adequacy of organ perfusion.

Resuscitation equipment should be available, and familiarity with the use of defibrillators and external pacing systems is imperative.

Oxygen delivery and consumption

Any patient with a compromised cardiovascular system is likely to have impaired tissue perfusion. Management should attempt to correct the tissue oxygen deficit when oxygen transport is limited by impaired cardiovascular function. Prompt and adequate prevention of tissue hypoxia increases the chances of avoiding organ dysfunction and failure.

Oxygen delivery

This is the amount of oxygen delivered to the tissues by the blood and depends on blood flow (cardiac output) and the amount of oxygen carried in the blood (haemoglobin concentration and oxyhaemoglobin saturation, with a small amount dissolved in plasma that is usually disregarded) Therefore, if cardiac output, arterial oxyhaemoglobin saturation, and total haemoglobin level are known, the tissue oxygen delivery of blood can be calculated:

$$\text{oxygen delivery}\left(DO_2\right)=CO\times\left(1.34\times Hb\times SaO_2\right)\times 10$$

where CO is cardiac output (measured in L/min), Hb is the haemoglobin content of the blood (g/100 ml), S_aO_2 is the percentage of arterial Hb that carries oxygen (1.34 ml O_2 is carried by 1g Hb), and the factor 10 is used to convert ml of O_2 per 100 ml blood to ml/L. Normal DO_2 for the resting adult is approximately 1000 ml/min.

When oxygen has been extracted from the blood by the tissues, an oxygen reserve remains in the venous blood. If the tissue demand for oxygen increases, the venous oxygen reserve will be utilized if the oxygen supply does not improve to meet the increased demand. The venous saturation thus drops. Measurement of central venous saturation (or mixed venous saturation from a pulmonary artery catheter) can be used to monitor this. The normal value for mixed venous saturation is approximately 70%, assuming arterial saturation is in the normal range of 95–98%. Blood for measuring central venous saturation ($S_{cv}O_2$) is usually drawn from an internal jugular or subclavian venous catheter; as this samples blood draining from the upper body, the normal value of $S_{cv}O_2$ is approxiamtely 5% higher than mixed venous saturation (S_vO_2).

An additional mechanism to improve energy production is to increase anaerobic metabolism. Though not as efficient as aerobic metabolism, it does not require any oxygen. Lactic acid is a by-product of anerobic metabolism, so a rising blood lactate or increasing acidosis can be used as markers to indicate deterioration in tissue oxygenation and guide treatment. However, although sensitive, these markers are not very specific for decreased tissue oxygenation.

Oxygen consumption

This is the amount of oxygen used by the tissues over one minute (VO_2). It can be calculated by measuring the arteriovenous oxygen difference (i.e. the difference in oxygen content between arterial and venous blood) (see Box 5.5):

$$\begin{aligned}&\text{Venous oxygen reserve}=\\&\text{Oxygen consumption}=\text{arterial oxygen delivery}\\&\qquad\qquad-\text{venous oxygen reserve.}\\&\qquad=CO\times 1.34\times Hb\\&\qquad\quad\times\left(SaO_2-SvO_2\right)\times 10.\end{aligned}$$

Box 5.5 Oxygen delivery, consumption, and demand

- Oxygen delivery (DO_2): the amount of blood pumped to the tissues by the heart
- Oxygen consumption (VO_2): the amount of oxygen consumed by the tissues
- Oxygen demand: the amount of oxygen required by the tissues to function aerobically.

The normal range in an adult is 225–275 ml/min.

Blood taken from the pulmonary artery is considered true mixed venous blood and the percentage oxygen saturation of this blood is termed the mixed venous oxygen saturation (S_vO_2). Venous blood is aspirated from the pulmonary artery and a sample is taken from an arterial line. The oxygen saturation of both are measured in a co-oximeter. This can then be used to calculate the oxygen extraction ratio (O_2ER), which is the amount of oxygen extracted by the peripheral tissues divided by the amount of oxygen delivered:

$$O_2ER = \frac{\text{arterial} - \text{venous } O_2\text{saturation}}{\text{arterial } O_2\text{saturation}}$$

The normal value of O_2ER in an adult is about 20–25%.

Factors increasing the O_2 extraction ratio are:

- decreased cardiac output
- increased oxygen consumption (not compensated by improved oxygen delivery)
- anaemia
- decreased arterial oxygenation.

DO_2 and VO_2 can be adjusted for the patient's size by dividing by their body surface area to produce the oxygen delivery index (DO_2I) and the oxygen consumption index (VO_2I). The normal range for the oxygen consumption index is 125–165 ml O_2/m^2.

Methods of increasing oxygen delivery

Physiological responses

When the body's requirement for oxygen increases (e.g. during exercise), this need stimulates mechanisms in the respiratory and circulatory systems that will effectively increase oxygen delivery to the tissues.

In the **respiratory system** respiratory effort is increased to augment oxygen intake and CO_2 elimination.

In the **circulatory system**:

- venous return (and thus preload) is increased
- heart rate is increased (due to adrenergic stimulation)
- contractility is increased (due to adrenergic stimulation).

All of these mechanisms serve to increase cardiac output.

Clinical interventions

Critically ill patients are often unable to increase oxygen delivery sufficiently by their own physiological mechanisms. If delivery does not match consumption, specific cardiovascular and respiratory interventions (see Table 5.17) can be instituted (see Table 5.17).

When oxygen transport is limited by cardiac output (e.g. cardiogenic shock), oxygen consumption by the tissues is initially maintained by increased oxygen extraction from the blood. The normal S_vO_2 is 70–75%, but if increased oxygen extraction occurs it may drop well below 50%. This is associated with a serious disturbance in the oxygen supply–demand relationship.

Cardiac disorders

Hypotension

There is no precise level of BP that can define hypotension. It depends on the patient's age, clinical condition, and premorbid state (e.g. history of chronic hypertension). A patient is usually considered hypotensive when the MAP falls below 60 mmHg, or when the MAP is ≥40 mmHg below normal. It is important to note that impaired organ perfusion can still be present despite a normal or elevated BP and, conversely, that perfusion may be adequate despite a low BP. See Box 5.6 for causes of hypotension.

The aims of treatment of hypotension should be to:

- establish and treat the cause
- maintain or improve tissue oxygenation by increasing cardiac output, haemoglobin, and/or arterial oxygen saturation, where appropriate

Table 5.17 Interventions to improve oxygen delivery

System	Manipulation	Rationale	Intervention
Cardiovascular	Optimize preload Reduce afterload Increase contractility Increase heart rate (if bradycardic)	Blood flow to the tissues will be increased	Serial fluid challenges until no further increase in SV (Starling curve) Nitrates or other arterial vasodilators, e.g. sodium nitroprusside Inotropes (e.g. dobutamine, epinephrine) Pacing or drugs (e.g. atropine)
Haemoglobin	Keep level >70 g/L (may need to be higher if patient has cardiorespiratory compromise)	Oxygen-carrying capacity of the blood will be augmented	Transfuse blood
Respiratory	Maintain oxygen saturation >95% Respiratory support if patient is fatigued or hypoxaemic	Increase amount of oxygen carried by Hb Work of breathing may in itself increase oxygen demand	Increase inspired oxygen concentration Provide ventilatory support (e.g. use of NIV, invasive ventilation) or alter current ventilator settings. Hyperoxygenate prior to suction procedures, if necessary

- maintain tissue perfusion pressure (if necessary) by increasing systemic BP.

Ensure that the BP recording is correct. If a cuff is being used, confirm that it is the right size and correctly applied to the arm. Repeat the measurement. If an arterial line is being transduced, check for damping of the trace (e.g. air bubbles in the circuit), kinking (e.g. wrist movements), the position of the transducer relative to the left atrium, and that it is zeroed correctly. If doubt exists regarding transducer accuracy, confirm a low reading by a cuff measurement.

Treatment strategies and choice of drugs may vary amongst different ICUs and will be influenced by the methods of monitoring that are available. However, the underlying principles of management will be the same.

If there is evidence of tissue hypoperfusion (see Box 5.7), the BP should be restored by one or more of the following:

Box 5.6 Causes of hypotension

- Hypovolaemia
- Cardiogenic: heart failure, tachy/bradyarrhythmias, valvular stenosis/incompetence
- Obstructive: cardiac tamponade, massive pulmonary embolism, tension pneumothorax
- Loss of arterial tone: sepsis/inflammation, anaphlyaxis

Box 5.7 Manifestations of organ hypoperfusion

- Kidneys: oliguria
- Skin: pallor, cool peripheries
- Brain: confusion, drowsiness, agitation, syncope
- Metabolic: acidosis, hyperlactataemia
- Compensatory tachycardia

- ensuring circulating volume is adequate before vasoactive drugs are used
- administering inotropic drugs to attain adequate cardiac output and organ perfusion in low output states.
- administering vasopressor drugs, rather than inotropes, in the hypotensive patient with a high cardiac output and low systemic vascular resistance (e.g. most cases of sepsis, anaphylaxis).
- specific treatment where appropriate (e.g. drainage of a tension pneumothorax).

Hypovolaemia as a cause of hypotension

Management of hypovolaemia

The underlying cause must be identified and treated. The usual pointers are tachycardia, hypotension (postural before supine), oliguria, and a decreased cardiac output. However, the young fit patient can compensate by increased vasoconstriction and can often maintain a normal BP until the hypovolaemia is well advanced. It is therefore important not to rely solely on BP as an indicator of shock.

Immediate treatment is by rapid administration of fluid guided by monitored haemodynamic variables. If there is no stroke volume measuring technique in situ, intravascular fluid status can be guided by CVP measurements. Fluid challenges (200–500 ml) should be repeated until the CVP rises by ≥3 mmHg 5–10 min after the challenge has been completed. If the CVP rises ≥3 mmHg and MAP remains <60 mmHg in the presence of oliguria, cardiac output monitoring may provide additional valuable information. No response in stroke volume to a fluid challenge, in the absence of continued bleeding, suggests that vasoactive drugs such as inotropes will be necessary. Heart rate, blood pressure, urine output, and level of consciousness/orientation can also provide a guide to improvement in organ perfusion.

The fluid used to restore intravascular volume is partly related to local custom; however, blood will be needed if the Hb level drops too low and clotting products such as fresh frozen plasma will be needed for severe coagulopathy. The choice of crystalloid and colloid remains contentious, but there is no strong evidence supporting any particular fluid for initial resuscitation. Currently, starches are not recommended in many national guidelines because of multi-centre trial data showing lack of outcome efficacy over crystalloids and suggestion of harm. Millilitre for millilitre, colloid has a quicker and longer-lasting effect than crystalloid, but high volumes may induce a coagulopathy. If hypovolaemia is due to major haemorrhage, fluid should be given until blood is available. Group-specific or O rhesus-negative blood, in conjunction with clotting products such as fresh frozen plasma, platelet transfusions, and cryoprecipitate, should be used if haemorrhage is particularly severe. Fluids should be administered rapidly, under pressure if necessary, and continued until organ perfusion and blood pressure are maintained at adequate values.

If hypovolaemic hypotension is due to excessive fluid loss from vomiting, large nasogastric aspirates, diarrhoea, or pooling of extravascular fluid, colloid or crystalloid can be given rapidly as a series of fluid challenges. Blood pressure, urine output ± stroke volume ± CVP ± PAWP should be checked after each challenge. If the CVP, PAWP, and BP remain unchanged and the stroke volume (if measured) continues to rise, fluid challenges should be given repeatedly until adequate pressures and organ perfusion are achieved. Following initial resuscitation, the hourly fluid requirements of the patient should be regularly reviewed and a crystalloid solution given to replace losses, with further challenges as needed. However, it is important not to cause fluid overload as this can also be deleterious. See Box 5.8 for causes of hypovolaemia.

Box 5.8 Causes of hypovolaemia

- Haemorrhage (e.g. trauma, dissecting/ruptured aortic aneurysm, bleeding ulcers)
- Fluid loss (e.g. vomiting, diarrhoea, burns)
- Pooling of fluid in extravascular spaces (e.g. increased capillary permeability secondary to an insult, ileus following bowel surgery)
- Inadequate fluid input
- Relative vasodilatation and loss of peripheral vascular tone (e.g. as in sepsis)

Cardiogenic causes of hypotension

These include arrhythmias (e.g. tachyarrhythmias, heart block), pump failure, intracardiac shunts, and valvular dysfunction. If hypotension is secondary to a tachy- or bradyarrhythmia, the arrhythmia should be treated promptly to restore the circulation.

Cardiogenic shock results from failure of the heart to maintain adequate organ perfusion (see later for more details). Such patients will require intensive monitoring and complex treatment strategies. The initial treatment for cardiogenic hypotension is with inotropes to restore an adequate perfusion pressure. However, fluid challenges should also be considered as hypovolaemia often coexists.

Treatment of the severely hypotensive patient should not be withheld while monitoring devices are being inserted/applied. Empirical 'best guess' therapy may be needed in the interim. Fluid should be given by repeated challenges if hypovolaemia is suspected or more loading of the ventricle is needed (e.g. post pulmonary embolus or right ventricular infarction). Dobutamine and epinephrine are inotropic drugs commonly given and dosages are titrated according to response. If systemic vascular resistance is high, a vasodilator (e.g. glyceryl trinitrate (GTN)) may be infused and titrated according to changes in pressure, flow, organ perfusion, and symptomatic response. Reducing afterload is an important means of improving cardiac efficiency since peripheral resistance, and hence left ventricular work, is decreased. Cardiac over-distension should also be treated by decreasing venous return. Care must be taken to ensure that the intravascular volume is maintained while vasodilators are given, otherwise further hypotension may result.

Obstructive causes of hypotension

These include cardiac tamponade, pneumothorax, and pulmonary embolus. The cause must be identified and treated to restore blood pressure and organ perfusion.

'Inflammatory' causes of hypotension

Infection or other insults, such as burns, pancreatitis, and trauma, will stimulate a generalized inflammatory response resulting in loss of peripheral vascular tone and increased capillary leak. The resultant vasodilatation, relative hypovolaemia, loss of vascular tone ('hyporeactivity'), and, possibly, myocardial depression from circulating toxins and mediators produces hypotension.

The management of sepsis is aimed at identification and treatment of the infection, plus restoring and then maintaining organ perfusion and tissue oxygenation. Monitoring of vital signs will usually show low central venous, pulmonary artery wedge, and systemic arterial pressures, low SVR, tachycardia, pyrexia, and a high cardiac output. These represent a hyperdynamic circulation and are frequently, but not always, seen in such patients. The skin may feel hot to the touch and the patient may have a bounding pulse.

A minority of such patients may present with hypotension but have a low cardiac output. This may be due to pre-existing poor cardiac function or to inflammatory-mediator-induced myocardial depression.

Fluid resuscitation is usually the first-line treatment. However, for severe hypotension, empirical therapy with norepinephrine or epinephrine may also be needed, while adequate monitoring is being inserted, to rapidly restore a satisfactory perfusion pressure.

Fluid restoration has the aim of optimizing stroke volume. Large volumes may be required and infusion should continue until no further improvement in stroke volume is seen. Because of capillary leak, intravascular volume expansion may still be required, even if there is evidence of oedema. If respiratory function is severely compromised with coexisting ARDS, it may be necessary to institute vasopressors at an earlier stage and to restrict the amount of fluid given.

If the patient remains hypotensive after fluid resuscitation, vasopressors will be required; high dosages are often necessary. Norepinephine (or high-dose dopamine) is the current drug of choice as it is an effective vasoconstrictor. Other options include vasopressin or its synthetic analogue terlipressin. If myocardial dysfunction is present and afterload is raised, epinephrine, dobutamine, levosimensdan, or milrinone may be of benefit as they increase myocardial contractility. Care should be exercised with dobutamine, levosimendan, and milrinone as they may cause excessive vasodilatation.

Anaphylaxis as a cause of hypotension

The acute reaction to an allergenic substance can cause severe hypotension or even cardiovascular collapse. Severe anaphylactic reactions may require full cardiorespiratory resuscitation. Allergenic substances (e.g. food, blood, drugs, insect stings) can result in degranulation of mast cells, releasing histamine and other mediators that cause vasodilatation, smooth muscle constriction, and increased capillary permeability. Hypotension is caused by loss of vascular tone, vasodilatation, and loss of fluid from the capillaries. Hypotension and tachycardia may be severe. There may be dyspnoea and cyanosis due to bronchospasm or laryngeal obstruction, skin flushing, urticarial rash, soft tissue swelling, nausea, vomiting, and diarrhoea. Immediate treatment is to provide respiratory support if required, epinephrine, and fluid infusion. Epinephrine (0.5–1 mg) is given intramuscularly but may be given intravenously in situations where severe shock may impede absorption from muscle. For this reason, epinephrine should not be given subcutaneously. An intravenous infusion may also be necessary. Hydrocortisone 200 mg and chlorpheniramine 10 mg are also given intravenously. Fluid should be given rapidly to correct hypovolaemia, ideally guided by stroke volume or CVP measurements. In their absence, treatment should be titrated against blood pressure, heart rate, urine output, and physical assessment.The causative agent should be identified to avoid re-exposure. If an anaphylactic reaction occurs during transfusion of blood or blood products, the bag of fluid should be retained and sent to the haematology and microbiology departments for analysis. A sample of the patient's blood should also be taken for subsequent analysis (see Chapter 10 for further details).

Summary of changes in haemodynamic parameters

Table 5.18 shows common changes seen in many patients, but these are by no means universal to all.

Hypertension

Hypertension can be defined as a sustained raised BP above that considered normal for the patient's age. 'Normal' BP is difficult to quantify as it is a statistical range of values based on the mean of the population. Chronic antihypertensive therapy is generally begun if the resting diastolic blood pressure is consistently above 90–95 mmHg. However, acute treatment may be started at lower pressures for specific conditions, such as dissecting aortic aneurysm, to minimize the risk of further deterioration.

Table 5.18 Hypotension: haemodynamic parameters

Cause of hypotension	CO	PAWP/CVP	SVR
Hypovolaemia	Decreased	Decreased	Increased
Cardiogenic	Decreased	Increased	Increased
Inflammatory	Increased	Decreased	Decreased
Anaphylactic	Increased or decreased	Decreased	Decreased

If the cause of the hypertension cannot be identified, it is termed 'primary' (or 'essential') hypertension. Secondary hypertension is when there is an identifiable cause (see Box 5.9). Blood pressure is regulated by multiple endocrine, neuronal, humoral, renal, and other factors that moderate vasomotor and vasoconstrictor responses. However, the mechanisms involved in causing primary hypertension remain complex and are not fully understood.

Hypertension may also be a natural response to pain and stress, and this will require the appropriate treatment (e.g. analgesia, anxiolysis).

Management of acute hypertensive crisis

If symptomatic (headaches, confusion, drowsiness, fits, agitation), the aim of treatment is to reduce BP urgently, yet smoothly, and not aim for an excessive fall. A mean BP of approximately 120–125 mmHg may be an appropriate initial target, though the rate of fall depends on the underlying condition. Guidelines recommend that this should be achieved over 2–3 hours for hypertensive encephalopathy, 6–12 hours for subarachnoid haemorrhage, and over days to weeks for strokes. However, recent data from the INTERACT2 study (Anderson *et al.* 2013) suggest that patients with intracerebral haemorrhage could benefit from more aggressive treament (lowering systolic BP <140 mmHg). However, the findings are contradicted by other studies, such as the SCAST study (Sanset *et al.* 2011). Nevertheless, sudden drops in blood pressure should be avoided. If the cause of the hypertension is raised intracranial pressure, the BP is usually allowed to remain high (but not excessively high) to maintain an adequate cerebral perfusion pressure.

Intravenous drug therapy is often required, and continuous BP monitoring is ideal. The choice of hypotensive drug will depend on the cause of the hypertension (see Box 5.10) and the urgency of treatment. Adequate pain relief should be confirmed. A commonly used antihypertensive agent in the ICU setting is sodium nitroprusside, which produces a rapid effect and can be finely controlled. Other alternatives include glyceryl trinitrate, a short-acting β-blocker such as esmolol, labetalol, and hydralazine, which can all be given by infusion. The drug dosage should always be titrated against response. Nifedipine was used previously, although sublingual administration has a variable absorption rate and a variable, often abrupt, hypotensive effect leading to complications.

Box 5.9 Causes of secondary hypertension

- Endocrine: phaeochromocytoma, primary aldosteronism, Cushing's syndrome, acromegaly
- Renal: chronic glomerulonephritis, chronic pyelonephritis, renal artery stenosis, polycystic disease, polyarteritis nodosa
- Pregnancy-induced
- Intracranial haemorrhage
- Coarctation of the aorta
- Drug-related, e.g. clonidine, monoamine oxidase inhibitors (MAOIs), antidepressants with tyramine-containing foods (e.g. cheese), sudden withdrawal of certain drugs (e.g. antihypertensives, opiates)

Box 5.10 Manifestations of hypertension

- Neurological: headache, dizziness, transient ischaemic attacks, focal disturbances, confusion, fits, coma (hypertensive encephalopthy)
- Cardiovascular: palpitations, left ventricular failure (causing pulmonary oedema), angina, myocardial infarction
- Renal: renal failure, proteinuria
- Other: retinopathy

Hypertensive encephalopathy

This can be caused by uncontrolled hypertension from any cause. There may be areas of cerebral infarction, haemorrhage, or transient ischaemia. Symptoms are initially severe headache and nausea, but this can progress to agitation, a deteriorating level of consciousness, seizures, and coma. If the hypertension is treated early, changes are often reversible.

Malignant hypertension

Malignant hypertension is a distinct pathological condition where there is progressive severe hypertension (diastolic pressure may exceed 140 mmHg). Patients can develop renal failure, heart failure, retinal haemorrhages, papilloedema, and hypertensive encephalopathy. If untreated, mortality is 90% within a year of onset. Treatment is strict bed rest and antihypertensive drugs (e.g. nitroprusside or labetalol) to reduce the blood pressure slowly, but not excessively, to a diastolic of 110–120 mmHg. Over-aggressive reduction may result in poor perfusion and stroke. See Box 5.11 for disorders which may cause an accute hypertensive crisis.

Box 5.11 Disorders that may cause an acute hypertensive crisis

- Malignant hypertension
- Phaeochromocytoma
- Pre-eclampsia/eclampsia
- Any cause of raised intracranial pressure
- Drug-related, e.g.withdrawal of clonidine, reaction of MAOIs with foods containing tyramine

Acute coronary syndrome (ACS)

ACS consists of a spectrum of three conditions.

- ST segment elevation myocardial infarction (STEMI).
- Non ST segment myocardial infarction (NSTEMI or non-STEMI, also known as non Q wave MI).
- Unstable angina: this covers a range of clinical states falling between stable angina and acute myocardial infarction. It is defined as episodes of angina on minimal effort or at rest. It may represent deterioration from stable angina.

Therapeutic decisions such as administering thrombolytic therapy or performing percutaneous coronary intervention (PCI) are based on this categorization.

Priorities of care for suspected ACS

Intervention should occur promptly while undertaking a rapid assessment of the patient, obtaining a brief but pertinent history, and performing appropriate assessment and investigations. Cardiorespiratory status must be adequately evaluated and resuscitation measures commenced as needed.

- Pain relief (sublingual or buccal GTN and/or IV opiate)—assess effectiveness and repeat as required ± an anti-emetic.
- Give a single loading dose of aspirin 300mg (unless contraindicated) if not already administered at home or by ambulance personnel.
- Resting 12-lead ECG. If regional ST segment elevation or presumed new left bundle branch block is present, follow protocol for STEMI. This will include urgent referral to the local cardiac centre for possible angiography and PCI. For NSTEMI and unstable angina follow local protocol if there is regional ST depression or deep T wave inversion until a firm diagnosis is available. This is likely to include heparin ± clopidogrel.
- Continuous ECG and pulse oximetry monitoring, regular BP recording. Assessment of haemodynamic status and correction of abnormalities. Repeat the ECG when chest pain occurs and at least at 6 hours and 12 hours after arrival.
- Wide bore peripheral venous access.
- Pulse oximetry—give supplemental oxygen if S_pO_2 <94% (if the patient is not at risk of hypercapnic respiratory failure), aiming for an S_pO_2 of 94–98%. Do not give too much oxygen as this can cause vasoconstriction of the coronary microcirculation.
- Investigations—take blood for troponin T or I test. With the older assays, samples needed to be taken at least 6 hours after the onset of symptoms and, if equivocal, repeated at 12 hours. The newer high sensitivity troponin I or T assays allow samples to be taken on admission. Again, repeat samples may be necessary if the result is equivocal, but at 3 or 6 hours. Also measure urea and electrolytes, full blood count, cholesterol and triglycerides, and blood glucose. Perform a chest X-ray to exclude complications

Box 5.12 **Other non-MI causes of chest pain**

- Angina
- Gastritis and peptic ulceration
- Pericarditis
- Pancreatitis
- Myocarditis
- Pneumonia
- Oesophagitis
- Pulmonary embolism
- Pleurisy
- Acute aortic dissection
- Chest wall—intercostal myalgia, costochondritis, pre-rash shingles

of ACS (e.g. pulmonary oedema) and other diagnoses (e.g. pneumothorax, pneumonia).

- Management of complications (cardiac arrest, pulmonary oedema, cardiogenic shock, life-threatening or haemodynamically compromising arrhythmias).
- Relief of patient anxiety and distress using skilled competent care and reassurance, and providing information appropriate to the situation.

See Box 5.12 for other non-MI causes of chest pain.

Myocardial infarction (MI)

Myocardial infarction is the development of necrosis caused by a critical imbalance of oxygen supply and demand to an area of myocardium. This usually results from plaque rupture and thrombosis formation in a coronary artery, resulting in an acute reduction in blood supply to a part of the myocardium (see Box 5.13). Up to 25% of myocardial infarctions are 'silent' with no chest pain or symptoms and are discovered on ECG or cardiac biomarker measurement. Risks factors for MI are shown in Box 5.14.

There are two types of acute MI.

- Transmural—damage extends through the entire thickness of the heart muscle from endocardium to epicardium and is usually the result of complete occlusion of the blood supply. This can be further categorized into anterior, posterior, and inferior depending upon which area of the heart is affected.
- Subendocardial—involves a small area of the subendocardial wall of the left ventricle, ventricular septum, or papillary muscles with multifocal areas of necrosis.

Box 5.13 **Causes of myocardial infarction**

- Rupture of atherosclerotic plaque within a coronary artery and thrombus formation
- Coronary artery spasm
- Ventricular hypertrophy
- Hypoxia (e.g. carbon monoxide poisoning)
- Drugs—cocaine, amphetamines, ephedrine
- Coronary abnormalities (e.g. aneurysm)
- Aortic dissection
- Increased afterload or inotropic effects which increase myocardial O_2 demand

Diagnosis of myocardial infarction

This is based on information derived from:

- assessment of the symptoms and physical state of the patient
- ECG changes
- cardiac biomarkers
- coronary angiography, echocardiography.

For the diagnosis of an acute, evolving, or recent MI the following criteria must be met.

- A typical rise and gradual fall of biochemical markers suggestive of myocardial damage (e.g. troponin),

Box 5.14 **Risk factors for myocardial infarction**

- Age—greater risk if >45 years
- Male—greater risk in males aged 40–70 years
- Smoking—especially in women taking the combined oral contraceptive pill
- Hypercholesterolaemia—especially if high levels of low density lipoprotein (LDL) cholesterol with low levels of high density lipoproteins (HDL)
- High triglycerides
- Diabetes mellitus
- Poorly controlled hypertension
- Chronic stress levels—type A personality
- Sedentary lifestyle
- Obesity (BMI >30)
- Family history of ischaemic heart disease
- Chronic kidney disease
- Excess alcohol consumption

together with evidence of ischaemia and at least one of the following:

- ischaemic symptoms (e.g. chest pain)
- development of pathological Q waves on the ECG
- ECG changes indicative of new ischaemia (new ST-T changes or new left bundle branch block)
- imaging evidence of new loss of viable myocardium or new regional wall motion abnormality.

Patient assessment

- **Pain**—classically, the patient presents with crushing central chest pain, with or without radiation of pain into the left arm, neck, or jaw. Unless relieved by medication, the pain usually lasts more than 30 min and is not eased by posture or food.
- **Skin**—may be sweaty, pale, grey or cyanosed, peripherally constricted.
- **Respiratory**—tachypnoeic or dyspnoeic, with possible evidence of pulmonary oedema.
- **Other physical signs**—nausea and vomiting may occur.
- **Anxiety**—usually appears distressed and anxious and may require considerable comfort and reassurance.
- **Confusion**—due to hypoxaemia or poor cerebral perfusion.
- **Blood pressure**—may be normal, elevated, or low.
- **ECG monitoring**—may show tachycardia and arrhythmias.
- **Urine output**—may be oliguric due to poor renal perfusion.
- **Blood glucose**—may be raised due to increased sympathetic activity.

Investigations

12-lead ECG

Less than half of patients with acute MI have clear diagnostic changes on their first ECG. Approximately 10% with proven MI fail to develop ST elevation. In most cases, however, serial ECGs over 3 days show evolving changes that follow a recognized pattern. Changes are seen in particular leads depending on the location of the infarction on the ventricular wall (see Table 5.19).The sequence of an evolving ST-elevation myocardial infarction (STEMI) is as follows:

- peaked T waves—present for only 5–30 min after the onset of infarction
- ST segment elevation—commencing about an hour after myocardial injury

Table 5.19 12-lead ECG changes in acute myocardial infarction

Wall affected	Leads
Anterior	V3 + V4, sometimes V2
Anterolateral	I, aVL, V3-V6
Anteroseptal	V1, V2, V3, sometimes V4
Extensive Anterior	I, aVL, and V1-V6
Inferior	II, III, aVF
Lateral	I, aVL, V5 + V6
Septal	V1 + V2
Apical	V3 + V4

- Q wave formation and loss of R wave
- T wave inversion.

Q waves represent necrosis of the myocardium and result from absence of electrical activity. They have to be ≥25% of the height of the partner R wave, and/or >0.04 sec in width and >2 mm in depth.

Posterior wall infarction does not produce Q wave abnormalities in conventional leads and is diagnosed by the presence of tall R waves in leads V1 and V2.

In the recovery phase of an acute infarction the ST segment normalizes, followed by the T wave; the Q wave usually persists. However, if the myocardium is reperfused early as a result of percutaneous coronary intervention or thrombolysis, myocardial tissue can recover and the Q waves disappear.

Cardiac biomarkers

These are substances released into the blood as a consequence of cardiac injury and can assist in the diagnosis of ACS in conjunction with ECG and clinical findings.

The most commonly used biomarker for cardiac injury are the troponins (I or T). These have supplanted older markers such as creatine kinase, myoglobin, and alanine aminotransferase (ALT). Additional markers that may be used to evaluate heart function are brain-type natriuretic peptide and highly selective C-reactive protein.

Troponin

Troponins are structural protein components of striated muscle. There are three types: troponins C, T, and I. Troponins T and I are found solely in cardiac muscle and are released following cardiac damage (from as little as 1 g of myocardial cell death). They will not rise unless myocardial injury has occurred. Troponin I rises after 3–6 hours and peaks at 20 hours. The new high sensitivity troponins (hsTnI and hsTnT) can detect significant injury with high reliability on admission to hospital. If the results are equivocal for any test, they can be repeated at 6–12 hours to exclude a myocardial infarct. Both troponins remain elevated for a much longer time than creatine kinase. Troponin I is detectable in the blood for up to 5 days and troponin T for 7–10 days following MI. This allows the diagnosis to be made, or excluded, in a patient who presents late with a history of chest pain.

Although elevation of troponin T or I is indicative of cardiac damage, this can also occur as a result of myocarditis, severe cardiac failure, cardiac trauma from surgery or road traffic accidents, sepsis, coronary artery spasm from cocaine, and pulmonary embolism, and in patients with chronic renal failure. In the last case, levels are sustained rather than rising and falling as in myocardial infarction.

The measurement of either cardiac troponin T or I is now considered the gold standard for the diagnosis of cardiac injury and can identify high risk patients who would likely benefit from prompt percutaneous coronary intervention.

Creatine kinase (CK)

CK is released from any damaged muscle cell and therefore is a marker for muscle injury. The CK enzyme consists of M (muscle type) and B (brain type) subunits, which combine to form three possible isoforms; CK-MM, CK-BB, and CK-MB. CK-MB is found in high concentrations within heart muscle, but also in lower concentrations in skeletal and smooth muscle and can give a false indication of myocardial injury (e.g. in rhabdomyolysis or trauma). A significant amount of myocardial damage is required to raise CK-MB to pathological levels. It takes 4–6 hours after the injury to reach significant levels and remains elevated in the blood for 3–5 days. It is normally present in healthy individuals but over a wide range (e.g. athletes have higher levels).

Myoglobin

Myoglobin is an oxygen-carrying protein found in all muscle cells (smooth, skeletal, and cardiac) and is released during muscle injury. It is released rapidly within 2–3 hours of injury and peaks at 8–12 hours. Levels return to normal within 24 hours. It is poorly specific for cardiac injury, but if levels do not rise within 3–4 hours of injury it is unlikely that myocardial damage has occurred.

B-type natriuretic peptide (BNP)

This hormone is released in response to stretching of the atrial muscle in the heart, and is usually caused by ventricular dysfunction or volume overload. It is used as a marker for heart failure, and high levels can identify those at higher risk of death in both ischaemic and sepsis-related failure.

Highly selective C-reactive protein (hs-CRP)

This protein is a marker for inflammation of the cardiovascular system. Although not a specific prognostic indicator for heart disease, there is an association between elevated levels and the development of heart disease or recurring coronary events.

Principles of care

The patient should be admitted to a high dependency area, such as a coronary care unit (CCU), although admission to an ICU may be warranted if complications are present.

The uncomplicated patient should initally be on strict bedrest with continuous ECG and regular BP monitoring for the first 24 hours. Both patient and family should be reassured and provided with information about rehabilitation and suggestions for lifestyle alteration. Blood glucose estimations should be performed regularly, as glucose intolerance and hyperglycaemia are frequent and poor control is associated with worse outcomes. Hyperglycaemia usually settles over the following week, although the patient may occasionally need either short- or long-term control with insulin or an oral hypoglycaemic. Pyrexia is also common for the first 2–3 days after MI and does not necessarily mean infection is present.

On day 2 the patient is allowed to mobilize slowly, if stable. Discharge to a general ward often takes place after 1–2 days. Most hospitals have their own mobilization regimens, with the patient being discharged after 7 days, by which time they will have climbed a staircase and performed a treadmill exercise test. After hospital discharge the patient will be advised to undertake a slowly increasing exercise regimen and will be followed up in cardiac rehabilitation classes and the outpatient clinic. Return to work is generally delayed for 2–6 months depending on the type of activity involved. Further investigations, such as angiography, may be indicated, particularly in a young person, if complications develop or the treadmill test is positive. Surgery or percutaneous coronary intervention may be recommended, as appropriate, if not already performed.

Therapies

The goals of therapy are restoration of normal coronary blood flow and maximum salvage of functional myocardium. Local and national guidelines and algorithms (e.g. National Institute for Clinical Excellence 2013) should be followed to ascertain what drugs should be given, as well as other management strategies. This depends on the risk of predicted adverse events and prognosis, as well the ability to perform rapid angiography and PCI. A general overview is given in the next section.

Management of non ST segment elevation myocardial infarction (NSTEMI) or unstable angina (UA)

Patients who present without ST segment elevation are suffering from either NSTEMI or unstable angina (UA). The distinction is ultimately made on the basis of the presence or absence of a biomarker of cardiac necrosis (e.g. troponin) in the blood.

Risk assessment

A formal assessment of the individual's risk of future adverse cardiovascular events should be made using an established scoring system such as the Global Registry of Acute Coronary Events (GRACE) score which grades the patient as being at low, intermediate or high risk.

Antiplatelet therapy

This prevents platelet aggregation and thrombus formation. Aspirin is given as a single loading dose of 300 mg at the onset of symptoms and continued indefinitely at a low dose of 75–100 mg (unless contraindicated). Clopidogrel is given to all patients (unless contraindicated) and continued for 12 months.

Glycoprotein 11b/111a inhibitors (e.g. eptifibatide, abciximab, or tirofiban) should be considered as they reduce the risk of subsequent cardiac ischaemic events in patients at high risk, or if the duration of risk is prolonged. They prevent platelet aggregation and thrombus formation by inhibition of the Gp11b/111a receptor on the surface of the platelet.

Clopidogrel may be given to patients who are unable to take aspirin or given in addition to aspirin if they are considered to be at high or medium risk of MI or death. It is given to all patients (unless contraindicated) who may undergo percutaneous coronary intervention (PCI) within 24 hours of admission to hospital.

Antithrombin therapy

This reduces the likelihood of thrombus formation. Low molecular weight heparin (LMWH) is given by subcutaneous injection and does not require monitoring by blood testing. The duration of effect is greater than that of unfractionated heparin, and the anticoagulation response is more predictable. LMWH also carries a reduced risk of causing immune-mediated thrombocytopenia. The dose may have to be adjusted for very obese patients and those with renal failure. Fondaparinux may be offered to patients who do not have a high risk of bleeding unless angiography is planned within 24 hours of hospital admission. Unfractionated heparin can be offered to patients as an alternative to fondaparinux if coronary angiography is planned or to patients with significant renal impairment. Bivalirudin may be considered as an alternative to heparin plus a glycoprotein 11a/111b inhibitor (GPI) if the patient is at intermediate or high risk of adverse cardiovascular events, is not receiving a GPI or fondaparinux, and is scheduled for angiography within 24 hours of admission. It is important to note that neither fondaparinux nor bivalirudin have specific antidotes so they should be avoided in patients at high risk of bleeding.

Intermediate and high risk patients

Coronary angiography must be performed to define the severity of coronary artery disease before PCI or coronary artery bypass grafting is considered. Angiography often requires further anticoagulation and is invasive. It may be undertaken early, deferred until later, or undertaken selectively if the patient has evidence of recurrent ischaemia despite appropriate medication therapy. It should be performed as soon as possible if the patient is clinically unstable or at high ischaemic risk. Otherwise, unless contraindicated, it should be performed within 96 hours of hospital admission if the patient is at high or intermediate risk of adverse cardiovascular events. It should also be offered to patients assessed as low risk but who susequently experience ischaemia.

Low risk patients

These are patients with a history of brief episodes of chest pain (<20 min) in whom an ECG taken during pain suggests accelerating unstable angina. Assessment of left ventricular function should be made in all patients who have suffered MI; this should also be considered for those with unstable angina. Non-invasive stress testing (treadmill exercise test or pharmacological stress testing with imaging) is recommended for patients at low risk who have been free from ischaemic pain at rest or with a low level of activity for a minimum of 12–24 hours. Ischaemia testing should be performed before (or soon after) hospital discharge on all patients whose condition has been managed conservatively and have not had coronary angiography.

Management of patients with ST segment elevation myocardial infarction (STEMI)

These patients are treated with thrombolytics or emergency angiography and PCI. Primary PCI is the treatment of choice (if interventional cardiology is available) as it is more effective in opening acutely occluded arteries and reduces the risk of adverse outcomes (e.g. reinfarction, stroke) and the need for coronary artery bypass graft (CABG). Speed of treatment is vital; the target is to perform primary PCI within 90 min of arrival or within 60 min for thrombolysis.

Thrombolysis

Thrombolytic drugs (e.g alteplase, reteplase, streptokinase, tenectoplase) break down the thrombus so that blood flow can be restored to the myocardium. If the area has fully infarcted, little can be achieved by thrombolysis. However, early administration may reverse, or at least minimize, the amount of permanently necrosed muscle. It is only suitable if given within 12 hours of onset of symptoms and the potential adverse risks must be considered before administration (see Box 5.15).

Indications for thrombolysis are:

- ST segment elevation ≥1 mm in two or more contiguous limb leads or ≥2 mm in precordial leads
- new, or presumed new, left bundle branch block and ST segment depression of ≥2 mm in V1 and V2 (true posterior infarction)
- chest pain of between 30 min and 12 hours' duration that is unrelieved by sublingual nitroglycerin(glyceryl trinitrate)

Box 5.15 **Contraindications for thrombolysis**

Absolute

- Haemorrhagic stroke or stroke of unknown origin at any time
- Ischaemic stroke within previous 6 months
- Central nervous system trauma or neoplasm
- Major surgery/trauma/head injury within preceding 6 months
- Gastrointestinal bleeding within last month
- Known bleeding disorder
- Aortic dissection
- Non-compressible puncture (e.g. liver biopsy, lumbar puncture)

Relative

- Transient ischaemic attack in preceding 6 months
- Oral anticoagulant therapy
- Pregnancy or within one week post-partum
- Refractory hypertension
- Advanced liver disease
- Active peptic ulcer
- Refractory resuscitation

Failure of thrombolysis is evident by failure of the ST segment elevation to resolve within 30-60 min of thrombolytic therapy. If the coronary artery remains occluded, a rescue PCI should be considered and performed within 12 hours of the onset of symptoms. If facilities for PCI are unavailable and thrombolysis has failed, or is contraindicated, consideration should be given to transferring the patient to another hospital where this can be carried out.

Arterial and/or central venous cannulation should not be delayed following commencement of thrombolysis if clinically indicated. Cannulation should be performed by an experienced operator, avoiding the subclavian route.

If considerable haemorrhage does occur from either attempted cannula insertion or other causes (e.g. peptic ulcer), this can often be reversed by stopping the infusion, giving fresh frozen plasma, and either (1) aprotinin 500,000 units over 10 min and then 200,000 units over 4 hours, or (2) tranexamic acid 10 mg/kg repeated after 6–8 hours.

Revascularization arrhythmias are common during thrombolysis. Over 90% of these are benign and do not require treatment. If these occur during infusion, temporary cessation may be all that is necessary. Allergic or anaphylactic reactions (e.g to streptokinase—hypotension and rash) are relatively rare and should be treated by stopping the infusion and giving hydrocortisone 200 mg IV, chlorpheniramine 10 mg IV, and ranitidine 50 mg IV. The circulation should be supported, if necessary, with the aim of restarting thrombolytic therapy.

Patients who have previously been treated with streptokinase should not be given it again between 5 days and 12 months of the first administration. This is because of a likelihood of resistance due to the formation of streptokinase antibodies, which may cause it to be ineffective. Further thrombotic events could be treated with tissue plasminogen activator (tPA)

Percutaneous coronary intervention (PCI)

This is defined as angioplasty and/or insertion of one or more coronary artery stents. Prior to angioplasty or stent insertion a pre-treatment bolus of nitoglycerin (glyceryl trinitrate (GTN)) can be given into the coronary artery. This allows assessment of the true size of the vessel, unmasks vasospasm, and reduces the risk of vasospastic reactions during the procedure.

Coronary angioplasty involves passing a balloon catheter (usually via the femoral artery) into a stenotic coronary artery. The balloon is then inflated, causing the atheromatous plaque to be crushed into the vessel wall. A stent can then also be introduced and is left behind as the catheter is withdrawn. The stent provides a mechanical framework that holds the artery open.

Stents may be bare metal (wire mesh) or drug-eluting (coated with drugs which are released slowly). The decision as to which type of stent is used depends on the size and shape of the narrowed part of the artery. Drug-eluting stents are used when the inside of the artery is less than 3 mm across, or the narrowed area is less than 15 mm long. There are several different drug-eluting stents, which contain different drugs; for example, the Cypher stent elutes sirolimus, while Taxus elutes paclitaxel. These help prevent restenosis by several different physiological mechanisms that rely on suppression of tissue growth at the stent site and local modulation of the body's inflammatory and immune responses. Angioplasty with stenting is superior to angioplasty alone.

PCI is not without risk, although major complications are uncommon. These include stroke, ventricular fibrillation, aortic dissection, and myocardial infarction (which may require emergency bypass surgery).

Complications of MI

Complications of MI include:

- arrhythmias
- heart failure/cardiogenic shock/left ventricular dysfunction
- hypertension
- post-infarction angina
- pericarditis ± tamponade
- rupture of papillary muscle, ventricular septal defect, LV aneurysm formation
- myocardial rupture.

Hypertension may occur for various reasons after MI including pain, anxiety, and excessive vasoconstriction, perhaps due to inappropriate use of diuretics. Treatment, if necessary, should aim to gradually reduce the BP.

Hypotension post-MI should not be automatically assumed to be due to pump failure. Other common causes include hypovolaemia secondary to excess diuretic usage, or it may be related to other drugs (e.g. β-blockade, ACE inhibition).

Post-infarction angina has to be treated aggressively and is an important indication for angiography with a view to either PCI or bypass surgery. This pain can usually be distinguished from pericarditis, which may occur either within a few days of the infarct or after a period of 2–6 weeks. This latter situation, known as Dressler's syndrome, is thought to be related to the formation of autoantibodies against the myocardium. Other causes and management of pericarditis are described later in this chapter.

Papillary muscle rupture results in disruption of the mitral valve. It usually presents with acute pulmonary oedema. Echocardiography will reveal severe mitral regurgitation and the damaged valve. The patient should be treated as for severe heart failure and also referred for urgent cardiac surgery. A ventricular septal defect may occur after septal infarction. It usually presents several days after the MI as acute heart failure. Colour-flow Doppler echocardiography will reveal the abnormal flow jet across the defect, while sampling of blood from the right atrium and right ventricle will reveal a 'step-up' in oxygen saturation due to the left-to-right shunt. Again, the patient should be treated for heart failure and also considered for urgent cardiac surgery.

Ventricular aneurysm formation usually develops over weeks to months after the infarction. Clues are persistent elevation of ST segments on ECG and a bulge in the cardiac contour on chest X-ray. Echocardiography or angiography will reveal the abnormal and often paradoxical movement of the aneurysmal area during the cardiac cycle and, possibly, an associated mural thrombus. Complications that may develop include arrhythmias, heart failure, and systemic embolization. Cardiac rupture is recognized, although is invariably a terminal event. Treatment depends on the size of the aneurysm and the degree of compromise or complications caused. It may be treated either conservatively or surgically (aneurysmectomy).

Secondary prevention of MI

Drug therapy

- Asprin should be given to all patients following MI (unless contraindicated) and continued at a low dose indefinitely. This reduces both reinfarction and long-term mortality.
- Clopidogrel should be continued, in addition to aspirin, for a year in patients with NSTEMI or unstable angina (unless contraindicated), and for those who have had a STEMI, especially following stent insertion. The precise duration of therapy is controversial so local guidelines should be followed.
- Beta-blockers should be given to patients following an acute MI (unless contraindicated) and commenced once the patient is clinically stable. These drugs decrease the rate and force of contraction, and decrease overall myocardial oxygen demand. They

reduce mortality, readmission, and reinfarction for both coronary artery disease and congestive cardiac failure. Possible contraindications include asthma, heartblock, bradycardia, hypotension, and cardiogenic shock. They should be continued indefinitely unless the patient has troublesome symptoms (e.g. severe fatigue, postural hypotension).

- Statins: measurement of blood lipids should be carried out within 24 hours of admission and statins commenced if levels are elevated (unless contraindicated). Nutritional assessment should also be performed.
- Angiotensin-converting enzyme (ACE) inhibitors (e.g. ramipril) or angiotensin II receptor antagonists (e.g. losartan) reduce cardiac work by their afterload-lowering properties and reduce wall stress within the heart, thereby limiting infarct expansion and excessive ventricular dilatation. They should be started once the patient is clinically stable (unless contraindicated) and continued indefinitely unless side effects supervene.
- Glycaemic control: tight control of blood glucose is important in patients with diabetes mellitus. Diabetics and patients who are not known to be diabetic but have new hyperglycaemia on admission following an acute MI, have a greater mortality than non-diabetics and those without elevation of glucose.
- Ongoing anticoagulation: warfarin therapy may be initiated in certain situations (e.g. post-infarction congestive cardiac failure or anterior MI with a high risk of left ventricular thrombus) This can be commenced once the patient is clinically stable and all diagnostic studies have been completed. It may be continued following an MI in patients already receiving anticoagulation for other conditions (e.g atrial fibrillation, valve replacement, systemic embolus). Patients who are intolerant of both aspirin and clopidogrel may be considered suitable for warfarin therapy.
- Aldosterone receptor antagonists (e.g. spironolactone) may be given to patients who have post-MI heart failure or left ventricular diastolic dysfunction. They should be commenced within 3–14 days of the infarct, preferably after ACE inhibitor therapy has started, but being aware of possible hyperkalaemia.
- Antihypertensive therapy: it is important that hypertension should be treated and BP maintained at or below 140/90 mmHg (lower if the patient has other comorbidities such as diabetes).

Cardiac rehabilitation

The aim of rehabilitation is to promote lifelong lifestyle changes that will reduce risk factors for coronary artery disease. This begins in hospital when the patient is medically stable with a structured individualized programme of assessment, education, and exercise. This continues in the community, usually for a further 3 months. A multidisciplinary approach is taken with particular risk factors being addressed.

- Tobacco use: smoking cessation advice and support to stop smoking using nicotine replacement therapy; advice to avoid passive smoking.
- Weight management: weight loss advice if overweight or obese; referral to dietician if necessary.
- BP control: monitoring, adherence to medication.
- Physical activity: individual exercise programme.
- Diet: low salt intake with regular fruit, vegetables, and fish, increased comsumption of omega-3-fatty acid (oily fish), alcohol in moderation.
- Adherence to secondary prevention medication: monitoring, education.
- Management of diabetes mellitus.
- Lipid control: diet, exercise, and medication.
- Psychological support: early detection of anxiety, fear, and depression (depression can affect one in four of patients following acute MI). The patient and family/carers should be given sensitive reassurance and explanation of the nature of the illness. Antidepressants may be necessary.
- Advice on return to work and driving. In the UK driving is not recommended for the first 4 weeks after MI.

Stable angina pectoris

The usual cause is critical narrowing of one or more coronary arteries leading to a myocardial oxygen debt and ischaemia during periods of increased demand such as exercise. Symptoms are relieved within about 5 minutes by rest or GTN. It is considered stable when the triggers, ease of relief, and duration and frequency of symptoms are predictable and there is no recent myocardial damage. Rarer causes include aortic stenosis or hypertrophic obstructive cardiomyopathy, where both aortic and coronary blood flow may be severely compromised), hypertensive heart disease, and severe anaemia (where the oxygen-carrying capacity of the blood is significantly reduced). Significant arrhythmias may compromise cardiac output, leading to angina. Prinzmetal angina is chest pain occurring at rest but due to coronary artery spasm.

Risk factors include smoking, diabetes, hypertension, obesity, raised cholesterol and other lipids, and a family history of coronary heart disease. The long-term prognosis is variable and depends on the severity of disease, left ventricular function, exercise tolerance, and comorbidities. It can result in unstable angina and MI, and a reduced quality of life and general health.

Pain

The typical pain is described as a constricting discomfort in the front of the chest, shoulders, neck, jaw, or back. Assessment should include the severity, location, duration, radiation, and frequency, and any factors that provoke or alleviate the pain. It is not usually sharp, stabbing, or influenced by respiration and lasts only a few minutes.

Investigations

- Full blood count—to exclude anaemia.
- Urea and electrolytes—to identify renal impairment, electrolyte abnormalities.
- Lipid profile—to identify hyperlipidaemia.
- Fasting blood sugar—to identify impaired glycaemia or diabetes.
- Resting 12-lead ECG—this may indicate ischaemia or previous MI but may not be conclusive. It should considered in addition to the clinical history, presence of cardiovascular risk factors, and history of ischaemic heart disease.
- Exercise tolerance testing (exercise ECG).
- Myocardial persfusion scintography—for patients unable to tolerate exercise testing or who have pre-existing ECG abnormalities.
- Coronary angiography—usually performed on patients at high risk, those who continue to have symptoms despite optimal medical management, or where the diagnosis is unclear. CT coronary angiography may be performed in those deemed low to intermediate risk.

Management

Drug therapy

Patients are usually treated with one of the following drugs, but sometimes two are given in combination. For example, if anginal symptoms are not controlled on β-blockade, a calcium-channel blocker can be added.

- Beta-blockers—these are used as first-line therapy for relief of symptoms. They improve the oxygen supply–demand balance by reducing heart rate and blood pressure, decreasing end-systolic stress and contractility, and prolonging diastole, thus increasing coronary blood flow. If β-blockers are contraindicated, patients should be treated with calcium-channel blockers, long-acting nitrates or the potassium-channel opener nicorandil.
- Calcium-channel blockers (e.g. verapamil, amlodipine)—these inhibit calcium transport and induce smooth muscle relaxation. They are generally as effective as β-blockers in reducing anginal symptoms.
- Potassium-channel activators (e.g nicorandil).
- Nitrates—these act on vascular smooth muscle and produce venous and arterial dilatation, reducing preload, afterload, and oxygen demand. Sublingual GTN spray or tablets should be used for immediate pain relief and before activities known to precipitate angina. Nitrate intolerance can be avoided by taking long-acting preparations (e.g. isosorbide mononitrate) at staggered intervals.

All patients with stable angina due to atherosclerotic disease should also receive long-term aspirin (to prevent new vascular events) and statins (to lower blood lipids). ACE inhibitors may also be considered.

Heart failure

The commonest cause of acute heart failure is pump failure due to myocardial ischaemia or infarction. However, other causes should be considered, as many have specific treatments (Table 5.20). Some pathologies will result in high-output cardiac failure (e.g. thyrotoxic crisis, beriberi, severe anaemia). The body's response to a fall in cardiac output is sympathetic induction of vasoconstriction and tachycardia. However, this will increase the workload and thereby exacerbate the strain on a damaged heart.

BP is initially maintained in the face of a falling cardiac output by vasoconstriction. A normal value may camouflage a barely adequate (or inadequate) cardiac output. Indeed, there may be an exaggerated vasoconstrictor response, which, with coexisting anxiety, may cause an initial elevation in BP, a further increase in LV afterload, and a greater reduction in cardiac output. Only when this vasoconstrictor reflex response fails will the BP fall. When organ hypoperfusion coexists, this is termed cardiogenic shock.

The consequences of an inadequate cardiac output are clinically manifest through inadequacies of forward blood flow and increased retrograde venous congestion. Left-sided retrograde congestion results in an increase in left atrial and pulmonary venous pressures and increasing hydrostatic pressures within the lung, thereby forcing water from intravascular to interstitial compartments. When the lymphatics' absorptive capacity is exceeded pulmonary oedema ensues with resulting dyspnoea and orthopnoea. Gas exchange is impaired

Table 5.20 Heart failure: causes and treatment

Cause	Specific treatment
Myocardial infarction	Thrombolysis, PCI, early surgical revascularization
Drugs (e.g. β-blockers, verapamil)	Specific 'antagonists', e.g. glucose–insulin–potassium
Dysrhythmias	Appropriate anti-dysrhythmic agents or pacemaker insertion
Valve dysfunction	Valve replacement, valvuloplasty (NB: antibiotics for endocarditis)
Ventricular septal defect	Surgery
Pericardial tamponade	Drainage, pericardiotomy
Constrictive pericarditis (e.g. TB)	Surgery
Haemorrhage and anaemia	Resuscitation and transfusion, correction of cause
Pulmonary embolus	Thrombolytics, embolectomy
Cardiomyopathy, myocarditis	Specific (e.g. immunosuppression)
Hypertension	Antihypertensives, treat cause if found
Thyrotoxic crisis	Iodine, propranolol, steroids, carbimazole
Wet beri-beri (i.e. vitamin B1 deficiency resulting in heart failure)	Thiamine replacement

with resulting hypoxaemia. Right-sided retrograde congestion causes a raised CVP, hepatic congestion with elevated liver enzymes and bilirubin, and, eventually, progression to dependent oedema.

The combination of hypoxaemia, lactic acidosis, increased extravascular lung water, respiratory muscle fatigue (resulting from poor perfusion), and anxiety will cause tachypnoea and an increase in the work of breathing, accounting for up to 30% of total cardiac work. Either the left and/or right heart may be affected by the disease process. A worsening of lung disease may cause acute right ventricular decompensation. Myocardial ischaemia/infarction may affect predominantly one ventricle. The normal co-relationship between ventricular filling pressures no longer, holds. For example, with right ventricular infarction there may be high right-sided pressures (CVP) but low left-sided filling pressures (PAWP).

Ventricular compliance will also be affected; this worsens due to a variety of factors including myocardial ischaemia, increased afterload, and fluid overload. As a consequence, the ventricle becomes stiffer, altering the intraventricular pressure–volume relationship such that a higher filling pressure is required to achieve the same end diastolic volume (LVEDV). For the same filling pressure the LVEDV will thus be smaller and the stroke volume lower. Monitoring the patient using filling pressures alone (i.e. CVP and PAWP) is thus unhelpful.

Finally, the patient's fluid balance status in acute heart failure is often misjudged. The clinical or radiological presence of pulmonary oedema does not imply total body fluid overload. By the time the patient arrives in hospital in acute pulmonary oedema, they may well be in negative fluid balance through a combination of sweating, mouth breathing, vomiting and inadequate fluid intake. The fluid is thus in the wrong compartment and requires redistribution rather than removal. The fall in cardiac output and intravascular volume leads to a drop in renal blood flow, stimulating the renin–angiotensin–aldosterone system to produce still more vasoconstriction and oliguria.

With time, secondary hyperaldosteronism will promote fluid retention and an increase in circulating blood volume. The threshold of lymphatic drainage of pulmonary interstitial fluid will be raised and higher pulmonary arterial hydrostatic pressures will be tolerated. However, in the acute phase, the intravascular compartment is often contracted, a situation which may be further aggravated by fluid restriction and diuretic usage.

Assessment

Physical assessment

- **Skin**: cyanosis, pallor, and sweating may be apparent. Inadequate forward blood flow resulting in organ hypoperfusion produces cold shut-down peripheries.

Peripheral oedema (leg or sacral) may be seen with right-sided heart failure.

- **Respiration**: the patient is often tachypnoeic and may produce blood-stained frothy sputum as a result of pulmonary oedema. Wheeze ('cardiac asthma') may be a presenting feature.
- **General**: the patient may show signs of generalized weakness and fatigue.
- **Auscultation**: the apex beat of the patient's heart is often displaced, and a gallop rhythm (due to a third and/or fourth heart sound) may be heard on auscultation. In left heart failure end-inspiratory crackles ('crepitations') may be heard at the lung bases.

Physiological assessment

- **CVP** will be high with right-sided heart failure.
- **PAWP** will be elevated in left-sided heart failure.
- **BP** may be low, normal, or high.
- **Heart rate**: tachycardia will usually be evident unless bradycardia is the main cause of failure.
- **Renal function**: urine output may be reduced and renal dysfunction evident from blood urea and creatinine levels.
- **Lactic acidosis** is produced because of insufficient tissue oxygen delivery to meet cellular needs.

Neurological/psychological assessment

Mental obtundation (drowsiness, confusion or agitation) may be seen3 as a result of poor cardiac output and cerebral hypoperfusion

Investigations

Urgent investigations include 12-lead ECG, chest X-ray, and appropriate blood investigations such as urea and electrolytes, haemoglobin, glucose, and cardiac enzymes. Troponin T or I should be measured if there is a suspicion of myocardial injury. Brain-type natriuretic peptide (BNP) should also be measured. This is released into the bloodstream from the ventricle when it is excessively stretched. Although plasma BNP levels rise in other conditions, such as pulmonary embolus, a high level does suggest heart failure. A high degree of elevation is a poor prognostic factor in chronic heart failure; it may be useful as a therapeutic endpoint for such patients.

Pulmonary oedema has a characteristic chest X-ray appearance with upper lobe blood diversion, increased fluid in the lymphatics (Kerley B lines) and the lung fissures, pleural effusions, and cardiomegaly. A 'bat's wing' appearance due to an engorged vasculature may be seen at the pulmonary hilum.

Echocardiography should be performed and may show regions of the ventricular wall that move poorly, irregularly, or not at all, or other causes such as pericardial tamponade or valvular dysfunction.

Priorities of care

These are aimed at restoring an adequate circulation as quickly as possible.

- Administration of high flow, high concentration oxygen.
- Preload and afterload reduction (by vasodilators, opiates, and, for intravascular overload, diuretics).
- If required, augmentation of cardiac output by inotropes or mechanical support including invasive or non-invasive mechanical ventilation, intra-aortic balloon pulsation (IABP), and ventricular support devices.
- Reassurance, information, and comfort.

Principles of care

Monitoring

This depends on the severity of the failure and usually consists of a minimum of continuous ECG monitoring, pulse oximetry, and frequent BP monitoring. In progressively more severe cases, invasive arterial pressure monitoring, CVP monitoring, and CO monitoring may be required. Mixed (or central) venous saturation are also reasonable indicators of oxygen supply–demand balance. If more sophisticated monitoring is in place, treatment can be titrated more precisely to achieve adequate organ perfusion. However, whether this achieves any improvement in outcome has not been formally demonstrated.

Rest

The heart can be 'rested' by reducing excessive degrees of preload and afterload, by reducing the work of breathing using mechanical ventilatory support, and by insertion of an IABP or other cardiac support device.

Optimizing intravascular fluid volume

The PAWP provides a rough guide to left ventricular filling, while the CVP offers the same for the right heart. Abnormal elevations in PAWP/CVP are seen in heart failure and may indicate the need for preload reduction, albeit acknowledging that the decrease in ventricular compliance will increase filling pressures though not necessarily filling volumes. Patients with chronic heart failure will often run a high filling pressure in the non-acute situation, sometimes >25–30 mmHg. Likewise, treatment with vasoconstrictors will further increase tone and reduce ventricular compliance, thereby elevating the PAWP/CVP still further for the same end-diastolic volume. Thus, rather than routinely aiming for a target figure of, say, 14–18 mmHg for PAWP (or 10–12 mmHg for CVP), the filling pressure should be used in conjunction with stroke volume to monitor dynamic challenges such as a fluid challenge. Because of the potential alterations in ventricular compliance, and vasoconstriction induced by coexisting hypovolaemia (e.g. excessive diuretics) and inotropes, a fluid challenge should be contemplated even when the PAWP/CVP is 'normal' or even raised. No rise in stroke volume and a rise in PAWP/CVP >3 mmHg following a 200–250 ml challenge suggests that optimal filling of the intravascular compartment has been achieved. The patient is very unlikely to decompensate with a single fluid challenge, and the circulating volume should be optimized before introducing other drugs. A fall in blood pressure on a low vasodilator infusion dose suggests underfilling of the left ventricle. A fluid challenge should not be withheld even in patients with poor gas exchange, as patients generally die from organ hypoperfusion rather than hypoxaemia.

Supporting the cardiac output

Failing the measures just described, the heart can be 'driven' by inotropes, although this should not be more than necessary to maintain adequate organ perfusion. No target figure of cardiac output exists. In general, the cardiac index (output indexed for body surface area) should exceed 2.2 L/min/m^2 (approx 3.5 L/min), but this is a very rough guide. More relevant is the worsening or improvement in base deficit and lactic acidaemia, the production of adequate urine, good cerebration, etc. Mixed (S_vO_2) or central ($S_{cv}O_2$) venous oxygen saturations are sensitive guides to the ability of the cardiorespiratory system to meet whole-body oxygen demands. In low output states the tissues compensate for the decrease in oxygen delivery by extracting more oxygen and the S_vO_2 falls. In severe heart failure this can drop below 30–40%, indicating virtually maximal extraction with very little reserve held. An S_vO_2 of 60% is a useful goal in the haemodynamic management of severe heart failure.

Reducing ventricular afterload

The SVR is usually raised in heart failure and thus cardiac workload is increased. Reducing afterload will reduce cardiac work. Cardiac output is usually augmented by vasodilatation, though further filling may be necessary. Likewise, for right ventricular failure, manipulation of pulmonary vascular resistance will allow optimization of right ventricular output.

Therapies

The standard textbook approach consists of oxygen, low dose opiates, diuretics, and nitrates. These may be preceded or followed by inotropes, depending on the presence or persistence of a low cardiac output/low BP state. Diuretics cause an initial vasodilatation followed, 20–30 min later, by a diuresis. Although the vasodilatation is beneficial, the diuresis is not if the patient is not fluid overloaded. Falls in cardiac output following diuretic treatment of heart failure are well documented. Although symptomatic relief is quickly afforded with the initial vasodilatation and improvement in output, the ensuing diuresis may result in significant hypovolaemia with vasoconstriction, increased cardiac work, a fall in output, and reduced perfusion. This will lead to a metabolic acidosis and compensatory tachypnoea and oliguria. The tachypnoea and oliguria may be mistaken for worsening pump failure, resulting in the administration of additional, and larger, doses of diuretic, which compound the problem further.

Diuretic therapy should not be totally discounted. It does have a role in certain situations, notably true intravascular volume overload (e.g. excessive IV infusion), or total body fluid overload as may often be found with chronic heart failure. Furthermore, patients on long-term diuretic therapy will often require continuation to maintain an adequate diuresis. Cessation, if indicated, should be gradual. For those patients not on diuretics, an effective diuresis may frequently be achieved by small intravenous doses (i.e. 10–20 mg furosemide).

Nitrates can be given rapidly by either oral or sublingual nitrolingual spray while an infusion is being prepared. Nitrates have both preload- and afterload-reducing properties which are dose dependent. Tolerance will develop by 24 hours, necessitating higher doses to achieve a similar effect. A drop in BP on a low dose infusion is suggestive of hypovolaemia.

No drug used to increase cardiac contractility is a pure inotrope—all have additional vasodilator or vasoconstrictor properties to a greater or lesser degree. Falls in blood pressure are occasionally seen with dobutamine and, more commonly, with phosphodiesterase inhibitor inodilators such as enoximone and milrinone. Reductions in dose, or fluid challenges, may be required to restore the BP to satisfactory levels. The advantage of dobutamine over the currently available phosphodiesterase inhibitors is its much shorter half-life. Epinephrine, dopamine, and norepinephrine all possess vasoconstrictor properties. A balance has to be achieved between adequate vasoconstriction to maintain a reasonable coronary perfusion pressure and excessive vasoconstriction which will increase cardiac work and myocardial oxygen consumption, possibly resulting in a fall in cardiac output. As norepinephrine and higher doses of dopamine have more of a vasoconstrictor effect than epinephrine, they should generally be used in heart failure states only in combination with dobutamine or a vasodilator. Levosimendan, a calcium sensitizer, improves ventricular contractility and vasodilates peripherally without having a major impact on cardiac work.

CPAP or BiPAP reduces the work of breathing, improves oxygenation, and has beneficial effects on preload and afterload in heart failure. Mechanical ventilation, with or without the addition of PEEP, also reduces the work of breathing and allows the use of heavy sedation, thereby reducing demands placed upon the heart. It will also reduce right and left ventricular preload and left ventricular afterload. In an overfilled state, cardiac output is augmented by the use of non-invasive or invasive mechanical ventilation; however, a fall in output may occur if the patient is hypovolaemic.

Intra-aortic balloon counterpulsation and ventricular assist devices can also be considered, although their availability tends to be restricted to specialist centres. (See Table 5.21 for a summary of the management of heart failure.)

Indications for surgery are few. Some centres in the United States and Germany have shown significant improvements in outcome for post-infarction ventricular failure by salvaging ischaemic but not yet necrosed myocardium through either immediate angioplasty or surgery. A permanently damaged myocardium will not improve following revascularization. Other surgically remediable causes include papillary leaflet rupture of the mitral valve, aortic stenosis, and ventricular septal defect. Surgery may be required for uncommon pathologies such as constrictive pericarditis and hypertrophic obstructive cardiomyopathy.

Pericarditis

Pericarditis is an inflammation of the pericardium due to a variety of causes:

- myocardial infarction: either within 1-2 days, or Dressler's syndrome
- malignancy (primary or secondary)
- radiotherapy
- trauma
- heart surgery and post pericardiotomy syndrome
- metabolic disorders (e.g. uraemia, hyperthyroidism)
- connective tissue disorders (e.g. SLE, rheumatoid arthritis, sarcoidosis, scleroderma)
- infection (bacterial, viral, fungal, tuberculous)
- medication reactions (e.g to phenytoin, hydralazine, procainamide).

Table 5.21 Directed management of heart failure

Physiological derangement	Directed management
Vasoconstriction (indicated by low cardiac output, normal or high BP)	If evidence of hypovolaemia (low PAWP/CVP), give fluid challenges to optimize stroke volume If BP/PAWP high, commence (or increase) nitrate (or other vasodilator) infusion
Low CO and BP despite optimizing fluid and nitrates	Consider obstructive cause, e.g. pulmonary embolus Commence dobutamine or epinephrine ± more vasodilator therapy Consider IABP, invasive/non-invasive mechanical ventilation
S_vO_2 <60% ± signs of inadequate organ perfusion persisting despite optimizing ventricular filling and attempted normalization of afterload	Inotropes ± inodilators, ± mechanical ventilation, ± IABP, ± ventricular assist device
Total body fluid overload, or intravascular volume overload	Diuetics: initially at low doses, taking care not to cause hypovolaemia; increase as necessary. Haemofiltration if poor response to diuretics
Poor urine output.	Exclude hypovolaemia Treat low output state as above Consider further elevation in mean systemic BP Has an ACE inhibitor been administered? If so, consider stopping because of renovascular disease Consider diuretics (initially at low doses) or haemofiltration

Assessment

Physical assessment

- **Pain**: usually presents as a sharp constant central chest pain eased by sitting forward and worsened by deep inspiration or coughing. It may radiate to the neck, arm, shoulder, or occasionally abdomen. It is not related to food or eased by nitrates.
- **Auscultation** may reveal a pericardial friction rub—a scratchy noise heard throughout the cardiac cycle caused by the inflamed surfaces rubbing together.
- **Pulsus paradoxus**: a raised jugular venous pressure (JVP) and muffled heart sounds may be present with severe constrictive pericarditis or a significant pericardial effusion.

Physiological assessment

- **Heart rate**: tachycardia may be evident.
- **Pyrexia** may be present.

Pericardial tamponade presents with signs of poor forward flow and right heart congestion, or with cardiac arrest.

Investigations

The ECG classically reveals concave-upwards ST segment elevation in all leads with no reciprocal changes in the opposite leads. The chest X-ray and echo usually reveal no abnormality unless a pericardial effusion, constrictive pericarditis, or associated myocarditis is present. A significant pericardial effusion produces a globular cardiac contour on X-ray. Fluid in the pericardial space may be visualized by echo. With constrictive pericarditis, small heart chambers and restricted filling are seen. Calcification may be visible in long-standing TB pericarditis.

Principles of care

- Bed rest.
- Non-steroidal anti-inflammatory drugs (NSAIDs).
- Treat the underlying cause wherever possible.

Steroids are rarely indicated except in immunologically-mediated causes. Complications of pericarditis include cardiac tamponade (see next section) and constrictive pericarditis. Constrictive pericarditis occurs when chronic inflammation of the pericardium causes thickening and scarring such that the heart cannot expand when blood enters it. Occasionally, pericardiotomy (cutting a small hole in the pericardial sac) or, rarely, pericardiectomy may be performed. During a pericardiectomy the pericardium is completely stripped away, but this is a high risk procedure. Most patients are managed medically.

Pericardial tamponade

A build-up of blood or fluid in the pericardial space prevents the ventricles from expanding fully, leading to decreased ventricular filling. With each successive diastolic period, less and less blood enters the ventricles, and the increasing pressure on the heart forces the septum to bend towards the left ventricle, causing decreased stroke volume. This causes obstructive shock and is a life-threatening condition; unless treated it will result in cardiac arrest (usually pulseless electrical activity (PEA)).

Causes of pericardial tamponade

- Pericarditis.
- Dissecting aortic aneurysm.
- Trauma to the heart.
- Myocardial infarction.
- Heart surgery.

Symptoms

- Hypotension due to decreased stroke volume.
- Jugular venous distension due to impaired venous return to the heart.
- Muffled heart sounds due to the sound-damping effect of fluid inside the pericardium.
- Pulsus paradoxus (a drop of at least 10 mmHg of arterial BP on inspiration).
- ST segment changes; there may also be low voltage QRS complexes.
- Symptoms of shock (tachypnoea, tachycardia, breathlessness, decreased level of conciousness).

Investigations

If time allows, echo is the diagnostic tool of choice. Chest X-ray will show a globular heart.

Management

Treatment is by percutaneous pericardiocentesis where a needle is inserted into the pericardium and the fluid is removed. In emergency situations this is done 'blind' (if time allows, it is done under echo or fluoroscopic screening). The patient is laid resting semi-supine and, after cleansing of the site and injection of local anaesthetic, a long 18-gauge catheter connected to a syringe is introduced by the side of the xiphisternum under the costal margin and advanced in the direction of the scapula. An ECG V lead can be attached to the needle to detect when the myocardium is being penetrated (ST segment changes or multiple ventricular ectopics are often seen). When fluid is aspirated the catheter should be advanced no further. At this stage, a three-way tap can be attached and total drainage performed. Alternatively, a guide wire may be advanced through the cannula into the pericardial space, the cannula removed, and a pigtail catheter placed over the guide wire. Specimens should be sent for culture and cytology where appropriate. Blood may be aspirated (haemopericardium), particularly after trauma, cardiac surgery, or malignancy. This differs from blood aspirated from within the heart chamber as it does not clot. If in doubt, the catheter may be transduced to see whether a characteristic right ventricular pressure waveform is seen. Further details on pericardial tamponade are given in Chapter11.

Complications of needle pericardiocentesis include damage to the ventricle or a coronary artery, arrhythmias, or pneumothorax.

Infective endocarditis

This is infection of the endocardial surface of the heart, which includes the heart valves (native or prosthetic), endoventricular septum, chordae tendineae, mural endocardium, and intracardiac devices (e.g. pacemakers, defibrillators). The heart valves are predominantly affected. Endocarditis is caused mainly by bacteria but, occasionally, by other infective agents. All cases develop from non-bacterial thrombotic endocarditis (a sterile platelet/fibrin vegetation) which provides a site for adhesion and invasion by micro-organisms. In acute infective endocarditis these arise as a result of trauma (pacing wires, catheters, etc.) or turbulence to the endothelial surface of the heart. A transient bacteraemia (e.g. from invasive procedures, dentistry, recreational drug use, urinary tract infection) then delivers the organism to the vegatation and if a heart valve is involved, the organism invades the valvular leaflets. Heart valves that have previously been damaged (e.g. by rheumatic fever) or are prosthetic allow an increased risk of attachment, but half of all cases occur on previously normal valves. Left-sided heart valves are more commonly affected, except in intravenous drug abusers who usually have right-sided heart valve lesions, particularly tricuspid. Since heart valves do not receive a dedicated blood supply, local defensive immune responses cannot be initiated and drug therapy has difficulty reaching them. Severe valvular insufficiency can result, leading to intractable congestive heart failure and myocardial abcesses.

The developing disease produces further clinical features of embolic or immunological origin. These include:

- emboli of the middle cerebral artery causing hemiplegia
- renal infarction
- splenic infarction
- retinal artery occlusion causing blindness
- coronary artery embolus causing myocardial infarction
- pulmonary embolus
- acute meningitis
- immune-mediated vasculitis
- interstitial nephritis or proliferative glomerulonephritis from circulating immune complexes causing renal failure
- immunologically mediated synovitis causing musculoskeletal symptoms
- immune-mediated myocarditis causing palpitations
- deposition of immune complexes in disc spaces causing back pain
- skin lesions.

Assessment

Patients may present with one or more of the following:

- fever, malaise, weight loss, night sweats, finger clubbing, anaemia
- heart murmur
- petechiae (affecting conjunctival, oral mucosa, hands, feet, abdominal wall, chest)
- retinal haemorrhages
- Osler's nodes (small tender red nodules on fingers and toes)
- splinter or subungual haemorrhages
- signs and symptoms of embolic or immunological manifestations
- splenomegaly.

Specific investigations

- Echocardiography may reveal vegetations on the affected valves; however, these have to be large enough to be visualized (usually >3 mm). Trans-oesophageal echocardiography is a more sensitive technique for detecting vegetations.
- Blood cultures.
- Blood and urine tests for antigen (e.g. staphylococcal, streptococcal), acute phase titres.

Management

- Antibiotic treatment has to be aggressive and prolonged. Two agents are often used in combination,
- Replacement of the damaged valve may be necessary. Traditionally, this was delayed until a course of antibiotics had been given, but surgical practice is now becoming more aggressive.
- Specific complications such as renal and heart failure and embolic events require treatment.
- Guidelines now recommend antibiotic prophylaxis is no longer offered routinely for defined interventional procedures (National Institute for Health and Clinical Excellence 2008).

Valvular heart disease: stenosis

Valvular stenosis predominantly affects the aortic and mitral valves and occurs when the valve opening is smaller than normal because of stiff, fused or damaged leaflets.

Mitral stenosis results from narrowing of the mitral valve orifice so that it is more difficult for blood to flow from the left atrium into the left ventricle during ventricular diastole. This high resistance causes the left atrium to enlarge over time because it has to generate higher than normal pressures when it contracts against the stenotic valve. The consequent manifestations include reduced cardiac output, tachycardia, congestive heart failure, and pulmonary oedema. As the left atrium enlarges, it is also more prone to develop atrial fibrillation with the additional risk of systemic embolism.

Aortic stenosis is characterized by the left ventricular pressure being much greater than the aortic pressure during left ventricular ejection. Because the ventricle is required to generate greater pressures this leads to left ventricular hypertrophy and diastolic dysfunction (impaired filling). Elevated LVEDP causes blood to back up into the left atrium and pulmonary veins which increases left atrial pressure and pulmonary artery wedge pressure, resulting in congestive cardiac failure and pulmonary oedema. The left atrium becomes enlarged and hypertrophies. In calcific aortic stenosis the calcification can progress and extend to the electrical conduction system, resulting in heart block.

Causes of mitral stenosis

- Rheumatic fever.
- Congenital.
- Calcification of mitral valve leaflets.

Causes of aortic stenosis

- Age-related calcification.
- Bicuspid aortic valve.
- Rheumatic fever.

Assessment

Aortic stenosis (AS) may present with angina, symptoms of heart failure, low output (including syncope: 'Stokes–Adams attacks'), or sudden death. Mitral stenosis (MS) usually presents with symptoms of heart failure including fatigue and breathlessness.

Characteristic murmurs are heard for AS (ejection systolic murmur) and for MS (mid-diastolic rumbling murmur); their absence or prolongation may indicate increasing severity. The pulse pressure is usually narrow with AS.

Investigations

- ECG: P mitrale (broad notched P wave) in several leads in AS. No specific changes occur in MS but heart block and left ventricular hypertrophy may be seen.
- Echocardiography may show left ventricular hypertrophy, a thickened and immobile aortic valve, and a dilated aortic root in AS. With MS the left atrium may be dilated. Doppler flow across the stenosed valve shows turbulent flow and a high pressure gradient.
- Chest X-ray may show left atrial enlargement in mitral stenosis, and a calcified aortic valve, enlarged left ventricle, and enlarged atrium in aortic stenosis. Pulmonary oedema may be apparent.
- Cardiac catheterization provides definitive diagnosis

Management

- Heart failure is treated in conventional fashion. Excessive arterial dilation should be avoided in severe aortic stenosis as this can precipitate collapse.
- Hypertension should be aggressively controlled.
- Angina is treated with nitrovasodilators, β-blockers, and/or calcium-channel blockers.
- Surgery is needed for severe cases—either valve replacement or, less commonly nowadays, percutaneous valvuloplasty by balloon catheter. Transcatheter aortic valve implantation (TAVI) is an increasingly popular means of valve replacement in patients deemed high risk for traditional valve replacement

as it can be performed under local anaesthetic in the catheter laboratory.
- Anticoagulation therapy for atrial fibrillation for prophylaxis against emboli.

Valvular heart disease: incompetence (regurgitation)

This may be due to direct valve damage (e.g. endocarditis) or functional, i.e. secondary to ventricular dilatation. Valve leaflets are stiff, misshapen, or incorrectly supported and thus do not seal. Regurgitant flow occurs, either back into the atria during systole with mitral and tricuspid incompetence, or back into the left ventricle during diastole with aortic incompetence.

Causes of valvular incompetence

Aortic incompetence:

- rheumatic heart disease
- endocarditis
- ankylosing spondylitis
- Marfan's syndrome
- aortic dissection
- syphilis.

Mitral incompetence:

- rheumatic heart disease
- mitral valve prolapse
- ruptured chordae tendinae or papillary muscle (after MI or trauma)
- functional (due to dilated ventricle)
- endocarditis
- cardiomyopathy.

Tricuspid incompetence:

- rheumatic heart disease
- functional (due to dilated ventricle)
- endocarditis (especially drug abusers).

Assessment

Incompetence results in a decrease in forward flow with symptoms of low output (e.g. fatigue) and an increase in retrograde congestion. This may result in breathlessness for left-sided lesions, and hepatic congestion and peripheral oedema for right-sided lesions.

Investigations

Characteristic murmurs are heard for aortic regurgitation (high-pitched early diastolic murmur), mitral regurgitation (pan-systolic murmur), and tricuspid regurgitation (pan-systolic murmur, louder on inspiration). The chest X-ray may show cardiomegaly. A wide pulse pressure with a collapsing pulse is seen with aortic regurgitation, and a pulsatile liver is seen with tricuspid regurgitation. Echocardiography is diagnostic.

Management

- Conventional treatment for heart failure.
- Digoxin and anticoagulation if atrial fibrillation is present.
- Surgery—valve replacement or repair.

Cardiomyopathy

This is an idiopathic heart muscle disease not related to ischaemia. There are three types of cardiomyopathy.

- Congestive (also called dilated). The walls of the heart chambers dilate to hold a greater volume of blood than normal. Causes include coronary artery disease, infection, non-infectious inflammatory conditions, alcohol and other drugs or toxins, nutitional and metabolic disorders, and pregnancy.
- Hypertrophic (HCM). A portion of the myocardium becomes hypertrophied without obvious cause (though it is often congenital). The normal alignment of the muscle cells and electrical function of the heart then becomes disrupted. It may be obstructive (hypertrophic obstructive cardiomyopathy (HOCM)) or non-obstructive, depending on whether the distortion of normal heart anatomy causes an outflow obstruction of blood from the left ventricle. It is a significant cause of sudden unexpected death in any age group, and is frequently asymptomatic until sudden death occurs.
- Restrictive. The walls of the atria and ventricles are rigid and the heart is restricted from stretching and filling with blood properly. Preload and end-diastolic volume are reduced. Diastolic dysfunction and heart failure subsequently develop. Cause include cardiac amyloidosis, haemochromatosis, sarcoidosis, and post-radiation fibrosis.

Assessment

The presentation of cardiomyopathy is often mistaken for another cause, for example:

- heart failure (congestive)
- constrictive pericarditis (restrictive)
- angina (HOCM)
- syncope (HOCM)

- palpitations may be experienced and a late systolic murmur heard due to outflow obstruction of the left ventricle (HOCM)
- dyspnoea (HOCM).

Investigations

Definitive diagnosis is usually made by echocardiography. Myocardial biopsy may be performed.

Management

- Treatment of heart failure.
- Treatment of any arrhythmias.
- Surgery (e.g. myomectomy) or transplantation may be necessary.
- Patients will require counselling and education regarding the disease and its prognosis.
- Family members should be screened if a hereditary cause is suspected.

Myocarditis

This is characterized by inflammation of myocytes due to infectious, toxic, or autoimmune causes (e.g Coxsackie virus, diphtheria, rheumatic fever, connective tissue diseases such as SLE, and drugs). This can lead to ventricular dysfunction and dilated cardiomyopathy. Many patients present with a non-specific illness (myalgia, mild dyspnoea, fatigue), but some may present acutely with congestive cardiac failure. More than half of patients have a viral illness with cardiac symptoms occuring about 2 weeks after the viraemia.

Assessment

- Fever.
- Dyspnoea on exertion or symptoms of heart failure (orthopnoea, shortness of breath at rest).
- Fatigue, malaise, arthralgia, fibralgia.
- Chest pain—pleuritic, stabbing, sharp precordial pain. Pericarditis may be present.
- Palpitations.
- Syncope—may indicate atrioventricular block. The patient is at risk of sudden death.

Investigations

- Chest X-ray is often normal, but may show cardiomegaly if congestive cardiac failure is present. There may be pleural effusions and pulmonary oedema.
- Echocardiography may show impaired left ventricular and diastolic function, impaired ejection fraction, segmental wall abnormalities, and pericardial effusion.
- MRI may show patchy areas of inflammation and can be used for later guided endocardial biopsy.
- ECG may show sinus tachycardia, ST segment elevation without reciprocal depression, decreased QRS amplitude and transitory Q waves. Conduction disturbances (Mobitz types I and II, or complete heart block, or left or right bundle branch block) may be present.
- Specific blood tests: cardiac troponin I is positive in 35% of patients. Antinuclear antibody (ANA) and other tests for collagen vascular disease should be performed if a systemic disorder is suspected.
- Endomyocardial biopsy: if unexplained heart failure with haemodynamic compromise.

Management

Treatment is bed rest and conventional treatment of heart failure or angina, if present. The patient should be continuously monitored. Placement of a temporary cardiac pacemaker may be required for Mobitz type II or complete heart block. Patients usually recover spontaneously, but may progress to severe irreversible heart failure requiring mechanical support ± cardiac transplantation.

Other types of heart muscle disease

Symptoms are usually those of congestive cardiomyopathy with features of heart failure:

- hypertension
- haemochromatosis
- alcohol
- sarcoidosis
- post-partum
- Friedrich's ataxia
- diabetes
- myotonic dystrophy
- hyper- and hypothyroidism
- radiation and cytotoxic drugs such as adriamycin.

Aortic aneurysm

A tear in the intimal lining of the aortic vessel wall allows blood to track into the media. The blood may track along the media dissection, either up or down the aorta, occluding branch vessels. Rupture may occur through the outer adventitial layer. Atheroma is the commonest underlying pathology, and this may be accelerated by hypertension and hyperlipidaemia. Other causes include congenital conditions such as Marfan's syndrome and connective tissue disorders. A major cause is direct trauma (see Chapter 11).

Assessment

Physical assessment

- **Pain:** a tearing pain of abrupt onset in the chest or upper abdomen radiating through to the back is the classic mode of presentation.
- **Neurological symptoms:** syncope, headache, stroke, or paraplegia.
- **Pulses:** one or more of the major pulses may be absent or asymmetric.
- **Signs of acute aortic incompetence** may be present if the ascending aorta is involved. Angina may also be present due to occlusion of the origins of one or more coronary arteries.

Physiological assessment

- Collapse may occur.
- Angina may also be present due to occlusion of the origins of the coronary vessels.

Investigations

- Chest X-ray may reveal mediastinal widening.
- ECG is usually unremarkable, although ischaemic changes may be present due to occlusion of the origins of one or more coronary arteries.
- CT scan or angiography will delineate the extent of the aneurysm (see Fig 5.43).

Priorities of care

- Management of cardiovascular compromise, including immediate surgery if necessary.
- Pain relief (opiates are usually given).
- High flow, high concentration oxygen.
- BP should be aggressively controlled using an intravenous infusion of sodium nitroprusside, glyceryl trinitrate or a short-acting β-blocker (esmolol) or combined α- and β-blocker (labetalol). Ideally, systolic BP should be decreased below 100 mmHg to reduce shear stresses on the damaged aorta.

Principles of care

- Continuous BP monitorng.

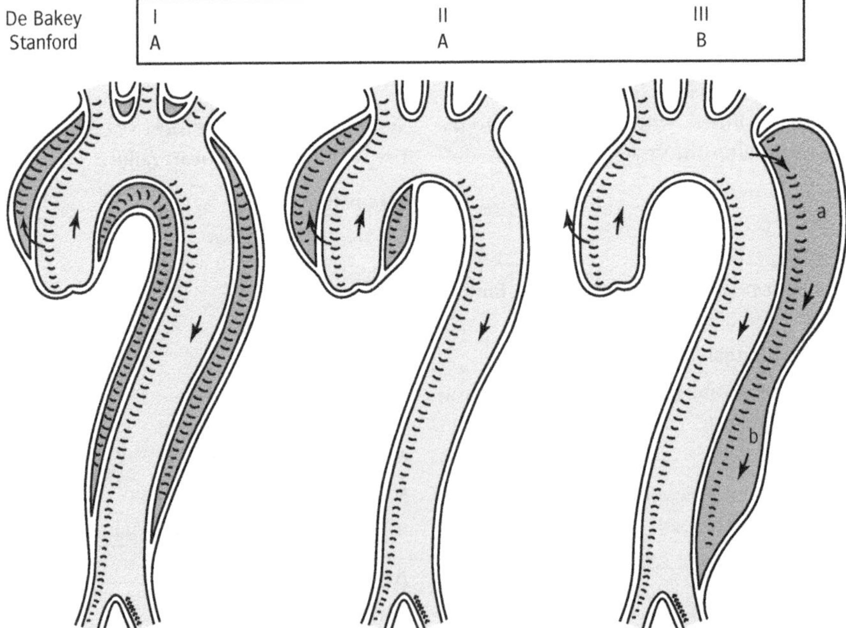

Figure 5.43 Schematic drawing of aortic dissection showing DeBakey and Stanford classification.

Reproduced with permission from Ebel R, Alfonso F, Boileau C *et al.*, Diagnosis and management of aortic dissection. Recommendations of the Task Force on Aortic Dissection, European Society of Cardiology. *European Heart Journal*, Volume 22, Issue 18, pp.1641–1681. Copyright © 2001 Oxford University Press and European Society of Cardiology

- Urinary catheter—to measure urine output. Oliguria suggests that the lowering of blood pressure may be excessive while anuria is suggestive of aneurysmal involvement of the renal arteries.

The regional cardiothoracic unit should be contacted if a thoracic aortic aneurysm is suspected. The patient should be transferred promptly for any further investigations and surgery, as necessary. Ascending aortic aneurysms often require surgery, while those involving the descending aorta are often managed conservatively in the first instance. Radiological placement of stents is another option that may be considered. A risk of surgery or stent placement is occlusion of feeder vessels to the vertebral artery resulting in paraplegia.

Pulmonary embolus

Detachment of part or all of a thrombus, usually from the deep veins of the legs or pelvis, or from within the right heart, passes into the pulmonary vasculature, blocking forward blood flow. The extent of flow obstruction depends on the size (or multitude) of clots, thereby giving rise to signs and symptoms of major (massive) or minor pulmonary embolism (PE). The patient may have recently undergone a long flight, surgery, or be undergoing a prolonged period of immobilization. There may be signs and symptoms of deep venous thrombosis.

Assessment

- Sudden onset of dyspnoea and tachypnoea due to hypoxaemia, metabolic acidosis, and heart failure.
- Chest pain—often pleuritic in nature.
- Cough, haemoptysis.
- With massive pulmonary embolus there may be cyanosis, collapse, and cardiovascular instability (hypotension, tachycardia, raised CVP) due to decreased blood flow through the lungs to the left side of the heart.

Investigations

- CT pulmonary angiography (CTPA) is the definitive investigation.
- Chest X-ray—often normal in the early stages. With massive PE, reduced vascularity is seen in the affected area. A wedge-shaped pulmonary infarct may be seen after several days. CXR can also rule out other causes (e.g congestive cardiac failure, rib fractures).
- ECG may show signs of right ventricular strain. The classic signs are a large S wave in lead I, a large Q wave in lead II, and an inverted T wave in lead III (S_1, Q_3, T_3). The most common ECG changes are sinus tachycardia, right axis deviation, and right bundle branch block.
- Arterial blood gas analysis may show a low P_aO_2 ± a low P_aCO_2 and a metabolic acidosis, but may be normal with small emboli.
- An isotope ventilation/perfusion (V/Q) scan provides an indication of the likelihood of a PE by revealing a ventilated but non-perfused area of lung. This may be multiple. Results are often equivocal, especially if the CXR is abnormal for any reason.
- Doppler studies of the legs—performed to detect deep vein thrombosis.
- Echocardiography—dysfunction of the right side of the heart may be seen with massive PE, indicating severe obstruction of a pulmonary artery.

Priorities of care

- Urgent resuscitation is needed if cardiovascular collapse has occurred. Fluid loading is an important initial step, even though the CVP may be elevated. However, it is important not to overload the right ventricle with too much fluid.
- The patient may prefer to lie flat to improve symptoms of dyspnoea by increasing their venous return.
- Mechanical ventilation may be necessary, but this may cause cardiovascular collapse and/or worsening of gas exchange due to loss of preferential shunting of blood through ventilated areas.
- Anticoagulation is the mainstay of treatment. Heparin, low molecular weight heparins (e.g. enoxaparin or dalteparin), or fondaparinux are administered initially while warfarin loading is commenced. There should be a 3 day overlap of the initial anticoagulant with warfarin to ensure that adequate warfarin anticoagulation levels are achieved.
- Thrombolytic therapy—massive embolism causing haemodynamic instability (shock and/or hypotension) is an indication for thrombolysis. An alternative, especially if thrombolysis is contraindicated, is removal or disruption of large clots either radiologically or surgically. There is a risk of bleeding or stroke with thrombolysis, and the benefit–risk ratio seems at present to be only justified for massive pulmonary embolus. Some authorities argue that the long-term risk of pulmonary hypertension and right heart failure is increased in intermediate PE if thrombolysis is not used.
- A filter ('umbrella') can be placed radiologically in the inferior vena cava to prevent further clots

passing from pelvis or leg veins into the lung. This is particularly useful in patients who cannot be anticoagulated. The filter can be removed after several months once the risk of new PE is adjudged to be low

Shock

Shock is defined as a state of impaired cellular delivery or utilization of oxygen. This, results in a tissue oxygen debt producing a range of metabolic, biochemical, and physiological sequelae including metabolic acidosis and organ dysfunction (e.g. oliguria, confusion). Though hypotension is often present, shock can exist in the presence of a normal (or even elevated) BP. On the other hand, the patient may have a low BP without being shocked.

An alternative way of considering the pathophysiological mechanisms underlying shock is to consider the three components of tissue oxygen delivery (namely cardiac output, arterial oxygen saturation, and haemoglobin concentration) and, secondly, the ability of the cell to use oxygen—predominantly by the mitochondria to generate energy in the form of ATP. Thus shock can be due to one or more of the following:

- circulatory hypoxia (low cardiac output)
- hypoxic hypoxia (decreased oxyhaemoglobin level)
- anaemic hypoxia (decreased haemoglobin)
- cellular dysoxia (mitochondrial impairment), e.g. sepsis, carbon monoxide poisoning, cyanide poisoning).

Clinical forms of shock can be subdivided into cardiogenic, inflammatory, hypovolaemic, anaphylactic, neurogenic, and obstructive.

Cardiogenic shock

This is the most severe manifestation of decreased (left or right) ventricular pump function, and usually occurs after extensive injury to the myocardium (e.g. ischaemia, myocarditis), but can also be due to other conditions (e.g. severe valvular regurgitation). Stroke volume and cardiac output are greatly reduced. There may also be a tachy- or bradyarrhythmia, occurring either as the primary cause or as a secondary response. Intracardiac filling pressures are usually increased. The body initially attempts to compensate for the decrease in cardiac output by vasoconstriction and diversion of blood away from 'non-essential' organs and tissues. However, at a certain point, these reflexes will fail and the BP falls, further compromising organ perfusion. In particular, an underperfused myocardium will impair cardiac contractility and promote further tissue damage. This may increase the size of any new infarction, causing yet further decreases in cardiac output. The usual appearance of cardiogenic shock is a low pressure, low output circulation with or without pulmonary oedema (see section on heart failure).

Inflammatory shock (including septic shock)

This occurs as a result of an extrinsic insult (e.g. infection, trauma, burns) triggering an exaggerated generalized inflammatory response that leads to the clinical and pathological sequelae of organ dysfunction and failure. Sepsis (the systemic inflammatory response to infection) remains the most common single cause but 40–50% of patients do not have an identifiable septic focus or a positive blood culture. The circulation is affected by this systemic inflammation through vasodilatation, vascular hyporeactivity (decreased responsiveness to catecholamines such as norepinephrine), increased capillary leak, and myocardial depression. The classical manifestation of inflammatory shock is a low pressure, high output 'hyperdynamic' circulation; however, excessive hypovolaemia and myocardial depression may occasionally produce a low pressure, low output circulation. Further details are given in Chapter 10.

Hypovolaemic shock

Hypovolaemia results from excessive fluid loss (e.g. haemorrhage, vomiting, diarrhoea, burns) or inadequate fluid intake. This then leads to organ hypoperfusion. As with cardiogenic shock, the body initially attempts to compensate for the low output state by vasoconstriction and redistribution of blood flow. The usual cardiovascular effects are tachycardia, hypotension, oliguria, decreased cardiac output, and a high SVR. Further details are given in Chapter 11.

Anaphylactic shock

An anaphylactic reaction is a potentially life-threatening systemic response that occurs after re-exposure to an antigen. Anaphylactic shock usually occurs within seconds to minutes of exposure to the stimulus. The patient may present with rapid onset cardiovascular collapse, with or without myocardial depression, angioedema, laryngeal obstruction, or severe bronchospasm. This can lead to death within minutes. A fuller explanation is given in Chapter 13.

Neurogenic shock

Patients with injury to the cervical or high thoracic cord may have reduced sympathetic outflow between the T1 and L2 segments causing vasodilatation, hypotension, and bradycardia. Further details of this type of shock are given in Chapter 8.

Obstructive shock

This occurs when an acute pathology (or decompensation of a chronic illness) causes obstruction to flow in a major vessel or within the heart. Examples include pulmonary embolus, tension pneumothorax, and pericardial tamponade.

Specific cardiac interventions

Pacing

Pacing refers to the technique of stimulating a myocardial contraction using a small current electrical energy delivered to the heart. Pacing may be either temporary or permanent.

There are two types of pacing electrode:

1. **Unipolar** has only one conducting wire and electrode. Electrical current returns to the pacemaker via body fluids. These are used with permanent pacing systems.
2. **Bipolar** has two conducting wires and two electrodes. The impulse passes down one wire to (usually) the distal electrode. The circuit is then completed via the second electrode and wire back to the pacemaker.

Pacing routes

Transvenous endocardial

The wire passes down a vein (usually jugular or subclavian) to the endocardial surface of the septal region of the right ventricle. It is a bipolar electrode wire in which an inflatable balloon may be incorporated to aid flotation of the catheter during 'blind' placement. Placement of pacing wires without balloons is usually carried out under X-ray imaging (fluoroscopy). The wire is advanced through the right atrium into the right ventricle where it is positioned against the ventricular septal wall. Positioning is confirmed using ECG monitoring. Right atrial stimulation produces large P waves and right ventricular stimulation produces large widened QRS complexes occurring at the rate set on the pacing box. A pacing spike (a deflection of the ECG trace) is seen prior to each stimulated complex. The voltage threshold should then be checked for good electrode placement, suggested by a threshold of less than 0.5 V.

Epicardial

Electrodes are sutured onto the pericardial surface of the heart during cardiac surgery. One or two epicardial electrodes may be used. If only one is used, a skin surface electrode is used to complete the circuit.

External (transcutaneous)

Adhesive skin electrodes with a large surface area are placed on the patient's chest and back. Three ECG electrodes are connected from the external pacer to the usual positions on the patient's chest. Current is passed between the skin electrodes, inducing a paced heartbeat. This is the method of choice in an emergency as it is rapidly placed and effective, requiring little operator skill. However, it is not particularly pleasant for the awake patient and it may be difficult to achieve an output in very muscular or obese patients, despite a high current and changing the location of the surface electrodes.

Trans-oesophageal

This is a difficult and unreliable method of pacing in an emergency, which uses an electrode placed in the patient's oesophagus.

Modes of pacing

Most temporary pacemakers are only capable of single-chamber demand or fixed-rate pacing. More advanced models have the ability to synchronize pacing in dual chambers, but these are generally placed in the catheter laboratory or during cardiac surgery.

Fixed rate

The heart is stimulated at a fixed rate per minute and will not alter in response to any intrinsic activity. This is rarely used unless there is no evidence of any underlying rhythm, as arrhythmias may result if the pacing beat occurs close to the patient's intrinsic beat.

Demand

An impulse is initiated if a preset interval elapses without an intrinsic stimulation of the ventricle. The interval is determined by the rate at which the pacemaker is set. For example, a setting of 60 bpm on the pacemaker will only initiate pacing if the patient's own rate falls below 60 bpm.

Synchronous

Electrodes placed in both right atrium and ventricle will allow synchronization of the stimulus in both cardiac chambers. For example, a sensing electrode in the atrium will sense an atrial contraction and stimulate a ventricular beat via a pacing electrode sited in the ventricle. This allows atrial contraction to fulfil its role of optimally filling the ventricle.

AV sequential

Stimulation of both atria and ventricles can be accomplished when necessary with a set interval between atrial and ventricular stimulation. This allows optimization of atrial filling for ventricular contraction.

- Fixed-rate pacing would be designated V00 or A00 under the Inter-Society Commission for Heart Disease (ICHD) code because the atrium or the ventricle is the chamber paced, but there is no sensing in either chamber and therefore no response to sensing.
- Ventricular demand pacing would be designated VVI because the ventricle is the paced chamber, the ventricle is the sensed chamber and the pacemaker is inhibited by the sensed beat.
- Atrial synchronized pacing would be designated VAT because the ventricle is the paced chamber, the atrium is the sensed chamber, and the ventricular pacemaker is triggered by the sensed atrial beat (P wave) (see Tables 5.22 and 5.23).

Overdrive pacing for terminating tachycardias

Pacing at rates of 10–15 beats above the spontaneous rate may suppress ventricular or atrial arrhythmias. Arrhythmias suitable for overdrive pacing are paroxysmal supraventricular tachycardias, atrial flutter, and ventricular tachycardia. However, it is not effective in slowing sinus tachycardia or atrial fibrillation.

Table 5.22 Types of pacing

Type of pacing	Indications
Ventricular demand (VVI)	Emergency situations, life-threatening bradycardias
AV sequential (DVI)	Impaired AV conduction with atrial bradycardia
Atrial synchronous	Normal sinus rhythm with impaired AV conduction
Ventricular inhibited (VDD) or AV universal (DDD)	Different functions according to underlying problem

Table 5.23 The ICHD pacemaker code

Chambers paced (i)	0	None
	A	Atrium
	V	Ventricle
	D	Dual (atrium and ventricle)
Chambers sensed (ii)	0	None
	A	Atrium
	V	Ventricle
	D	Dual (atrium and ventricle)
Mode of response (iii)	0	None
	T	Triggered
	D (dual)	Triggered and inhibited

Note: Other categories for programmable and antitachycardia functions are available but are not relevant for temporary pacing in the ICU.

Published with permission of the Publisher. Original source: Robledo Nolasco R, Ruiz Soto JC. A simple new code for multisite cardiac pacing and implantable cardioverter defibrillator. *Arch. Cardiol. Mex.*, 2006, Volume 76, pp. 27–9.

Care of the patient with a pacemaker

Electrical safety

The pacing wire provides a direct efficient conduction route for electrical current into the heart. This is a particular problem with older forms of temporary pacing generator. Therefore contact with any poorly insulated source of electrical current could prove dangerous to the patient. Any connections between pacemaker and pacing wire should be securely fixed and, if necessary, protected with gauze or tape.

Monitoring

In the acute setting the patient with temporary pacing should be monitored with the ECG lead which gives the clearest picture. The paced rhythm can be clearly seen as either a negative or positive 'spike' on the ECG. Any failure in pacing will cause an absence of the spike or a spike without a following QRS complex. Note that battery failure can be a cause of loss of pacing. Pacing box batteries should always be checked prior to use and if failure is suspected.

Failure to capture

Absence of a QRS complex following a spike is known as 'failure to capture'. This can be due to an increase in threshold (see below) or displacement of the pacing electrode. An increase in delivered current may overcome an increase in threshold, or the pacing wire may have to be re-sited or replaced.

Pacing threshold

This is the minimum level of current required to consistently pace the heart. This is measured when the pacemaker is first attached and should be <1.0 mA (milliampere) or <0.5 V (depending on the device used). It should then be checked daily or if there is a change in monitored rhythm. Ideally, the pacemaker current should be set at 2–3 times the threshold to allow for minor variations and the usual increase in threshold level that occurs over a period of days after pacing is initiated. The threshold increase is thought to be due to fibrosis at the electrode tip.

Implantable cardioverter–defibrillators (ICDs)

These are used in patients at risk of sudden death from sustained ventricular tachycardia (VT) or fibrillation (VF), such as those with familial cardiac disease (such as long QT syndrome, hypertrophic cardiomyopathy, or Brugada syndrome), those who have survived cardiac arrest due to VT or VF, and those with previous myocardial infarction with ventricular arrhythmias and low ejection fraction. ICDs are small battery-powered impulse generators implanted beneath the skin in the pectoral region of the chest and are similar in size to a permanent pacemaker. Leads connect the device, via a vein, to electrodes positioned in the apex of the right ventricle and, by recognizing the rate and cycle length, are programmed to deliver a shock when set parameters are exceeded. Current devices not only defibrillate, but can act as pacemakers if bradycardia develops, initiate pacing pulses to end an episode of VT, and give low energy cardioversion shocks for persisting VT. It can be quite painful when a shock is discharged, but no harm will come to anyone touching the patient at the time a shock is delivered.

Problems associated with ICDs

- Failure to deliver a shock. This can be caused by failure to sense, fracture of the leads, electromagnetic interference, device malfunction, inadequate energy output or a rise in defibrillation threshold caused by antiarrhythmic drugs, myocardial infarction or scarring at the lead implantation site, and lead dislodgement.
- Inappropriate shocks, i.e. shocks not precipitated by accurate detection of VT or VF, may occur when atrial arrhythmias (e.g atrial fibrillation) accelerate the ventricular rate beyond the programmed limit for delivery of a shock. They may also result from sinus tachycardia, supraventricular tachycardia, or ventricular over-sensing.
- Patients must avoid strong electromagnetic fields (e.g. MRI, large generators) as these interfere with the sensing circuitry.
- ICDs do not prevent all sudden deaths. The device may properly deliver the shock when triggered but is not effective at resolving it.

Synchronized electrical cardioversion

Here, a DC electrical discharge is synchronized with the R wave of the QRS complex. This synchronization avoids energy delivery near the T wave which coincides with a vulnerable period for induction of ventricular fibrillation. Transient delivery of the electrical current causes a momentary depolarization of most cardiac cells, allowing the sinoatrial node to resume normal pacemaker activity. It is used :

- on patients who are unstable and have a ventricular rate >150 bpm (e.g. hypotensive)
- on patients with stable ventricular tachycardia (VT) that does not respond to medication
- electively for haemodynamically stable patients with fast atrial fibrillation/flutter or supraventricular tachycardia (SVT).

Two types of defibrillator are available: monophasic and biphasic. Biphasic defibrillators need less energy to convert an arrhythmia than monophasic models. For example, to treat fast atrial fibrillation a monophasic defibrillator would require a setting of 100–200 J whereas a biphasic defibrillator would need only 75 J.

The technique

The procedure should be fully explained to the patient and intravenous access established. Emergency airway management equipment should be available at the bedside. Connect the patient's cardiac monitor to the cardioverter–defibrillator (or connect the ECG leads directly to the monitor on the defibrillator). Ensure that a good ECG trace is seen on the screen and that the negative and positive deflections are not too small. The patient should be given adequate IV sedation (e.g. propofol or midazolam) because delivery of the shock can be painful. The defibrillator is placed in 'synchronized' mode which permits a search for the R wave; these will be indicated on the monitor by an arrow or line. The energy requirement is selected, usually starting at 50–100 J, depending on the arrhythmia). Two pre-gelled pads are placed in position on the chest and the paddles placed firmly against the chest wall. Ensure that no-one is touching the patient, bed, or attached equipment as there is a risk of their receiving a shock. Manual button depression by the operator will cause the cardioverter to discharge the electrical current. The button should be held down until the shock is delivered as there may be a brief delay as it waits for the next R wave.

If the patient converts to a normal organized rhythm, monitor vital signs and administer anti-arrhythmic medication as required (e.g. amiodarone). If the patient does not convert, repeat the steps but use increasing amounts of energy (100 J → 200 J→ 300 J → 360 J for monophasic defibrillators) Remember to press the synchronization button again before each shock is delivered and confirm that the patient's R wave is being captured. If the patient develops VF the defibrillator should be switched out of synchronization mode and conventional defibrillation carried out as per resuscitation guidelines.

Anti-arrhythmic drugs

Only those anti-arrhythmic drugs particularly relevant to the critically ill patient will be detailed in this chapter. Anti-arrhythmic drugs are categorized into four classes (I–IV), determined by their action on the electrophysiological mechanisms of the myocardial cell:

Class I Class IA drugs lengthen the effective refractory period by (1) inhibiting the fast sodium current and thus the speed of action potential, and (2) prolonging the duration of the action potential.

Class IB drugs inhibit the fast sodium current while shortening the duration of the action potential. This action is selective on diseased or ischaemic tissue and is thought to promote conduction block, thereby interrupting re-entry (e.g. lidocaine, mexiletine, phenytoin).

Class IC drugs possess three major electrophysiological effects: (1) powerful inhibition of His–Purkinje conduction with QRS widening; (2) marked inhibition of fast sodium channels with depression of speed of action potential; (3) shortened action potential in the Purkinje fibres only, leaving the surrounding myocardium unaltered (e.g. flecainide).

Class II These drugs inhibit the sympathetic nervous system and include β-adrenergic blockers. These antagonists also act on myocardial β-adrenergic receptors in the myocardium and block their effect (e.g. esmolol, metoprolol).

Class III These agents lengthen the duration of the action potential and hence the effective refractory period. They also homogenize the pattern of the action potential throughout the myocardium but with relatively little negative inotropic effect (e.g. amiodarone).

Class IV These drugs inhibit slow channel-dependent conduction through the AV node (e.g. adenosine, diltiazem, verapamil).

Amiodarone

This is a complex anti-arrhythmic drug sharing at least some of the electrophysiological properties of all four classes of anti-arrhythmics. Amiodarone lengthens the effective refractory period by prolonging the duration of the action potential. It also has a powerful class I effect, inhibiting sodium channels.

Indications

Control of ventricular tachyarrhythmias, recurrence of paroxysmal atrial fibrillation or flutter, paroxysmal supraventricular tachycardias, and Wolff–Parkinson–White syndrome.

Dosage

In life-threatening arrhythmias, amiodarone 300 mg IV may be given over 10–15 min followed by an infusion of 10–20 mg/kg over 24 hours. The loading dose is essential for rapid action. Otherwise, for less dangerous arrhythmias, 300 mg can be infused through a central venous catheter over an hour, followed by a further 900 mg over the next 23 hours. The daily dose is reduced thereafter.

Side effects

In higher doses, pneumonitis may occur, potentially leading to pulmonary fibrosis. Torsades de pointes may result from QT prolongation plus hypokalaemia. Amiodarone has a complex effect on the metabolism of thyroid hormones, the main action being inhibition of peripheral conversion of T_4 to T_3, and thus hypothroidism. It can cause phlebitis if infused peripherally, Nausea can occur in 50% of patients with cardiac failure.

Precautions

A pro-arrhythmic effect may occur if given with other drugs prolonging the Q–T interval. Amiodarone will prolong the prothrombin time and may cause bleeding in patients on warfarin. It also potentiates the effect of digoxin.

Lidocaine (lignocaine)

This class IB agent acts preferentially on ischaemic myocardium and is more effective in the presence of a high plasma potassium level.

Indications

Emergency treatment of ventricular arrhythmias. Suppression of ventricular arrhythmias such as those associated with myocardial infarction and cardiac surgery.

Dosage

An initial loading dose of 100 mg IV is given followed by an infusion of 1–4 mg/min. This is gradually decreased after 24–30 hours. The dose should be decreased in the elderly, where lidocaine toxicity develops rapidly.

Side effects

Relatively few side effects are seen, though high infusion rates may result in drowsiness, speech disturbances, and dizziness. If toxicity develops there may be seizures, agitation, loss of consciousness, respiratory depression, and cardiac arrest.

Precautions

Clearance of lidocaine via the liver may be reduced if the patient is receiving cimetidine, propanolol, or halothane. Lidocaine metabolites circulate in high concentrations and may contribute to toxic and therapeutic actions. Drugs that induce hepatic enzymes, such as barbiturates, phenytoin, and rifampicin, may require an increase in dosage requirements. It is contraindicated in second- or third-degree heartblock, severe sinoatrial block, and bradycardia.

Adenosine

This has multiple effects including opening of potassium channels and inhibition of sinoatrial and atrioventricular nodes. Opening of K^+ channels produces an indirect Ca^{2+} antagonist effect due to a change in polarity away from that required to open the slow Ca^{2+} channel.

Indications

It is chiefly used in paroxysmal supraventricular tachycardia and is particularly effective in treating re-entrant tachycardias via the AV node.

It is also used as a useful diagnostic test to distinguish between VT and SVT with aberrant conduction. If it is effective in slowing the tachycardia, the arrhythmia is usually SVT with aberrant conduction. Occasionally, adenosine is effective in some types of VT.

Dosage

A rapid IV bolus of 3–6 mg is given initially; if not effective within 1–2 min a further IV bolus of 12 mg is given. The 12 mg dose may be repeated once. The effect is almost instantaneous, but will last no longer than 10–30 sec.

Side effects

These include dyspnoea due to bronchoconstriction, and flushing and headache due to vasodilatory effects. Transient new arrhythmias may occur at the time of chemical cardioversion. Occasionally, the induced heart block may be prolonged. The patient should be warned of a transient sensation of impending death.

Precautions

Adenosine should not generally be used in patients with asthma, second- or third-degree heart block, or sick sinus syndrome. The dose should be reduced if the patient is on dipyridamole therapy because of the inhibitory effect of dipyridamole on adenosine breakdown. Caffeine and theophylline will competitively antagonize adenosine.

Verapamil

This inhibits the action potential of the upper and middle nodal regions where depolarization is calcium mediated. Thus it is able to terminate tachycardias of re-entry origin believed to be the cause of most paroxysmal SVTs. It increases AV nodal block and the effective refractory period of the AV node, and will reduce the ventricular rate in atrial fibrillation or flutter.

Indications

It is used in supraventricular tachycardias and chronic atrial fibrillation or flutter, especially where myocardial depression is not a problem.

Dosage

A slow bolus of 5–10 mg IV over at least 1 min can be repeated 10 min later if necessary. Calcium gluconate or chloride (5–10 ml, 10% solution) should be available for rapid administration (or pre-treatment) if there is a negative inotropic effect associated with the verapamil bolus.

Side effects

These include hypotension and bradycardia. Its vasodilatory effects produce flushing, headaches, and dizziness. Rarely, there is facial, epigastric, and gingival pain, hepatotoxicity, and transient confusion.

Precautions

Verapamil should not be give to patients with AV nodal disease, sick sinus syndrome, or myocardial depression. It should be given with caution if the patient has been treated with β-adrenergic blockers or other anti-arrhythmics.

Magnesium sulphate

Magnesium is important for preserving the electrical stability and function of myocardial cells. Low serum or intracellular magnesium is associated with an increased risk of tachyarrhythmias.

Its actual mechanism of action is unclear, but could be direct inhibition of potassium efflux from the cell, altered cellular calcium metabolism, decreasing peripheral vascular resistance, or stimulating a membrane-stabilizing enzyme.

Indications

Recurrent ventricular arrhythmias have been terminated with IV magnesium sulphate. It is also used as a preventative measure in patients following acute myocardial infarction or with heart failure, though no outcome benefit has been shown in large multi-centre studies. However, the use of magnesium is considered a relatively safe intervention which may be used when other anti-arrhythmic agents have failed, or when there is reason to suspect magnesium depletion.

Dosage

Optimal dosage and frequency has still not been fully determined. A dose of 10–20 mmol over 5–10 min (or more rapidly in emergencies), followed by a further 20–40 mmol given over 5–10 hours, is often used.

Side effects

Flushing, sweating, and a sensation of heat may occur with rapid IV injection.

Precautions

Serum magnesium levels should be monitored and kept below 2.7 mmol/L as higher levels are associated with bradycardia, prolonged PR intervals, and AV block. Since magnesium is excreted via the kidneys, magnesium levels should be closely monitored in patients with renal impairment.

Drugs commonly used in the treatment of low cardiac output and/or hypotension

Inotropic drugs can be termed either positive or negative in relation to their effect on heart muscle. Positive inotropes increase the contractility of the myocardium and hence the stroke volume (e.g. epinephrine). Negative inotropes decrease the contractility of cardiac muscle (e.g. β-blockers). Chronotropic drugs are those that increase heart rate (e.g. atropine).

The effect of the drugs used depends on their specific site of action.

- Inotropes increase cyclic AMP and calcium levels within the heart or vascular smooth muscle cell.
- Dopaminergic receptors.
- Phosphodiesterase inhibitors (e.g. milrinone)—these also increase cardiac contractility by elevating cAMP, albeit through preventing its metabolism.
- Calcium sensitizers (e.g. levosimendan)—augmented by enhancing the sensitivity of troponin to Ca^{2+} and thus the cardiomyocyte's contractile apparatus.
- An alternative is to use a high-dose glucose–insulin–potassium infusion, which enhances glucose entry into the cells and accelerates glycolysis as an alternative energy source. This enhances ventricular contractility, and the heart pumps more efficienctly.

Alpha-adrenergic receptors

There are two main types of α-adrenergic receptor: α_1 and α_2. The principal effect of α-receptors is to cause vasoconstriction of vascular smooth muscle.

- Alpha_1 receptors are the post-junctional receptors of vascular smooth muscle.

- Alpha$_2$ receptors are found in vascular smooth muscle and the pre-junctional receptors of nerve fibres. They inhibit release of norepinephrine.

Beta-adrenergic receptors

There are two main types of β-receptor: β_1 and β_2. The principal effects are to cause increase heart rate and contractility (β_1) and vasodilatation (β_2).

- β_1 receptors are found in the sinoatrial node and myocardium
- β_2 receptors are found in arterioles of heart, liver, and skeletal muscle, and in the smooth muscle of the bronchioles.

Beta-blockers should be given with caution to patients with asthma or a history of obstructive airways disease since there is a potential risk of inducing bronchospasm. The use of β-blockers may also mask the compensatory physiological responses to hypoglycaemia and sudden haemorrhage (tachycardia and vasoconstriction), so care should be taken with diabetics and patients with blood loss. Beta-blockers may also compromise blood flow in patients with peripheral vascular disease. While caution should be applied to the use of β-blockers in acute heart failure, large studies have shown a clear outcome benefit when given to patients with stable chronic heart failure or stabilized acute heart failure.

Beta$_2$-adrenergic agonists (e.g. salbutamol) depress plasma potassium and raise glucose levels; therefore these should be monitored in patients receiving such drugs. Dosages should be titrated according to response. In general, begin at the lowest dose and increase gradually according to effect. Observe for side effects, particularly arrhythmias and tachycardias. Infusions should not be discontinued abruptly but weaned gradually.

Dopamine

The cardiovascular effects of dopamine are dose dependent. At low dose (1–3 μg/kg/min) it stimulates dopaminergic receptors, having a diuretic effect and vasodilating the splanchnic circulation. At 5–10 μg/kg/min it mainly stimulates β-receptors, increasing contractility and coronary blood flow, but with little effect on heart rate. BP may sometimes fall slightly due to the decrease in systemic vascular resistance. At higher doses (>10 μg/kg/min) the α-adrenergic effects predominate with vasoconstriction, causing an increase in BP. These doses are approximate; some patients may react differently at lower doses.

Dopamine is administered as a continuous intravenous infusion via a flow-regulated pump. It should always be administered through a central vein because of its peripheral vasoconstrictor action. Extravasation can cause ischaemic tissue necrosis and skin sloughing. Side effects include tachycardia, arrhythmias, angina, abdominal pain, digital ischaemia, nausea, and vomiting.

Dobutamine

This positive inotrope and mild chronotrope is used to increase cardiac output in patients with low output cardiac failure (e.g. myocardial infarction, cardiogenic shock, following cardiac surgery). It directly stimulates myocardial β_1-receptors, increasing stroke volume and heart rate. Systemic vascular resistance and the left ventricular filling pressure also decrease as it has some β_2-mediated vasodilating properties.

Because of its short half-life of approximately 2 min, it is administered as a continuous IV infusion, ideally centrally, but can be given via a peripheral vein if necessary. Dosage is 2.5–20 μg/kg/min titrated according to response.

Side effects are dose related and include tachycardia, arrhythmias, headache, and chest pain. Hypotension can occur, predominantly due to its vasodilating effects. Tachycardia and arrhythmias are related to increases in AV conduction, especially if the patient is hypovolaemic. Those with atrial fibrillation may develop rapid ventricular responses. Use with care in patients with myocardial infarction as tachycardia may precipitate angina and intensify ischaemia.

Downregulation of the β-adrenoreceptor may occur if dobutamine is continuously infused for longer than 72 hours; larger doses may be required to maintain the same effect.

Dopexamine hydrochloride

Dopexamine is an arterial vasodilator and positive inotrope, and causes splanchnic vasodilation. It stimulates β_2-adrenergic and peripheral dopaminergic receptors. Dopexamine is administered by continuous infusion into a central or large peripheral vein. Its half-life is 6–11 min. The dose ranges from 0.5 to 2 μg/kg/min, and should be increased in increments of 0.5–1 μg/kg/min at intervals of not less than 15 min.

Side effects include tachycardia (dose-related), nausea, vomiting, tremor, and headaches. Tachycardia may precipitate angina or intensify cardiac ischaemia.

Epinephrine (adrenaline)

Epinephrine is a positive inotrope that affects both α- and β-receptors. Low doses have predominantly β-adrenergic effects while higher doses have more α-adrenergic vasoconstricting effects. It increases heart rate, cardiac output, systolic blood pressure, and myocardial oxygen consumption. When administered as an intravenous bolus it causes a rapid rise in BP by increasing the strength of ventricular contraction, increasing heart rate, and causing constriction of the arterioles of the skin, mucosa, and splanchnic areas of the circulation. However, by infusion there may be a decrease in peripheral resistance due to its action on β_2-receptors. This vasodilator effect may predominate, so any increase in BP is a result of cardiac stimulation and increase in cardiac output. Peripheral resistance may rise or be unaltered owing to a greater ratio of α to β activity in different vascular areas.

Although splanchnic blood flow is increased, renal blood flow can be decreased by up to 40%.

Epinephrine causes an increase in blood glucose by antagonizing the effects of insulin. It is also a bronchodilator and can be used in asthma or severe bronchospasm from anaphylaxis. It can cause a lactic acidosis, but this is usually due to a non-harmful accelerated aerobic glycolysis rather than being secondary to poor tissue perfusion.

When administered as an infusion it should be given via a central vein as extravasation can cause local necrosis. Dosage is titrated according to response, starting at 0.01 µg/kg/min by continuous infusion or 0.05–1 mg for bolus doses. Side effects include tachycardia, palpitations, myocardial ischaemia, and headache.

Milrinone

Milrinone is a phosphodiesterase inhibitor with positive inotropic and vasodilator properties.

Indications

Milrinone is used for the short-term treatment of patients with acute decompensated heart failure. In addition to increasing myocardial contractility, it improves diastolic function, as evidenced by improvements in left ventricular diastolic relaxation.

The duration of therapy should depend upon patient responsiveness.

Side effects

Supraventricular and ventricular arrhythmias can occur, including non-sustained ventricular tachycardia. Milrinone produces a slight shortening of AV node conduction time, indicating a potential for an increased ventricular response rate in patients with atrial flutter/fibrillation.

Hypotension, headaches, hypokalaemia, nausea, vomiting, diarrhoea, tremor, and thrombocytopenia may also occur.

Precautions

Milrinone should not be used in patients with aortic or pulmonary stenosis. Potassium loss due to excessive diuresis may predispose digitalized patients to arrhythmias. Therefore hypokalaemia should be corrected by potassium supplementation in advance of or during use of milrinone.

Furosemide should not be injected into an intravenous line of an infusion of milrinone as immediate precipitation will occur.

Dosage and administration

Milrinone is administered intravenously, often with a loading dose of 50 µg/kg given slowly over 10 min followed by continuous infusion (maintenance dose) using a controlled infusion device (0.375–0.75 µg/kg/min). The loading dose is more likely to produce hypotension and tachycardia and can be omitted.

The infusion rate should be adjusted according to haemodynamic and clinical response. Reductions in infusion rate may be necessary in patients with renal impairment. It has a long half-life of several hours, so other drugs may be needed to counteract any hypotension.

Norepinephrine (noradrenaline)

Norepinephrine acts predominantly on α-adrenergic receptors and increases BP by increasing peripheral resistance. Cardiac output usually falls as a result. Hepatic, renal, and splanchnic flows are decreased, but coronary blood flow may be increased due to the increase in diastolic pressure. It decreases insulin secretion, leading to an elevated blood glucose.

Norepinephrine is administered by continuous intravenous infusion via a flow-regulated pump. It should only be infused into a central vein. The dosage is titrated according to response, starting at 0.01 µg/kg/min. Side effects include arrhythmias, chest and abdominal pain from excessive vasoconstriction, digital ischaemia, and headache.

Vasopressin

Vasopressin has a direct vasoconstrictor effect on systemic vascular smooth muscle. Although it is the synthetic version of antidiuretic hormone, patients in septic shock receiving the drug often increase their urine output due to improvement in blood pressure and an improved blood pressure/flow gradient across the glomerulus. Vasopressin is an important adjunct therapy for the management of septic shock in patients who do not respond to catecholamines. A large multicenter study (Russell *et al*, 2008) reported an outcome improvement with low dose vasopressin in patients on low doses of norepinephrine, but no difference in those on high dose norepinephrine. There was also a suggestion of a beneficial synergistic effect between vasopressin and hydrocortisone. Higher doses of vasopressin, with or without steroids, are currently being investigated in a UK multi-centre trial (VANISH—VAsopressin versus Noradrenaline as Initial therapy in Septic Shock).

Complications with vasopressin (skin, mesenteric, and coronary artery vasoconstriction leading to ischaemia or infarction) generally relate to dosage and the patient's cardiac output. It should generally be avoided in low cardiac output states. Vasopressin should be started at a rate of 0.01 IU/min and then increased according to response up to 0.04 IU/min (or higher,with caution).

Terlipressin is an alternative option. This synthetic analogue of vasopressin has a longer duration of action than vasopressin (half-life 50 min compared with 6 min for vasopressin). There are no official recommendations for the use of terlipressin in septic shock mainly because of the lack of large multicentre studies. It can be given by small boluses (e.g. 0.25 mg repeated at 30 min intervals to a maximum of 2 mg) or by an infusion.

Levosimendan

This drug has a direct effect on the heart by increasing the sensitivity of troponin to calcium within the cardiomyocyte. For the same level of intracellular calcium (and thus the same level of cardiac work, as the intracellular calcium level dictates the work of the cardiomyocyte) more actin–myosin cross-bridges are formed, producing an increased contraction. It also has a vasodilating action through its effects on opening the ATP-sensitive potassium channel in vascular smooth muscle, thereby causing relaxation.

The drug is given by an infusion ranging from 0.05 to 0.2 μg/kg/min. A loading dose of 6–12 μg/kg can be given over 10 min for a faster onset of action, but this is more likely to cause hypotension so can be omitted.

Glucose–insulin–potassium (GIK)

This stratagem has been used for the last four or five decades as a means of increasing cardiac output. Although the precise mechanisms of action are not confirmed, it is postulated that increased substrate (glucose) provision and accelerated glycolysis augment cardiac efficiency and enhance contractility. Very large doses of insulin are given (the literature reports up to 22 U/kg/hour (!) but are usually in the range 0.5–2 U/kg/hour. Glucose and potassium need to be coadministered to prevent hypoglycaemia and hypokalaemia due to movement of glucose and potassium into the cell.

Table 5.24 summarizes the drugs used in hypotension.

Intravenous drugs for the treatment of hypertension

Sodium nitroprusside

Sodium nitroprusside acts directly on vascular smooth muscle causing predominantly arteriolar vasodilation. It has an immediate effect but a short duration of action; therefore it is administered by continuous infusion. It should be administered via a flow-regulated pump and through a dedicated catheter lumen. Intra-arterial pressure monitoring is considered essential as sodium nitroprusside can cause profound hypotension. Cardiac output usually increases due to the decrease in systemic vascular resistance. The drug causes cerebral vasodilation and may increase intracranial pressure in normocapnic patients.

Dosage is 0.5–1.5 μg/kg/min initially and is then adjusted according to response. The usual range is 0.5–8 μg/kg/min. Side effects include headache, dizziness, nausea, palpitations, and retrosternal pain. When sodium nitroprusside is metabolized it forms cyanide ions and has the potential to produce cyanide toxicity. This is related more to the rate of the infusion than to the total dose given, and the rate should not exceed 8 μg/kg/min. Ideally, it should not be given for more than 24–36 hours. A rising, and unexplained, metabolic acidosis may be due to cyanide accumulation.

The solution and tubing must be shielded from light. The drug is excreted renally but is removed by haemodialysis.

Table 5.24 **Summary of drugs used in the treatment of hypotension**

Drug	Primary action	CVS effect
Dopamine	Positive inotrope Vasoconstrictor at high dose Vasodilator at low dose	Increases cardiac output Increases SVR (high dose) Decreases SVR (low dose)
Dobutamine	Positive inotrope (NB: May vasodilate)	Increases cardiac output Decreases SVR
Dopexamine	Positive inotrope Vasodilator	Increases cardiac output Decreases SVR
Epinephrine	Positive inotrope Vasoconstrictor	Increases cardiac output Increases SVR
Glucose–insulin–potassium	Positive inotrope	Increases cardiac output
Levosimendan	Positive inotrope Vasodilator	Increases cardiac output Decreases SVR
Norepinephrine	Vasoconstrictor Some inotropic properties	Increases SVR Often decreases CO
Vasopressin	Vasoconstrictor (in sepsis)	Increases SVR Often decreases CO
Terlipressin	Vasoconstrictor (in sepsis)	increases SVR Often decreases CO

Glyceryl trinitrate (nitroglycerin)

Nitrates cause vasodilation of veins at lower doses. At higher doses, both arteries and veins are vasodilated. Nitrates allow a smooth reduction in blood pressure. As they cause cerebral vasodilatation, they may raise intracranial pressure. Duration of action is 2–5 min. It can be given as a sublingual spray or small bolus doses, but is more usually given as an intravenous infusion via a volumetric pump. It can be given into a peripheral vein at a dose range of 5–200 μg/min.Side effects include headache, tachycardia, and nausea. Tolerance ('tachyphylaxis') will develop within 24 hours, requiring increasing doses to achieve the same effect.

Hydralazine

Hydralazine acts on vascular smooth muscle, predominantly arteriolar, causing peripheral vasodilation. It decreases systemic vascular resistance and can cause a compensatory tachycardia with an increased cardiac output. This tachycardia may precipitate pre-existing angina. It can be given as a repeated slow bolus injection, or a continuous infusion via a volumetric pump.

Dosage is 20–40 mg when given as an intravenous bolus (and repeated as necessary), or a continuous infusion at 200–300 μg/min initially and then 50–150 μg/min. It is incompatible with dextrose solutions as contact with glucose causes rapid breakdown of hydralazine. Side effects include nausea, vomiting, headache, tachycardia, palpitations, and flushing.

Phentolamine

Phentolamine acts by blocking α-adrenergic receptors. This causes vasodilation and a reflex tachycardia. It increases respiratory tract secretions, salivation, insulin secretion, and gut motility. Phentolamine is particularly useful when hypertension is due to a phaeochromocytoma, a reaction between foods containing pressor amines and monoamine oxidase inhibitors, or clonidine withdrawal.

It can be given as a slow bolus injection or continuous infusion via a volumetric pump. Dosage is 5–10 mg when given as a bolus intravenously (and repeated as necessary), or a continuous infusion at a rate of 5–60 mg over 10–30 min and thereafter at 0.1–2 mg/min.

Side effects include tachycardia, arrhythmias, dizziness, nausea, vomiting, and diarrhoea.

Labetalol

Labetalol acts by blocking both α- and β-adrenoceptors, although β-blockade predominates at higher doses. It blocks the α-adrenoceptors in the peripheral arterioles and therefore lowers systemic vascular resistance. The concurrent β-blockade protects the heart from the reflex sympathetic drive that can be induced by this vasodilation. There is little change in cardiac output.

It can be administered as a repeated slow bolus injection or as a continuous infusion via a volumetric pump. In a hypertensive crisis, when the blood pressure needs to be reduced urgently, 50 mg may be given as an intravenous bolus over at least 1 min. This may be repeated at 5 min intervals, not exceeding 200 mg in total. By intravenous infusion the rate is variable according to the cause of the hypertension and can be up to 160 mg/h.

Side effects include headache, rashes, difficulty in micturition, nausea, and vomiting. It can cause severe postural hypotension. There may be a small decrease in heart rate but severe bradycardia is unusual.

Propanolol

Propanolol is a β-adrenoceptor antagonist. It is a negative inotrope, reduces heart rate, and increases peripheral resistance. It is administered as a slow bolus injection of 1–10 mg, repeated as necessary. Side effects include bradycardia and bronchospasm. It may also block the sympathetic response to hypoglycaemia by impairing the gluconeogenetic response. Heart failure and heart block may be precipitated and peripheral vascular disease exacerbated.

Esmolol

Esmolol acts by β-adrenoceptor blockade but has a very short half-life (approximately 5 min) so can be readily titrated. It decreases heart rate and cardiac output. It is administered by continuous infusion via a volumetric pump at a rate of 50–150 μg/kg/min. Side effects include bronchospasm, nausea and vomiting, and bradycardia.

Clevidipine

Clevidipine is a calcium-channel antagonist that lowers blood pressure by decreasing systemic vascular resistance without affecting cardiac filling pressures. It is an emulsion given as an intravenous infusion. Onset of action is rapid and of short duration; therefore it can be easily titrated for blood pressure control. Initial dosage is 1–2 mg which can be doubled at short intervals. An increase of approximately 1–2 mg/h will generally produce a decrease of 2–4 mmHg in systolic pressure. Hypotension and reflex tachycardia may occur during upward titration and it can exacerbate heart failure. Other side effects include nausea, vomiting, headache, shortness of breath, and chest discomfort.

References and bibliography

Alpert, J.S., Thygesen, K., Antman, E., Bassand, J.P. (2000). Myocardial infarction redefined—a consensus document of The Joint European Society of Cardiology/American College of Cardiology Committee for the redefinition of myocardial infarction. *Journal of the American College of Cardiology*, **36**, 959–69.

Anderson, J., Adams, C., Antman, E., *et al.* (2007). ACC/AHA 2007 guidelines for the management of patients with unstable angina/non-ST elevation myocardial infarction: A report of the American College of Cardiology/American Heart Association Task Force on Practice Guidelines. *Journal of the American College of Cardiology*, **50**, e1.

Anderson, C.S., Huang, Y., Wang, J.G., *et al.* (2008). Intensive Blood Pressure Reduction in Acute Cerebral Haemorrhage Trial (INTERACT): a randomised pilot trial. *Lancet Neurology*, **7**, 391–9.

Anderson, C.S, Huang, Y., Arima, H., *et al.* (2010). Effects of early intensive blood pressure-lowering treatment on the growth of haematoma and perihaematomal edema in acute intracerebral haemorrhage: the Intensive Blood Pressure Reduction in Acute Cerebral Haemorrhage Trial (INTERACT) *Stroke*, **41**, 307–12.

Anderson, C.S., Heeley, E., Huang, Y., *et al* (2013). Rapid blood pressure-lowering in patients with acute intracerebral haemorrhage. *New England Journal of Medicine*, **368**, 2355–65.

Aviles, R.J., Askari, A.T., Lindahl, B., *et al.* (2002). Troponin T levels in patients with acute coronary syndromes, with or without renal dysfunction. *New England Journal of Medicine*, **346**, 2047–52.

Bassand, J.P., Hamm, C.W., Ardissino, D., *et al.* (2008). Guidelines for the diagnosis and treatment of non-ST-segment elevation acute coronary syndromes. *European Heart Journal*, **28**, 1598–660.

Chan, D., Ng, L.L. (2010) Biomarkers in acute myocardial infarction. BMC Medicine, **8**, 34.

Davis, T., Bluhm, J., Burke, R., *et al.* Institute for Clinical Systems Improvement (2012). *Diagnosis and Treatment of Chest Pain and Acute Coronary Syndrome (ACS)*. http://bit.ly.ACS1112 (accessed 5 September 2016).

Deeks, E.D., Keating, G.M., Keam, S.J. (2009). Clevidipine: a review of its use in the management of acute hypertension. *American Journal of Cardiovascular Drugs*, **9**, 117–34.

Delinger, R.P., Levy, M.M., Carlet, J.M., *et al* (2008) Surviving Sepsis Campaign: international guidelines for management of severe sepsis and septic shock. *Intensive Care Medicine*, **34**, 17–60.

Diaz, R., Paolasso, E.C., Piegas, L.S., *et al.* (1998). Metabolic modulation of acute myocardial infarction: the ECLA glucose–insulin–potassium pilot trial. *Circulation*, **98**, 2227–34.

Ebel, R., Alfonso, F., Boileau, C., *et al.* (2001). Diagnosis and management of aortic dissection. Recommendations of the Task Force on Aortic Dissection, European Society of Cardiology, *European Heart Journal*, **22**, 1641–81.

Ebell, M.H., Flewelling, D., Flynn, C.A. (2000). A systematic review of troponin T and I for diagnosing acute myocardial infarction. *Journal of Family Practice*, **49**, 550–6.

Frontera, J. (2013). Blood pressure in intracerebral haemorrhage. How low should we go? *New England Journal of Medicine*, **368**, 2426–7.

GUSTO Investigators (1993). An international randomised trial comparing four thrombolytic strategies for acute myocardial infarction. *New England Journal of Medicine*, **329**, 673.

Hagen, P.J., Hartmann, I.J., Hoekstra, O.S., *et al.* (2003). Comparison of observer variability and accuracy of different criteria for lung scan interpretation. *Journal of Nuclear Medicine*, **44**, 739–44.

ISIS-4 (1995). A randomised factorial trial assessing early captopril, oral mononitrate, and intravenous magnesium sulphate in 58,050 patients with suspected acute myocardial infarction. *Lancet* **345**, 669–85.

Mousavi S. (2013). Vasopressin and septic shock. *Journal of Pharmaceutical Care*, **1**, 65–73.

NICE (National Institute for Health and Clinical Excellence). (2003). *Guidance in the Use of Coronary Artery Stents*. Technical Guideline 71, NICE, London.

NICE (National Institute for Health and Clinical Excellence) (2006). *Arrhythmia—Implantable Cardioverter Defibrillators*. Technology Appraisal, NICE, London.

NICE (National Institute for Health and Clinical Excellence) (2007). *MI: Secondary Prevention in Primary and Secondary Care for Patients Following an MI*. Clinical Guideline 48, NICE, London

NICE (National Institute for Health and Clinical Excellence) (2008). *Prophylaxis Against Infective Endocarditis*. Clinical Guideline 64, NICE, London.

NICE (National Institute for Health and Clinical Excellence) (2010a). *The Early Management of Unstable Angina and Non-ST Segment Elevation Myocardial Inf*arction. Clinical Guideline 94, NICE, London.

NICE (National Institute for Health and Clinical Excellence) (2010b). *Assessment and Diagnosis of Recent Onset Chest Pain or Discomfort of Suspected Cardiac Origin*. Clinical Guideline 95, NICE, London.

NICE (National Institute for Health and Clinical Excellence) (2013). Myocardial infarction with ST segment elevation. Clinical Guideline 167, NICE, London.

NICE (National Institute for Health and Clinical Excellence) (2015a). *Clinical Knowledge Summaries: MI—secondary prevention*. http://cks.nice.org.uk/mi-secondary-prevention (accessed 5 September 2016).

NICE (National Institute for Health and Clinical Excellence) (2015b). *Clinical Knowledge Summaries: Angina*. http://cks.nice.org.uk/angina (accessed 5 September 2016).

Rehberg, S., Westphal, M., Ertmerc, C. (2012). Vasopressin therapy in septic shock. In *Annual Update in Intensive Care and Emergency Medicine* (ed. J.-L. Vincent), pp. 76–84. Berlin: Springer-Verlag.

Robledo Nolasco, R., Constancio Ruiz Soto, J. (2006) A simple new code for multisite cardiac pacing and implantable cardioverter defibrillator. *Archivos de Cardiologia de México*, **76**, 127–9.

Russell, J.A., Walley, K.R., Singer, J., *et al.* (2008). Vasopressin versus norepinephrine infusion in patients with septic shock. *New England Journal of Medicine*, **358**, 877–87.

Sanset, E., Bath, P., Boysen G., *et al.* (2011) The angiotensin-receptor blocker candesartan for treatment of acute stroke (SCAST): a randomised, placebo-controlled, double blind trial. *Lancet*, **377**, 740–50.

Shulman, R., Paw, H. (2013). *Handbook of Drugs in Intensive Care*. Cambridge: Cambridge University Press.

Swedberg, K., Held, P., Kjekshus, J., *et al* (1992). Effects of the early administration of enalapril on mortality in patients with acute myocardial infarction. Results of the Cooperative New Scandinavian Enalapril Survival Study II (CONSENSUS II), *New England Journal of Medicine*, **327**, 678–84.

van de Werf, F., Bax, J., Betriu, A., *et al.* (2008). Management of acute myocardial infarction in patients presenting with persistent ST segment elevation. *European Heart Journal*, **29**, 2909–45.

West, J., Dollery, C., Naimark, A. (1964) Distribution of blood flow in isolated lung; relation to vascular and alveolar pressures. *Journal of Applied Physiology*, **19**, 713–24.

White, H.D., Chew, D.P. (2008) Acute myocardial infarction. *Lancet*, **372**, 570–84.

Woods, K., Fletcher, S., Roffe.,C., *et al.* (1992). Intravenous magnesium sulphate in suspected acute myocardial infarction: results of the second Leicester Intravenous Magnesium Intervention Trial (LIMIT-2), *Lancet*, **339**, 1553–8.

Worsley, D.F., Alavi, A. (1995). Comprehensive analysis of the results of the PIOPED Study. Prospective Investigation of Pulmonary Embolism Diagnosis Study. *Journal of Nuclear Medicine*, **36**, 2380–7.

CHAPTER 6
Cardiac arrest and cardiopulmonary resuscitation

Introduction

Cardiac arrest is generally fatal. Of 23,554 in-hospital resuscitations in the UK, 45% achieve a return of circulation for >20 min, but only 18% live to hospital discharge (Nolan *et al.* 2014). Patients who arrest in critical care areas may do better, with a reported survival to discharge of 25% (Dumot *et al.* 2001). This may be related to rapid recognition and ready availability of skilled clinicians and the necessary equipment for advanced life support.

In the hospital setting an important focus should be on early recognition of deterioration and appropriate interventions to prevent arrest. Most cardiac arrests in hospital are to some extent predictable, often associated with acute exacerbations of severe chronic disease and, especially, with worsening respiratory or circulatory failure. Indeed, most hospital arrests are preceded by such warning signs as hypoxaemia, hypotension, or reduced consciousness (Kause *et al.* 2004; Harrison *et al.* 2006). Nevertheless, critical care staff should be trained and practiced in cardiopulmonary resuscitation (CPR) for those occasions when cardiac arrest does occur. An important emphasis should be placed on identifying those patients at particular risk, and understanding potentially reversible causes relevant to individual patients. Unfortunately, resuscitation knowledge and skills can decline in as little as six weeks following training (Yang *et al.* 2012). Many of the necessary skills, such as external chest compression (ECC), are practical functions that should be practised frequently using training manikins to aid retention.

This chapter outlines the pathophysiology associated with cardiac arrest, reviews management of arrest, and examines techniques and drugs used in CPR. Finally, the care of the patient and family following both successful and unsuccessful resuscitation is discussed. The definitive reference for this text is the latest European Resuscitation Council guideline. These guidelines can be downloaded in their entirety from the European Resuscitation Council website at www.cprguidelines.eu/.

Definition of cardiac arrest

Cardiac arrest is the cessation of cardiac output—when the heart stops pumping blood—signalled by loss of consciousness, loss of normal breathing, and the absence of a pulse. Hypoperfusion then causes tissue ischaemia and can rapidly result in irreversible damage to brain, heart, and other vital organs.

Cardiac arrest rhythms

Cardiac arrest is associated with four cardiac rhythms: ventricular fibrillation (VF) and pulseless ventricular tachycardia (VT) are usually caused by a primary myocardial pathology (ischaemia or a conduction pathway defect), while asystole and pulseless electrical activity (PEA) have a wide variety of causes. VF and pulseless VT should be treated with defibrillation, but asystole and PEA are non-shockable rhythms. The rhythm may change several times during cardiac arrest. PEA is the term for any cardiac rhythm that is capable of producing a cardiac output but is not doing so in a particular case.

Asystole and PEA are the initial rhythms seen in the majority of cardiac arrests (72%) and are associated with very poor outcomes; only 10% survive to hospital discharge (Nolan *et al.* 2014). Cardiac arrests beginning in asystole or PEA that later turn into VF/pulseless VT have even worse outcomes (Meaney *et al.* 2010). Cardiac arrests where the initial rhythm is VF or pulseless VT are much less common, with 49% of such cases surviving to discharge (Nolan *et al.* 2014). Immediate recognition and treatment are essential; without effective management, VF will rapidly degenerate into a small amplitude waveform (so-called 'fine VF') and then to electrical standstill (i.e. asystole).

Various types of tachyarrhythmia and bradycardia can also significantly compromise cardiac output, evidenced by adverse signs such as heart failure and shock with hypotension, reduced consciousness, and myocardial ischaemia. Without prompt treatment, such cases will almost certainly progress to actual cardiac arrest.

Pathophysiology of cardiac arrest

Reduced or complete loss of blood flow and oxygen supply to the tissues causes the following.

1. Rapid depletion of high energy phosphates such as adenosine triphosphate (ATP) in myocardial cells. These are not replenished due to lack of oxygen and absence of aerobic metabolism.
2. Failure of pacemaker activity, electrical impulse conduction, and myocardial contractility due to lack of ATP (energy currency).
3. Complete loss of electrical activity. Note: it is possible for electrical dysfunction to be the primary cause.

Following cardiac arrest, peripheral blood vessels are initially vasoconstricted by the release of endogenous catecholamines (up to 300× normal levels) acting on alpha$_1$-adrenergic receptors in arterial vascular smooth muscle. This is followed by a fall in systemic vascular resistance caused by loss of blood flow and vasodilation due to ischaemia, hypoxia, and hypercapnia, with a downregulation of vascular alpha-receptor responsiveness to catecholamines (Lindner 1991). Vasodilation also produces a rapid equilibration of arterial and venous pressures, so the usual pressure gradient across the circulation is lost.

Once external chest compressions are commenced, a reasonably strong pulse may be felt. However, the actual cardiac output associated with external cardiac compressions (ECC) is only 20–30% of normal (Peters and Ihle 1990); the palpated 'pulse' is most likely a pulse pressure wave transmitted down the arteries as a result of chest compression. These are more readily felt in atherosclerotic arteries which are less elastic and so more likely to transmit pressure waves. The relatively low cardiac output produced by even good quality ECC means that inadequately oxygenated tissues rely on anaerobic glycolysis for some ATP generation, with lactic acidosis resulting as a consequence. Ischaemic tissue continues to generate CO_2 but this accumulates as the lack of an adequate blood flow does not effectively transport it away. Impaired ventilation and reduced pulmonary elimination of CO_2 compound these processes, resulting in a respiratory acidosis. Effective ventilation may restore arterial pH to normal relatively quickly, but venous pH will still generally remain low due to pulmonary hypoperfusion and high levels of venous CO_2 (von Planta 2005).

Assessment and confirmation of cardiac arrest

The clinical signs of cardiac arrest are absence of normal signs of life. Many critical care patients will already be unresponsive due to their underlying critical illness or drug-induced coma, and will frequently be mechanically ventilated using modes that continue regardless of complete loss of respiratory drive. Thus cardiac rhythms incompatible with life and loss of the arterial blood pressure waveform may be the first signs of cardiac arrest in the critical care patient. However, it must be remembered that monitors are not infallible. Cardiac monitoring can be disturbed by patient movement or lead disconnection, while the arterial pressure waveform can be altered or completely lost by kinking, blockage, or disconnection, or by excessive damping of the system. Therefore a diagnosis of cardiac arrest should be confirmed by hands-on assessment of the presence or absence of signs of life—in this case the presence of a carotid or femoral pulse.

Cardiac arrest is characterized by the following.

1. Loss of consciousness:
   - test by shaking the patient's shoulders and calling 'are you alright?' or similar phrase.
2. Minimal or absent respirations:
   - open the airway (if appropriate), and look, listen, and feel for breathing for no more than 10 seconds. In the unconscious patient, gasping and grossly abnormal breathing are early signs of cardiac arrest. There may be no initial change in the appearance of a mechanically ventilated patient.
3. Absent pulse:
   - peripheral arteries may be vasoconstricted, so palpate a central pulse (carotid or femoral) for up to 10 sec to check whether the pulse is present or not. Experienced critical care staff ought to be able to check breathing and a pulse at the same time.
4. An ECG exhibiting any of the arrhythmias listed in Table 6.1 with loss of the arterial pressure waveform.

See Box 6.1 for factors associated with sudden ventricular dysrhythmias.

Even if there is some doubt about whether or not cardiac arrest has definitely occurred, the nurse should never

Table 6.1 Dysrhythmias in cardiac arrest

	Ventricular fibrillation (VF)	Pulseless ventricular tachycardia (VT)	Pulseless electrical activity (PEA)	Asystole
Definition	Sudden loss of coordinated electrical activity leading to random contraction of individual myocardial fibres	Repetitive electrical discharge from a ventricular ectopic focus	Organized electrical activity without effective myocardial contraction	Complete absence of electrical activity
ECG trace	Rapid irregular activity without identifiable rate or recognizable shape	Rapid, broad, complex QRS complexes, usually 150–220/min	Visible QRS complexes	No recognizable electrical activity, although agonal (dying) beats are sometimes seen
Arterial pressure trace	None	None	Usually none, although occasional very low pressure waveforms may be seen	None

Box 6.1 Factors associated with sudden ventricular dysrhythmias

Drug toxicity

- Digoxin (often precipitated by hypokalaemia and hypomagnesaemia)
- Amphetamines
- Tricyclic antidepressants
- Adrenergic drugs
- Cocaine

Electrolyte disturbance

- Hypokalaemia
- Hypomagnesaemia
- Hypercalcaemia

External factors

- Unsynchronized cardioversion attempt
- Exacerbating factors of myocardial ischaemia (hypoxaemia (carbon monoxide poisoning, hypoperfusion due to hypovolaemia, ventricular failure, rapid tachycardia)

hesitate to shout for help, call 'cardiac arrest', or use an emergency buzzer if any signs of possible cardiac arrest are seen. Unless it is known that there are staff present with all the skills needed to undertake the full range of advanced life support interventions, a call for the hospital cardiac arrest team must be made immediately. All nurses should know the phone number used locally: '2222' is the standard number for in-hospital use in the UK.

Aims of management

1. To obtain help immediately—and have a defibrillator brought to the bedside.
2. To start CPR instantaneously, beginning with 30 chest compressions and continuing chest compressions with minimal interruptions thereafter.
3. To connect a monitor and/or defibrillator as soon as possible, with prompt assessment of the cardiac rhythm. VF and pulseless VT should be defibrillated as soon as they are identified.
4. To establish and maintain a patent airway, and ventilation, with 100% high flow oxygen.
5. To achieve venous access, preferably at more than one site. Ideally, blood samples should be taken for urgent analysis of blood gases, and glucose, electrolytes, full blood count, clotting studies—as an important abnormality (e.g. hypoxaemia, hyperkalaemia, haemorrhage) may be responsible for the arrest.
6. To continue chest compressions and ventilation until spontaneous cardiac output is restored.
7. To stabilize and optimize breathing and circulation when spontaneous cardiac output is restored.

The overall aim of resuscitation is the return of an adequate spontaneous circulation with little or no cerebral dysfunction. The intervention can only be considered successful if the patient is able to return home with intact cerebral function. Unfortunately, the probability of a successful outcome decreases with the length of time taken to restore cardiac output.

Cardiac arrest algorithm

Two fundamental treatment pathways are used in cardiac arrest (see Figure 6.1). The main difference is that if the cardiac rhythm is VF/pulseless VT, early defibrillation is an essential intervention; while defibrillation is not useful and should not be employed in PEA/asystole. In all cases, CPR, with good quality chest compressions and effective ventilation, is required to circulate oxygenated blood to vital organs. CPR is performed in 2 min

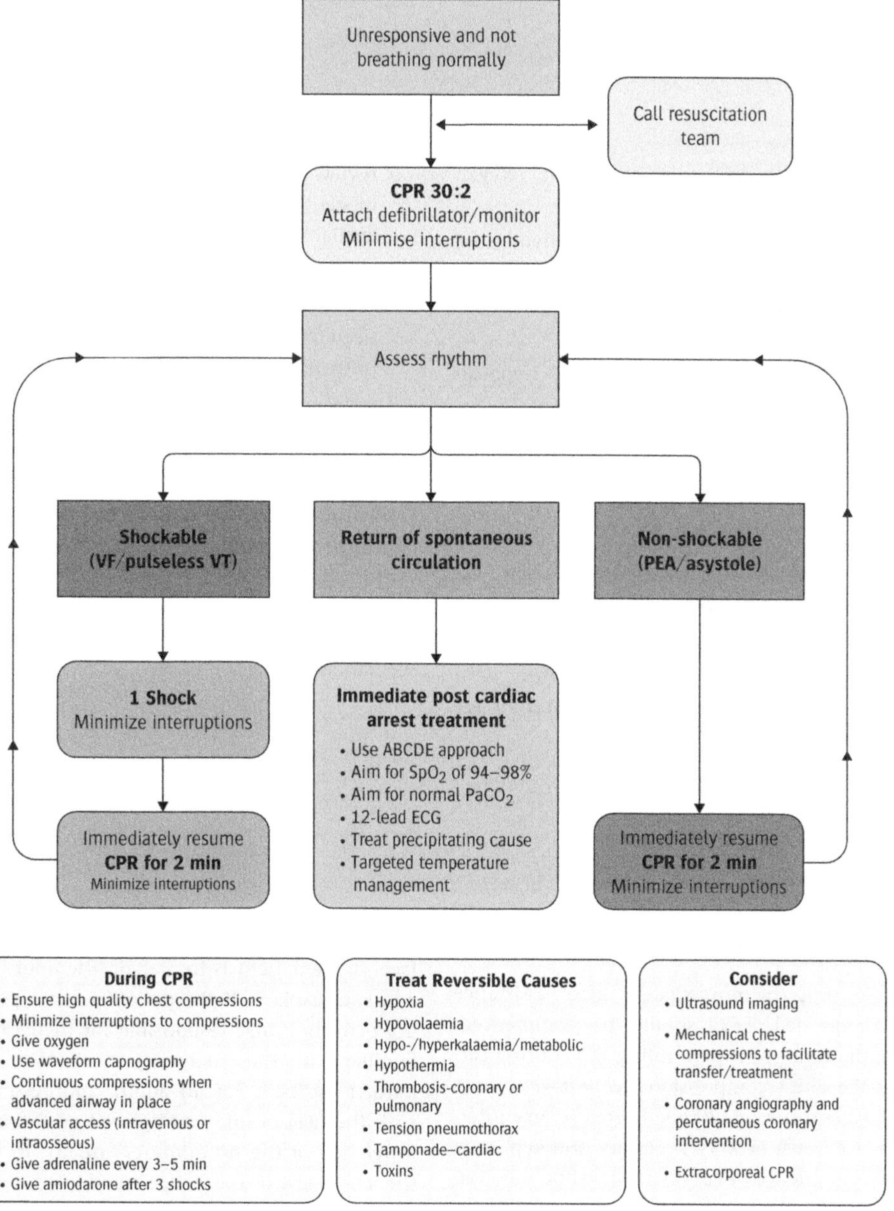

Figure 6.1 Adult Advanced Life Support algorithm.
Reproduced with the kind permission of the Resuscitation Council (UK).

cycles with short breaks in between to check for signs of life and review the cardiac rhythm. Epinephrine is recommended for all patients in PEA/asytole (administered as soon as possible) and all patients remaining in VF/pulseless VT after three shocks have been delivered. Other drugs are only given for particular problems, such as amiodarone for persistent VF/pulseless VT. As well as ensuring that these key processes are maintained, the resuscitation team must also consider and identify possible causes of the cardiac arrest that might respond to specific treatments. This is guided by review of the '4 Hs and 4 Ts' which are common and potentially reversible causes of collapse (Soar *et al.* 2015). The nurse caring for an arrested patient has a key role in considering their past history and current problems to help clarify the most likely causes of arrest.

Reversible causes of cardiac arrest and possible actions

- Hypoxia:
  - check air entry, tracheal tube placement, oxygen supply, etc.
- Hypovolaemia, e.g. haemorrhage, severe dehydration, diarrhoea/vomiting, severe sepsis.
  - ensure adequate fluid replacement/attempts to control haemorrhage are instigated.
- Hypo/hyperkalaemia—or hypoglycaemia, hypocalcaemia, or other metabolic disorder:
  - take bloods and check serum electrolyte levels, give iv potassium chloride/glucose/calcium chloride/ magnesium sulphate etc as necessary.
- Hypothermia:
  - institute rewarming with warmed fluids (e.g., via IV/NG/bladder routes), and/or warm air devices.
- Tension pneumothorax:
  - auscultate and palpate chest, decompress with needle thoracocentesis and then pleural drainage system if required.
- Cardiac Tamponade:
  - review patient presentation, perform needle pericardiocentesis/cardiothoracic surgical intervention as available
- Toxins (i.e. poisoning) including medications:
  - review patient presentation and drug chart, consider need for drug screen, identify any possible antidotes or treatment of anaphylaxis.
- Thrombosis (or embolism), usually in the pulmonary circulation, or in a coronary or cerebral vessel:
  - review patient presentation, consider thrombolysis.

Transthoracic echocardiography is a useful adjunct to clinical examination which can be performed during resuscitation in order to identify potentially treatable causes of cardiac arrest, including hypovolaemia, tension pneumothorax, cardiac tamponade, and thrombosis/embolism.

Resuscitation techniques

External chest compression (ECC)

At the same time or immediately after assistance has been summoned, ECC should be commenced. Maximizing the time spent performing ECC during cardiac arrest—the chest compression fraction—improves survival (Christenson *et al.* 2009). Therefore any interruptions to ECC must be very necessary and kept very brief. Ideally, a sequence of compressions should be followed by rescue breaths. If ventilation is not possible for any reason, compression-only resuscitation is better than nothing (Perkins *et al.* 2015). ECC should be performed with the patient flat on their back and on a firm surface. If the patient is in a chair, the floor is the nearest and easiest place. If the patient is on a pressure-relieving bed, the nurse responsible for their care should be familiar with the emergency mechanism to flatten or harden the bed. For an adult, compressions are done with the heel of one hand placed on the middle of the lower half of the sternum—essentially, in the centre of the chest—with the other hand placed on top. The arms should be straight and the shoulders above the patient's chest (see Figure 6.2). Compressions should continue at a rate of 100–120/min to a depth of 5–6 cm,

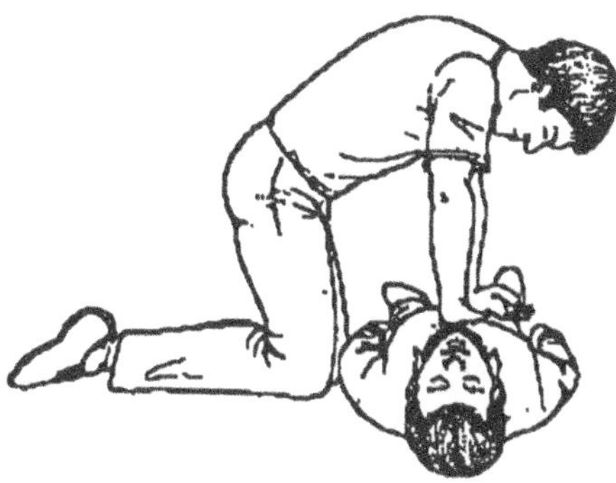

Figure 6.2 Hand position for chest compression
Reproduced from Handley A.J. and Swain A. (ed.) (1994). *Advanced Life Support Manual* ((2nd edn). Reproduced with the kind permission of the Resuscitation Council (UK).

with the patient's chest allowed to recoil completely between compressions.

The ratio of compressions to ventilations is 30:2 when the patient is not intubated; i.e. ECC is paused after each sequence of 30 compressions to allow two breaths to be given using a bag–valve–mask system. Compressions do not need to be synchronized with ventilations when a definitive sealed airway is established (i.e. by endotracheal intubation) or when a supraglottal airway device is placed. Here, ECC can be maintained while breaths are delivered at a rate of 10/min. It can be useful if the person performing ECC counts aloud to help synchronization with ventilation in the non-intubated patient, especially towards the end of each sequence: '26, 27, 28, 29, 30'. The individual providing ventilation is then prepared and prompted to immediately deliver the breaths. In addition, if ECC is discontinued for any other reason (e.g., to check the cardiac rhythm or to defibrillate) counting should continue with the word 'off' after each number (e.g. 'one–off, two–off, three–off, four–off', etc.). This reminds the team that no circulatory support is being provided for this period and may help ensure that time 'off the chest' is minimized.

Compressions should continue even when the defibrillator is being charged, with the aim of reducing the pre-shock pause to less than 5 sec, and resumed immediately after any shock is given (unless there are very obvious signs of life). There should be no pause to check the cardiac rhythm at this point. Few people can maintain effective compressions for more than about 2 min. The resuscitation team should be organized to change the person performing ECC after each cycle (which lasts 2 min), but with minimal delay.

See Box 6.2 for further information on chest compressions.

Box 6.2 Mechanisms of external chest compression generated cardiac output

There are two proposed mechanisms by which blood flow is generated during chest compression (Babbs 2005). The first is the 'cardiac pump' theory, put forward by Kouwenhoven *et al.* (1960) in a landmark early paper about ECC. This theory suggests that ECC produces compression of the heart itself between the depressed sternum anteriorly and the vertebrae posteriorly. Compression increases pressure inside the heart, and blood is forced out of the right side of the heart into the pulmonary arteries and out of the left side of the heart into the aorta. Backflow through the venae cavae and the pulmonary veins is prevented by competent intracardiac and venous valves. Cardiac filling then takes place during relaxation as the reduction in pressure draws blood back into the heart. Again, retrograde flow is prevented by venous valves. In this theory, an increased rate of compressions will improve cardiac output as each compression can only deliver a set amount of blood (i.e. that contained within the heart itself).

The second suggested mechanism is the 'thoracic pump' theory, which holds that the whole chest acts as a pump during ECC. Here, compression raises intrathoracic pressure resulting in blood flow from the pulmonary vasculature (which acts as a relatively large capacity reservoir) into the left side of the heart, forcing blood already there out through the aorta. This can only work if both the mitral and aortic valves are open. Retrograde flow from the lungs is prevented by partial closure of the pulmonary valve and the venae cavae valves, and by collapse of veins which are then resistant to flow. Cardiac filling occurs during relaxation as the release of pressure in the intrathoracic space brings blood from the superior vena cava through the right side of the heart to fill the pulmonary vessels. If this theory is correct, increasing depth and time of compression to increase intrathoracic pressure will improve cardiac output because an increased volume of blood will be squeezed from the pulmonary circulation. This would explain the improvement in cardiac output seen with asynchronous ventilation and compression, particularly if there are high ventilation pressures involved.

In both theories, the cause of flow is increased pressure with cardiac and venous valves acting to ensure one-way flow. Normal arterial resistance to flow is not present because of the loss of peripheral tone caused by hypoxia, ischaemia, and acidosis. Arterial and venous pressures equilibrate, and therefore forward blood flow (arterial to venous) must be generated by a pressure difference between aorta and right atrium. Both mechanisms may play a part at different times in different patients. However, research mainly indicates that the thoracic pump theory is likely to be more important.

1. The tricuspid and mitral valves are usually found to be open during ECC.
2. During chest compression with a flail segment, the arterial pressure does not increase until the segment is stabilized (by intermittent positive pressure ventilation).
3. There have been case reports of some cardiac output being maintained at the onset of VF by repeated coughing which increases intrathoracic pressure.

Mechanical aids to chest compression

Even good quality manual ECC achieves no more than 30% of normal cardiac output (Peters and Ihle 1990). This deficit has encouraged the development of several types of mechanical device designed to improve the quality of chest compressions. Some deliver automatic compressions (and decompression) that can relieve a member of staff from performing manual ECC. Some of these mechanical aids are described below.

Active compression–decompression (ACD) devices

The concept underpinning ACD devices comes in part from reports of successful CPR being performed with toilet plungers pushed against the chests of victims of cardiac arrest. Essentially, a large suction cup with a handle can be used to compress the chest and then actively lift, expand, and decompress the chest. Venous return to the heart is augmented during thoracic decompression, so that there is a greater pre-load available for output on compression. Purpose-made hand-held ACD devices may incorporate a built-in pressure gauge so the user can see the pressures being exerted, and a metronome to guide compression rate (e.g. the CardioPump, manufactured by Advanced Circulatory Systems). Other devices are strapped onto the patient's chest and include an electrically or compressed gas driven piston to deliver compressions, and sometimes a decompression component as well (e.g. the Lund University Cardiac Arrest System (LUCAS) from Physio-Control).

Another approach is the 'load-distributing band' CPR (e.g. the Zoll Medical Corporation AutoPulse). Here, a close-fitting band of material is placed across the chest and connected to a backboard, with the material automatically tightened and relaxed to deliver chest compressions.

Various mechanical aids to chest compression are already being used in a wide range of out-of-hospital and in-hospital settings, and there are some promising reports (Deakin *et al.* 2010). As yet, these devices are less frequently employed in the critical care unit. No particular approach or specific device is endorsed in the current resuscitation guidelines (Soar *et al.* 2015). Soar *et al.* (2015) emphasize that effective use of these devices needs training and practice, and that some studies have shown negative consequences such as delays and interruptions in CPR (e.g. Wang *et al.* 2007). A Cochrane Review of the research published in 2009 found most studies to be poor quality and/or contradictory (Brooks *et al.* 2011). The authors concluded that it could not be stated that mechanical aids were either beneficial or harmful. Several trials are under way that may clarify the situation in the next few years.

The precordial thump

The precordial thump—a blow to the lower third of the patient's sternum using the lateral aspect of a closed fist—is rarely effective and is employed less and less. This must not delay getting help and a defibrillator to the bedside, but could be attempted in the first seconds of a witnessed cardiac arrest when VT or VF is seen on the monitor. Excessive force is not required, but rather a sharp blow using the weight of a swing of the forearm from the elbow. The impact of this mechanical energy acts like the electrical energy of a defibrillatory shock, albeit with relatively low level energy. This may occasionally reorganize the chaotic electrical activity of VF so that sinus or other effective rhythm is restored.

Defibrillation

Defibrillation is the passage of a current of electricity through a fibrillating heart. The current acts to depolarize myocardial cells, allowing them to uniformly repolarize. Normal physiological cardiac pacemaker mechanisms may then regain control over initiation and conduction of organized depolarization through the standard conduction pathways.

The defibrillator stores and delivers pre-set amounts of direct current electrical energy through two paddles or pads placed on the patient's chest. The electrical energy is measured in joules (J). Older defibrillator models deliver a single directional monophasic waveform (a current flowing in one direction from one paddle or pad to the other). Monophasic defibrillators are no longer manufactured, but are still in use in some services. Modern defibrillators produce biphasic waveforms which deliver a current that flows first in one direction and then reverses to the opposite direction for the remainder of the electrical discharge. This is associated with a reduced defibrillation threshold so lower levels of energy are needed. This may cause less collateral damage to the heart. There is also a longer refractory period that may help to block recurring fibrillation.

Defibrillation can be delivered either with paddles pressed against gel pads, or through multi-function hands-free adhesive pads that can be used for cardiac monitoring, defibrillation, and pacing when necessary. To monitor the cardiac rhythm via paddles, some machines must be set to 'paddles', while others automatically monitor through the paddles until switched to an ECG lead setting. These differences mean that nurses must familiarize themselves with whichever equipment is used locally. Automated external defibrillators (AEDs) are now commonly used in some hospitals and many public places, such as railway stations, airports, shopping malls, and large institutions. They are not used in critical care units as manual defibrillators are generally considered more versatile if used by staff with advanced life support skills. Some defibrillators may have both manual and AED functions, thus increasing the options available, but this does mean that there are more switches and settings with which staff must be familiar.

The chances of successful defibrillation of VF/pulseless VT rapidly decrease in a short time. A 12% reduction in survival is reported with each minute that passes without a shock (Perkins *et al.* 2015). Getting access to a defibrillator in a critical care area should not be a problem. If nurses are trained in advanced life support, there is no reason why they should not defibrillate, as immediate defibrillation of VF and pulseless VT improves outcomes. In the UK, it has been said that the 'extension of nursing skills, e.g. to the use of airway adjuncts, intravenous cannulation, rhythm recognition, manual defibrillation, and administration of specific drugs in resuscitation, should be encouraged' (Royal College of Anaesthetists *et al.* 2008). However, not all hospitals support nurses in these roles.

The person defibrillating must take responsibility for the safety of others when preparing and delivering the shock, and should also ensure that these processes are as swift as possible so that there are minimal pauses in ECC.

Defibrillation procedure

Cardiac arrest must be confirmed, the resuscitation team called, and external chest compressions begun while the defibrillator is attached.

Defibrillators with paddles need to be used with gel pads. These act as conductors providing an efficient electrical pathway to the patient, reducing the risk of current passing through less efficient pathways such as air or bare skin. One pad should be placed below the right clavicle (collar bone) and the other on the left side of the chest, centred on the fifth intercostal space in the midaxillary line. Hands-free adhesive pads have the same purpose and are sited at the same points. Diagrams showing placement positions are often on the pads and/or defibrillator (Figure 6.3). While the pads are placed, any metal objects on the patient's upper body should be removed, as these can preferentially conduct electrical current and cause burns, and the patient will receive a reduced amount of charge. Glyceryl trinitrate patches must also be removed because of their potential to explode.

Once the defibrillator is connected to the patient, ECC is briefly halted so that the cardiac rhythm can be positively identified. If VF or pulseless VT is present, ECC must be recommenced while the patient is quickly prepared for defibrillation.

The person defibrillating should then dial in the appropriate energy level on the defibrillator. Different

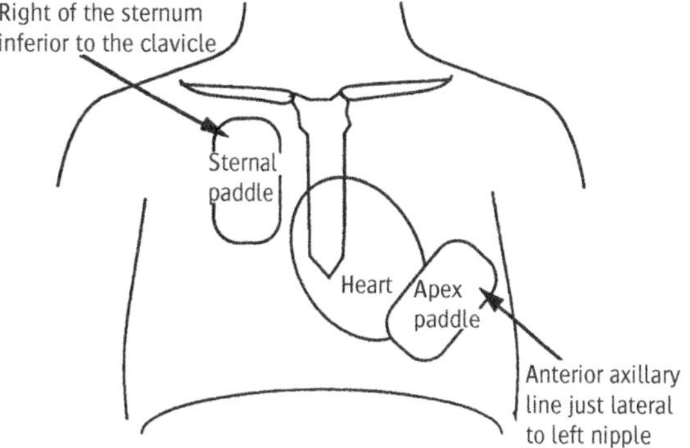

Figure 6.3 Paddle/pad positions for defibrillation.

hospitals and different machines have different guidelines, so the local policy must be known. Energy levels are commonly set at 150 J for biphasic machines and higher for monophasic devices. If in doubt, the highest energy level available should be used. A warning to 'stand clear' must be clearly stated while the defibrillator is switched to charge, so that the whole team—apart from the individual performing ECC—moves away from the patient. Ensure that no other person is in contact with the patient or any conducting surfaces such as the metal bed frame or a drip stand. Any oxygen delivery system that might leak oxygen near the patient must also be removed as poorly placed paddles may cause sparking and fire if fuelled by oxygen; although this is very rare. There are no reports of fire when adhesive pads have been used (Soar *et al.* 2015). Only when the defibrillator is charged should the person performing ECC be required to immediately 'stand clear' and the shock be delivered.

CPR must then be restarted straight away, with no pause to check a pulse or look at the cardiac monitor, and continued for 2 min when the cardiac rhythm is assessed again. If VF/pulseless VT is still present, a second shock should be given, as before, with CPR immediately recommenced and then halted after 2 min to check the rhythm. A third shock is given if the patient remains in VF/pulseless VT and CPR is performed again, continuing in the same pattern as required. Either spontaneous circulation will be restored, although this is less likely as time passes, or it will be decided that further treatment is futile.

Alternatively, if a rhythm potentially compatible with a cardiac output is seen after 2 min of CPR, a central artery (carotid and/or femoral) should be palpated for a pulse. If no pulse is found, which must then mean that the patient is in PEA, CPR is again performed for 2 min, followed by reassessment of the rhythm, continuing with more 2 min cycles of CPR until the patient recovers or a considered decision to stop is made. Asystole is managed in the same way as PEA.

'Stacked' shocks

As just described, the standard treatment for VF/pulseless VT cardiac arrests is single shocks separated by 2 min periods of CPR. There are some very specific circumstances when *three* 'stacked' shocks are given one after other as quickly as possible at the beginning of a VF/pulseless VT arrest. These are when a monitored patient is seen to arrest (which may well be the case in the critical care unit), in the first days after cardiac surgery, or in the cardiac catheter laboratory. Following this sequence of stacked shocks, 2 min of CPR should be completed and the rhythm then reassessed, after which the arrest is managed as previously described. Importantly, when three stacked shocks are used in this way and the patient remains in VF/pulseless VT, the three shocks are effectively counted as the first single shock for the purposes of the resuscitation protocol. This means that CPR, another shock, CPR and one more shock are given before epinephrine—and amiodarone—are administered to the patient in ongoing VF/pulseless VT.

Airway management—non-intubated patients in cardiac arrest

If there is no artificial airway of any kind in place, the patient's own airway must be assessed for patency and then kept open. The suggested methods for opening the airway are the head tilt–chin lift manoeuvre (Figure 6.4) or the jaw thrust, both of which should pull the base of the tongue away from the back of the throat. Head tilt–chin lift involves placing two fingers of one hand under the point of the chin and the other hand over the forehead. The head is then tipped back, pulling the chin upwards. The airway should be cleared of any obvious obstructing material using a Yankauer sucker. Well-fitting dentures are left in place to improve the seal around the mouth for ventilation, but loose-fitting or broken dentures should be removed. A simple airway adjunct, such as an oropharyngeal (Guedel) airway, is useful for maintaining airway patency and can be inserted once the airway is clear, with bag–valve–mask ventilation then performed.

Ventilation is much easier with placement of a supraglottic airway device, such as a laryngeal mask airway (LMA) or an i-gel®. These devices can be inserted 'blind', meaning that direct visualization of the airway with

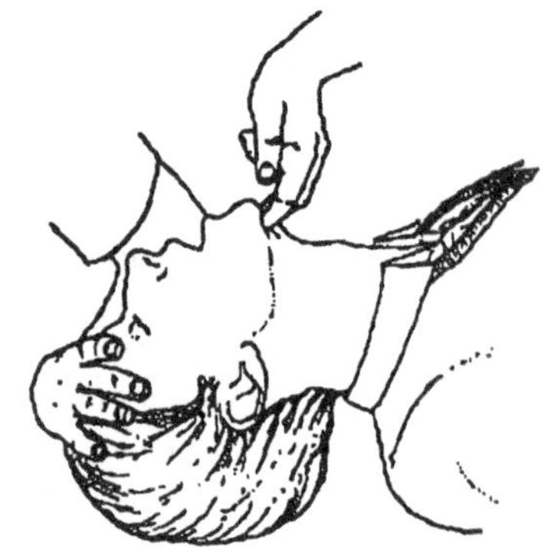

Figure 6.4 Opening the airway

Reproduced from Handley A.J. and Swain A. (eds) (1994). *Advanced Life Support Manual* (2nd edn). Reproduced with the kind permission of the Resuscitation Council (UK).

laryngoscopy is not required. The LMA looks like a conventional endotracheal tube at the proximal end with a large inflatable elliptical cuff at the other, distal, end. The LMA is placed through the mouth into the pharynx until the cuff is at the level of the larynx—essentially pushed, not forced, as far as it will go. When inflated, the cuff forms an airtight seal around the posterior perimeter of the larynx, allowing ventilation of the lungs. The insertion technique is more easily learned than endotracheal intubation, although supraglottic airway devices may not be completely effective in preventing pulmonary aspiration and will tend to leak if ventilation pressures are high. A more recent development is the i-gel which is quite similar to the LMA in appearance, with a large, soft, flexible cuff, and is inserted in a similar way. However, the i-gel® cuff does not require inflation. As with the LMA, the i-gel® is quite easy to place and provides a reasonably well sealed airway, but is less effective than an endotracheal tube (ETT).

If the patient is not already intubated, insertion of a cuffed ETT is generally considered the optimal method of ensuring and protecting a patent airway. However, intubation can be very difficult, especially in emergency situations, and frequent failures to properly site the ETT in cardiac arrest situations have been reported (Soar *et al.* 2015). Therefore it is now recommended that a carbon dioxide detector measuring expired CO_2 be used to help check that the ETT is correctly positioned, preferably with a continuous waveform display (see Box 6.3). In addition, although more or less continuous chest compressions are a priority in cardiac arrest, these are sometimes reduced in strength or stopped completely by someone asking for the patient to be kept still for the process of intubation. The latest guidelines state that ECC should not be halted for more than 5 sec (Soar 2015). Therefore, if good ventilation is being maintained with a bag–valve system, especially through a supraglottic airway device, there may be little value in attempting endotracheal intubation. However, if there is a high risk of aspiration or ventilation is problematic, intubation by a skilled and practised individual—usually an anaesthetist—with full consideration of the risks and benefits is probably the best option. A pillow can be placed under the patient's shoulders and occiput to extend the head and facilitate placement of a tube in the trachea.

Airway control—already intubated patients

Many critical care patients will already have an endotracheal or tracheostomy tube in place. If there is any doubt about the patency of the tube, a suction catheter should be inserted to check for any blockage and, if possible, remove it. If there is an immovable obstruction or doubt about the position of the tube in the trachea it should be removed as a manner of urgency. This should only be done by nurses in the unlikely event that there are no medical staff available. These patients will probably need to be re-intubated as quickly as possible but may be maintained in the short term by airway manoeuvres and bag–valve–mask ventilation. If the tube is patent, the patient should be ventilated on 100% oxygen during the arrest; however, once stabilization is achieved the FiO_2 should be reduced promptly to maintain normoxaemia

Box 6.3 End-tidal carbon dioxide monitoring (capnography)

It is now recommended that a carbon dioxide detector measuring expired CO_2 (end-tidal CO_2 ($ETCO_2$)) is used to help check that the ETT is correctly positioned, preferably with a continuous waveform display (Deakin *et al.* 2010). If the ETT is not in the trachea, a few ventilations will soon eliminate any residual CO_2 that may be present, so the $ETCO_2$ reading will be zero or nearly zero. In contrast, an ETT correctly placed in the respiratory tract accesses a steady source of CO_2 from the lungs so there should always be CO_2 evident on expiration. This assumes that there is at least some blood flow through the chest. If pulmonary blood flow is low or non-existent, there will be little or no CO_2 transported to the lungs for detection. In cardiac arrest, this blood flow can only be generated by ECC.

It follows that as $ETCO_2$ correlates with pulmonary blood flow, monitors displaying continuous $ETCO_2$ (capnographs) help monitor the quality of ECC in real time. Good quality ECC should produce a cardiac output that delivers venous blood containing CO_2 to the lungs. Effective ventilation then enables this CO_2 to be eliminated on expiration. A near normal $ETCO_2$ is an indicator that reasonable blood flow is being achieved. The waveform should show $ETCO_2$ rising with each expiration, and falling on inspiration. Any subsequent obvious rise in $ETCO_2$ levels is indicative of a marked improvement in blood flow, which may be the first sign of a return of spontaneous circulation. In contrast, a consistently low $ETCO_2$ (e.g. <2 kPa/15mmHg) is suggestive of poor blood flow that could be improved by trying to optimize the quality of ECC.

as continued high levels of arterial oxygen are associated with worse outcomes.

Ventilation

In a cardiac arrest situation the patient should be ventilated with 100% oxygen to optimize P_aO_2 and arterial oxygen saturation. Proper equipment should be available in the critical care unit, so the patient can be ventilated via a tight-fitting anaesthetic mask attached to a bag connected to 100% oxygen. The bag should not be a rebreathing bag, as this will increase P_aCO_2, but rather a bag with a one-way valve such as a self-inflating bag–valve system, ideally with a reservoir attached to maximize the FiO_2. Bag–valve–mask ventilation is a skill that requires practice on training manikins and can be done very poorly by novices. A two-person technique is likely to be more effective, with one person holding the mask in place while the other ventilates (Soar *et al.* 2015).

Positioning of head and neck is important. A non-intubated patient should have no pillow under the head and the neck should be flexed with the head tipped back. To ventilate via a mask, head tilt is maintained by lifting the lower jaw forward at the angles of the jaw using the fingers, while the thumbs press the seal of the mask to the face. It may be useful to begin with two relatively slow breaths, giving a volume sufficient to cause the chest to visibly rise. It is vital that chest movement is observed as it may be the only indicator that the airway is patent and an adequate tidal volume can be delivered. Once established, ventilation is continued using breaths with an inspiratory time of about 1 sec, aiming for normal-sized chest movements at a rate of 10 per minute. It is easy for the stress of the cardiac arrest situation to result in over-enthusiastic delivery of ventilation; gas may be propelled into the oesophagus and stomach with possible regurgitation and aspiration of stomach contents.

If the patient is intubated, the ventilator provides more reliably effective ventilation than use of a bag–valve system. Typically, the ventilator should be set to deliver 15 breaths/min with a tidal volume of 6–7 mL/kg of bodyweight, PEEP of 5 cmH_2O and FiO_2 1.0. The FiO_2 should then be rapidly reduced to a more normal level once the patient is stabilized. The ventilator alarms may need to be silenced throughout the resuscitation attempt. However, if there is any doubt about the efficacy of the ventilator it is safest to switch to the self-inflating bag while investigating any problems with the ventilator. Pneumothorax should be considered if airway pressures suddenly increase in the ventilated patient who has a cardiac arrest.

Management of cardiac arrest

Attention to detail and a series of rapid coordinated actions are essential in a situation which is highly stressful and has great potential for ineffective disorganization. Management of cardiac arrest requires an optimum number of people. Too few staff will mean unnecessary delays in instituting treatments, but too many will increase confusion and may physically impede access to the patient. An effective team usually needs no more than 4-5 individuals, or perhaps six in complex cases (see Box 6.4). Personnel involved in resuscitation should be trained in advanced life support (ALS), or at least in immediate life support, with management of the arrest following a standard protocol. Training should include practice of key skills to a clear standard and simulated cardiac arrest scenarios with expert feedback on performance.

It is crucial that staff attending a cardiac arrest function as an integrated team. Team composition will vary considerably, but certain skills are essential, including performance of good quality ECC and manual ventilation. UK standards suggest that the team should contain at least two doctors trained in ALS (Royal College of Anaesthetists *et al.* 2008), preferably a senior acute care physician or critical care doctor, and an anaesthetist. Between them, the team should be capable of:

- defibrillation
- advanced airway management, i.e. tracheal intubation
- intravenous (i.v.) cannulation—even in difficult cases—including central venous access, and intraosseous (i.o.) access if the iv route is not possible
- drug administration by i.v. and i.o. routes
- other advanced skills such as external cardiac pacing or pericardiocentesis
- understanding of requirements for post-resuscitation care.

One individual should be designated 'team leader'. Ideally, this individual should not take a hands-on role

Box 6.4 **Roles during cardiac arrest**

Nurse 1 (nurse caring for the patient)

Recognize the cardiac arrest, alert other team members, begin CPR, inform team of the patient history and preceding events, record what happens during the resuscitation process, protect the patient's dignity and rights, speak to the family with the doctor.

Nurse 2 (back-up)

Bring emergency equipment, prepare defibrillator and defibrillate if appropriate, draw up drugs and infusions, administer drugs as prescribed, record events and interventions, take over CPR from Nurse 1 when required.

Team leader

This is usually the senior doctor on the critical care unit, or the duty CCU or medical registrar, or, if no senior medical staff are present, the nurse-in-charge.

Re-confirm cardiac arrest and the cardiac arrhythmia, direct overall resuscitation management, decide on interventions, assess response, defibrillate if appropriate (if no other staff available), may obtain (central) venous access if needed, prescribe drugs, ensure CPR is being done correctly and that ECC is rotated so fatigue is not a problem, call in outside help if necessary, decide on endpoint if resuscitation seems to be futile, talk to the patient's family.

Anaesthetist

Intubate if necessary, secure airway, ventilate by hand or attach to mechanical ventilator; if necessary, assist with ECC, obtain (central) venous access if required.

A fifth person, probably a doctor, is often a helpful addition to the team, particularly if venous or intra-osseus access is required, or other interventions are needed.

but, if possible, stand back slightly to get an overview. Decisions on interventions should be made by the team leader, so all information pertaining to the situation should be passed to them to aid decision-making.

In most cases, a nurse with specialist knowledge or training is included on the resuscitation team. In the critical care unit the nurse caring for the patient can add all-important knowledge of the patient. A back-up nurse can provide assistance as necessary. This back-up should reflect the experience and skills of the nurse assigned to the patient. A junior nurse will require experienced back-up, while an experienced nurse can be assisted by a junior who can learn from the experience. The nurse-in-charge of the unit should be fully aware of the situation, but may not necessarily need to remain with the patient provided that back-up is appropriate.

Venous and intra-osseus access

Intravenous cannulation is crucial in cardiac arrest, both to administer drugs and to obtain blood samples for laboratory analysis. Most critical care patients will already have IV access. If not, one and ideally two cannulae should be inserted, preferably short devices with a large diameter (14 or 16 gauge). A central venous catheter (CVC), directly accessing the central circulation, would be better for rapid distribution of any drug. The critical care patient may have a CVC in place but, if not, the difficulties of CVC insertion and the likelihood that chest compression will be disturbed mean that peripheral sites are best used in the first instance.

If venous access has not been achieved within 2 min, intraosseus (IO) access should be obtained so that drugs and fluids can be delivered into bone marrow, which connects to the central circulation (Resuscitation Council UK 2011). Few nurses are familiar with this technique, although it is relatively easily learned and is becoming more widely used. Various purpose-made IO devices are available, including hand-held, spring-loaded, and battery-powered models. At the very least, critical care nurses should be familiar with the equipment used locally and be able to assist with insertion, for example by flexing the patient's knee and holding the leg still for insertion. The most commonly used insertion site is near the top of the tibia, 2–3 cm below the tibial tuberosity. The IO needle is used to puncture the thin layer of skin found there and then advanced with a controlled twisting motion until resistance ceases, at which point the tip of the device should be in the cortex of the bone. It should then be possible to aspirate blood; if not, the needle may be blocked by bone marrow, which can be cleared by a 10 mL 0.9% NaCl flush. Once inserted and secured, standard preparations and doses of drugs can be administered through the IO device. It should be removed when IV access is eventually achieved.

Please note that drug administration via a tracheal tube is no longer recommended; experience has shown it to be unreliable.

Agents used in resuscitation

Oxygen

Even good quality ECC produces a low cardiac output, so every effort should be made to maximally saturate the haemoglobin that is being circulated. Therefore 100% oxygen should be used during CPR. However, if a resuscitation is successful and the patient is then stabilized, the FiO_2 should be titrated to achieve a saturation no more than 94–98% as there is observational data showing higher levels of blood oxygen are associated with worse outcomes (Kilgannon *et al.* 2011).

Drug therapies

Many drugs have been used in cardiac arrest in the past, mostly with little or no real evidence of benefit. The lack of good evidence and the value of simplifying treatments when possible have resulted in just seven drugs being recommended for use in the most recent guidelines (Soar *et al.* 2015). Even now, there is no definitive evidence that giving a vasopressor (including epinephrine) or any anti-arrhythmic drugs improves long-term outcomes, although there are reports of short-term benefits and animal studies that support their use (Soar *et al.* 2015). The seven drugs now listed in the guidelines include intravenous fluid and thrombolytic agents. Where possible, prefilled drug syringes should be used so that no time is lost in drawing up medications. A 0.9% NaCl bolus or a continuous 0.9% NaCl infusion should be used to flush each drug into the central circulation.

Epinephrine (adrenaline)

This is the main drug used to support the circulation in both shockable and non-shockable cardiac arrest. The essential treatment of PEA/asystole is good quality CPR, but epinephrine should be given as soon as possible once ECC has begun. For patients with VF or pulseless VT, the priority is CPR and defibrillation, but epinephrine is administered if the patient still remains in cardiac arrest after three shocks. Epinephrine has mixed α- and β-adrenergic actions. Its α effects are predominantly responsible for aiding resuscitation by causing systemic vasoconstriction that increases diastolic blood pressure and coronary and cerebral perfusion. Beta-receptor actions have chronotropic and inotropic effects on the heart and some vasodilator effect on coronary arteries, but can also cause undesirable side effects such as increasing myocardial oxygen demand and reducing sub-endocardial blood flow (by increasing myocardial muscle tension which compresses coronary blood vessels). The recommended dose is 1 mg IV (10 ml 1:10,000 solution) every 3–5 min. It is generally given in alternate cycles, i.e. about every 4 min. The 10 mL 1:10,000 dilution is used instead of a 1 mL 1:1000 dilution as the larger volume ensures that most of the drug will enter the circulation even without a flush,

Amiodarone

This potent ventricular and supraventricular anti-arrhythmic has replaced lidocaine (lignocaine) as a treatment for VF and pulseless VT as there is evidence of better survival, at least in the short term (Dorian *et al.* 2002). Amiodarone prolongs the duration of the action potential, equalizing the length of repolarization in all myocardial cells and increasing the effective refractory period. It is the first-line agent for VF/pulseless VT that persists after three shocks, and should be given immediately after the epinephrine has been administered. The initial dose is a 300 mg bolus given over a few minutes. Amiodarone can be given into a peripheral cannula in the arrest situation, although ideally it should be administered through a central line as extravasation can cause local tissue damage. Another bolus dose of 150 mg can be given if VF/pulseless VT continues despite further shocks, followed by a 900 mg intravenous infusion given over 24 hours.

Magnesium

Magnesium suppresses myocardial irritability and prevents tachyarrhythmias but evidence of its value in cardiac arrest is inconclusive, except in cases of hypomagnesaemia. It may work by directly inhibiting potassium efflux from the cell, by altering cellular calcium levels, or by stimulating a membrane-stabilizing enzyme (Herroeder *et al.* 2011). In cardiac arrest, magnesium (given as magnesium sulphate) can be considered for ventricular tachycardia (VT) or supraventricular tachycardia (SVT), especially when associated with hypomagnesaemia, and particularly for cases of torsades de pointes (polymorphic VT with an axis that shifts from positive to negative). If the rhythm is pulseless VT, magnesium may be given following amiodarone. In PEA, it could be used when the rhythm is an SVT. Magnesium can also be employed as part of the treatment of digoxin toxicity. The initial dose is 2g/4 ml (or 8 mmol) 50% magnesium sulphate given IV over 1–2 min. This may be repeated after 10 min. Side effects are rare.

Calcium

Calcium is essential in myocardial excitation–contraction coupling, in increasing contractility, and in enhancing ventricular automaticity during asystole. These effects are potentially useful in resuscitation, though calcium may prevent reperfusion of ischaemic areas of the brain and heart due to vascular spasm related to intracellular calcium overload. Furthermore, cytoplasmic calcium accumulation is associated with cell death. Therefore calcium is only recommended in specific circumstances, for example where hypocalcaemia or blockade of calcium channels (e.g. verapamil toxicity) may be the cause of PEA, or with known or suspected hypermagnesaemia and hyperkalaemia. The dose is 10 ml of 10% calcium chloride IV (6.8 mmol). Calcium chloride is used in preference to calcium gluconate as the number of free calcium ions produced is three times greater for the same volume of drug.

Sodium bicarbonate ($NaHCO_3$)

Sodium bicarbonate is now only used in resuscitation for specific cases of hyperkalaemia or tricyclic antidepressant overdose, and not to treat acidaemia, as was the case in previous years. Serum bicarbonate levels will almost always be low in cardiac arrest as it is a natural buffer of the excess acid production. While seemingly logical to give sodium bicarbonate, research shows administration actually increases venous CO_2 levels, resulting in worse intracellular and respiratory acidosis. This is because bicarbonate (HCO_3^-) in the blood combines with hydrogen ions (H^+) to form H_2CO_3 (carbonic acid), which then dissociates into H_2O and CO_2. The CO_2 in the blood rapidly diffuses into cells where it recombines with H_2O to form H_2CO_3. This creates a paradoxical intracellular acidosis, even though extracellular acidosis—indicated by the serum pH—may be improved (Weil *et al.* 1986). Mixed venous acid–base values are a much better indicator of tissue acid–base. In a study of patients in cardiac arrest, Weil *et al.* (1986) found that the average arterial pH was 7.41 and P_aCO_2 was 4.26 kPa, yet average mixed venous pH was 7.15 and mixed venous CO_2 was 9.86 kPa.

Sodium bicarbonate does have a role in the treatment of severe hyperkalaemia (serum potassium ≥6.5 mmol/L) as it may help shift potassium back into the cells. It is also used in the management of peri- and cardiac arrest associated with overdose of tricyclic antidepressants (e.g. amitriptyline). These drugs can cause a widening QRS complex and VT; administration of bicarbonate to achieve a relatively high arterial pH of 7.45–7.55 may decrease the development of more malignant cardiac rhythms (Truhlář *et al.* 2015). The dose of sodium bicarbonate is 50 mmol (50 ml 8.4% solution) given IV.

Intravenous fluids

A 0.9% NaCl infusion can provide a flush for IV drugs, and dilution if necessary. If hypovolaemia is suspected, crystalloids (0.9% sodium chloride or Hartmann's solution), colloid or O rhesus-negative blood (for severe blood loss) may be infused to restore normovolaemia.

Thrombolytic agents

Thrombolytics (e.g. tenecteplase, alteplase) are not recommended for routine use in cardiac arrest, but can be considered if pulmonary embolus is a likely cause of the arrest. These agents do not act very quickly, so at least an hour of CPR may be necessary to enable thrombolysis to succeed.

Lengthy resuscitation

If a protracted resuscitation is needed, the team must plan to ensure that fatigue does not become a problem (e.g., by getting new staff to perform ECC), and that there are sufficient supplies of drugs, particularly epinephrine. A continuous iv infusion of epinephrine delivering 250 mcg/min may be useful (equivalent to 1 mg every 4 minutes).

Care of the successfully resuscitated patient

If not there already, it is usual for patients in the post-arrest period to be admitted to the critical care unit for stabilization and optimization. Continuing care and attention over the following days can make a significant difference to recovery. Review of almost 110,000 resuscitated patients found significant differences in post-cardiac arrest outcomes in different institutions, and it was suggested that more highly resourced, modern and aggressive approaches produced better results (Carr *et al.* 2009). The decision to transfer to critical care should be made by the resuscitation team leader in consultation with the critical care team and medical staff primarily responsible for the patient. Exceptions may be patients who have experienced VF/pulseless VT in a coronary care unit where immediate defibrillation has swiftly restored cardiac output and consciousness is not impaired, or subsequent recognition that the patient has an end-stage disease where escalation of care is inappropriate.

Even if a spontaneous circulation is restored, the post-arrest patient is likely to be unstable and susceptible to complications, including another cardiac arrest, especially if the resuscitation was a lengthy process. The so-called 'post-cardiac arrest syndrome' is a function of the disease state that led to the arrest and to the effects of ischaemia followed by reperfusion. Even with the most effective CPR, the patient will have suffered a period of relative ischaemia that will most affect organs that are particularly dependent on a continuous supply of oxygen. This includes the heart, which even if beating, is very likely to have impaired function for at least a few days. The brain is particularly vulnerable because of its high energy requirements and its minimal substrate reserves for anaerobic metabolism. Thus there is a high risk of cerebral and other tissue injury that tends to be exacerbated by ongoing stress responses, systemic inflammation, immunological disturbances, and disordered blood clotting. These damaging processes may be apparent simply as common and treatable abnormalities such as hyperglycaemia and acidosis. Therefore a detailed systematic review and consideration of all fundamental physiology is required after cardiac arrest.

Once obvious signs of life have been seen and a pulse able to generate an adequate blood pressure is palpated or witnessed on the monitor, a structured review of the patient's airway, breathing, circulation, disability, and exposure for full examination should be performed, informed by consideration of possible causes of the arrest (see Box 6.5).

Targeted temperature control (previously known as therapeutic hypothermia)

There is generally believed to be a benefit in preventing fever after the insult of cardiac arrest, but the ideal body temperature in this situation is unknown. A recent large multicentre trial randomized victims of out-of-hospital cardiac arrest to be cooled to either 33°C or 36°C and found that there was no difference in mortality (49% died overall) or survivors' neurological function (52% had poor function) (Nielsen *et al.* 2013). It is possible that other patient groups—for example, those who arrest during hospital admission—might have different characteristics and different ideal body temperatures in the post-resuscitation period.

'Targeted temperature control' is currently recommended for all adults who have an out-of-hospital cardiac arrest with an initial rhythm of VF/pulseless VT and remain unconscious after resuscitation (Nolan *et al.* 2015). It should also be considered for cases where the initial rhythm was non-shockable, or when the arrest happened in hospital. The process involves maintaining, or cooling, the body to a core temperature of 32–36°C with the objective of reducing its metabolic demands in order to optimize neurological recovery from the insult of cardiac arrest.

Cooling method

Temperature control can be achieved using external methods —for example, ice packs, cooling blankets, heat exchange cooling pads—and/or internal techniques—for example, administration of IV cold fluid or placement of an endovascular cooling device (NICE 2011).

Typically, the aim is to achieve a core temperature below 36°C within 4 hours. Cooling may be rapidly instigated with 30 mL/kg of IV cold crystalloid (from a refrigerator) given over an hour, and then continued and maintained for 24 hours with one of the methods of surface cooling. The patient's temperature can be monitored with a nasopharyngeal or bladder catheter. Short-acting IV sedative agents (e.g. propofol) and muscle relaxant (e.g. pancuronium) are given to dull awareness

Box 6.5 Patient review and initial management after resuscitation

- Check that there is air entry to both lungs (which also indicates that the airway is patent) and ventilation is adequate.
- In the first instance, confirm that the patient is ventilated on 100% oxygen and attach a pulse oximeter, if not already in place.
- Measure the blood pressure either with a sphygmomanometer or by using the arterial trace. The goal is to achieve a cardiac output and blood pressure that will avoid further ischaemia and preserve cerebral perfusion pressure. Careful management of the circulation will be required, and haemodynamic monitoring should be put in place if not already present.
- Take an arterial blood gas sample and measure blood gases, serum lactate, electrolytes, blood glucose, haemoglobin, and relevant cardiac enzymes as appropriate.
- Confirm with medical staff whether the patient is to be extubated, if they seem capable of adequate spontaneous ventilation, or needs continuing invasive respiratory support. If so, this may require sedation, at least for a period.
    - If the patient is not awake enough to breathe normally, or was previously ventilated, mechanical ventilation to ensure normal levels of oxygenation and normocapnia should be delivered. Once the patient is stabilized, the FiO_2 should be promptly titrated down to achieve arterial oxygen saturations of 94–98%.
- Record a 12-lead ECG. Acute myocardial infarction should usually be treated by percutaneous coronary intervention (PCI) or thrombolysis as soon as possible.
- Obtain a chest X-ray to check for fractured ribs, possible pneumothorax, possible aspiration, position of the ET tube, any central venous lines, nasogastric tube, etc.
- Review fluid balance and urine output. Urinary catheterization will almost certainly be necessary, if not already in place.
- Any IV cannulae sited during the arrest should be checked to ensure that an aseptic technique was used, and if in doubt replaced. Intra-osseous devices should be removed as soon as IV access is in place.
- Check the patient's drug chart to check which medications should be continued, which may need to be stopped, and if any should be added.
- Consider results of blood tests; highlight and correct significant abnormalities as relevant and possible.
- Other tests may be required to determine the cause of the arrest (e.g. echocardiogram, pulmonary angiogram).

and prevent shivering. Active cooling may be discontinued after 24 hours, and the patient allowed to slowly re-warm over no less than 8 hours.

Care of the family

Once the patient is stable, attention can be turned to the patient's family. Although they should have been updated during the cardiac arrest, they will still require a full explanation of what has happened. If the patient arrested on the ward and is transferred to critical care, then the family must be informed about what this entails. It can be helpful to have a nurse from the ward who knows the patient's family present to provide a known point of contact for them. A senior member of the medical staff and a nurse should explain what has occurred, giving as much information as the family can absorb. Much of it will require repetition as the stress of the situation will reduce the ability to fully understand and retain what is said. Care must be taken to avoid jargon and emotive terms such as 'shocked out of VF'.

Ethics of resuscitation

An important concern for all those involved with resuscitating patients is that inappropriate CPR simply prolongs the act of dying rather than offering a real chance of survival (see British Medical Association

2016). Resuscitation attempts do not allow a peaceful and dignified death. They can remove the family and loved ones from the scene and just create a technical intervention-dominated setting for what may be the patient's final minutes. CPR is appropriate if the patient has a reasonable chance of recovery from cardiac arrest and there is no end-stage disease underlying the event, but if it is carried out in the wrong circumstances it has little benefit for the patient or family.

Clinicians are not obliged to provide treatment that they do not believe will provide clinical benefit. However, there are two situations where assessment is particularly difficult. The first is the resuscitation of 'out-of-hospital' victims whose medical history and circumstances are unknown to the team. In this case, CPR is always attempted. The second scenario is the hospital in-patient who has an end-stage chronic disease or malignancy but who has not been assessed by the medical team for a possible 'do not attempt cardiopulmonary resuscitation' (DNACPR) decision despite clearly being unsuitable for CPR. In these cases, CPR will still be initiated by junior staff who do not have the seniority to make any other decision. Following resuscitation, the patient may be in need of organ support; unless senior medical staff are involved, they may be admitted inappropriately to the critical care unit. There is little that can be done about the first situation, but the frequency of the second situation can be limited by raising awareness and emphasizing the responsibility of senior medical staff. All clinical staff should be familiar with local policies on DNACPR decisions and related issues; ideally, assuming that there is time, the whole team should be asked for their opinion on these critical matters. Discussion of prognosis and what is appropriate/inappropriate treatment in a terminal end-stage illness is crucial, both with the patient and, unless the competent patient requests otherwise, with their next-of-kin/legal guardian. The option of a written advance decision by the patient to refuse or limit CPR may also be brought into the discussion if appropriate (British Medical Association *et al.* 2016). An informed decision communicated to all personnel caring for the patient will prevent inappropriate resuscitation attempts.

- Decisions about CPR must be made on the basis of an *individual* assessment of each patient's case.
- Advance care planning, including making decisions about CPR, is an important part of good clinical care for those at risk of cardiorespiratory arrest.
- Communication and the provision of information are essential parts of good quality care. There should be clear communication with the patient him/herself and, unless the patient requests otherwise, with those close to him/her. Discussions and decisions about resuscitation and DNACPR should also be documented and communicated to all those involved in the patient's care.
- It is not necessary to initiate discussion about CPR with a patient if there is no reason to believe that the patient is likely to suffer a cardiorespiratory arrest.
- Where no explicit decision has been made in advance, there should be an initial presumption in favour of CPR.
- If CPR would not restart the heart and breathing, it should not be attempted.
- Where the expected benefit of attempted CPR may be outweighed by the burdens, the patient's informed views are of paramount importance. If the patient lacks capacity, those close to them should be involved in discussions to explore the their wishes, feelings, beliefs, and values.
- If a patient with capacity refuses CPR, or a patient lacking capacity has a valid and applicable advance decision refusing CPR, this should be respected.
- A DNACPR decision does not override clinical judgement in the unlikely event of a reversible cause of the patient's respiratory or cardiac arrest that does not match the circumstances envisaged.
- DNACPR decisions apply only to CPR and not to any other aspects of treatment.

Resuscitation from cardiac arrest can produce four results:

- complete recovery
- partial recovery
- prolonged survival
- death.

The two extremes of complete recovery or death do not involve the moral problems associated with the grey areas of partial recovery and prolonged survival. The worst scenario is to leave a patient in the so-called 'persistent vegetative state' where all higher neurological function is lost and the patient remains alive but functioning purely on brainstem reflexes (see Chapter 8). These patients may end up in the ICU post-arrest and the problem of how far to continue treatment then ensues. Assessment of neurological function is extremely difficult with no clearly identifiable marker of neurological dysfunction at this level. There is no simple formula that can be applied, and each patient has to be assessed as an individual by the team as a whole. It is also appropriate to discuss the situation with the family. However, they should never be made to feel that withdrawal of treatment is their decision because of the enormous potential for guilt that this could evoke. Ultimately, the decision must be made by the ICU consultant in conjunction with the patient's own consultant and the intensive care team.

References and bibliography

Babbs, C.F. (2005). Chest compression technique. In *Cardiopulmonary Resuscitation* (eds J.P. Ornato, M.A. Peberdy). Totowa, NJ: Humana Press.

British Medical Association, Resuscitation Council (UK), Royal College of Nursing (2016). *Decisions Relating to Cardiopulmonary Resuscitation*. British Medical Association, London / Resuscitation Council (UK), London / Royal College of Nursing, London.

Brooks, S.C., Bigham, B.L., Morrison, L.J. (2011). Mechanical versus manual chest compressions for cardiac arrest. *Cochrane Database of Systematic Reviews*, (1), CD007260.

Carr, B.G., Goyal M, Band, R.A., *et al.* (2009). A national analysis of the relationship between hospital factors and post-cardiac arrest mortality. *Intensive Care Medicine*, **35**, 505–11.

Christenson, J., Andrusiek, D., Everson-Stewart, S., *et al.* (2009). Chest compression fraction determines survival in patients with out-of-hospital ventricular fibrillation. *Circulation*, **120**, 1241–7.

Dorian, P., Cass, D., Schwartz, B., *et al.* (2002). Amiodarone as compared with lidocaine for shock-resistant ventricular fibrillation. *New England Journal of Medicine*, **346**, 884–90.

Dumot, J.A., Burval, D.J., Sprung, J., *et al.* (2001). Outcome of adult cardiopulmonary resuscitations at a tertiary referral center including results of 'limited' resuscitations. *Archives of Internal Medicine*, **161**, 1751–8.

Harrison, G.A., Jacques, T., McLaws, M.L., *et al.* (2006). Combinations of early signs of critical illness predict in-hospital death—the SOCCER study (Signs of Critical Conditions and Emergency Responses). *Resuscitation*, **71**, 327–34.

Herroeder, S., Schönherr, M.E., De Hert, S.G., *et al.* (2011). Magnesium—essentials for anesthesiologists. *Anesthesiology*, **114**, 971–93.

Kause, J., Smith, G., Prytherch, D., *et al.* (2004). A comparison of antecedents to cardiac arrests, deaths and emergency intensive care admissions in Australia and New Zealand, and the United Kingdom—the ACADEMIA study. *Resuscitation*, **62**, 275–82.

Kilgannon, J.H., Jones, A.E., Parrillo, J.E., *et al.* (2011). Relationship between supranormal oxygen tension and outcome after resuscitation from cardiac arrest. *Circulation*, **123**, 2717–22.

Kouwenhoven, W.B., Jude, J.R., Knickerbocker, G.G. (1960). Closed chest cardiac massage. *JAMA*, **173**, 164–7.

Lindner, K.H. (1991). Vasopressor therapy in cardiopulmonary resuscitation. In *Update in Intensive Care and Emergency Medicine* (ed. J.-L. Vincent). Berlin: Springer-Verlag.

Meaney, P.A., Nadkarni, V.M., Kern, K.B., *et al.* (2010). Rhythms and outcomes of adult in-hospital cardiac arrest. *Critical Care Medicine*, **38**, 101–8.

NICE (National Institute for Health and Clinical Excellence) (2011). *Therapeutic Hypothermia Following Cardiac Arrest*. Interventional Procedure Guidance 386, NICE, London.

Nielsen, N., Wetterslev, J., Cronberg, T., *et al.* (2013). Targeted temperature management at 33°C versus 36°C after cardiac arrest. *New England Journal of Medicine*, **369**, 2197–206.

Nolan, J.P., Soar, J., Cariou, A., *et al.* (2015). European Resuscitation Council and European Society of Intensive Care Medicine Guidelines for Post-resuscitation Care 2015: Section 5 of the European Resuscitation Council Guidelines for Resuscitation 2015. *Resuscitation*, **95**, 202–22.

Nolan, J.P., Soar, J., Smith, G.B., *et al.* (2014). Incidence and outcome of in-hospital cardiac arrest in the United Kingdom National Cardiac Arrest Audit. *Resuscitation* **85**, 987–92.

Perkins, G.D., Handley, A.J., Koster, R.W., *et al.* (2015). European Resuscitation Council Guidelines for Resuscitation 2015: Section 2. Adult Basic Life Support and Automated External Defibrillation. *Resuscitation*, **95**, 81–99.

Peters, J., Ihle, P. (1990). Mechanics of the circulation during cardiopulmonary resuscitation. Pathophysiology and techniques (Part I). *Intensive Care Medicine*, **16**, 11–27.

Resuscitation Council UK (2011). *Advanced Life Support* (6th edn). London: Resuscitation Council UK.

Royal College of Anaesthetists, Royal College of Physicians of London, Intensive Care Society, Resuscitation Council UK (2008). *Cardiopulmonary Resuscitation Standards for Clinical Practice and Training*. http://www.rcoa.ac.uk/system/files/PUB-CardioResus_2.pdf (accessed 5 September 2016).

Soar, J., Nolan, J.P., Böttiger, B.W., *et al.* (2015). European Resuscitation Council Guidelines for Resuscitation 2015: Section 3. Adult Advanced Life Support. *Resuscitation*, **95**, 100–47.

Truhlář, A., Deakin, C.D., Soar, J., *et al.* (2015). European Resuscitation Council Guidelines for Resuscitation 2015: Section 4. Cardiac arrest in special circumstances. *Resuscitation*, **95**, 148–201.

Tunstall-Pedoe, H., Bailey, L., Chamberlain, D.A., *et al.* (1992). Survey of 3765 cardiopulmonary resuscitations in British hospitals (the BRESUS Study): methods and overall results. *BMJ*, **304**, 1347–51.

von Planta M (2005). Buffer therapy. In *Cardiopulmonary Resuscitation* (eds J.P. Ornato, M.A. Peberdy). Totowa, NJ: Humana Press.

Walters, J.H., Morley, P.T., Nolan, J.P. (2011). The role of hypothermia in post-cardiac arrest patients with return of spontaneous circulation: a systematic review. *Resuscitation*, **82**, 508–16.

Wang, H.C., Chiang, W.C., Chen, S.Y., *et al.* (2007). Video-recording and time-motion analyses of manual versus mechanical cardiopulmonary resuscitation during ambulance transport. *Resuscitation*, **74**, 453–60.

Weil, M.H., Rackow, E.C., Trevino, R., *et al.* (1986). Difference in acid–base state between venous and arterial blood during cardiopulmonary resuscitation. *New England Journal of Medicine*, **315**, 153–6.

Yang, C.W., Yen, Z.S., McGowan, J.E., *et al.* (2012). A systematic review of retention of adult advanced life support knowledge and skills in healthcare providers. *Resuscitation*, **83**, 1055–60.

Further reading

The *European Resuscitation Council Guidelines for Resuscitation 2015* and the *Consensus on CPR and ECC Science with Treatment Recommendations (CoSTR)* (summary of the scientific evidence supporting the guidelines) can both be downloaded from www.cprguidelines.eu/ (accessed 1 January 2016).

CHAPTER 7
Renal problems

Introduction

The kidneys perform several essential functions, including crucial roles in maintaining fluid, electrolyte, and acid–base balance, as well as the excretion of waste substances such as the products of nitrogen metabolism (urea and creatinine). This means that the consequences of kidney dysfunction can be widespread and devastating.

A small but significant group of patients come to the critical care unit with severe kidney problems—6% of critical care admissions in the UK (Kolhe *et al.* 2008)—and many more are at risk of developing kidney injury at some later time, most often due to circulatory failure. There are numerous precipitating factors, including:

- poor perfusion (e.g. haemorrhage, heart failure or sepsis causing reduced cardiac output, and/or hypotension)
- direct renal damage/trauma (e.g. from nephrotoxic drugs or urological surgery)
- multisystem diseases such as systemic lupus erythematosus.

Preservation of kidney function and early detection of any deterioration are key aspects of the care of the critically ill.

Functional anatomy and physiology

The main functions of the kidneys are listed in Box 7.1. These functions utilize processes of filtration, reabsorption, and secretion. Two other homeostatic mechanisms are integral to kidney function: the renin–angiotensin–aldosterone (RAA) and antidiuretic hormone (ADH) pathways.

The nephron

The functional unit of the kidney is the nephron. There are about one million nephrons in each kidney. The nephron consists of a glomerulus, a glomerular capsule (Bowman's capsule), a proximal convoluted tubule, a loop of Henle (descending and ascending limbs), a distal convoluted tubule, a collecting duct, and the connected blood supply (Figure 7.1). Cortical nephrons have glomeruli located in the cortex and short loops of Henle, while juxtamedullary nephrons have glomeruli in the juxtamedullary region and long loops of Henle extending into the medulla.

Blood supply

Blood enters the kidney via renal arteries that branch off the aorta. Each kidney receives approximately 625 ml blood per minute, which is about 25% of total cardiac output. The renal arteries divide into interlobar arteries that further divide into arcuate arteries, then into interlobular arteries, and finally into afferent arterioles. Blood flow in the renal cortex is greater than in the renal medulla.

Box 7.1 Functions of the kidney

- Production of urine
- Excretion of waste products
- Control and maintenance of fluid balance
- Maintenance of acid–base balance
- Control and maintenance of electrolyte balance
- Renin production
- Erythropoietin production
- Control of calcium reabsorption and vitamin D hydroxylation

The glomerulus

Afferent arterioles feed the glomerulus which is enclosed within the glomerular capsule. Glomeruli can be described as 'tufts' of capillaries. This arrangement allows a large surface area to be available for filtration. The capsule is double-walled, with the outer wall known as the parietal layer and the inner as the visceral layer. The two are separated by the capsular space. The visceral layer of the capsule and the endothelial layer of the glomerulus constitute the endothelial–capsular membrane, which rests on a layer of contractile mesangial cells. Modified cells, called juxtaglomerular cells, are situated around afferent and efferent arterioles. Parts of the distal tubules lie in close proximity to their originating arterioles. These tubule cells are collectively known as the macula densa. The juxtaglomerular cells and macula densa together form the juxtaglomerular apparatus which secretes renin.

Blood entering the glomerulus from the afferent arteriole is filtered by the endothelial–capsular membrane. This membrane is impermeable to molecules greater than 4 nm in size/70,000 daltons (Da) molecular weight.

Filtration depends on the size and shape of individual molecules, their electrostatic charge, and the opposing pressures within the glomerulus and capsule. Blood in the glomerulus creates a hydrostatic pressure (usually ~60 mmHg) that tends to force fluid out of the afferent vessels. This hydrostatic pressure is opposed by the pressure within the capsular space (~20 mmHg) and the osmotic pressure exerted by blood in the glomerulus (~30 mmHg). The filtration pressure is therefore (see Figure 7.2).

$$60\ \text{mmHg} - 20\ \text{mmHg} - 30\ \text{mmHg} = 10\ \text{mmHg}.$$

If the hydrostatic pressure of blood in the glomerulus falls until it is equal to or less than the sum of the capsular and osmotic pressures, filtration cannot occur. This may happen, for example, because of some haemodynamic compromise such as hypovolaemia. To help compensate for any reduction in the glomerular filtration rate (GFR), chloride reabsorption by the macula densa cells of the distal tubules is increased. This results in dilation of afferent arterioles so as to increase blood flow and thus GFR. The chloride also promotes renin secretion which causes constriction of efferent arterioles, increasing glomerular pressure, and, again, GFR.

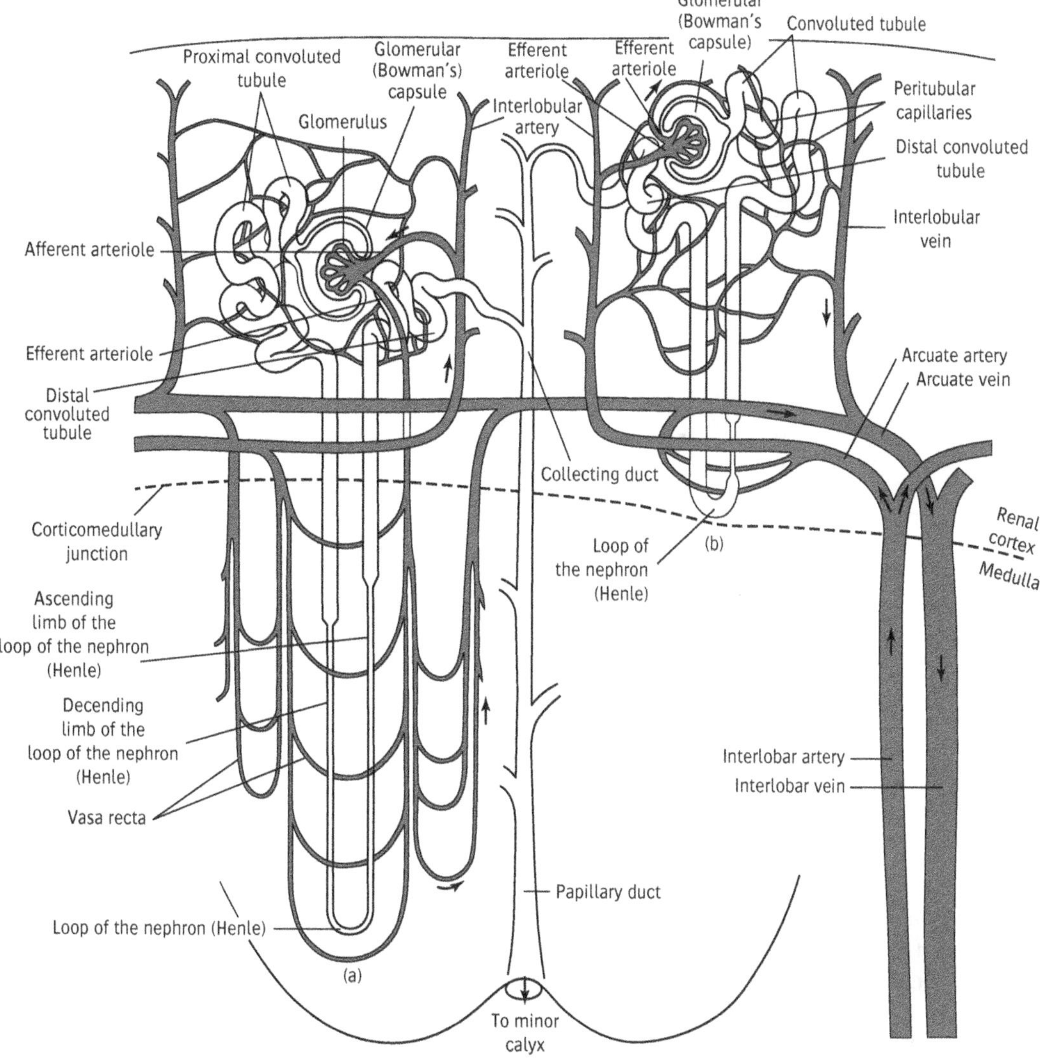

Figure 7.1 The nephron, showing glomerulus, proximal and distal tubules, and collecting duct, with blood supply.

Blood that is not filtered through the membrane leaves the glomerulus via the efferent arterioles. The efferent arterioles in the cortical region of the kidney divide to form peritubular capillaries around the convoluted tubules. The juxtaglomerular efferent arterioles also form peritubular capillaries, and, in addition, form a network of thin-walled vessels known as the vasa recta which reach down into the renal medulla. The peritubular capillaries and the vasa recta eventually join to form the interlobar veins and, finally, the renal veins.

The fluid that is filtered across the endothelial–capsular membrane is known as filtrate. It enters the next part of the nephron, the proximal convoluted tubule. At this stage the filtrate has an osmolality (see Box 7.2) of 300 mOsmol/L.

In the proximal tubule, various solutes are both actively and passively reabsorbed into the surrounding peritubular capillaries, reducing the filtrate by some 75–80%. When sodium (a positively charged ion) is reabsorbed from tubules and moved into the peritubular capillaries, blood within those capillaries becomes positively charged. Chloride (a negatively charged ion) follows, moving from the filtrate and into the capillaries to achieve electrostatic balance. The presence of sodium and chloride in peritubular capillary blood increases its osmolality; so water then moves from the filtrate in

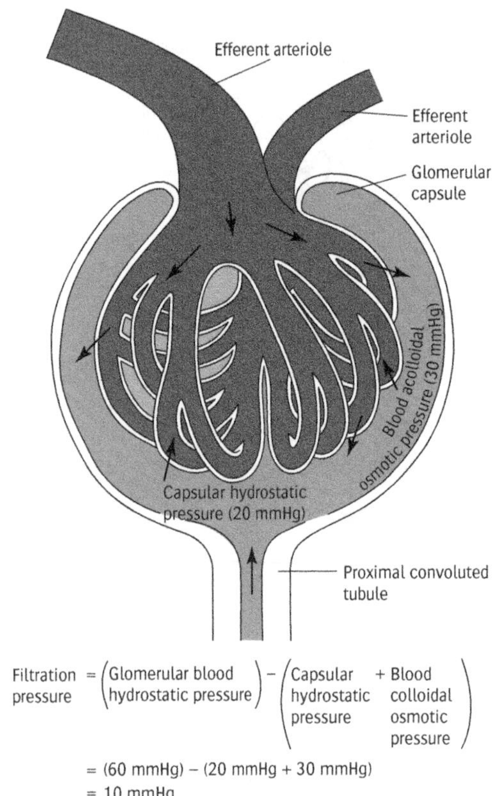

Filtration pressure = (Glomerular blood hydrostatic pressure) − (Capsular hydrostatic pressure + Blood colloidal osmotic pressure)

= (60 mmHg) − (20 mmHg + 30 mmHg)

= 10 mmHg

Figure 7.2 Glomerular capsule, showing fluid dynamics producing filtration pressure.

the proximal tubule and into the blood by osmosis (See Boxes 7.3 and 7.4)

Most water reabsorption occurs in the proximal tubule, which is always permeable to water. Therefore there is no control over water moving out of the tubule as such; it is governed by movement of sodium. After leaving the proximal tubule, filtrate enters the loop of Henle where more sodium, chloride, bicarbonate, and glucose are reabsorbed into the peritubular blood. The ascending limb of the loop is impermeable to water, but chloride ions are actively reabsorbed, moving from the filtrate, into the interstitial fluid, and into the peritubular capillaries. Blood in the capillaries then becomes negatively charged, and in order to equalize this sodium passively follows the chloride. This results in the filtrate becoming less concentrated, with osmolality reduced to approximately 100 mOsmol/L. Conversely, the interstitium surrounding the loop becomes hyperosmolar, to about 1200 mOsmol/L. The filtrate then enters the distal convoluted tubule where further solute reabsorption occurs, making the filtrate even more dilute. Various substances, including creatinine and some drugs, are secreted by the distal tubules into the filtrate for excretion at this point. The final part of the nephron is the collecting duct, running through the renal medulla, which takes the filtrate, now called urine, to the ureters.

The distal tubules and the collecting ducts are sites of action for RAA and ADH mechanisms (Figure 7.3 and Figure7.4). The RAA pathway regulates sodium reabsorption from the distal tubules and collecting ducts, with sodium reabsorption dependent on its concentration in the extracellular fluid. Because water accompanies sodium, extracellular volume is also affected. Therefore the RAA mechanism can alter sodium levels and blood volume. ADH also has a role in that it can modify water reabsorption from the distal tubules and collecting ducts.

Box 7.2 **Osmolality**

Osmolality is the osmotic pressure of a solution expressed in osmoles or milliosmoles per kilogram of water

Box 7.3 **Substances reabsorbed in the proximal tubule**

- Sodium (80%)
- Water (80%)
- Phosphate
- Chloride
- Glucose
- Bicarbonate
- Potassium
- Sulphate (100%)
- Amino acids
- Low molecular weight proteins

Box 7.4 **Osmosis**

Osmosis is the movement of a pure solvent (e.g. water) through a semi-permeable membrane, from a solution that has a lower solute concentration to one that has a higher solute concentration.

Decreased renal arterial pressure

Stimulates

Juxtaglomerular apparatus to secrete renin

Stimulates conversion of

Angiotensinogen to angiotensin I

Conveted to

Angiotensin II (causes arterial vasoconstriction and increases filtration pressure)

Stimulates

Adrenal cortex to increase aldosterone secretion

Stimulates

Increased sodium reabsorption from distal tubules and collecting ducts

Results in

Increased blood volume and restoration renal arterial pressure

Figure 7.3 Renin–angiotensin–aldosterone pathway.

Increased osmolality of the blood

Stimulates

ADH release from posterior pituitary gland

Increases

Permeability of distal and collecting tubules

Causes

Reabsorption of water

Increases

Concentration of water in the blood

Inhibits

Secretion of ADH

Figure 7.4 Antidiuretic hormone pathway.

Concentrating abilities of the kidney

As solutes are reabsorbed, filtrate becomes progressively more dilute during its passage through the nephron. The impermeability of the ascending limb of the loop of Henle to water and the control of water reabsorption exercised by ADH in the distal tubules and collecting ducts further ensures a dilute filtrate by the end of the nephron. At the same time, reabsorption of solutes results in fluid in the interstitium becoming more concentrated, particularly in the medulla of the kidney. However, there are situations, such as dehydration, where dilute urine is undesirable. The ability to vary the concentration of urine according to different circumstances depends on the maintenance of a hyperosmolar medullary interstitium. As described in the previous section, chloride and sodium reabsorption in the ascending limb of the loop of Henle increases the concentration of solutes in the interstitium and this is then carried down into the medulla by blood flow in the vasa recta. Osmolality in the medulla is further increased by the movement of sodium and chloride out of the collecting ducts. Separately, ADH can promote movement of water out of the collecting ducts, resulting in a high urea concentration within the ducts, so urea then moves by diffusion (see Box 7.5) out of the ducts and into the surrounding interstitium. Therefore the

Box 7.5 Diffusion

Diffusion is the process by which particulate matter in a fluid moves from an area of higher concentration to one of lower concentration, resulting in an even distribution of particles.

concentration of urea in the interstitium is greater than that in the loop of the nephron, so urea moves into the loop, again by diffusion. When filtrate (containing the diffused urea) reaches the ascending limb of the loop and the distal tubule, water—but not urea—is removed under the control of ADH, resulting in additional concentration of urea in the collecting ducts. The counter-current mechanism here further assists in maintaining medullary osmolality.

The loop of Henle essentially consists of two parallel tubes with fluid flowing in opposite directions (counter-current flow). The descending limb of the loop is impermeable to solutes but permeable to water. This allows water to move by osmosis into the relatively more concentrated interstitium, thus increasing the concentration of the filtrate. This process continues in a cumulative fashion through the descending limb, with the filtrate eventually reaching an osmolality of 1200 mOsmol/L. Further on, sodium and chloride move from the ascending limb into the interstitium of the medulla. As this part of the loop of Henle is impermeable to water, the filtrate then becomes progressively less concentrated, falling to about 200 mOsmol/L at the cortex. The accompanying vasa recta are similar to the loop in that there are ascending and descending limbs. This arrangement also plays a part in keeping medullary fluid concentrated. As blood moves (within the vasa recta) towards the medulla, solutes enter the blood from the interstitium.

When the now concentrated blood moves into the ascending vasa recta and then towards the cortex, solutes diffuse back into the interstitium. This counter-current mechanism works partly because of sluggish blood flow within the vasa recta; but if that flow increases (e.g. due to expansion of blood volume), medullary osmolality can be disrupted, decreasing water absorption and resulting in a dilute urine.

Acid–base balance

Acid–base balance is also discussed in Chapter 4.

An acid is a substance that can provide hydrogen ions (H^+), while a base (an alkali) is a substance that can accept hydrogen ions. Even in extremely acid solutions, the concentration of H^+ ions is so small that absolute values are inconvenient to use as a measure. Because of this, the pH scale is employed to indicate H^+ ion concentration. The pH value is the negative logarithm of the H^+ concentration, meaning that a change of one pH unit represents a 10-fold change in the H^+ concentration in the opposite direction. That is, if the H^+ concentration rises (creating stronger acid) the pH value falls, and if the H^+ concentration falls, the pH value rises.

The pH of blood is normally maintained in the range 7.35–7.45 by buffers in the blood (e.g. bicarbonate), and also by lung and kidney functions. An increase in arterial blood pH above 7.45 constitutes an alkalaemia, while a pH below 7.35 is termed acidaemia. Alkalosis or acidosis can be respiratory, metabolic, or mixed in origin (see Table 7.1 and also Chapter 4 for descriptions of respiratory acidosis and alkalosis). In addition to an altered pH, metabolic acidosis is characterized by a fall in bicarbonate (<22 mmol/L) and metabolic alkalosis by raised bicarbonate (>26 mmol/L).

Table 7.1 Causes of metabolic acidosis and alkalosis

Metabolic acidosis	Acute and chronic kidney failure
	Ingestion of acids (e.g. salicylates)
	Loss of small bowel or biliary fluid
	Tissue ischaemia/necrosis
	Diabetic ketoacidosis
	Drugs, poisons (e.g. excessive normal saline administration (causing hyperchloraemic acidosis), methyl alcohol)
Metabolic alkalosis	Excessive sodium bicarbonate
	Ingestion of alkali
	Loss of gastric acid (e.g. copious vomiting/ nasogastric drainage)
	Excessive citrate infusion
	Liver failure

Blood buffers

Blood buffers provide a rapid response to changes in pH but the effects only last for a relatively short time. The most important buffer in extracellular fluid is bicarbonate (HCO_3^-), which buffers hydrogen ions to form carbonic acid (H_2CO_3). Carbonic acid easily dissociates into water (H_2O) and carbon dioxide (CO_2), allowing the carbon dioxide to be eliminated by the lungs:

$$HCO_3^- + H^+ \leftrightarrow H_2CO_3 \leftrightarrow H_2O + CO_2.$$

Plasma proteins can also act as buffers, although their effect is small compared with that of the bicarbonate system. Haemoglobin is important as it is present in erythrocytes which are prime sites for carbonic acid formation; thus the haemoglobin is immediately available to buffer hydrogen ions in that situation.

The strong ion theory of acid–base balance (physiochemical approach to acid–base balance)

The conventional Henderson–Hasselbalch model of acid–base balance assumes that pH is a function of the relative levels of bicarbonate and PCO_2. This is challenged by the more recent, physiochemical, Stewart's strong ion theory. Stewart's theory suggests that three independent variables determine plasma pH by altering the degree of water dissociation into hydrogen ions. These three variables are the strong ion difference (SID), PCO_2, and the combined total charge from weak acids, inorganic phosphate, and serum proteins (known as ATOT). Strong ions are those that fully dissociate in biological solutions; in humans, these are principally sodium (Na^+) and chloride (Cl^-). Other, less important, strong ions are potassium (K^+), magnesium (Mg^{2+}), calcium (Ca^{2+}) and sulphate (SO_4^{2-}). A decrease in SID, an increase in PCO_2, and an increase in ATOT all have acidifying effects (Adrogué *et al.* 2009).

Renal component in acid–base balance

A low blood pH stimulates tubular cells to secrete hydrogen ions into the filtrate. To maintain electrostatic balance, sodium (Na^+) diffuses from the filtrate and into the tubular cells where it combines with bicarbonate to produce sodium bicarbonate ($NaHCO_3$). The bicarbonate is absorbed into the blood and is then available to act as a systemic buffer. This mechanism, in conjunction with the excretion of excess hydrogen ions, gives the kidney an important role in counteracting acidosis. Similar processes occur with ammonia and phosphate (see Figure 7.5).

Acute kidney injury

'Acute kidney injury' (AKI) has supplanted the term 'acute renal failure' (Schrier 2010), and is now the standard label for an abrupt deterioration in kidney function that leads to inadequate clearance of metabolic waste as well as other features, usually,but not always, including oliguria. AKI actually encompasses a continuum of kidney dysfunction, most simply identified by a rapid increase in serum creatinine and/or oliguria (urine volume <0.5 ml/kg/hour); and also by a variety of fluid balance, electrolyte, and acid–base disturbances. As glomerular filtration falls, metabolic waste products such as urea and creatinine accumulate in the blood, resulting in increased plasma concentrations of these substances. AKI can develop and progress in a few hours, but prompt attention to risk factors for AKI and careful monitoring of urine output and blood results can enable early interventions that prevent progression to severe or life-threatening disease. Nonetheless, up to two-thirds of critical care patients suffer these types of problem, and 5% end up having renal replacement therapy, up to 60% of whom do not survive (Hoste and Schurgers 2008).

Definitions

Acute kidney injury is defined by[1]

- serum creatinine increased by ≥26 μmol/L in 48 hours, or
- serum creatinine increased to ≥1.5 times the patient's baseline value in a week (i.e. a 50% increase), or
- urine output <0.5ml/kg/h for over 6 hours (Mehta *et al.* 2007).

This profile equates to Stage 1 of the AKI continuum.

Stage 2 (more severe) AKI is signified by serum creatinine increased by 2–2.9 times the baseline, or urine output <0.5ml/kg/h for >12 hours.

Stage 3 (most severe) AKI is signified by serum creatinine increased to >354 μmol/L or ≥3 times the baseline

[1] Data from the Kidney Disease Improving Global Outcomes, KDIGO Clinical Practice Guideline for Acute Kidney Injury, *Kidney International Supplements*, Volume 2, Issue 1. 2002, KDIGO, http://www.kdigo.org/).

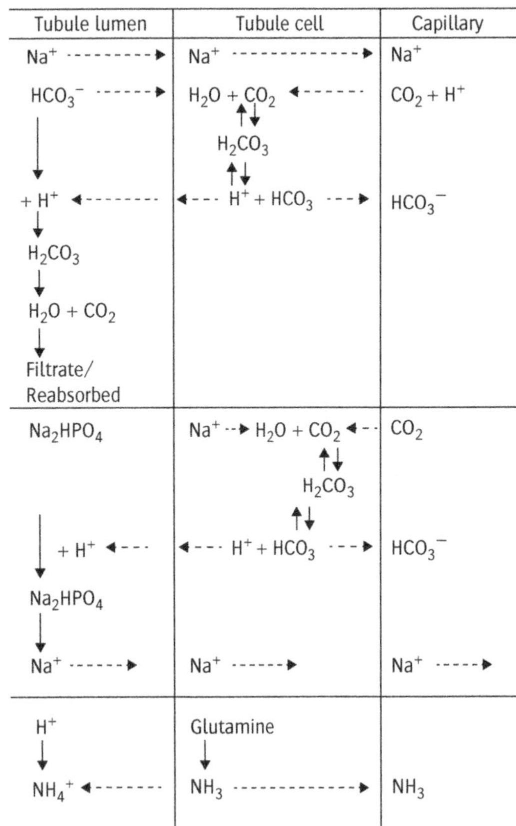

Figure 7.5 Diagrammatic representation of renal control of acid–base balance with bicarbonate, phosphate, and ammonia.

value or by urine output <0.3ml/kg/h for more than 24 hours, or, more subjectively, by the commencement of renal replacement therapy (Lewington and Kanagasundaram 2011).

Critically ill patients with AKI may be seen either

- in single organ failure—that is, only the kidneys are dysfunctional, while other body systems are operating normally, or
- in multi-organ failure that includes the kidneys.

Most AKI in critically ill patients is associated with multi-organ failure. There may well be a background of chronic kidney disease as well.

Causes of acute kidney injury

There are many potential causes of acute kidney injury. It is useful to classify these in three main categories.:

1. Pre-renal factors, i.e. renal hypoperfusion due to hypovolaemia and/or reduced blood flow and/or systemic hypotension.

Table 7.2 Pre-renal causes of acute kidney injury

Cause	Examples
Hypovolaemia	Hypovolaemia, burns, gastrointestinal losses, renal losses, third-space losses (e.g. SIRS/sepsis, pancreatitis)
Cardiogenic factors	Arrhythmias, heart failure, valvular dysfunction
Obstructive shock	Pericardial tamponade, pulmonary embolism

2. Intrinsic renal factors—essentially to do with the kidney itself (e.g. due to nephrotoxic medications).
3. Post-renal factors related to problems with the outflow of urine from the kidney, e.g. obstruction by kidney stones or an enlarged prostate gland.

More details are given in Tables 7.2, 7.3, and 7.4 for more detail.)

A good blood supply is crucial for the kidneys. Critically ill patients very often have some type of circulatory failure, so pre-renal factors are the most common cause of AKI in this group. It follows that optimization of cardiac output is the key treatment in these cases, usually with fluid loading in the first instance. Intrinsic causes result in damage to the kidney itself and are less likely to be improved by fluid therapy.

Mechanisms of acute kidney injury

A sustained fall in renal blood flow leads to reduced glomerular filtration, smaller urine volumes, and less urea and creatinine clearance. However, tubular function and concentrating ability are still maintained at this stage, so urine osmolality, urea, and creatinine concentrations can be increased (and urine sodium decreased). If renal perfusion is restored at this point, progression to more severe AKI can be avoided. If renal perfusion is not restored, GFR and urine output reduces further, and significant tubular damage occurs. Concentrating ability is lost with a resulting loss of sodium reabsorption.

However, it should be noted that a few patients maintain normal or near normal urine output despite significantly decreased renal perfusion and GFR. This presentation probably reflects less severe pathology, and is associated with lower mortality than oliguric cases (Avila *et al.* 2009).

There are several theories about what happens to the nephron following an ischaemic insult to the kidney. Some or all of the following may coexist in AKI.

Table 7.3 Intrinsic causes of acute kidney injury

Acute tubular necrosis	Unrelieved pre-renal causes Acute haemorrhage Haemoglobin/myoglobin Pancreatitis Septic abortion Eclampsia Post-operative Cardiogenic shock Burns Nephrotoxins (e.g. radiographic contrast, heavy metals, organic solvents, aminoglycosides, amphotericin) Systemic lupus erythematosus
Cortical necrosis	Nephrotic syndrome Renal artery occlusion/emboli Renal vein thrombosis Disseminated intravascular coagulation Acute pyelonephritis Hepatorenal syndrome Glomerulonephritis Polyarteritis nodosa Post-streptococcal infection Goodpasture's syndrome Granulomatosis with polyangiitis (Wegener's granulomatosis) Infective endocarditis Henoch–Schönlein purpura Snake venom
Acute interstitial nephritis	Penicillins (e.g. ampicillin, benzylpenicillin, methicillin) Cephalosporins (e.g. cefuroxime, ceftazidime) Sulphonamides Rifampicin Diuretics (thiazides, furosemide) Non-steroidal anti-inflammatory drugs (e.g. indomethacin, diclofenac)

Tubuloglomerular feedback

During periods of renal hypoperfusion, cortical blood flow tends to be reduced relative to medullary blood flow; probably as a protective mechanism for the medulla which normally operates on the verge of hypoxia anyway. This action also decreases the oxygen demand necessary for solute reabsorption as GFR falls.

Table 7.4 Post-renal causes of acute kidney injury

Intra-ureteral	Calculi Papillary necrosis Crystals (e.g. uric acid) Tumour Blood clot
Extra-ureteral	Retroperitoneal fibrosis Tumour Aneurysm
Bladder obstruction	Prostatic hypertrophy Bladder tumour Blood clot Calculi Functional neuropathy
Urethral obstruction	Stricture Meatal stenosis Phimosis

Note: intra-abdominal hypertension (increased abdominal pressure) caused by ascites or other pathology may result in abdominal pressures exceeding renal perfusion pressure and thus reducing renal function

However, if the mechanism fails, medullary ischaemia occurs and solute, particularly chloride, reaching the macula densa activates the tubuloglomerular feedback mechanism. A consequence of this is vasoconstriction which, in turn, further reduces GFR.

Reduced glomerular permeability

Local stimuli (including angiotensin II, thromboxane, and histamine) cause glomerular mesangial cell contraction which serves to reduce permeability and the area available for filtration.

'No reflow' phenomenon

Endothelial cell swelling resulting from ischaemic injury prevents reperfusion of the microcirculation even when renal blood flow is restored. (The efferent arterioles of the cortical glomeruli supply blood to the medulla. These arterioles divide and form the vasa recta, which are resistance vessels with the ability to control medullary blood flow. The ascending vessels have very thin walls and are susceptible to compression by swollen tubules in the vicinity.)

Tubular obstruction

Obstruction of the tubules by debris causes a rise in intratubular pressure until glomerular filtration stops.

Filtrate 'back-leak'

Damaged tubular basement membrane allows filtrate to escape so the GFR is further reduced. Various mediators produced in the kidney have additional effects, e.g. prostaglandins (PGI_2 and PGE_2). These cause vasodilatation, promote mesangial cell relaxation, and inhibit platelet aggregation, all of which may have some benefit. Conversely, thromboxane (TxA_2) causes vasoconstriction and glomerular cell contraction (reducing filtration surface area), as well as promoting platelet aggregation.

Nitric oxide (NO)

NO helps regulate blood flow in resistance vessels (including the vasa recta) by vasodilatation. Physiological antagonists to NO are the endothelins that promote vasoconstriction, and, in response to ischaemia, mesangial cell contraction.

Reperfusion of previously ischaemic tissue (reperfusion injury)

The restoration of oxygen delivery, the accumulation of calcium, and the correction of acidosis promotes phospholipid activity and oxygen radical formation. This can damage cell membranes, increase intracellular calcium, and reduce ATP synthesis and mitochondrial respiration, all of which contribute to cell death. These processes may be part of the reason why there is often continuing deterioration in kidney function despite restoration of renal blood flow.

Table 7.5 Investigation of acute kidney injury

Urine	Urinalysis
	Urine microscopy, culture, and sensitivity
	Electrolytes, osmolality, urea, and creatinine
	Creatinine clearance
	Urine/plasma ratios of urea, sodium, and osmolality
	Myoglobinuria
Blood	Full blood count
	Coagulation screen
	Electrolytes, urea, creatinine, calcium, phosphate, magnesium, glucose
	Arterial blood gases
	Liver function tests
	Creatine kinase
	Autoantibodies (e.g. ANCA for granulomatosis with polyangiitis, polyarteritis nodosa or anti-glomerular basement membrane antibody for Goodpasture's syndrome)
Imaging	Plain abdominal and chest X-ray
	Renal ultrasound
	Urography
	Isotope renography
	Computed tomography (CT) scan
Other	12-lead ECG
	Renal biopsy

Investigation and diagnosis of acute kidney injury

Clinical assessment and any investigations should, in the first instance, be used to identify the cause of AKI (pre-renal, intrinsic, or post-renal) so as to enable prompt and suitable treatment (see Table 7.5).

A history should be taken and physical examination performed if not already done (see Table 7.6). Coexisting diseases which affect the kidneys may be identified. Cardiovascular disease, liver disease, diabetes mellitus, and, obviously, chronic kidney disease are particular risk factors. It is important that a chronological sequence of events is established and a drug history obtained; a range of medications can affect the kidney or its blood supply (e.g. angiotensin-converting enzyme inhibitors such as enalapril or captopril). Physical examination can reveal signs and symptoms of established kidney dysfunction, including uraemia, anaemia, coagulopathy, and fluid overload.

Urinary investigations

The simple urine dipstick can give urinary pH, glucose, ketones, bilirubin, urobilinogen, protein, and blood. The presence of protein may indicate an underlying glomerulonephritis or interstitial nephritis. Blood may indicate haemoglobin or myoglobin in the urine (i.e. intravascular haemolysis or rhabdomyolysis, respectively).

Urine can also be examined directly for red and white blood cells or, after centrifugation, for casts and crystals (see Box 7.6).

The creatinine clearance test uses a 24-hour collection of urine and a plasma sample collected in the same period to measure the quantity of blood plasma cleared of creatinine per minute. This is an indicator of glomerular filtration. It is calculated as follows:

Table 7.6 History and physical examination

History	Taken from patient, family members, case notes, and the referring team, including: (1) coexisting diseases (e.g. heart failure, hypertension, vascular disease, diabetes) (2) potentially nephrotoxic medications (e.g. non-steroidal anti-inflammatory drugs, aminoglycosides) (3) history of trauma
Physical examination	(1) Signs and symptoms of uraemia (e.g. drowsiness, coma, nausea, vomiting, pruritis) (2) Bruising, possibly indicating platelet dysfunction (3) Signs of metabolic acidosis hyperventilation or 'air hunger' (4) Pericarditis (5) Joint pain (6) Signs of fluid overload (e.g. raised jugular venous pressure, peripheral and/or pulmonary oedema)

$$\text{Creatinine clearance} = \frac{\text{urinary creatinine concentration (mmol/l)} \times \text{urine volume (ml/min)}}{\text{Plasma creatinine concentration } (\mu\text{mol/l})}$$

Normal creatinine clearance is generally in the range 70–130 ml/Smin, with lower values indicating less effective kidney function. Muscle mass (usually calculated in terms of body surface area), age, gender, and ethnicity all influence creatinine production and creatinine clearance, and these can also be factored in. For example, African Caribbean people tend to have proportionally greater muscle mass than other ethnic groups and therefore produce more creatinine. This needs to be considered when analysing creatinine levels, and this is routinely done.

Box 7.6 Microscopic examination of urine

- Acute nephritis: white blood cells and white blood cell casts
- Acute tubular necrosis: tubular epithelial cells and casts
- Glomerulonephritis: granular and red cell casts

Table 7.7 Diagnostic urinary indices for oliguria

Test	Pre-renal	Renal
Specific gravity	>1020	1010
Osmolality (mOsmol/kg)	>500	250–300
Sodium (mmol/L)	<15	>40
Urea (mmol/L)	>250	<160
Urine:plasma osmolality ratio	>1.3:1	<1.1:1
Urine:plasma urea ratio	>10:1	<4:1
Urine:plasma creatinine ratio	>40:1	<20:1

Table 7.7 gives urinary values for oliguria secondary to either pre-renal or renal factors. This differentiation is not always clear; many patients fall between the two categories, especially in cases of AKI where there is no oliguria. Interpretation of these values is also more difficult if the patient has pre-existing kidney disease and/or has received diuretics, as these can affect tubular concentrating function and urinary electrolyte excretion.

Serum creatinine and urea and electrolytes should be measured. Even if the GFR is normal, serum urea can be raised due to:

- increased protein catabolism, as seen in burns, fever, and after surgery or trauma
- increased protein intake, e.g. in gastrointestinal bleeding when there is increased reabsorption of amino acids
- dehydration.

Therefore uraemia is a less reliable indicator of kidney function than creatinine concentration, although it is also the case that both plasma urea and creatinine concentrations may remain within the normal range of values until GFR falls by 50% or more. Creatinine production is related to lean body mass (except in rhabdomyolysis), so plasma creatinine is reduced in the very young, the elderly, and those with alcoholism and chronic wasting diseases. These patients may have significant kidney disease without a marked rise in serum creatinine and, although kidney function declines with age, serum creatinine may not change much in old age either because there is often a reduction in muscle mass as well.

Blood gas analysis in AKI will often reveal a metabolic acidosis with reduced bicarbonate and a base deficit—and low pH. Acidosis can lead to further complications, such as hyperkalaemia. This is because about 95% of total body potassium is usually located in the intracellular compartment, but if there are more than the usual quantities of hydrogen ions in the cells because of developing acidosis, intracellular potassium will be forced out into the extracellular fluid compartment to maintain ionic balance. (Normally, together with other cations such as calcium and magnesium, potassium maintains osmotic pressure in the intracellular fluid compartment.) The relatively small amounts of potassium usually found in the extracellular compartment are important in neuromuscular and cardiac function; but excessive extracellular potassium is dangerous because, for example, it causes life-threatening dysrhythmias.

Calcium levels tend to fall as phosphate levels rise in AKI. (In health, the kidneys produce 1a-hydroxylase which converts 25-hydroxycholecalciferol into 1,25-dihydroxycholecalciferol. This in turn promotes reabsorption of calcium from bone and decreases urinary calcium excretion.)

A summary of relevant blood investigations is given in Table 7.8.

Radiological investigations

These include the following.

- Renal ultrasound—useful for detecting obstruction or estimating kidney size. Chronic kidney disease reduces kidney size.
- Urography—also used to check kidney size and to detect obstruction or suspected trauma.
- Isotope renography—investigating kidney function, size, vasculature, and outflow.
- Computed tomography (CT) scanning—often used as an alternative to arteriography or venography, and if retroperitoneal disease is suspected.
- Plain abdominal X-ray—to detect renal calculi.
- Renal biopsy is performed if an episode of AKI is unexplained and a histological diagnosis is required; but is not advisable if the patient only has one kidney. Any clotting disorders should be corrected prior to biopsy and the patient closely monitored afterwards for signs of bleeding.

Table 7.8 Blood tests in acute kidney injury

Test	Normal value	Values in acute kidney injury
Full blood count	Haemoglobin (Hb): 120–180 g/L	Hb normal or low with anaemia or dilutional effect
	White blood cells (WBC): (4–11) × 10^9/L	WBC normal or raised if accompanying inflammatory or septic processes
Platelet count	150–400 × 10^9/L	Usually normal (but may be decreased, e.g. in systemic lupus erythematosus)
Sodium	132–144 mmol/L	Normal, high, or low
Potassium	3.3–4.7 mmol/L	Normal, high, or low
Urea	2.5–6.6 mmol/L	Raised
Creatinine	55–120 µmol/L	Raised
Phosphate	0.8–1.4 mmol/L	Usually raised
Glucose	Fasting <5.5 mmol/L	Normal
Osmolality	285–295 mOsm/L	Usually raised
Magnesium	0.75–1.0 mmol/L	Variable
Calcium	2.12–2.62 mmol/L	Normal or low

Priorities of care

As with all cases, the first priorities are management of airway, breathing, and circulation.

Airway

Uraemia can depress consciousness, so the ability to maintain a patent airway may be lost. Simple airway adjuncts have their place in these cases, but endotracheal intubation is frequently required. A neurological assessment should be performed when any patient is admitted to the critical care unit, and neurological observations recorded regularly thereafter.

Breathing

Respiratory function may be affected by pulmonary oedema due to fluid overload, coexisting pulmonary insufficiency (e.g. with the development of acute respiratory distress syndrome), or the neuronal effects of uraemia. If the patient is severely acidotic, rapid deep Kussmaul breathing may be observed in an effort to compensate. This excessive work of breathing is tiring and may eventually necessitate intubation and mechanical ventilation if the acidosis cannot be corrected. Respiratory rate and pattern should be assessed on admission and at routine intervals, together with continuous pulse oximetry and periodic arterial blood gas analysis. The patient's pulmonary secretions should be appraised, particularly to detect pulmonary oedema, pulmonary haemorrhage (in the presence of coagulopathy), or 'pulmonary–renal syndromes' such as granulomatosis with polyangiitis (inflammation of blood vessels) or Goodpasture's syndrome.

Circulation

ECG and blood pressure monitoring are standard practice, but a more advanced method of haemodynamic monitoring will also be needed. At the very least, a central venous catheter should be placed, and, if available, oesophageal Doppler or some other device used to monitor cardiac output and guide fluid management. The aim is to ensure that there is an adequate circulating volume and effective perfusion pressure.

Insertion of any intravascular lines should be performed under strict aseptic conditions to prevent infection, and also with due consideration of any clotting disorders. Bleeding in uraemic patients is common, primarily due to defects in platelet adhesion and aggregation. If at all possible, a full blood count, clotting studies, and bleeding time should be checked and treated before any invasive procedure. A one-off dose of DDAVP (l-desamino-8-d-arginine vasopressin/desmopressin) can give a short-term improvement in platelet function in the presence of uraemia by enhancing factor VIII and von Willebrand factor (Hedges *et al.* 2007).

Hyperkalaemia is identified by blood test and sometimes by tall peaked T waves and other changes seen on the ECG. A serum potassium 5.5–5.9 mmol/L is described as mild elevation, 6.0–6.4 mmol/L as moderate elevation, and ≥6.5 mmol/L as severe elevation. This is when peaked T waves and other ECG abnormalities, including a prolonged QRS complex, are most likely to be seen. Severe hyperkalaemia can cause fatal dysrhythmias such as ventricular tachycardia and ventricular fibrillation, so must be treated swiftly. If toxic ECG changes are seen, 10 ml of intravenous 10% calcium chloride should be given to stabilize the myocardial cell membrane. Then, reduction of serum potassium can be achieved with (Resuscitation Council UK 2011):

- 50 ml IV of 50% glucose containing 10 units of soluble insulin over 15–30 min and repeated as necessary (insulin promotes intracellular movement of potassium and thereby lowers the serum level)
- nebulized salbutamol by inhalation (up to 4 × 5mg doses), and
- if the patient is acidaemic, 50 mmol IV sodium bicarbonate (50 ml of 8.4% solution).

Renal replacement therapy will be needed if these measures are unsuccessful.

Principles of care

Monitoring urine output

A falling urine output is usually the first indicator of a potential renal problem. In an adult, an hourly volume of 0.5 ml/kg is the minimum acceptable volume. Catheterization and hourly recording of urine volumes must be done. The drainage bag tubing should be supported or fixed to the patient's leg to prevent drag on the urethra.

If a catheter is already in place, the possibility of catheter blockage should be excluded by bladder irrigation and, if necessary, the catheter replaced. If the patient has been admitted after urological surgery or trauma, obstruction by blood/blood clots or an anastomotic leak/ureteric rupture is possible. Any nephrostomy tubes, ureteric stents, or urostomies should be checked for blockage. However, if the patient is genuinely anuric, a urinary catheter may be a focus for infection and should be removed.

If the circulating blood volume has been optimized but the patient is still oliguric, any other fluid intake should be restricted to replace any urine output plus insensible losses only. This may be difficult as strict fluid restriction often precludes provision of adequate nutrition. Renal replacement therapy is often implemented to deal with this.

Care should be taken when administering hypertonic solutions, such as sodium bicarbonate, mannitol, or 10–50% glucose, especially if the patient is oliguric, as the hypertonicity will draw extravascular fluid into the circulation which may result in intravascular overload.

Avoidance of pre-renal factors

It is essential that the patient has an adequate circulating blood volume. Tachycardia, hypotension, and cool peripheries are signs that extra fluid is required. If so, one or more fluid challenges should be administered (e.g. 250–500 ml Hartmann's solution) (see discussion of fluid challenge in Chapter 5). The ventricular filling pressure (e.g. as indicated by central venous pressure/pulmonary artery wedge pressure) or the stroke volume/cardiac output should be measured before and after each fluid bolus. If, 5–10 min after fluid is given, the filling pressure rises by more than 3 mmHg and remains at that level, the patient probably has an adequate circulating volume. However, if there is little or no increase, optimal filling may not have been achieved and further fluid should be administered. Alternatively, a flow monitor (e.g. oesophageal Doppler) that measures stroke volume and cardiac output can be used to optimize fluid loading (see Chapter 5).

The urine output should be reassessed once an adequate circulating volume has been achieved; if there is no improvement and the patient remains tachycardic and/or hypotensive, inotropes and/or a vasodilator may be required to increase cardiac output. During this phase, cardiac output studies are useful to determine the effect of inotropes and other drugs. Circulating blood volume and cardiac output should then be continuously monitored and optimized throughout the patient's illness (see Box 7.7).

> **Box 7.7 Avoidance of pre-renal kidney injury**
>
> Ensure that there is adequate circulating volume, cardiac output, and organ perfusion pressure

Diuretic therapy

It seems logical to give diuretics to treat oliguria. In particular, loop diuretics (e.g. furosemide), and also osmotic diuretics (e.g. mannitol), have been much used in the past, and sometimes in the present. These drugs can promote diuresis, which should be useful as urine flow could remove debris obstructing the tubules and also prevent filtrate 'back-leak'. In addition, furosemide is known to reduce active sodium transport and therefore renal oxygen demand in critical illness (Swärd *et al.* 2005). However, despite these apparent advantages, and a certain amount of complex and contradictory research (e.g. Karajala *et al.* 2009; Grams *et al.* 2011), there is no strong evidence to show any clinical benefit from routine use of any diuretic in AKI (Kellum *et al.* 2011). Indeed, some studies have reported harm. Administration of mannitol can increase extracellular fluid volume, but may also cause pulmonary oedema. If a diuresis is promoted, fluid and solute loss can cause hypovolaemia and reduced renal perfusion. One group of patients given a continuous infusion of furosemide aimed at preventing kidney dysfunction after cardiac surgery had significantly higher urine outputs but also significantly raised creatinine levels and a greater incidence of AKI compared with those just given placebo (Lassnigg *et al.* 2000).

The international Kidney Disease: Improving Global Outcomes (KDIGO) expert group has concluded that diuretics have no value in the prevention or treatment of AKI, except perhaps in cases of symptomatic fluid overload (KDIGO 2012).

Nutrition

The patient suffering from AKI is often extremely catabolic with muscle tissue rapidly broken down to provide an energy source; so early nutrition is a priority. The oral or (more often) the enteral route is preferred as there are fewer metabolic complications and the risks associated with parenteral nutrition are avoided (e.g. intravenous feeding line related sepsis). Enteral nutrition also helps maintain gut integrity and may reduce translocation of bacteria and endotoxins.

The main principles of nutrition in critical illness are broadly similar for patients with kidney dysfunction. The aim is to correct any significant nutritional deficiencies and meet energy requirements, generally with a calorific intake of 25–35 kcal/kg/day (Lewington and Kanagasundaram 2011). If renal replacement therapy (RRT) is used, it can usually be manipulated to create space for whatever fluid volumes are required. RRT is likely to remove amino acids, protein, and other important nutritional substrates (e.g. electrolytes such as potassium, magnesium, and phosphorus and water-soluble B group vitamins), so regular blood tests to measure levels of these elements in the body are essential. Tailored supplementation can then be provided as needed. Periodic review by a specialist dietician is recommended.

Skin integrity

There is a high risk of skin damage in this group of patients. AKI is most often caused by hypoperfusion, where intense peripheral vasoconstriction occurs as a compensatory mechanism. In addition, these patients frequently require inotropes and vasoactive drugs that further decrease blood supply to the skin and underlying tissue. They are also often oedematous which makes the skin even more vulnerable. Furthermore, the time spent inserting lines, performing fluid resuscitation, and invasive monitoring can mean that the patient remains in the same position for long periods.

The patient should be examined and assessed for the risk of developing pressure ulcers as soon as possible following admission. This should be documented, along with a preventative strategy or a treatment programme appropriate to the risk or the sore involved. It may be necessary to use a pressure-relieving mattress or bed if the patient is particularly vulnerable or is too unstable to withstand frequent changes of position. Care should also be taken with skin underlying ECG electrodes, lines, any tapes, or similar devices as it could easily break down in the presence of poor perfusion. The patient may experience skin irritation arising from azotaemia (high blood levels of nitrogenous waste products), so the nurse should ensure that the patient does not scratch him/herself in a way that disrupts skin integrity.

Renal replacement therapy

The indications for commencing renal replacement therapy of one type or another are not absolute and considerable leeway is possible. The clinical and biochemical indicators suggested by the UK Renal Association (Lewington and Kanagasundaram 2011) include:

- urine output <0.3ml/kg/hour for 24 hours (equating to Stage 3 AKI, which is also defined by serum creatinine increased to >354 μmol/L or to ≥3 times the baseline value)
- fluid overload or the need to create space for nutrition
- severe uraemic symptoms (e.g. encephalopathy, pericarditis
- poisoning
- correction of high/low body temperature
- refractory metabolic acidosis (e.g. pH <7.15)
- hyperkalaemia (serum potassium >6.5 mmol/L) unresponsive to medical management.

The overall aims of any form of renal replacement therapy are:

- to relieve fluid overload, restore and maintain fluid balance
- to remove waste products (particularly urea and creatinine)
- to correct and maintain metabolic and electrolyte balance.

Types of renal replacement therapy

- Intermittent haemodialysis (IHD)
- Slow continuous ultrafiltration (SCUF)
- Continuous arteriovenous haemofiltration (CAVH)
- Continuous venovenous haemofiltration (CVVH)
- Continuous venovenous haemodialysis (CVVHD)
- Continuous venovenous haemodiafiltration (CVVHDF)
- High volume haemofiltration (HVHF)
- Peritoneal dialysis(PD) and continuous ambulatory peritoneal dialysis (CAPD)
- Combinations of IHD and continuous methods such as haemofiltration

Continuous venovenous methods are the techniques most used in the critical care unit.

Physiological principles common to all renal replacement therapies

Diffusion

Diffusion is the movement of solutes across a semi-permeable membrane from an area of high concentration to an area of low concentration. A concentration gradient is always necessary for diffusion to occur. Molecules with a smaller molecular weight will move across a semi-permeable membrane more readily than those with a larger molecular weight; a semi-permeable membrane has a defined pore size and any molecule exceeding this will not be able to pass through. Diffusion will be affected by the resistance offered by the membrane; this is related to the thickness, size, and shape of the pores. In addition, artificial membranes used in renal replacement therapy tend to become less efficient over time as a biofilm of protein and other material accumulates within the filter. Diffusion is utilized in peritoneal dialysis, haemodialysis, and haemodiafiltration (see Figure 7.6).

Diffusion

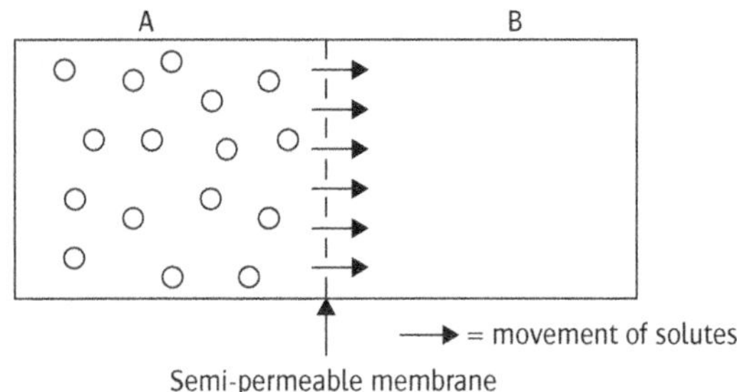

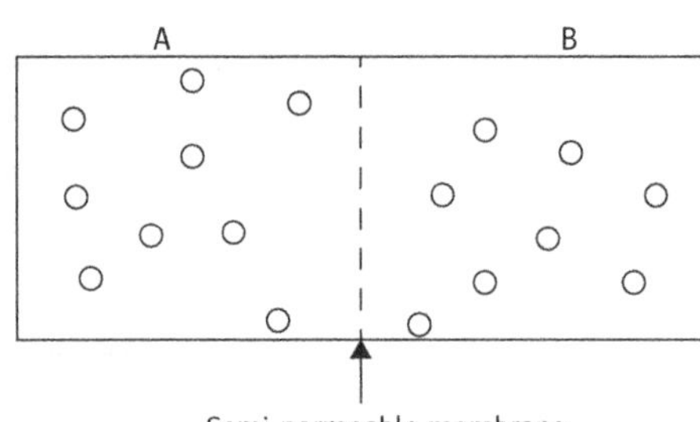

Figure 7.6 The movement of solutes across a semi-permeable membrane.

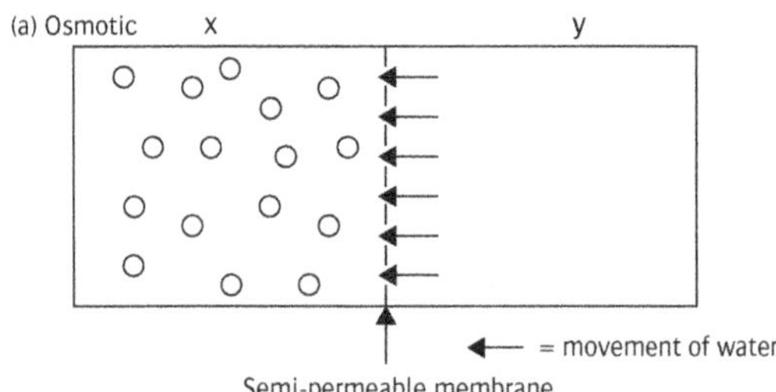

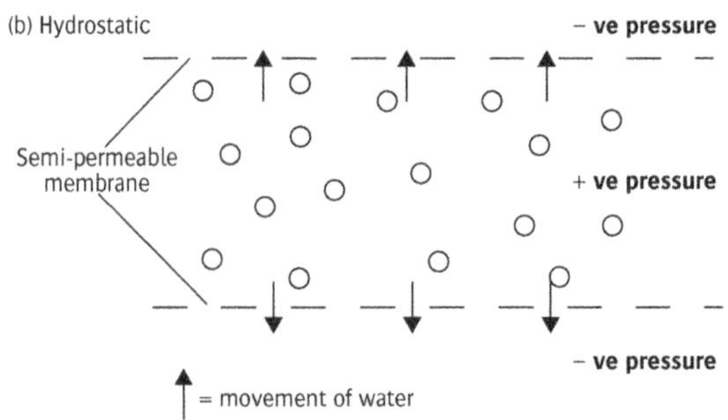

Figure 7.7 Ultrafiltration: (a) osmotic; (b) hydrostatic.

Ultrafiltration

Ultrafiltration is a method of convective transport when there is bulk movement of water across a semi-permeable membrane, together with any solutes that can penetrate that membrane. Water molecules are small and can pass through all semi-permeable membranes. The driving force for ultrafiltration can be either an osmotic gradient or hydrostatic pressure (see Figure 7.7).

1. Osmotic ultrafiltration occurs when water is drawn across a semi-permeable membrane from a hypotonic solution into a hypertonic solution. The osmotic 'pull' is generated by the concentrated solute in the hypertonic solution. Osmotic ultrafiltration is utilised in peritoneal dialysis.

2. Hydrostatic ultrafiltration is seen when water is forced across a semi-permeable membrane by a hydrostatic pressure exerted across the membrane. Hydrostatic ultrafiltration is utilized in haemofiltration and haemodialysis.

The ultrafiltration coefficient K_{UF} indicates the permeability of a particular semi-permeable membrane. It is defined as the number of millilitres of fluid per hour that will be transferred across the membrane per mmHg pressure gradient across the membrane.

Extracorporeal methods of renal replacement therapy

Most critical care units offer vascular forms of RRT using venovenous systems. Haemodialysis and haemofiltration work differently, but both use some similar processes and materials.

Buffers

To enable effective treatment of the metabolic acidosis that frequently accompanies AKI, a buffer must be provided in either the dialysate fluid or the replacement fluid used for RRT. Lactate-based solutions were previously used (on the basis that lactate is metabolized by the liver to bicarbonate); but now that manufacture of stable bicarbonate solutions has been achieved, bicarbonate itself is recommended as a buffer (Lewington and Kanagasundaram 2011; KDIGO 2012) (see Table 7.9).

Table 7.9 Dialysate/replacement fluid: typical composition

	Lactate buffered solution	Bicarbonate buffered solution
Fluid volume	5 L	5 L
Sodium	140 mmol/L	140 mmol/L
Potassium	0 mmol/L	0–4 mmol/L
Calcium	1.75 mmol/L	1.75 mmol/L
Magnesium	0.75 mmol/L	0.5 mmol/L
Chloride	115 mmol/L	109.5 mmol/L
Lactate	30 mmol/L	NA
Bicarbonate	NA	35 mmol/L
Glucose	5.55 mmol/L	0–5.55 mmol/L

Artificial kidneys/filters

A range of artificial kidneys/filters are available, with different properties and potential problems. Essentially, they all consist of a densely packed set of fine semi-permeable tubules through which blood is pumped, allowing the removal of plasma, water, and some other substances through the membrane. This effluent can then be drained from the system. Key issues for consideration are:

- the biocompatibility of the material used in the filter membrane
- the efficiency of the filter, which is particularly related to its flux property (i.e. its degree of permeability).

Concerns about biocompatibility have arisen from observation of complement activation, cytokine generation, and white cell and platelet activation during RRT, all of which can lead to pulmonary and other organ dysfunction. These problems have been most associated with the earlier generation of filters made from cellulose or some variant such as cuprophane. Modified cellulose or synthetic membranes (e.g. polysulfone, polyacrylonitrile) are less prone to such disturbances.

The modern standard artificial kidney has a hollow fibre design. Flat plate designs are now outmoded. Hollow fibre models enable a relatively large membrane surface area to be contained within a reasonably small volume device; products vary, but a standard haemofilter is usually a slim cylinder no more than 30 cm long but still able to provide a membrane surface area of at least 1.2 m^2. Filter membranes are typically permeable to molecules up to 50,000 Da. This should be seen in relation to the molecular weights of urea (60 Da), creatinine (113 Da), and albumin 60,000 Da.

Vascular access

Early RRT systems used blood taken from an arterial cannula. This meant that movement of blood around the circuit was governed by the patient's arterial pressure, which was problematic in several ways, especially if the patient was hypotensive (see Table 7.10).

Modern RRT equipment incorporates dedicated blood pumps to move blood around the circuit, so venous access can be used. This is a safer and more effective method for the critically ill patient. A double-lumen Y-shaped cannula with two distal ports is commonly used, inserted into a large vein (e.g. the femoral, subclavian, or internal jugular vein). The internal jugular vein is usually preferred; a cannula sited there is less likely to be kinked or infected than one in the femoral vein, and is less of a risk than subclavian vein cannulation which can

Table 7.10 Vascular access in renal replacement therapy

Access	Use	Comment
Separate artery and vein cannulation	Non-blood pump method (less than ideal)	Femoral approaches commonly used Renders patient immobile as blood flow obstructed if legs bent
Arteriovenous shunt (e.g. Scribner): radial artery cephalic vein or post tibial artery/ long saphenous vein	Pumped and non-pumped methods	Provides good blood flow Cannot be changed along with other patient lines if sepsis suspected
Double-lumen: jugular vein approach	Pumped methods	Provides good blood flow Position often uncomfortable for patient Can be difficult to fix to the skin due to position
Double-lumen: subclavian vein access	Pumped methods	Provides good blood flow Allows greater patient mobility Potential insertion complications: pneumothorax, brachial plexus injury, thrombosis/stenosis
Double-lumen: femoral vein access	Pumped methods	Provides good blood flow if legs straight No proven increased risk of infection Difficult site to expose for continuous observation

cause pneumothorax and other complications. If possible, ultrasound imaging should be used to aid insertion of the cannula. One arm of the Y-shaped cannula allows blood to be taken from the patient, while the other arm enables blood to be simultaneously pumped back into the vein at a separate location further along the vessel (Figure 7.8). This is to prevent 'access recirculation', i.e. the immediate extracorporeal recirculation of blood that has just been returned from the RRT system (because the concentration gradients will then be reduced and therefore the treatment will be less effective).

Anticoagulation

Most forms of extracorporeal circulation require some form of anticoagulation to help prevent the platelet and coagulation system activation that occurs as a result of contact with a foreign surface (i.e. the circuits and filter). Inadequate anticoagulation allows clotting to occur in the circuit, particularly in the filter, which will eventually stop the extracorporeal circulation of blood altogether. Replacing a clotted filter is time-consuming, expensive, and decreases the effectiveness of the therapy, but does not usually present a direct hazard to the patient—other than the loss of blood left in the circuit (up to 200 ml) and the consumption of endogenous clotting products. However, too much anticoagulant can be very dangerous. The patient's clotting function must be carefully monitored. Any signs of bleeding from vascular access sites, the gastrointestinal tract, or mucus membranes should be viewed with suspicion and investigated further.

There are methods used during intermittent HD that allow anticoagulation-free dialysis and are sometimes successful in continuous methods such as haemofiltration. These techniques are primarily dependent on the individual patient's endogenous coagulation function. Patients with coagulopathy or thrombocytopenia may not need anticoagulation at all.

Careful monitoring of coagulation and anticoagulation during RRT is essential. The data obtained must be considered in relation to the type and dose of anticoagulants used, and also with reference to other laboratory results such as full blood count. Values vary somewhat between centres as different methods of analysis give different results. Some critical care units have bedside testing equipment, but most will need to send blood samples to the hospital's main laboratory. Tests include the following.

1. Activated clotting time (ACT). A blood sample is added to a tube containing an activating agent that accelerates the clotting process. This is placed in a machine that automatically tilts/rotates the tube and detects clot formation. During HD, ACT is normally maintained between 200 and 250 sec, and during haemofiltration at approximately 150–220 sec (baseline, 120–150 sec).

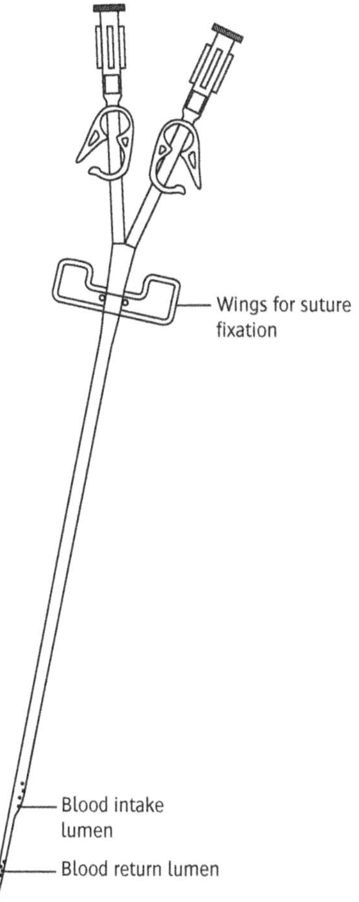

Figure 7.8 Double-lumen vascular cannula for veno-venous haemo(dia)filtration

2. The activated partial thromboplastin time (APTT) is the time taken for a fibrin clot to form in a plasma sample after precise quantities of a partial thromboplastin reagent (phospholipid), a contact factor activating agent, and calcium chloride have been added. APTT is generally used for routine monitoring of the effects of heparin administration in RRT. It should be checked 4-6 hours after starting a heparin infusion. The aim is usually for APTT to be approximately 1.5 times the control value.

Regular checking of platelet levels is also important; a platelet count <60 × 103 mm^{-3} indicates that active anticoagulation may not be needed (Intensive Care Society 2009).

Types of anticoagulant

Heparin is the most frequently used anticoagulant. However, it is a difficult agent to titrate, particularly because its effects vary hugely between individuals and even in the same individual over time. The half-life of heparin can range from less than 30 min to more than 3 hours for no predictable reason. When necessary, protamine sulphate can be given as an antidote to heparin overdose.

The most common type of heparin used is mixed molecular weight (5–30 kDa) unfractionated heparin (UFH) (Lewington and Kanagasundaram 2011). UFH is not completely cleared across artificial membranes because of its high negative charge and protein binding. Low molecular weight heparin (LMWH, 4.5–6 kDa) is occasionally used, as in theory it presents fewer haemorrhagic risks to the patient. However, LMWH has not been shown to give better outcomes than UFH and is also much harder to monitor; it requires an anti-factor Xa assay which is not performed as an urgent/emergency procedure in most hospitals.

Typically, heparin is infused proximal to the filter at 5–10 IU/kg/hour. This may be preceded by a loading dose of 2000–5000 IU. If the patient has adverse reactions to heparin (e.g. thrombocytopenia) or is at risk of bleeding (e.g. following surgery), epoprostenol (PGI_2) or alprostadil (PGE_1) can be used, infused at 2.5–10 ng/kg/min. These prostaglandins act by inhibiting platelet aggregation. This allows the dose of heparin to be decreased or stopped completely. A small group of patients given heparin can develop heparin-induced thrombocytopenia syndrome (HITS) which puts them at risk of potentially life-threatening thrombosis. In these cases, all heparin must be stopped, including that in flush lines. There is a lower incidence of HITS associated with LMWH than with unfractionated heparin, but LMWH does not completely remove the risk of HITS. Heparin-coated circuits are available as an adjunct or substitute for systemic heparinization, but have not been shown to improve outcomes.

Another alternative in HITS is a synthetic heparinoid such as danaparoid or fondiparinux, although they sometimes react with heparin-induced antibodies. If the platelet count does not improve within 3 days, further investigation and/or a different method of anticoagulation should be considered (Lewington and Kanagasundaram 2011). These drugs are normally excreted by the kidneys and so are likely to accumulate in AKI.

Direct thrombin inhibitors are also available (e.g. hirudin), but some patients develop antibodies to these which can extend the drug action for several days, especially if renal clearance is impaired. There is no agent that can reverse this process and so prolonged bleeding may result (Lewington and Kanagasundaram 2011).

Another option for patients at risk of bleeding is regional citrate anticoagulation (Oudemans-van Straaten and Ostermann 2012). This is widely used in the USA but less so in other countries. Citrate added proximal to the filter chelates ionized calcium, i.e. binds calcium so that it is not available to the coagulation cascade and therefore clotting is inhibited. Citrate also has the potential advantage of being metabolized to bicarbonate by the liver. The patient is likely to require infusions of calcium replacements after the filter to prevent hypocalcaemia. Monitoring of APTT, ionized calcium levels, pH, and sodium levels is necessary.

Haemofiltration

Principles

Haemofiltration is a convective process in which there is mass movement of plasma water and solutes across the semi-permeable artificial membrane in an extracorporeal circuit. The blood circulated through the filter exerts a hydrostatic pressure on one side of the membrane that moves plasma, water, and solutes to the other side where the water and solutes become 'filtrate'. This is hydrostatic ultrafiltration. The constant draining of the filtrate compartment ensures a negative pressure on that side so that a pressure gradient from the blood side of the membrane is maintained. The volume of filtrate removed by haemofiltration can be controlled by a volumetric pump. This is usually integrated into the purpose-built haemofilter machine.

Most of the protein and cellular constituents of blood cannot move across the membrane because they are too large. However, haemofiltration is not a selective process, and the removal of waste products can only be achieved by the removal of an accompanying load of water and other solutes. Some of these losses may be undesirable; and volumes of filtrate can be considerable (sometimes over 2 L/hour), so intravenous fluid must be concurrently replaced to maintain fluid balance and cardiovascular stability. This replacement fluid should be isotonic and also aim to replace the key solutes lost as filtrate (see Figure 7.9).

Pre-filter or post-filter fluid administration

Replacement fluids can be infused into the RRT circuit either before or after the filter. Pre-filter administration is also known as pre-dilution, and may reduce solute clearance through the filter membrane precisely because the blood and the solutes in it are diluted. The advantage of pre-dilution is that because it reduces the haematocrit of the blood, filter life may be prolonged and anticoagulation requirements reduced (Uchino *et al.* 2003). This could be particularly useful for RRT patients with a tendency to clot the filter.

Haemofiltration dose

Exchanges of 1–2 L (giving 1–2 L of filtrate) are typically prescribed in continuous haemofiltration. Alternatively, this can be prescribed as a weight-adjusted dose of 25 ml/kg/hour. It has been suggested that there might be advantages to higher doses (high volume haemofiltration), but two recent studies of large groups of critically ill patients, the ATN Study (VA/NIH Acute Renal Failure Trial Network 2008) and the RENAL Study (RENAL Replacement Therapy Study Investigators 2009), showed no significant benefit to doses of 35 ml/kg/hour and 40 ml/kg/hour versus 20 ml/kg/hour and 25 ml/kg/hour, respectively. However, it is important to note that the

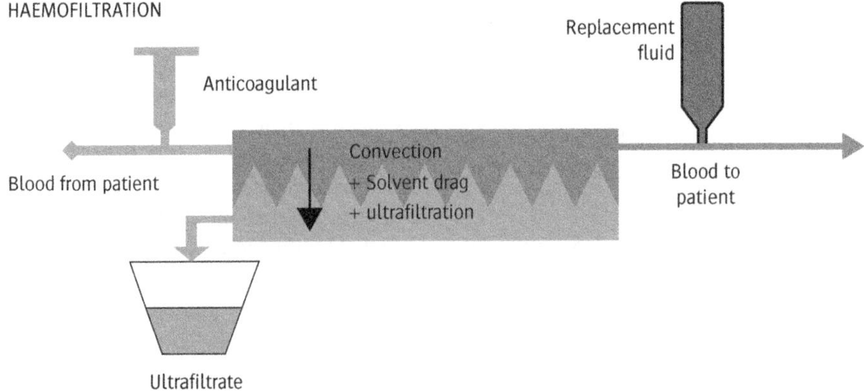

Figure 7.9 Continuous venovenous haemofiltration.

Reproduced with permission from Singer, M and Webb, A.R, *Oxford Handbook of Critical Care* (3rd edn). Copyright (2009) with permission from Oxford University Press

prescribed dose is very often *not* delivered, for example because the RRT system malfunctions or the therapy is interrupted for the patient to undergo some procedure or transportation away from the critical care unit. UK guidelines recommend that a minimum dose of 25 ml/kg/hour is maintained, but emphasize that it may be necessary to prescribe a higher dose (~30 ml/kg/h) to allow for interruptions and ensure that 25 ml/kg/h exchanges are actually delivered 24 hours a day (Lewington and Kanagasundaram, 2011).

Some authorities maintain that there are subgroups of patients who are still likely to benefit from high volume RRT. There is a particular interest in this approach for patients with AKI and severe sepsis/septic shock; several small *un*controlled trials have reported improved survival of such patients using haemofiltration at doses ranging from 40 to 115 ml/kg/hour (Rimmelé and Kellum 2011). Research is ongoing in this field.

Advantages of continuous haemofiltration

- Haemofiltration allows continuous control of uraemia and fluid balance which promotes cardiovascular stability.
- It does not require specialist renal staff or equipment/water supplies.
- It can be performed in the critical care unit, negating the need to transfer critically ill patients to renal centres.

Disadvantages of haemofiltration

- The process is relatively inefficient: a haemofiltration removal rate of 1 L/h equates to a creatinine clearance of 16 ml/min. Nonetheless, this is still adequate for most patients.
- Because it is relatively inefficient, haemofiltration needs to be a continuous process. Thus restricts the patient's mobility. Maintenance of the RRT system and the close monitoring required also necessitates frequent activity that can disrupt rest and sleep.
- Continuous anticoagulation has to be administered (and monitored), albeit at relatively low doses.
- Removal and replacement of large volumes of fluid is labour intensive and open to potential error.

Types of haemofiltration

Venovenous haemofiltration

CVVH is preferred to CAVH in critical illness, not least because much higher filtration rates can be obtained with the use of dedicated roller pumps to move blood around the extracorporeal circuit in purpose-built machines. Once blood pumps are included in these circuits, monitoring devices and alarms must also be incorporated. Either a double-lumen cannula sited in a large vein or two separate venous cannulae for blood access and return are employed.

Venovenous haemodiafiltration (CVVHD)

CVVHD adds another mechanism to those used in CVVH, with a dialysate solution run through the artificial kidney on the opposite side of the membrane to the blood, in a counter-current direction. Filtration still occurs because a pressure gradient still exists (albeit to a lesser degree), but diffusion is also utilized to facilitate the removal of solutes, particularly those that are of relatively small size (see Figure 7.10).

CVVHD can achieve the same clearance as CVVH with less filtrate, although the nurse will have the

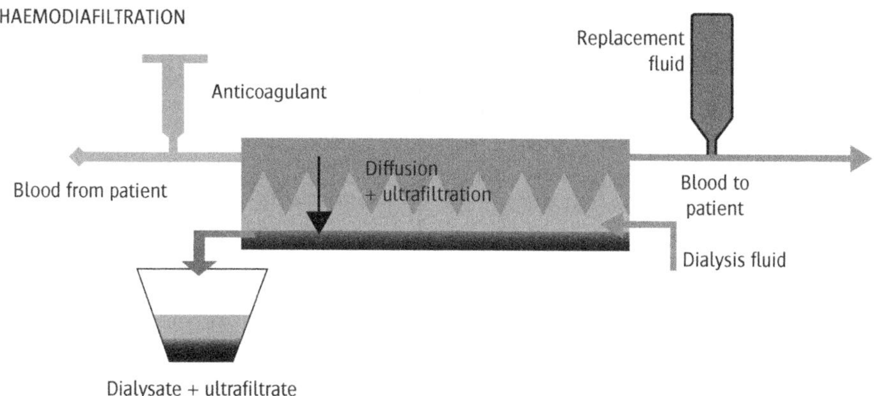

Figure 7.10 Continuous veno-venous haemodiafiltration

additional tasks of handling the infusion and drainage of dialysate fluid. CVVHD can also be more costly than CVVH because of the extra fluid required.

The dialysate fluid used is generally the same as the replacement fluid. Dialysate flow rates are usually set at up to 2 L/h, depending on the clearance of solutes desired.

CVVH and CVVHD are the main types of RRT used in the UK, Europe, and Australia, but it is not clear which is most effective; the choice of method is based at least in part on the nature of the local experience, equipment, and other resources. A pragmatic approach is to begin treatment with CVVH as it is somewhat easier and more economical, and then switch to CVVHD if CVVH proves to be ineffective for a particular patient.

Mechanised haemo(dia)filtration

A number of purpose-built haemofiltration machines delivering safe, accurate, semi-automated RRT are available from different manufacturers, although patients needing RRT are at high risk of serious complications—and death—so it is crucial that staff are well trained and vigilant. The precise mechanisms of these machines vary somewhat but are all based on the same principles

Fluid balance

Some haemofiltration machines operate on specific time cycles over a number of hours, while others operate on an hourly basis. Whichever time period is used, the patient's entire fluid intake (nutrition, drugs, infusions) must be balanced against any losses, including the filtrate. A target fluid balance (either positive or negative) is determined on the basis of clinical assessment of intravascular and total body fluid volume status. This needs to be reviewed at least once daily. Most machines incorporate pumps for replacement fluid and dialysate fluid, as well as the blood pump and filtrate pump. Fluid balance recordings must be carefully checked and documented to avoid accidental hypo- or hypervolaemia. Critically ill patients are prone to significant fluid shifts and periods of vasoconstriction and vasodilatation, so prescribed fluid balance objectives may become inappropriate. If haemodiafiltration is used, the volume of dialysate infused must be subtracted from the effluent fluid drained to obtain the actual filtrate volume. See Boxes 7.8 and 7.9 for examples of calculating replacement values.

Haemodynamic monitoring

Continuous ECG and blood pressure monitoring are essential, primarily to detect signs of hypovolaemia (i.e. tachycardia and hypotension). If significant hypovolaemia occurs, an increase in the core–peripheral temperature gradient and a decrease in cardiac filling pressures (e.g. central venous pressure) will also be seen.

Prior to use, the RRT circuit has to be primed (usually using a litre bag of heparinized saline solution) to

Box 7.8 Calculating replacement values: example 1

Intake

Enteral feed: 120 ml

Fentanyl: 5 ml

Insulin: 2 ml

Total: 127 ml

Output

Wound drain: 50 ml

Filtrate: 1500 ml

Total: 1550 ml

The time cycles are hourly and the patient is prescribed to have a neutral balance at the end of each cycle. Therefore the volume of replacement fluid needed during the cycle is 1423 ml (1550–127 ml).

Box 7.9 Calculating replacement values: example 2

Intake

Parenteral feed: 100 ml

Epinephrine: 5 ml

Propofol: l5 ml

Insulin: 3 ml

Total: 123 ml

Output

Nasogastric tube: 50 ml

Filtrate: 1800 ml

Total: 1850 ml

The time cycles are hourly and the patient is prescribed to have a balance of −100 ml at the end of each cycle. The volume of replacement fluid needed during the cycle is 1850−123 = 1727 ml to achieve a neutral balance, and therefore 1727−100 = 1627 ml to achieve a negative balance of 100 ml/h.

remove air, coat the circuit with heparin, and flush the artificial kidney. There are then two options when commencing the treatment. One is to attach the patient to both ends of the circuit from the beginning, which results in the patient receiving the prime solution from the RRT circuit (up to 200 ml). This may be undesirable if the patient is severely overloaded. More commonly, hypovolaemia can ensue as the patient loses blood into the extracorporeal circuit but initially only has the crystalloid prime solution returned to them. The second option is to start by only attaching the 'arterial' end (the access limb) of the circuit, allowing the patient's blood to move into the circuit and expel the prime solution before attaching the 'venous' connection (the return limb). This method is more likely than the double-connection technique to lead to relative hypovolaemia due to loss of blood into the RRT circuit without any of the fluid in the circuit being returned to the patient. Therefore, if the single-connection approach is used, it is advisable to have an intravenous fluid infusion ready to be given in case hypovolaemia becomes apparent. Even when the RRT is established, hypovolaemia may occur if the patient's fluid requirements change.

Dysrhythmias can occur with hypovolaemia, as well as with hypo/hyperkalaemia. Serum potassium values should be checked at least four-hourly, especially if haemofiltration is used. Electrolyte balance is less of a problem with haemodiafiltration as a balanced dialysate solution is used. For instance, serum potassium levels can equilibrate with potassium levels in the dialysate fluid if this contains potassium; i.e. if the dialysate fluid contains 4.5 mmol/L of potassium and the serum potassium falls below that value, potassium will diffuse across the artificial membrane into the blood until the serum potassium has also reached 4.5 mmol/L. If the patient's potassium rises above 4.5 mmol/L, the reverse process takes place. The same principle applies to all serum constituents which can diffuse across the artificial membrane. Notably, sodium losses during haemofiltration may exceed sodium intake, so additional sodium may have to be infused, but in haemodiafiltration, the sodium levels can be maintained by diffusion from the dialysate as described previously.

The patient's central temperature should be monitored and maintained at >36°C. Circulating blood outside the body tends to cool it, as does the infusion of large volumes of replacement and dialysate fluid. Replacement fluid and dialysate fluid can be warmed prior to infusion if necessary, and some machines incorporate a blood-warming device. Conversely, in the pyrexial patient, infusion of unwarmed replacement fluid can be useful. It is important to appreciate that an underlying pyrexia may be masked by the cooling effect of continuous RRT.

Nursing interventions

Rest and sleep

One significant disadvantage of continuous RRT is that constant attention to the patient and the attached equipment is needed, day and night. This is unavoidable, but all possible measures should be taken to allow the patient as much rest and sleep as possible. It is possible in theory to halt RRT overnight, but this has to be weighed against the time, costs, and reduced efficiency of changing the extracorporeal circuit every 24 hours.

Psychological care

The sight of what look like large volumes of blood in an extracorporeal circuit may be taken for granted by critical care staff, but can be alarming for both patient and relatives. RRT and the anxiety it may cause should be anticipated, so that the possibility of haemofiltration being used as a treatment is explained to the patient and relatives prior to its commencement to avoid the 'sudden' appearance of yet another piece of machinery. Giving the patient and relatives prior warning also gives them the message that staff are thinking ahead and know how the patient's critical illness is likely to develop.

Changing the circuit

There is no definitive evidence about how often the RRT circuit ought to be changed. Manufacturer's advice regarding the individual components of the RRT system and local policies (e.g. with respect to infection control) should be used as guidance. Typically, changes are performed at least every 72 hours or when there is:

- significant reduction in performance of the RRT
- suspected or known bacteraemia
- evidence of a large clot in the filter (clots in the circuit tend to consume platelets and may provide a medium for bacterial growth).

Ideally, the change of circuit should be arranged so as to return the residual volume of blood in the circuit back to the patient. This is done by disconnecting the 'arterial' limb of the circuit from the patient and attaching it to a bag of 0.9% sodium chloride. The saline solution is then allowed to run through the circuit, pushing the residual blood back into the patient via the still attached 'venous' limb. If the circuit needs to be changed due to clotting, the cause of clotting must be investigated prior to the connection of a new circuit. If clotting tests show that inadequate anticoagulation

Table 7.11 Problems associated with renal replacement therapy

Problem	Cause	Action
Filtrate volumes in excess of ability to concurrently replace fluid	Can be experienced with new circuits. Usually settles down after 3–4 h.	The filtrate outflow line can be partially clamped. Blood flow rate can be reduced but should be maintained above 100 ml/min.
Filtrate volumes decreasing	Inadequate blood flow (slow blood pump speed, obstructed access). Clotting in the artificial kidney.	The filtrate outflow line can be partially clamped. Blood flow rate can be reduced but should be maintained above 100 ml/min. In pumped methods: (a) check blood pump speed (>100 ml/min); (b) check vascular access. Clotting: see below.
Clotting of the circuit	Low blood flow, intermittent blood flow (from poor access), cool blood, inadequate anticoagulation, inadequate priming technique, low blood antithrombin III level.	It is possible to continue RRT with some clot present provided that: (a) sufficient volumes of filtrate are produced for control of uraemia; (b) any clots do not encourage further clinically significant platelet adherence (shown by a continuing low serum platelet count and spontaneous bleeding from line sites); (c) the patient is not bacteraemic (clots in the kidney provide a medium for bacterial growth). If indicated, the circuit should be changed.

was the cause, the rate of heparin infusion should be increased. This usually means that more frequent clotting tests will be needed for a period thereafter. Clotting in the artificial kidney and venous bubble trap may be detected by pressure increases in the venous pressure monitor (Table 7.11).

In pumped methods of RRT, blood flow must be maintained at >100 ml/min to avoid clotting in the artificial kidney and also to ensure adequate clearance of metabolic waste. After beginning treatment with a blood flow of 100 ml/min, it is standard practice to increase the flow rate to 150-250 ml/min to ensure optimal performance of the system (KDIGO 2012). While the speed of blood flow through the circuit at any one time is important, so is the consistency of that speed. For example, if vascular access is via a femoral vein cannula and the patient frequently bends their legs, the flow of blood from the femoral vein will be very variable and likely to precipitate clotting in the artificial kidney. Such reductions in blood flow from the patient can be detected by an arterial pressure monitor built in to the haemofilter machine. In addition, if blood flow is severely obstructed, the nurse may see air being sucked into the 'arterial' section of the circuit by the blood pump. Frequent problems of this kind should prompt review of the access site. Blood flow can also be interrupted because of cannula movement when the patient is repositioned. This problem can sometimes be minimized by temporarily slowing the blood pump speed for the duration of the procedure on the basis that a constant relatively slow blood flow is preferable to no blood flow at all.

If clotting occurs soon after connecting the patient to the haemofilter circuit and there is no other obvious problem, it is likely that the priming technique has been inadequate. One of the functions of priming is to flush the sterilizing and stabilizing materials used in manufacture out of the artificial kidney, and to open up the pores in the semi-permeable membrane. If this has not been done properly, diffusion through the membrane will be impaired and the filter will be more likely to clot. If clotting is a continual problem, it is possible that the patient has low plasma levels of antithrombin III which will disrupt the pathway through which heparin acts. Antithrombin III itself or fresh frozen plasma (which contains a quantity of antithrombin III) can be given in these cases, or an alternative anticoagulant such as prostacyclin can be administered—although this will probably be less effective. Failure to establish the cause of repeated clotting of the circuit or filter can be expensive, time-consuming, and, most importantly, allows only intermittent control of uraemia. Many critical care units now use standardized protocols to guide management of anticoagulation during RRT (e.g. Figure 7.11).

Monitoring anticoagulation

If unfractionated heparin is used, samples for clotting tests (systemic APTT or ACT) should be taken from the

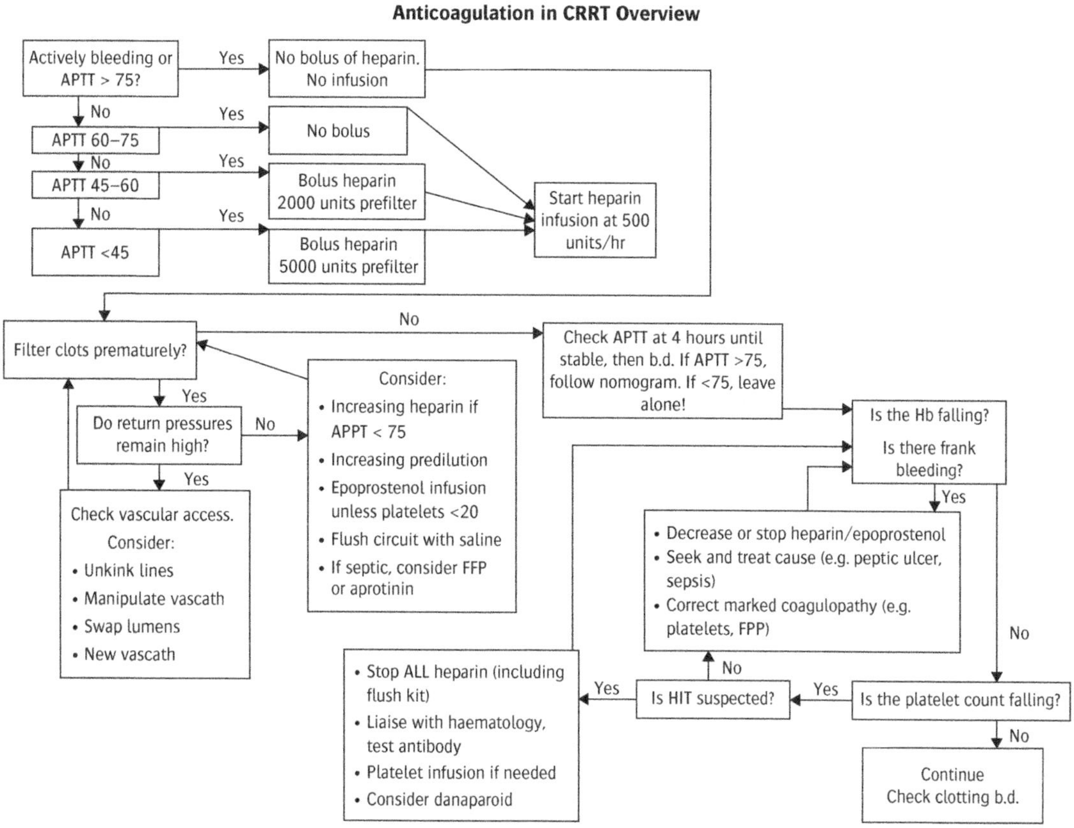

Anticoagulation in CRRT Overview

Actively bleeding or APTT > 75?
Yes
No bolus of heparin. No infusion
No
APTT 60–75
Yes
No bolus
No
APTT 45–60
Yes
Bolus heparin 2000 units prefilter
No
APTT <45
Yes
Bolus heparin 5000 units prefilter
Start heparin infusion at 500 units/hr
Filter clots prematurely?
No
Check APTT at 4 hours until stable, then b.d. If APTT >75, follow nomogram. If <75, leave alone!
Yes
Do return pressures remain high?
No
Consider:
• Increasing heparin if APPT < 75
• Increasing predilution
• Epoprostenol infusion unless platelets <20
• Flush circuit with saline
• If septic, consider FFP or aprotinin
Yes
Check vascular access.
Consider:
• Unkink lines
• Manipulate vascath
• Swap lumens
• New vascath
Is the Hb falling?
Is there frank bleeding?
Yes
• Decrease or stop heparin/epoprostenol
• Seek and treat cause (e.g. peptic ulcer, sepsis)
• Correct marked coagulopathy (e.g. platelets, FPP)
No
No
• Stop ALL heparin (including flush kit)
• Liaise with haematology, test antibody
• Platelet infusion if needed
• Consider danaparoid
Yes
Is HIT suspected?
Yes
Is the platelet count falling?
No
Continue
Check clotting b.d.

Figure 7.11 Anticoagulation algorithm.
University College Hospital, Critical Care Unit.

circuit distal to the haemofilter. (The heparin will have been infused at a proximal position to the filter.)

Safety

The importance of complete understanding of the practicalities of the RRT used and constant vigilance throughout the treatment cannot be overemphasized. The cannulae, circuits, and haemofilter machine are made to be as safe as possible, but RRT systems can be relatively complex. Complications are not uncommon and can be life-threatening; for example, an undetected disconnection at some point in the extracorporeal circuit can lead to exsanguination and/or air embolism. If air is entrained, the patient should be immediately placed in a head-down position and, if possible, on the left side. This is because air always moves to the top of any fluid medium. The priority is to prevent air entering the pulmonary circulation.

The vascular access device should be inspected regularly. The circuits should be supported to avoid undue tension being placed on the cannula(e), and the circuits and haemofiltration machine positioned to avoid being an obstacle to other equipment, especially emergency items, as the need to reach something quickly could result in inadvertent removal of cannulae or circuits.

Infection

Critically ill patients with AKI are generally immunocompromised to a greater or lesser degree. Strict aseptic methods must be used when inserting and manipulating vascular access devices and lines—and when priming or breaking the circuit (e.g. when setting up infusions of replacement or dialysate fluid).

The skin is the most common source of micro-organisms in catheter-associated bacteraemias. The vascular access device should be sutured in place and anchored with an adherent sterile transparent dressing for ease of viewing. If a local site infection is suspected, a swab should be taken for microbiological analysis and, unless there is a good reason not to, the catheter should be removed and a new venous access created at a different site. If a septic focus is suspected, the catheter tip and blood cultures should also be sent for analysis.

Drug removal

Renally excreted drugs can accumulate in AKI, while, in addition to waste products and other solutes, many therapeutic drugs are removed by RRT. Some drugs interact with the artificial kidney itself. Protein-bound drugs are less likely to be removed by the haemofilter because of the size of the drug–protein complex. It is particularly important to appreciate that levels of antibiotics can be significantly altered by AKI and RRT. If possible, a critical care pharmacist should advise on drug dosing (Intensive Care Society 2009). If an individual patient's GFR is unknown, drug prescription can be done on the basis that GFR will be about 10 ml/min for the patient with AKI, increasing to up to 50 ml/min if RRT is used. These factors should be remembered when titrating vasoactive drugs, sedatives, muscle relaxants, or analgesics, when the patient's requirements may seem unusually high. Plasma levels of aminoglycoside antibiotics (e.g. gentamicin) and other drugs which can be monitored (e.g. digoxin) should be regularly checked to ensure therapeutic levels.

Intermittent haemodialysis (IHD)

IHD is rarely used in UK, European, or Australian critical care units, but is often employed in the USA. The main principles are the same as those employed in CVVD: blood is pumped into an extracorporeal circuit where it is anticoagulated before passage through an artificial kidney or dialyser containing multiple hollow fibres or sheets that form semi-permeable membranes. Within the artificial kidney, dialysate fluid is pumped on the opposite side of the semi-permeable membrane to the blood, in a counter-current direction. Waste products move from the blood, across the membrane, and into the dialysate by diffusion.

A key difference from CVVD (and CVVHD) is that blood flows of up to 600 ml/min are used in haemodialysis. The clearance of small molecules is governed by the concentration gradient across the membrane and can also be enhanced by increasing the counter-current dialysate flow up to 500 ml/min. Water is removed by ultrafiltration with the exertion of a pressure across the semi-permeable membrane (so-called 'transmembrane pressure' or TMP). TMP is created by generating a positive pressure in the blood compartment and manipulating dialysate inflow and outflow to produce a relatively negative pressure on the dialysate side of the membrane.

Very large quantities of fluid are required for haemodialysis (in the range of 120 L per session), although there are systems that can recycle spent dialysate by passing it through a sorbent cartridge. This is an expensive option, but reduces the total volume of fluid required. Dialysate fluid must of course be sterile and contain appropriate levels of electrolytes and other solutes. These solutions are made up to suit the individual patient and their blood profile at a particular time, although this is a labour-intensive process.

Advantages of haemodialysis

- Its high intensity means that it is the most effective method of clearing waste products.
- An intermittent technique is used, and anticoagulation is only required during the procedure.
- The patient can be mobile between dialysis sessions.
- The intermittent nature is less demanding of nursing time when the treatment is not performed.

Disadvantages of haemodialysis

- Nursing staff need to be specifically trained in the technique.
- During a 2–4 hour period of HD, enough fluid has to be removed to allow nutrition and other infusions to be given throughout the period before the next treatment (usually 24–72 hours).
- The patient may develop a negative fluid balance at the end of dialysis, with the potential for significant fluid shifts leading to haemodynamic instability—especially in critical illness.
- Haemodialysis provides only episodic control of uraemia.
- Hypoxaemia, hypotension, and complement activation are associated with cheaper types of membrane and buffer solutions, all of which are undesirable in the critically ill patient.
- The equipment and water supply required can be expensive.

Nursing interventions

As with continuous RRT, there is a focus on detection and early treatment of complications. The dialysis machine incorporates various monitoring and alarm systems which must be observed, recorded, and acted on as necessary.

Complications

Some complications of haemodialysis are similar to those of CVVH and CVVHD, but can be more extreme in nature as haemodialysis is a more aggressive treatment that changes the patient's physiology more quickly.

Hypotension

Hypovolaemia and hypotension in the patient receiving haemodialysis may occur due to rapid and excessive removal of fluid. The acetate that is sometimes used as a buffer can also precipitate vasodilatation and hypotension. Critically ill patients receiving haemodialysis should have continuous blood pressure monitoring.

Cardiac dysrhythmias

Dysrhythmias caused by hypovolaemia or hypo/hyperkalaemia can occur, as they can in CVVH. Continuous ECG monitoring is required.

Hypoxaemia

Dialyser membranes have been known to cause hypoxaemia, probably secondary to cytokine activation, oxygen removal, and shunting. Continuous pulse oximetry, supported by arterial blood gas analysis when appropriate, should be performed during dialysis.

Muscle cramps, nausea, and vomiting

The aetiology of cramps, nausea, and vomiting is not completely understood but they are experienced by many patients receiving haemodialysis. The critically ill patient, who may be sedated, can present with signs of restlessness, agitation, and tachycardia, and, if so, the possibility of cramps or nausea should be considered. Common predisposing factors to cramps are hypotension, dehydration, and low plasma sodium.

Disequilibrium syndrome

Disequilibrium syndrome is a rare but potentially serious complication of haemodialysis. It is believed to be caused by the rapid removal of urea and 'uraemic toxins' during dialysis, which results in a much decreased concentration of these substances in the plasma when compared with the cerebrospinal fluid (CSF). The osmotic gradient that then develops between the plasma and CSF allows water to move into the CSF and brain tissue, causing headache, vomiting, restlessness, convulsions, and even coma. The severely uraemic patient should not experience a reduction in plasma urea of greater than 30% in the first treatment to avoid this complication.

Acute haemolysis

This can be caused by overheated, hypotonic, or contaminated dialysate fluid. The patient may complain of back pain, tightness in the chest, and dyspnoea. Blood in the venous circuit may take on a 'port wine' appearance in colour. If haemolysis is not detected, hyperkalaemia can result from the release of potassium from haemolysed red cells.

Plasma estimations of sodium, potassium, urea, and creatinine should be taken before and after dialysis, in addition to a coagulation screen. If possible, the patient should be weighed (perhaps on a 'weigh bed') before and after each session to estimate fluid status.

Continuous methods of RRT (primarily haemofiltration and haemodiafiltration) and haemodialysis are the most common forms of RRT used in critical care area units around the world (Legrand *et al.* 2013). Direct comparative evidence is lacking, but there is a consensus that continuous methods should be used for patients at risk from haemodynamic instability and also for those at particular risk from fluid shift, such as patients with acute brain injury (Lewington and Kanagasundaram 2011; KDIGO 2012). Less frequently used methods of RRT include slow continuous ultrafiltration (SCUF) and peritoneal dialysis (PD). As the phrase suggests, slow continuous ultrafiltration is a method of managing resistant fluid overload by gradual fluid removal through the haemofilter by convection. PD is relatively simple and inexpensive, but does not provide reliable control of uraemia, especially in the catabolic patient. Furthermore, PD can give rise to abdominal distension and restrict diaphragmatic movement so that ventilation is impaired, and is contraindicated in patients with abdominal pathology. Therefore it has little place in the care of the critically ill.

Disorders associated with renal dysfunction

Rhabdomyolysis

The relationship between skeletal muscle damage and impaired renal function was first noted in reports of air-raid casualties suffering crush injuries in the London Blitz (Bywaters and Beall 1941). Other causes include ingestion of toxins (e.g. alcohol, MDMA (ecstasy), heroin), and some prescription drugs (e.g. anti-psychotics, statins) (see Box 7.10).

Rhabdomyolysis has pre-renal, intrinsic renal (nephrotoxic), and post-renal (obstructive) effects. Damaged muscle releases potentially harmful quantities of myoglobin, which is the main cause of kidney injury (producing myoglobinuria), and also excessive creatine

Box 7.10 Causes of rhabdomyolysis

- Direct trauma, crush injury, burns
- Muscle compression from prolonged immobility (surgery, coma)
- Metabolic illness (diabetic metabolic decompensation)
- Hypokalaemia, hypophosphataemia
- Myxoedema
- Myositis
- Temperature extremes
- Toxins—alcohol, solvents, carbon monoxide, drug abuse (e.g. ecstasy, heroin)
- Muscular dystrophies
- Excessive muscle activity (e.g. prolonged seizures)

Box 7.11 Substances released by muscle

- Potassium → ηyperkalaemia
- Hydrogen ions → acidosis
- Phosphate → hyperphosphataemia
- Creatine → raised creatine kinase level
- Myoglobin → myoglobinuria

(elevating creatine kinase levels), hydrogen ions (causing acidosis), potassium (hyperkalaemia), and phosphate (hyperphosphataemia) (see Box 7.11). The phosphate chelates with calcium and this can cause hypocalcaemia, while increased leakage of salt and water may lead to hyponatraemia and hypovolaemia. Myoglobin (an iron-containing pigment found in skeletal muscle) is nephrotoxic, especially in the presence of acidosis and hypovolaemia. It can also obstruct the renal tubules.

Management of rhabdomyolysis

The principal aims are:

1. prevention of acute kidney injury
2. correction of electrolyte imbalances
3. prevention of further muscle damage.

Aggressive intravenous fluid therapy is required to optimize renal perfusion and to achieve a large diuresis so as to flush myoglobin from the renal tract; with the aim of producing ≥300 ml/h urine for ≥24 hours (Scharman and Troutman 2013). Alkalinization of the urine (pH >7) by giving IV sodium bicarbonate, with the objective of reducing oxidant damage, and use of mannitol and loop diuretics to promote urine flow may have some benefits, although the evidence for these methods is weak (Zimmerman and Shen, 2013). Care should be taken to maintain patency of the urinary catheter, especially if the urine contains excessive myoglobin. Hyperkalaemia in these cases is often resistant to dextrose and insulin therapy and therefore may be an early indication for haemodiafiltration. These patients are also highly catabolic, so adequate nutrition is a priority.

Careful attention must be given to any area of musculoskeletal damage, remembering that compartment syndrome may occur, when a muscle compartment is so compressed that neurovascular supply to distal areas is reduced and necrosis results. This has the potential for massive muscle and nerve damage. Compartment pressures may be monitored using an implanted needle connected to a manometer, with urgent fasciotomy indicated if pressures exceed 20–25 mmHg or other signs or symptoms of significant ischaemia are apparent. Any extremities affected should be regularly examined to check the quality of perfusion as indicated by strength of arterial pulses, skin colour, and temperature, and also the presence of swelling or any pain.

Hepatorenal syndrome

Hepatorenal syndrome (HRS) is a syndrome where renal failure resistant to volume expansion accompanies liver failure, particularly cirrhosis. The underlying mechanisms of HRS are not fully understood; the kidney structures and histology are essentially normal when examined. Pre-renal factors such as reduced circulating volume (e.g. due to haemorrhage), renal hypoperfusion (e.g. due to vasoconstriction of the renal cortical vasculature), infection (particularly bacterial peritonitis), and ascites are associated with the condition (Wadei and Gonwa 2013). Acute liver failure caused by hepatitis or paracetamol overdose may also lead to HRS.

HRS is characterized by low urinary sodium (<10 mmol/L) and increased urinary osmolality without proteinuria, i.e. the functions of sodium and water conservation are intact, unlike renal failure with coexisting liver disease where urinary sodium is >20 mmol/L. Type 1 HRS is mainly associated with some form of circulatory failure and an acute course with a doubling of serum creatinine to >220 μmol/L (>2.5 mg/dl) in <14 days, while type 2 HRS develops more slowly with less of an increase in creatinine and is more often associated with ascites. Both types of HRS significantly increase mortality; with type 1 having a particularly poor prognosis.

Management of HRS includes haemodynamic monitoring and fluid optimization (with administration of albumin in cirrhotic patients), RRT, treatment of liver failure, and control of ascites (Wadei and Gonwa 2013). Manipulation of vascular tone with vasoconstrictors such as vasopressin and its analogue terlipressin has been shown to improve renal function in several studies—but not survival as yet (Wadei and Gonwa 2013). A transjugular intrahepatic portosystemic shunt (TIPS) procedure to relieve portal hypertension in patients with cirrhosis and ascites may be beneficial in some cases.

Glomerulonephritis

The term glomerulonephritis encompasses a range of kidney disorders. The clinical presentation is variable and can be difficult to relate to histological findings. Circulating immune complexes that trigger systemic inflammation and complement activation are key factors. Circulating immunoglobulins are also a feature in a smaller number of cases. Some of the forms of glomerulonephritis encountered in critical care are outlined in the following sections.

Goodpasture's syndrome

This is a systemic autoimmune disorder also known as anti-glomerular basement membrane disease; it is seen more often in young men and diagnosed by a positive titre of anti-glomerular basement membrane antibody in the blood. It is frequently accompanied by haemoptysis (there may be pulmonary alveolar haemorrhage and bilateral lung opacities on chest X-ray), anaemia, proteinuria—and renal dysfunction. The pulmonary involvement can necessitate mechanical ventilatory support. Immunosuppression with steroids and cyclophosphamide together with plasmapheresis to remove circulating antibodies are the mainstays of treatment.

Vasculitis

Vasculitis may present as polyarteritis nodosa (when damaged arteries develop multiple small aneurysms) with diverse signs and symptoms including asthma, hypertension, neuropathy, abdominal pain, and skin rashes. Renal dysfunction can rapidly follow, with haematuria, proteinuria, and nephrotic syndrome. It is diagnosed by histology or raised P-ANCA. P-ANCA is the P form of antineutrophil cytoplasmic antibody in the blood.

Vasculitis can also accompany granulomatosis with polyangiitis (GPA), formerly known as Wegener's granulomatosis, in which blood vessels and the respiratory and renal tracts are all damaged by vasculitic lesions. Diagnosis is by histology or raised C-ANCA (the C form of ANCA).

Again, treatment of vasculitis is with steroids, cyclophosphamide, and plasmapheresis.

Systemic lupus erythematosus

Systemic lupus erythematosus (SLE) is the most frequently reported autoimmune disease in critical care (Quintero *et al.* 2013). A requirement for respiratory support is the most common reason for admission, but renal function is often impacted as well. Myocardial, cerebral, and hepatic involvement may also be seen, as well as thrombotic events. Females are affected more than males, with various presentations including fever, rashes, and arthritis. Diagnosis is by positive titre to double-stranded DNA antibody in the blood. Treatment consists of immunosuppression with steroids and blood purification with plasmapheresis.

References and bibliography

Adrogué, H.J., Gennari, F.J., Galla, J.H., *et al.* (2009). Assessing acid–base disorders. *Kidney International*, **76**, 1239–47.

Avila, M.O., Zanetta, D.M., Abdulkader, R.C., *et al.* (2009). Urine volume in acute kidney injury: how much is enough? *Renal Failure*, **31**, 884–90.

Bywaters, E.G., Beall, D. (1941). Crush injuries with impairment of renal function. *British Medical Journal*, **i**(4185), 427–32.

Grams, M.E., Estrella, M.M., Coresh, J., *et al.* (2011). Fluid balance, diuretic use, and mortality in acute kidney injury. *Clinical Journal of the American Society of Nephrology*, **6**, 966–73.

Hedges, S.J., Dehoney, S.B., Hooper, J.S., *et al.* (2007). Evidence-based treatment recommendations for uremic bleeding. *Nature Clinical Practice. Nephrology*, **3**, 138–53.

Hoste, E.A. and Schurgers, M. (2008). Epidemiology of acute kidney injury: how big is the problem? *Critical Care Medicine*, **36**(Suppl), S146–51.

Intensive Care Society (2009). *Recommendations for the Provision of Renal Replacement Therapy on Intensive Care Units in the United Kingdom*. Report, Intensive Care Society, London.

Karajala, V., Mansour, W., Kellum, J.A. (2009). Diuretics in acute kidney injury. *Minerva Anestesiologia*, **75**, 251–7.

KDIGO (Kidney Disease: Improving Global Outcomes): Acute Kidney Injury Work Group (2012). KDIGO clinical practice guideline for acute kidney Injury. *Kidney International Supplements*, **2**(1), 1–138.

Kellum, J.A., Unruh, M.L., Murugan, R. (2011). Acute kidney injury. *BMJ Clinical Evidence*, pii: 2001.

Kolhe, N.V., Stevens, P.E., Crowe, A.V., *et al.* (2008). Case mix, outcome and activity for patients with severe acute kidney injury during the first 24 hours after admission to an adult, general critical care unit: application of predictive models from a secondary analysis of the ICNARC Case Mix Programme database. *Critical Care*, **12** (Suppl 1), S2.

Lassnigg, A., Donner, E., Grubhofer, G., *et al.* (2000). Lack of renoprotective effects of dopamine and furosemide during cardiac surgery. *Journal of the American Society of Nephrology*, **11**, 97–104.

Legrand, M., Darmon, M., Joannidis, M., *et al.* (2013), Management of renal replacement therapy in ICU patients: an international survey. *Intensive Care Medicine*, **39**, 101–8.

Lewington, A., Kanagasundaram, S. (2011) *Acute Kidney Injury*. http://www.renal.org/Clinical/GuidelinesSection/AcuteKidneyInjury.aspx#downloads (accessed 1 June 2012).

Mehta, R.L., Kellum, J.A., Shah, S.V., *et al.* (2007). Acute Kidney Injury Network: report of an initiative to improve outcomes in acute kidney injury. *Critical Care*. **11**, R31.

Oudemans-van Straaten, H.M., Ostermann, M. (2012). Bench-to-bedside review. Citrate for continuous renal replacement therapy: from science to practice. *Critical Care*, **16**, 249.

Quintero, O.L., Rojas-Villarraga, A., Mantilla, R.D., *et al.* (2013). Autoimmune diseases in the intensive care unit: an update. *Autoimmunity Reviews*, **12**, 380–95.

RENAL Replacement Therapy Study Investigators (2009). Intensity of continuous renal-replacement therapy in critically ill patients. *New England Journal of Medicine*, **361**, 1627–38.

Resuscitation Council UK (2011). *Advanced Life Support* (6th edn). London: Resuscitation Council UK.

Rimmelé, T., Kellum, J.A. (2011). Clinical review: blood purification for sepsis. *Critical Care*, **15**, 205.

Scharman, E.J., Troutman, W.G. (2013). Prevention of kidney injury following rhabdomyolysis: a systematic review. *Annals of Pharmacotherapy*, **47**, 90–105.

Schrier, R.W. (2010). ARF, AKI, or ATN? *Nature Reviews Nephrology*, **6**, 125.

Swärd, K., Valsson, F., Sellgren, J., *et al.* (2005). Differential effects of human atrial natriuretic peptide and furosemide on glomerular filtration rate and renal oxygen consumption in humans. *Intensive Care Medicine*, **31**, 79–85.

Uchino, S., Fealy, N., Baldwin, I., *et al.* (2003). Pre-dilution vs. post-dilution during continuous veno-venous hemofiltration: impact on filter life and azotemic control. *Nephron Clinical Practice*, **94**, c94–8.

VA/NIH Acute Renal Failure Trial Network (2008). Intensity of renal support in critically ill patients with acute kidney injury. *New England Journal of Medicine*, **359**, 7–20.

Wadei, H.M., Gonwa, T.A. (2013). Hepatorenal syndrome in the intensive care unit. *Journal of Intensive Care Medicine*, **28**, 79–92.

Zimmerman, J.L., Shen, M.C. (2013). Rhabdomyolysis. *Chest*, **144**, 1058–65.

CHAPTER 8
Neurological problems

Introduction

There is limited scope within the confines of a single chapter to cover all the neurological conditions that the critical care nurse might meet. However, important aspects of neuroscience nursing and some of the more common conditions are covered. A brief overview of related basic anatomy and physiology is also included as revision for the reader.

An understanding of neurological conditions and their consequences and the ability to effectively monitor and detect changes in a patient's condition are crucial to patient outcome. Improving ICU care, in combination with good medical and nursing management, can prevent secondary brain injury and has been shown to improve outcome in this group of patients. While this chapter focuses mainly on acute nursing and medical management, it should be recognized that rehabilitation for these patients should start as soon as possible, even in the acute stage in critical care, and this requires a multidisciplinary approach.

Anatomy and physiology

The bony cranial vault, three layers of protective membranes (the meninges), and the cerebrospinal fluid (CSF) all physically protect the brain.

Meninges

The three layers of meninges are as follows (see Figure 8.1).

1. **Dura mater** (Latin for 'hard mother'). The dura is the outermost layer and is composed of tough fibrous connective tissue with outer (periosteal) and inner (meningeal) components. The dural layer extends into the cranial cavity to form the falx cerebri (between the two hemispheres) and the tentorium cerebelli (between the cerebellum and the occipital lobes). While neural tissue itself does not generally sense pain, the dura does.
2. ***Arachnoid mater*** (from the Greek for 'spider'). The arachnoid is the middle of the three meninges and adheres closely to the inner surface of the dura mater. It is a thin avascular spider-web-like membrane containing arachnoid villi—protrusions of arachnoid membrane into the superior sagittal sinus. The arachnoid villi act as one-way valves for the flow of CSF from the subarachnoid space to the venous sinuses.
3. **Pia mater** (Latin for 'tender mother'). The pia is the innermost layer and is composed of thin connective tissue. Unlike the dura and arachnoid layers, which closely follow the contours of the cranial vault, the pia mater follows the contours of the brain. As a result, the space between the arachnoid and pial layers (the subarachnoid space) contains cerebrospinal fluid and is not uniform; the larger spaces are called subarachnoid cisterns.

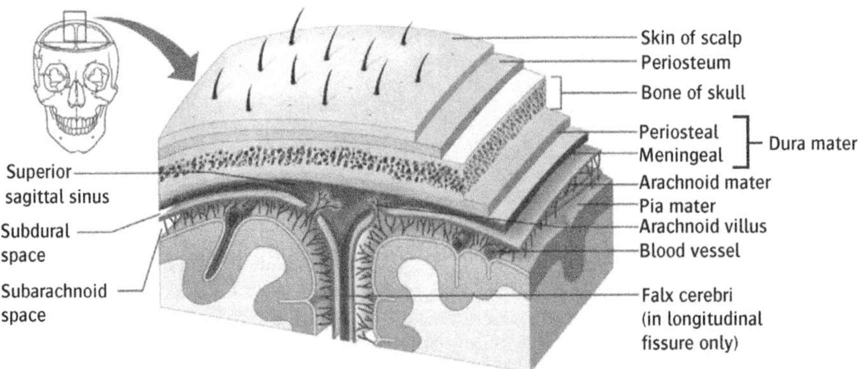

Figure 8.1 The meninges of the brain.

Reprinted from Marieb, E.N., *Essentials of Human Anatomy and Physiology* (9th edn), copyright (2009) printed and electronically reproduced by permission of Pearson Education, Inc.

Cerebrum

The cerebrum is divided into two hemispheres (Figure 8.2). The outermost (2–4 mm thick) is the cerebral cortex, or grey matter, which consists of nerve cell bodies. The cerebral cortex is necessary for conscious awareness, thought, memory, and intellect. All sensory input must reach the cerebral cortex (mostly via the thalamus) to be consciously perceived and interpreted, and passed on to the cortical motor areas for the appropriate

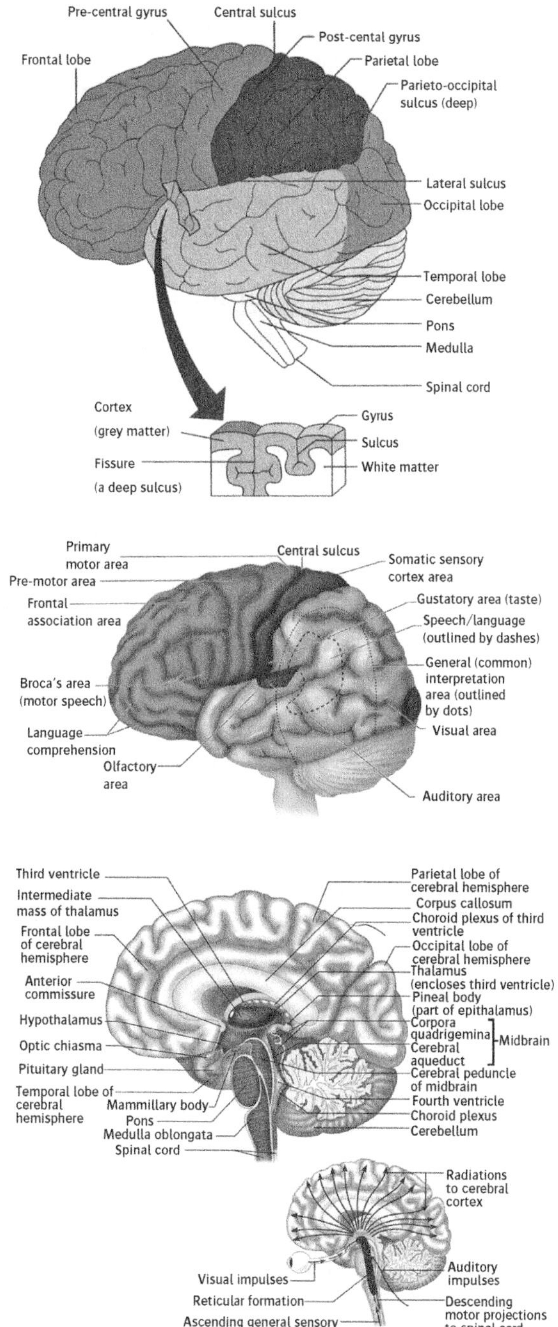

Figure 8.2 The cerebral hemispheres, cerebellum, and brainstem. (a) Left lateral view of major structural areas. (b) Functional areas of the cerebral hemisphere. (c) Midbrain structures, cerebellum, and brainstem.

motor response. Certain important areas of grey matter, such as the thalamus and basal ganglia (see later), are also found deeper in the brain tissue.

The white matter beneath the grey matter consists of axons that project from the cell bodies and carry messages between them. Many axons are surrounded by a layer of lipid or myelin sheath that acts as an electrical insulator, allowing rapid transmission of impulses. Ascending fibres taking sensory information to the cortex and descending fibres controlling movement cross over from one side to the other. Thus each cerebral hemisphere mostly perceives sensations and controls the movements of the opposite side of the body. In most individuals, cortical areas in the frontal, parietal, and temporal lobes of the left hemisphere are responsible for the comprehension and expression of language. Therefore the left hemisphere is said to be dominant for language.

Each hemisphere is divided into four lobes<

1. The **frontal lobe** is concerned with executive functioning. It contains important areas: the primary motor cortex, the pre-motor cortex, and the supplementary motor cortex and Broca's area for speech in the dominant hemisphere.
2. The **parietal lobe** deals mainly with functions connected with movement, orientation, and calculation, and contains the primary somatosensory cortex and association cortex.
3. The **temporal lobe** is concerned with sound, speech comprehension (dominant hemisphere), and some aspects of memory. It contains the primary auditory cortex and auditory association cortex (also known as Wernicke's area) in the dominant hemisphere.
4. The **occipital lobe** is made up almost entirely of visual processing areas including the primary visual cortex and the visual association cortex.

Cerebellum

The cerebellum (from the Latin 'little brain') modulates and regulates motor function. It is primarily concerned with coordination of movements on the same side. Cerebellar integrity is important for smooth, accurate, coordinated motor tasks and the maintenance of a stable posture.

Thalamus

The thalamus is an area of grey matter deep within the brain that acts as a relay station, modifying and directing incoming information to the appropriate area of the cerebral cortex for further processing. In turn, the cerebral cortex can modify the activity of the thalamus, thus influencing the messages sent.

Hypothalamus

The hypothalamus has been established as the master pacemaker, driving circadian rhythms in physiology and behaviour through autonomic and neuroendocrine modulation via the pituitary gland. The hypothalamus plays an important role in thermoregulation.

Basal ganglia

The basal ganglia control motor output for the body, head, and eyes, and work in conjunction with the supplementary motor area of the frontal lobes to plan movements prior to initiation.

Brainstem

The brainstem, comprising midbrain, pons, and medulla, has attachments for the cranial nerves III–XII (see Table 8.1). It also contains part of the reticular formation that controls the level of consciousness and the

Table 8.1 Cranial nerves

Cranial nerve	Main function(s)
Olfactory (sensory)	Smell
Optic (sensory)	Vision
Oculomotor (mixed—primarily motor)	Movement of eyelid and eyeball, pupil size and shape
Trochlear (mixed—primarily motor)	Movement of eyeball
Trigeminal (mixed)	Chewing, facial sensation
Abducens (mixed—primarily motor)	Movement of eyeball
Facial (mixed)	Facial expression, activates salivary and lacrimal glands, supplies taste buds of anterior tongue
Vestibulocochlear (sensory)	Hearing and balance
Glossopharyngeal (mixed)	Swallowing, gag reflex
Vagus (mixed)	Swallowing, speech, control of visceral organs
Accessory (mixed—primarily motor)	Movement of head and shoulders
Hypoglossal (mixed—primarily motor)	Swallowing

cardiovascular and respiratory systems. Ascending and descending fibres pass through the brainstem en route to the thalamus and spinal cord.

Communication within the central nervous system

Nerve cells, or neurons (Figure 8.3), are the structural and functional units of the nervous system. Their functions are to receive and integrate incoming information from sensory receptors or other neurons, and to transmit information to other neurons or effector organs. They generate and conduct electrical changes in the form of nerve impulses, and communicate chemically with other neurons at points of contact called synapses. The release of a neurotransmitter substance at these synapses is the essential link between neurons.

A neuron's chemical and physical environment influences both impulse conduction and synaptic transmission. Alkalosis (pH >7.45) results in increased excitability of neurons, while acidosis (pH <7.35) results in progressive depression of neuronal activity.

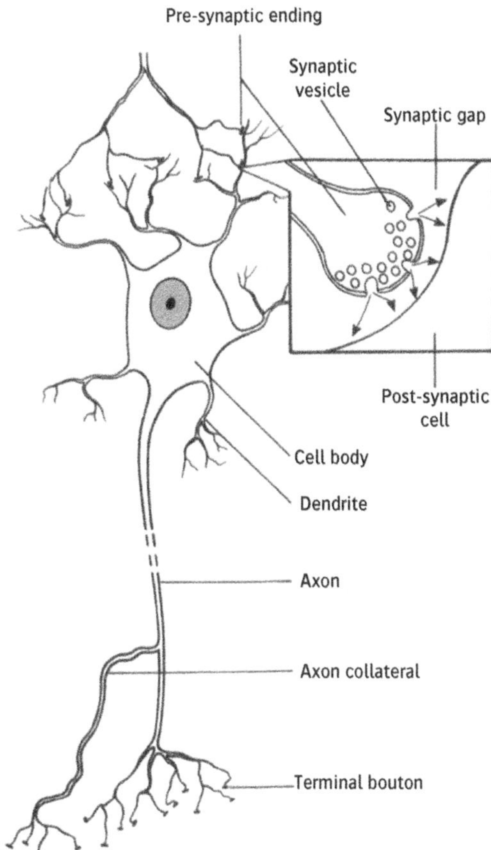

Figure 8.3 The basic structure of the neuron and synapse

This figure was published in *Neuroanatomy: An Illustrated Colour Text*, Crossman, A.R. and Neary, D, Copyright Elsevier (1998).

The other major cells within the central nervous system (CNS) are neuroglial cells (from the Greek word meaning 'glue') that provide support, insulation, and nourishment to neurons. Unlike neurons, the neuroglial cells do not have a direct role in information processing but take on various supporting roles essential for the normal functioning of neurons. There are four types of neuroglial cell:

- oligodendroglia form the myelin sheath around neuronal axons, which is important for the propagation of the nerve impulse (in the peripheral nervous system myelin is made by Schwann cells)
- astrocytes form tight junctions between neurons and the blood supply and therefore are essential to the 'blood–brain barrier'
- ependymal cells form the inner surface of the ventricles and the central canal of the spinal cord
- microglia have a phagocytic role when there is injury to the CNS.

Neurotransmitters

Numerous transmitter substances have been identified within the CNS (Table 8.2). These enable communication between brain cells and are localized in certain parts of the brain. They can excite, inhibit or enhance the actions of post-synaptic neurons. Examples include acetylcholine (ACh), various amino acids (e.g. glutamate, g-aminobutyric acid (GABA)) and catecholamines (noradrenaline, dopamine, serotonin).

Peptides

Numerous peptides are also stored and released at synapses (Table 8.3). They modulate the release and effects of other transmitters and include substance P, enkephalins and endorphins.

Ventricular system

The ventricular system consists of two C-shaped lateral ventricles (one per hemisphere), a narrow slit-like third ventricle (bounded on either side by the thalamus and hypothalamus), and a fourth ventricle (between the cerebellum and the brainstem at the level of the pons and medulla) (Figure 8.4). In adults, approximately 150 ml of CSF is in circulation, half around the brain and half around the spinal cord. CSF is constantly produced by the choroid plexus of the ventricles and fills the ventricular and subarachnoid spaces (about 500 ml

Table 8.2 Neurotransmitters

Neurotransmitter	Details
Acetylcholine (ACh)	ACh is the transmitter between neurons and striated muscle, and at autonomic ganglia. It produces an excitatory effect. Blockage of ACh receptors (AChR) in skeletal muscles at the neuromuscular junction occurs after administration of non-depolarizing neuromuscular blocking drugs (e.g. atracurium, vecuronium) and in myasthenia gravis.
Glutamate	Glutamate is widespread throughout the CNS and has an excitatory effect. It is important for learning and memory, and is implicated in epilepsy and excitotoxic cell death after brain injury.
Gamma-aminobutyric acid (GABA)	GABA has a high concentration in the thalamus, hypothalamus, and occipital lobes and is the most common inhibitory neurotransmitter. Some drugs (e.g. anti-anxiety drugs) enhance the action of GABA. Some of the drugs used to control epilepsy work by modifying the balance between glutamate and GABA.
Dopamine (DA)	DA is found mainly in the midbrain and basal ganglia and exerts a mostly inhibitory effect. It is involved in emotional responses and subconscious movement of skeletal muscles, and is implicated in Parkinson's disease, addiction, and schizophrenia.
Norepinephrine (NE)	NE is released at some neuromuscular and neuroglandular junctions and is mostly excitatory. It is highly concentrated in the brainstem and is involved in arousal, dreaming, and regulation of mood. Changes in NE levels are implicated in depressive illness
Serotonin (5-hydroxy-tryptamine, 5-HT)	Serotonin is concentrated in the brainstem and is mostly excitatory. It is involved in inducing sleep, sensory perception, temperature regulation, and control of mood. Like norepinephrine, serotonin is implicated in depressive illness

Table 8.3 Neuropeptides

Neuropeptide	Details
Substance P	Substance P is found in sensory nerves, spinal cord pathways, and parts of the brain associated with pain.
Enkephalins	Enkephalins are the body's own natural painkillers and are several times more potent than morphine.
Endorphins	Endorphins are concentrated in the pituitary gland and, like enkephalins, have morphine-like properties to suppress pain. Both enkephalins and endorphins inhibit pain impulses partly by suppressing substance P.

is produced daily). It is reabsorbed through the arachnoid villi in the sagittal sinus into the venous system. CSF cushions and protects the brain, acts as a pathway for nutrients and chemical mediators, and affects cerebral blood flow and pulmonary ventilation via pH levels.

Cerebral circulation

Arterial blood supply

There are two arterial systems: (i) the right and left internal carotid arteries, which supply the anterior two-thirds of the cerebral hemispheres, and (ii) the vertebrobasilar system, which supplies the posterior regions of the hemispheres, brainstem, and cerebellum (Figure 8.5). The anastamoses between the internal carotid and vertebrobasilar systems (at the anterior and posterior communicating arteries) form the circle of Willis.

Venous drainage

There are a series of external and internal veins that drain into the venous sinuses, formed by folds of the dura mater (Figure 8.6). The sinuses have no valves and therefore venous drainage is gravity-dependent. Superficial cerebral veins in the subarachnoid space drain the cerebral cortex and white matter and empty into the intracranial venous sinuses. The upper part of each hemisphere drains into the superior sagittal sinus, the middle part drains into the cavernous sinus, while the lower part drains into the transverse sinus.

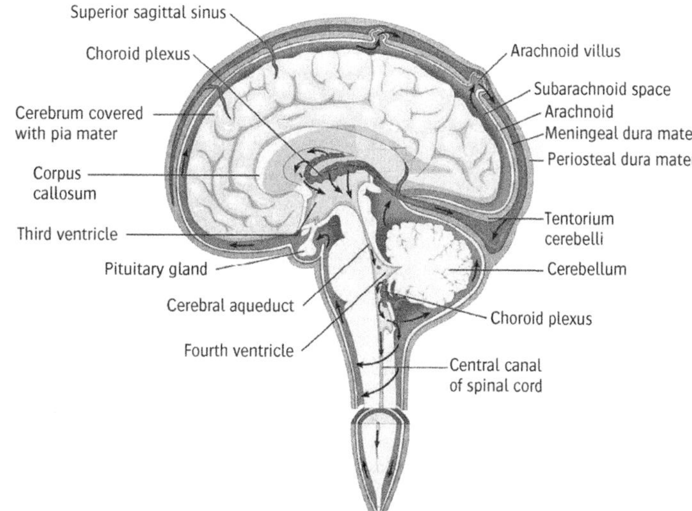

Figure 8.4 The ventricular system

Reprinted from Marieb, E.N., *Essentials of Human Anatomy and Physiology* (9th edn), copyright (2009) printed and electronically reproduced by permission of Pearson Education, Inc.

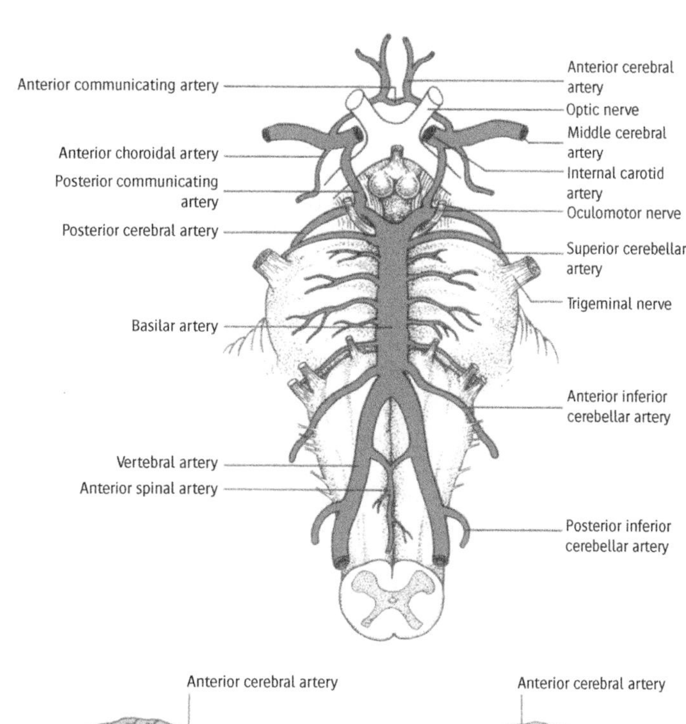

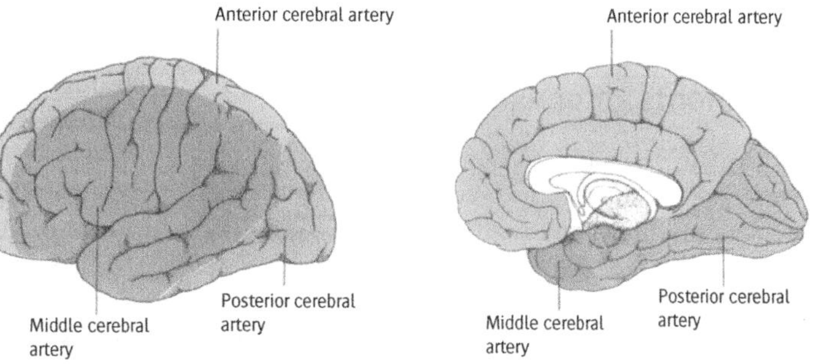

Figure 8.5 (a) Cerebral arterial blood supply (circle of Willis). (b) Cortical distribution

This figure was published in *Neuroanatomy: An Illustrated Colour Text*, Crossman, A.R. and Neary, D. Copyright Elsevier (1998).

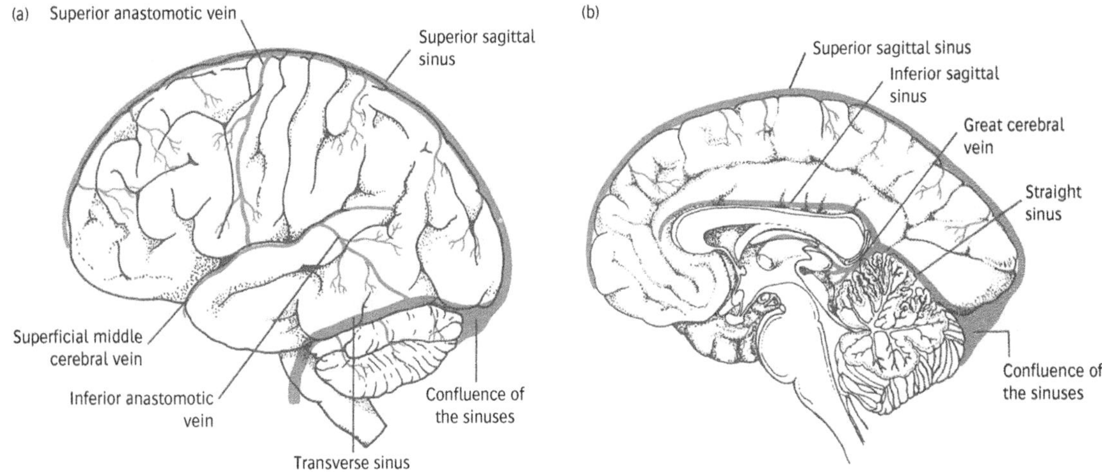

Figure 8.6 Cerebral venous drainage: (a) lateral view, (b) sagittal view.
This figure was published in *Neuroanatomy: An Illustrated Colour Text*, Crossman, A.R. and Neary, D, Copyright Elsevier (1998).

Spinal cord

This is continuous with the medulla oblongata of the brainstem and is surrounded and protected by the vertebral column and three layers of membrane (the meningeal dura, arachnoid, and pia mater). The spinal cord is divided into two almost symmetrical halves by anterior and posterior grooves. In its centre is the small central canal which is a continuation of the cerebral ventricular system. In contrast with the cerebrum and cerebellum, the grey matter (consisting of nerve cell bodies) in the spinal cord is innermost, while the white matter (containing ascending and descending nerve fibres) is on the outside.

Many functions within the spinal cord can operate in an automatic or reflex action. However, when information is conveyed to specific areas of the brain via the ascending nerve fibres, the brain can exert a controlling influence over these spinal mechanisms via the descending nerve pathways.

Neurological assessment

Despite continued developments in neuromonitoring, clinical observation remains the most sensitive measure of neurological function. Impaired consciousness is an expression of brain dysfunction as a whole, so changes in conscious level provide the best indication of the development of complications following brain injury.

Components of consciousness

This is a state of general awareness of oneself and the environment. It has two components, arousal and awareness, and these arise from the reticular activating system (RAS) in the brainstem and the cerebral cortex, respectively (see Figure 8.2). Consciousness depends on interaction between the neurons in the RAS and cortical neurons. The content of consciousness is determined by neurons in the cerebral cortex, while those in the RAS are responsible for the primitive state of arousal.

Arousal

Simply being awake is a primitive state managed by the RAS. This consists of neurons extending through the central core of the brainstem, with projections upwards to the cortex and downwards to the spinal cord. It receives auditory impulses, visual impulses, and impulses from the ascending sensory tracts. Because of its connections, it is ideal for governing arousal of the brain as a whole.

Unless inhibited by other brain areas (e.g. sleep-inducing areas), reticular neurons send a continuous stream of impulses to the cerebral cortex, maintaining the cortex in an alert conscious state. The RAS is the physical basis of consciousness. It is selective, forwarding only essential information to the cortex and filtering out unnecessary information. Certain drugs have a direct effect on the RAS; it is depressed by alcohol, sleep-inducing drugs, and tranquillizers, while some mood-enhancing drugs (e.g. LSD) cause heightened sensory arousal.

Awareness

Awareness is the more sophisticated part of consciousness, requiring an intact cerebral cortex to interpret the sensory input from the RAS and respond accordingly.

Assessing consciousness

Consciousness cannot be measured directly and can only be assessed by observing a person's behaviour in response to different stimuli. The response indicates the level at which sensory information has been translated within the CNS.

Levels of sensation

Sensory impulses terminating in the spinal cord can generate spinal reflexes without involving the brain, for example the brain-dead patient whose legs move when a peripheral painful stimulus is applied to them. Here the sensation is translated by the spinal cord which also generates the reaction. Sensory impulses reaching the lower brainstem cause subconscious motor reactions, for example non-purposeful decorticate (flexor) and decerebrate (extensor) motor responses). Impulses that reach the thalamus can be identified as a specific sensation (touch, pain, etc.) and localized crudely in the body, for example the patient flexing to painful stimuli. Only when sensory information reaches the cerebral cortex is there precise localization, for example the patient localizing to a painful stimulus. The sensory cortex identifies and localizes the source, while the motor cortex acts to remove the noxious stimulus.

Neurological assessment

Neurological assessment must include:

- assessment of conscious level (Glasgow Coma Scale)
- limb assessments
- pupil size and reaction to light
- vital signs.

The Glasgow Coma Scale (GCS)

Prior to the development of the GCS in 1974, level of consciousness was described in terms such as stupor, semi-coma, and deep coma. However, these terms were not clearly defined and there was considerable inconsistency between different observers. The GCS was designed to standardize observations using a simple system based on clearly definable criteria that could be reproduced objectively and reliably by a range of medical and nursing personnel, and 40 years on it has undergone a wide-ranging review to promote a more consistent and structured approach to assessment.

Conscious level is defined by three modes of behaviour: eye-opening, verbal response, and motor response. In each category, the response generated by different stimuli is assessed, with an increasing stimulus required to elicit a response indicating a decrease in the level of cerebral functioning. Each response is given a score and these are summed to range between 3 and 15 (Table 8.4). The best response in each category is recorded; therefore it provides a global assessment only.

Table 8.4 Glasgow Coma Scale and Score

Eye-opening	Score	Best verbal response	Score	Best motor response	Score
Spontaneous	4	Orientated	5	Obeys commands	6
To sound	3	Confused	4	Localizing	5
To pressure	2	Words	3	Normal flexion	4
	1	Sounds	2	Abnormal flexion	3
		None	1	Extension	2
				None	1

Adapted from *The Lancet*, Volume 304, Issue 7872, Graham Teasdale, Bryan Jennett, Assessment of coma and impaired consciousness: a practical scale, pp. 81–4, Copyright (1974), with permission from Elsevier.

The Glasgow Coma Scale is universally used to assess conscious level in the acute phase of brain injury and should be charted graphically to enable easy identification of any change in the patient's condition. It is more accurate in assessing altered levels of consciousness due to cerebral trauma than those due to medical causes.

Eye-opening

Eye-opening assesses arousal mechanisms and control of the eyes in the brainstem (see Box 8.1). Even when brain damage is severe, all patients who survive will eventually open their eyes (usually within 2–4 weeks). Spontaneous eye-opening merely indicates that the arousal mechanisms in the brainstem are active and does not necessarily mean that the patient is aware.

Verbal response

Verbal response assesses two elements of cerebral functioning, namely comprehension and transmission of sensory input, and the ability to articulate a reply. An orientated response shows a high degree of integration within the nervous system (see Box 8.2).

Motor response

This is the most important prognostic aspect of the Glasgow Coma Scale after traumatic brain injury (see Box 8.3). Here, the *best* response is recorded as an indication of the functional state of the brain as a whole. Only the response of the *upper limbs* is recorded, as this is more reliable than lower limb responses that could be purely spinal reflexes.

If the patient does not obey commands, motor activity has to be assessed by applying central pressure (e.g. pressure to the supra-orbital notch or trapezius pinch) and observing the response. The stimulus must be applied in a standard way and maintained until a maximum response is obtained. If there is no response to central stimulus, a peripheral stimulus should be applied.

Limb responses

A difference in responsiveness in one limb compared with the other indicates focal brain damage. Hemiparesis or hemiplegia usually occurs in the limbs on the opposite

Box 8.1 Assessment of eye-opening

- **Spontaneous**: observed before you approach the patient or speak to him/her.
- **To sound**: call the patient's name.
- **To pressure**: apply pressure to the side of the finger. (Central stimulus to the supra-orbital nerve will cause grimacing and eye closure.)
- **None**: ensure that the pressure is adequate.

Box 8.2 Assessment of verbal response

- **Orientated**: knows time, place, person. (Should know who he/she is, where he/she is, and why he/she is there, and know the month, year, season. If the patient answers one or more component wrongly then he/she must be recorded as confused.)
- **Confused**: talking in sentences but disorientated to time and place. (Patient attends to questioning but shows disorientation.)
- **Words**: utters occasional words rather than sentences. (These are often abusive words elicited by noxious stimuli rather than spontaneous.)
- **Sounds**: groans or grunts.
- **None**: if the patient has an ET tube or tracheostomy, T is recorded in this section.

Box 8.3 Assessment of motor response

- **Obeys commands**: 'Hold up your arms', 'Stick out your tongue'. (If you ask the patient to squeeze your hand, beware of the reflex hand grasp in unconscious patients.)
- **Localizing**: apply a pressure to the supra-orbital nerve until a response is observed. If the patient responds by bringing a hand up purposefully to the chin or above, this is localizing. (If there is trauma to the eyes, use the trapezius pinch.)
- **Normal flexion**: elbow bending is recorded as flexing to pain.
- **Abnormal flexion**: elbow flexion is accompanied by spastic flexion of the wrist.
- **Extension**: straightening of the elbow is recorded as extending.
- **None**: ensure that the stimulus is adequate.

side to the lesion (due to cross-over of nerve fibres in the medulla). However, it may also affect the limbs on the same side as the lesion because of pressure on the contralateral hemisphere (Kernohan's notch syndrome—a false localizing sign).

Pupillary response

Pupillary response to light depends upon intact afferent (optic nerve) and efferent (oculomotor nerve) function transmitting the light impulse from the retina to the midbrain and hence the pupillary musculature. A dilating pupil indicates an expanding lesion on the same side (ipsilateral since the oculomotor nerve does not cross over) and is an important localizing sign. As pupillary pathways are relatively resistant to metabolic insults, the presence or absence of the light reflex is the single most important sign potentially distinguishing structural from metabolic coma.

- Pupils should be assessed for size, shape, equality and reaction to light.
- Bilateral fixed and dilated pupils in a patient whose motor response is flexion or localizing suggests the recent occurrence of a seizure (or homatropine eye drops).
- Muscle relaxants do not affect pupil reaction. It is the only clinical sign of raised intracranial pressure (ICP) that can be tested i the patient who is paralysed and sedated. Since pupil abnormalities are a late sign of intracranial complications, such patients require ICP monitoring.
- Damage to the cervical cord or brachial plexus can cause inequality of the pupils due to Horner's syndrome.

Vital signs

Temperature

Temperature regulation may be disrupted due to damage to the hypothalamus. In the acute phase of brain injury hyperthermia should be treated since it will exacerbate cerebral ischaemia and adversely affect outcome.

Heart rate

ECG changes may occur in the acute stage following cerebral insult as a result of catecholamine release (the transient 'sympathetic storm'). These can include peaked P waves, prolonged QT interval, heightened T waves, and ST segment elevation or depression.

- Bradycardia (HR <50 bpm) is present in the later stages of raised ICP (compensatory phase—Cushing's response), or when there is an associated cervical injury.
- Tachycardia (HR >100 bpm) is present in the terminal stage of raised ICP.
- Arrhythmias are seen particularly with posterior fossa lesions or when there is blood in the CSF.

Blood pressure

In a normal brain a fall in BP does not cause a drop in cerebral perfusion pressure (CPP) since autoregulation results in cerebral vasodilation to protect brain tissue. However, following a cerebral insult when autoregulation may be impaired, hypotension may lead to brain ischaemia. Hypotension (defined as a systolic BP <90 mmHg) has been uniformly identified as the predominant factor in secondary brain injury and has the greatest association with morbidity and mortality.

- Hypotension is rarely attributable to cerebral injury itself, although this can occur in children. In severe brain injury it occurs as a terminal event when regulatory mechanisms in the medulla are no longer functioning because of inadequate perfusion.
- When hypotension and tachycardia are seen together the possibility of extracranial haemorrhage should be considered.
- Hypotension and bradycardia are seen with associated cervical spine injury due to autonomic dysfunction.
- Hypertension is associated with a rising ICP and is part of the Cushing's response, i.e. a rising BP with a widening pulse pressure, bradycardia, and decreasing respirations. This late response may not appear in some patients and is invariably preceded by a drop in GCS.

Respiration

Respiratory complications are common following cerebral insults. Patients often require advanced respiratory support even in the acute stage<

- The cerebral hemispheres regulate voluntary control over the muscles used in breathing.
- The cerebellum synchronizes and coordinates muscular effort.
- The brainstem regulates the automaticity of breathing.

An acute rise in ICP initially causes slowing of the respiratory rate. This indicates loss of cerebral and cerebellar control of breathing, with control being only at brainstem level. As ICP continues to rise, the rate becomes rapid, indicating that the brainstem is also affected.

Appropriate use of neurological assessment

Recording of neurological observations is only indicated when a patient has an injury or illness affecting the central nervous system. When the injury or illness involves the brain, observations must include the Glasgow Coma Scale and pupil and limb assessments. When it involves the spinal cord, limb assessments only need to be recorded (C1–T6, upper and lower limbs; T7 and below, lower limbs only). This applies even in high cervical spine surgery. The only exceptions are when there has been additional foramen magnum decompression or transoral access to the odontoid peg. In these cases, the GCS should also be documented in the first 12–24 hours post-surgery to detect haematoma formation or swelling that might cause brainstem compression or impede drainage of the fourth ventricle, leading to hydrocephalus. After this initial post-operative period limb assessments only are required.

The GCS was designed for the acute phase of brain injury when the patient's condition may fluctuate and there is an increased risk of secondary complications. It is not always an appropriate tool in chronic neurological conditions. Once the patient has passed the acute phase, when neurological observations need to be recorded less frequently than four-hourly, the appropriateness of using the GCS should be questioned.

Intracranial dynamics and possible changes following brain injury

Evidence for the changes in intracranial dynamics that can occur following brain injury is mainly derived from studies in traumatic brain injury (TBI). However, in practice, these are applied to guide the management of patients with other brain insults where raised intracranial pressure may be a component (e.g. subarachnoid haemorrhage, encephalitis).

Volume–pressure relationship

The Monro–Kellie hypothesis states that the sum of the intracranial contents of blood (10%), brain (80%), and cerebrospinal fluid (CSF) (10%) is constant. Since the skull is considered an enclosed and rigid container, an increase in volume of any one of the intracranial components must be offset by a decrease in one or more of the others, or ICP will rise. Under normal circumstances, a small increase in brain volume is compensated by translocation of CSF to the spinal CSF space and venous blood to the extracranial veins. However, once these compensatory mechanisms have been exhausted, even a small increase in volume will result in substantial ICP increases. Compliance (the change in volume for a given change in pressure) provides an index of compensatory reserve, with low values suggesting a diminished reserve (Figure 8.7).

After injury the brain's ability to react to volume changes may be impaired by several factors, including the failure of autoregulatory mechanisms (discussed later), disruption of the blood–brain barrier (BBB), and oedema. The point at which a critical volume is reached depends not only on the individual, but also on the speed of expansion.

Intracranial pressure (ICP)

ICP is defined as the CSF pressure within the lateral ventricles. The normal range in adults is 0–10 mmHg,

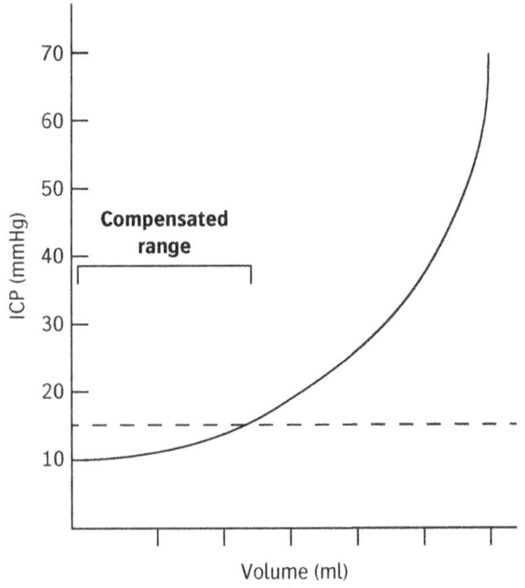

Figure 8.7 Volume–pressure curve.

with lower ranges (0–7 mmHg) in children. The volume of the intracranial components must be in a state of dynamic equilibrium to keep ICP constant. ICP rises transiently in response to actions such as coughing and sneezing without any adverse effect as compensatory measures quickly reduce it before any damage is caused by compromised blood flow. The duration of ICP >20 mmHg is strongly associated with increased morbidity and mortality. Table 8.5 shows potential causes of raised ICP.

Cerebral perfusion pressure (CPP)

CPP is the driving force for delivery of blood (and therefore oxygen and glucose) to the brain and is a marker of the adequacy of the cerebral circulation. CPP represents the pressure gradient across the brain; in its simplified form it can be calculated as the difference between the incoming mean arterial blood pressure (MAP) and the opposing ICP (CPP = MAP–ICP). In the healthy brain intrinsic autoregulatory mechanisms (discussed later) protect the brain tissue from damage during transient changes in MAP or ICP. After severe injury, changes in either MAP or ICP will alter CPP. In the initial stages following TBI, a low BP rather than a high ICP is the most frequent cause of an inadequate CPP.

Cerebral blood flow (CBF)

As the brain is mainly reliant on glucose as an energy source and has little storage capacity, neuronal function is critically dependent on CBF to meet its metabolic demands. The brain requires a constant supply of oxygen and glucose (see Box 8.4). Within limits, the vessels of the cerebral circulation can respond to meet these needs. The amount of blood delivered to the brain is highly regulated and is determined by several factors.

Table 8.5 Causes of raised ICP

Brain	Tumour Abscess Oedema
Blood	Haemorrhage Haematoma Restricted venous return Increased cerebral blood flow
CSF	Over-secretion (rare) Impaired circulation Impaired absorption

Box 8.4 Cerebral blood flow

- Normal CBF is 50–60 ml/100 g/min (750 ml/min for the entire brain which equals 15% of total resting cardiac output).
- Global CBF remains stable, but regional increases of 50–100% may occur locally during normal neuronal activity.
- Oxygen supply to the brain is about 80% of total body oxygen consumption.
- Each day the brain requires 1000 L of blood flow to obtain 71 L of oxygen and 100 g of glucose.
- Cessation of CBF causes unconsciousness within 5–10 sec due to lack of delivery of oxygen to the brain cells.
- If CBF <25–30 ml/100 g/min mental confusion and loss of consciousness will occur.
- If CBF <15 ml/100 g/min measurable electrical activity (EEG) is absent.
- If CBF <8 ml/100 g/min cellular alteration and cell death will occur.

Pressure autoregulation

Autoregulation is the intrinsic ability of cerebrovascular smooth muscle to maintain a relatively constant CBF over a wide range of perfusion pressures (50–150 mmHg). The cerebral vessels change diameter inversely with changing perfusion pressures. As CPP rises the vessels constrict to prevent damage to smaller vessels from higher pressures; as CPP falls the vessels dilate so that blood flow is kept constant. In hypertensive patients the autoregulatory pressure limits are higher (i.e. the autoregulation curve is shifted to the right).

After injury the autoregulatory response may be disrupted, with CBF and CPP becoming dependent upon the systemic circulation. The injured brain may also require the CPP to be above normal to maintain CBF, and it may be slower than normal to react to pressure changes. A shift to the right, increasing the lower and upper limits of autoregulation, occurs with chronic hypertension and sympathetic activation (e.g. shock or stress). A left shift, reducing the lower and upper limits, occurs with hypoxia, hypercarbia, and vasodilator therapy. Acute hypertension, i.e. a rapid increase in perfusion pressure to above the upper autoregulatory limit, may result in cerebral oedema secondary to increased microvascular pressures.

Metabolic regulation

Blood flow and metabolism in the normal brain are tightly coupled to ensure that cellular demands are matched by CBF. Although the exact mechanisms are not fully determined, concentrations of extracellular ions (e.g. hydrogen, calcium, and potassium) and metabolic products (e.g. adenosine, thromboxane, and prostaglandins) may act as local vasoregulators to match local blood flow to local metabolic demands. The normal cerebral metabolic rate for oxygen consumption ($CMRO_2$) is 3 ml/100 g/min.

Chemical regulation

Alterations in arterial oxygen partial pressure (P_aO_2) and arterial carbon dioxide pressure (P_aCO_2) can have a profound effect on CBF. Moreover, the effects of hypoxaemia and hypercapnia are additive; therefore a poorly ventilated and marginally oxygenated patient will have a dramatic increase in CBF.

1. **Oxygen**: CBF changes with arterial O_2 content to maintain the appropriate tissue O_2 tension for cerebral metabolism. The precise chemical mediator for this response is not known, though adenosine is thought to play an important role. CBF is not affected until the P_aO_2 falls below 7 kPa. At this point cerebral vasodilatation begins and CBF increases. At very high P_aO_2 (>40 kPa) there may be a slight decrease in CBF. Mild hypoxaemia (P_aO_2 <7 kPa) is associated with a twofold increase in CBF, while severe hypoxaemia is associated with a fivefold increase in CBF. Hypoxaemia (P_aO_2 <8 kPa) is the second most influential cause of secondary brain injury, after hypotension, and is associated with worse outcomes.
2. **Carbon dioxide**: P_aCO_2 is one of the most potent regulators of CBF. Unlike the response to oxygen, the CBF response to changes in P_aCO_2 is dramatic. Within the range of 3.3–10 kPa, for every 0.12 kPa change in P_aCO_2 there is a 1–2 ml/100 g/min change in CBF. Doubling P_aCO_2 doubles CBF, while halving P_aCO_2 halves the CBF. Hypercapnia increases CBF and cerebral blood volume (CBV) and decreases cerebral vascular resistance (CVR) (vasodilation), whereas the converse occurs with hypocapnia. These effects represent the most powerful stimulus to the cerebrovascular system and are probably due to changes in extracellular or interstitial H^+ concentration. However, after 6–8 hours the CBF returns to baseline values because the CSF pH gradually normalizes as a result of the extrusion of bicarbonate. Cerebrovascular reactivity to alterations in P_aO_2 and P_aCO_2 can be reduced or abolished during intracranial hypertension. This loss of reactivity, which is a bad prognostic sign, can be either global or focal.

Neurogenic regulation

Specific neuronal centres probably modify or facilitate autoregulatory responses. Some sympathetic and parasympathetic nerves and several neurotransmitters have been implicated.

Blood haemoglobin concentration

CBF can be influenced by blood viscosity, of which haematocrit is the single most important determinant. Blood viscosity increases logarithmically with increasing haematocrit; the optimal level is probably about 35%.

Blood–brain barrier (BBB)

The BBB is a specialization of the walls of brain capillaries that limits movement of blood-borne substances into the extracellular fluid of the brain and the CSF. Cerebral endothelial cells are joined by intracellular tight junctions that form a five-layered ring around all cerebral blood vessels, preventing any passage of molecules between individual cells. Injury to the brain can cause a breakdown of the BBB, allowing normally restricted substances to pass into the brain tissue.

Traumatic brain injury

Head injuries are the most common cause of death in young adults in the Western world, causing nine deaths per 100,000 population each year. This represents 1% of all deaths, but 15–20% of those between 5 and 35 years of age, and also carries a very significant impact on long-term disability. The immediate resuscitation and stabilization of patients with severe traumatic brain injury (TBI) and their subsequent intensive care management is aimed at preventing secondary brain injury

Pathophysiology

Injury to the brain following trauma includes both the immediate damage caused at the moment of impact, and secondary damage that develops during the first few hours or days after the impact (Table 8.6). Primary brain injury encompasses disruption of brain vessels, haemorrhagic contusions, and diffuse axonal injury (DAI); at present, there is no intervention to attenuate such injury. Secondary injury can be divided into intracranial and extracranial causes. Of these, the two main causes, associated with increased mortality and morbidity, are delay in appropriate surgical management and failure to correct systemic hypoxaemia and hypotension. The types of lesion that can occur in TBI are shown in Table 8.7.

Table 8.6 Primary and secondary brain injury

Primary brain injury	Disruption of brain vessels Haemorrhagic contusions Diffuse axonal injury (DAI)
Secondary brain injury	Extracranial causes: systemic hypotension, hypoxaemia, hypercarbia, disturbances of blood coagulation Intracranial causes: haematoma, brain swelling, infection

Intensive care management

Monitoring and assessment

Over and above the routine care given to critically ill patients, patients with TBI will require cerebral monitoring to allow measurement of CPP, estimation of CBF, and assessment of the adequacy of oxygen delivery to the brain. This allows therapy to be targeted to specific

Table 8.7 Types of lesion

Extradural haematoma (EDH)	This is an accumulation of blood in the extradural space between the inner side of the skull and the dura mater. Most (90%) are associated with skull fracture and are due to injury of the middle meningeal artery, therefore affecting the parietal and parieto-temporal areas. Outcome depends on the level of consciousness at the time of surgery, with mortality approaching 20% if unconscious.
Subdural haematoma (SDH)	This is an accumulation of blood between the inner side of the dura and the arachnoid layer due to tearing of cortical veins. As most patients with acute SDH have some kind of accompanying brain injury, their prognosis is worse than that of patients with an EDH. They can be classified as acute (ASDH) <3–4 days old, subacute 4–20 days old, and chronic >20 days old. A poor outcome is more likely if ASDH is bilateral, accumulates rapidly, or there is a delay of >4 hours in surgical management. Chronic subdural haematoma (CSDH) can occur many weeks after head injury.
Traumatic subarachnoid haemorrhage (SAH)	Traumatic SAH must be quantified on early CT scan since later scans underestimate its incidence and severity. Mortality and poor outcome is twice that seen in patients without the SAH component.
Intracerebral haematoma (ICH)	This usually affects the white matter or basal ganglia and can be the cause of delayed neurological deterioration.
Contusions and lacerations	Haemorrhagic contusions and lacerations are superficial areas of haemorrhage, usually affecting the cortex in the frontal and temporal lobes, which are sustained as the brain hits the bony protuberances of the skull at the site of impact (coup injury) and then the opposite side during deceleration (contrecoup injury).
Diffuse axonal injury (DAI)	This is the commonest cause of coma, vegetative state, and subsequent disability. It is attributed to tearing of nerve fibres at the junction between the grey and white matter because they decelerate at different velocities within the skull. This is likely to be a dynamic process at a cellular level that begins soon after trauma and may not be complete for 24 hours. Patients with severe DAI are often in deep coma in contrast with their CT scan appearance which can look quite normal and an initially normal ICP.
Skull fracture	This is evidence of major impact to the head and has an associated high incidence of intracranial haematoma. Clinical indicators of a basal skull fracture include peri-orbital bruising (panda eyes or racoon eyes) and retro-auricular (behind the ear) bruising (Battle's sign) and may be associated with a CSF leak from the nose (rhinorrhoea) or ears (otorrhoea). Most leaks close spontaneously.

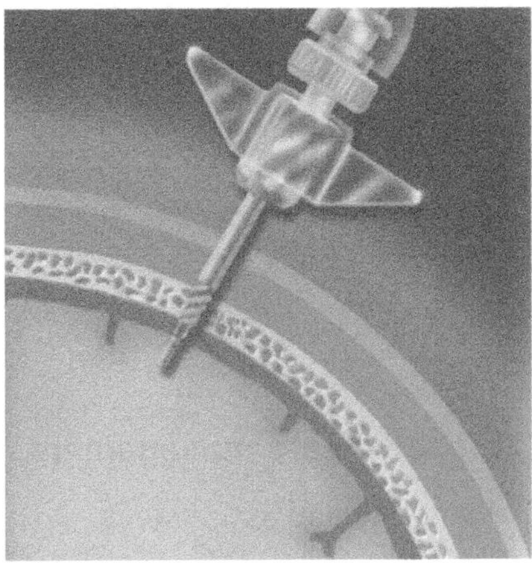

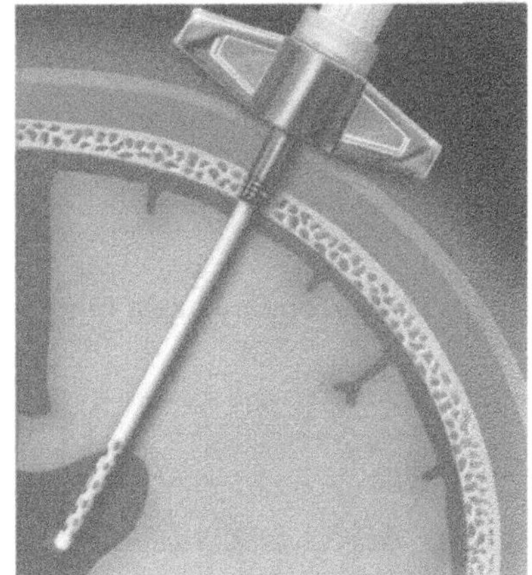

Figure 8.8 ICP monitoring (a) Intraparechymal (b) Intraventricular.
Permission granted by Integra LifeSciences Corporation, Plainsboro, New Jersey, USA.

changes in brain function and to ensure a balance between cerebral metabolic supply and demand:

- Intracranial pressure monitoring (Figure 8.8) provides a physiological variable that is not only useful for diagnosis and prognosis, but also serves as direct feedback to guide the treatment of cerebral perfusion. ICP can be measured using a subdural, intraparenchymal or intraventricular catheter. ICP monitoring is the only way to measure CPP accurately.
- Transcranial Doppler ultrasonography (TCD) provides an indicator of CBF and can provide a non-invasive assessment of CPP. TCD can also demonstrate loss of pressure autoregulation and CO_2 reactivity, which are indicators of poor prognosis after TBI.
- Jugular venous bulb oximetry ($S_{jv}O_2$) is used to assess the balance between cerebral oxygen supply and demand.
- Newer techniques for measuring the adequacy of cerebral oxygenation include near-infrared spectroscopy, tissue microprobes, and cerebral microdialysis.

Individual monitoring techniques provide information about specific aspects of cerebral function, but all have disadvantages and most suffer from significant artefact. Therefore decisions to treat are not usually based on a change in one variable alone. Monitoring of several variables simultaneously (multi-modality monitoring) allows cross-validation between monitor and artefact rejection, and greater confidence to make treatment decisions.

When clinical assessment is no longer possible because of sedation or pharmacological paralysis to facilitate ventilation, there is general agreement that ICP monitoring should be instituted in all patients with severe TBI (GCS <8). Uncontrolled intracranial hypertension remains an important cause of mortality and morbidity after severe TBI, and in more than one-third of patients ICP exceeeds 20 mmHg at some stage. While it has never been shown definitively that lowering ICP in patients with intracranial hypertension improves outcomes, an ICP >20 mmHg is the fourth most powerful predictor of outcome, after age, admission GCS, and pupillary signs. There is some evidence to suggest that treatment to reduce ICP should be initiated if the ICP is 20–25 mmHg. Both ICP and CPP are strongly associated with outcomes after TBI, with the worse outcomes occurring in patients with an ICP >20 mmHg and/or a CPP <60 mmHg.

One of the most controversial areas in the management of severe TBI is the level of CPP required to adequately perfuse the brain. While there is evidence that hypotension following TBI has an adverse effect on outcomes, there is less evidence to support the concept that induced hypertension, particularly if prolonged, is beneficial to the injured brain. A target CPP of 60mmHg is generally advocated.

ICP therapy

ICP therapy is indicated only if raised ICP has been demonstrated by monitoring, there is CT evidence of increased ICP, or there are clinical signs of developing intracranial herniation. Figure 8.9 illustrates the basic and advanced measures that should be taken to control ICP.

Sedation

It is common practice for severe TBI patients to be empirically managed with a protocol that includes the

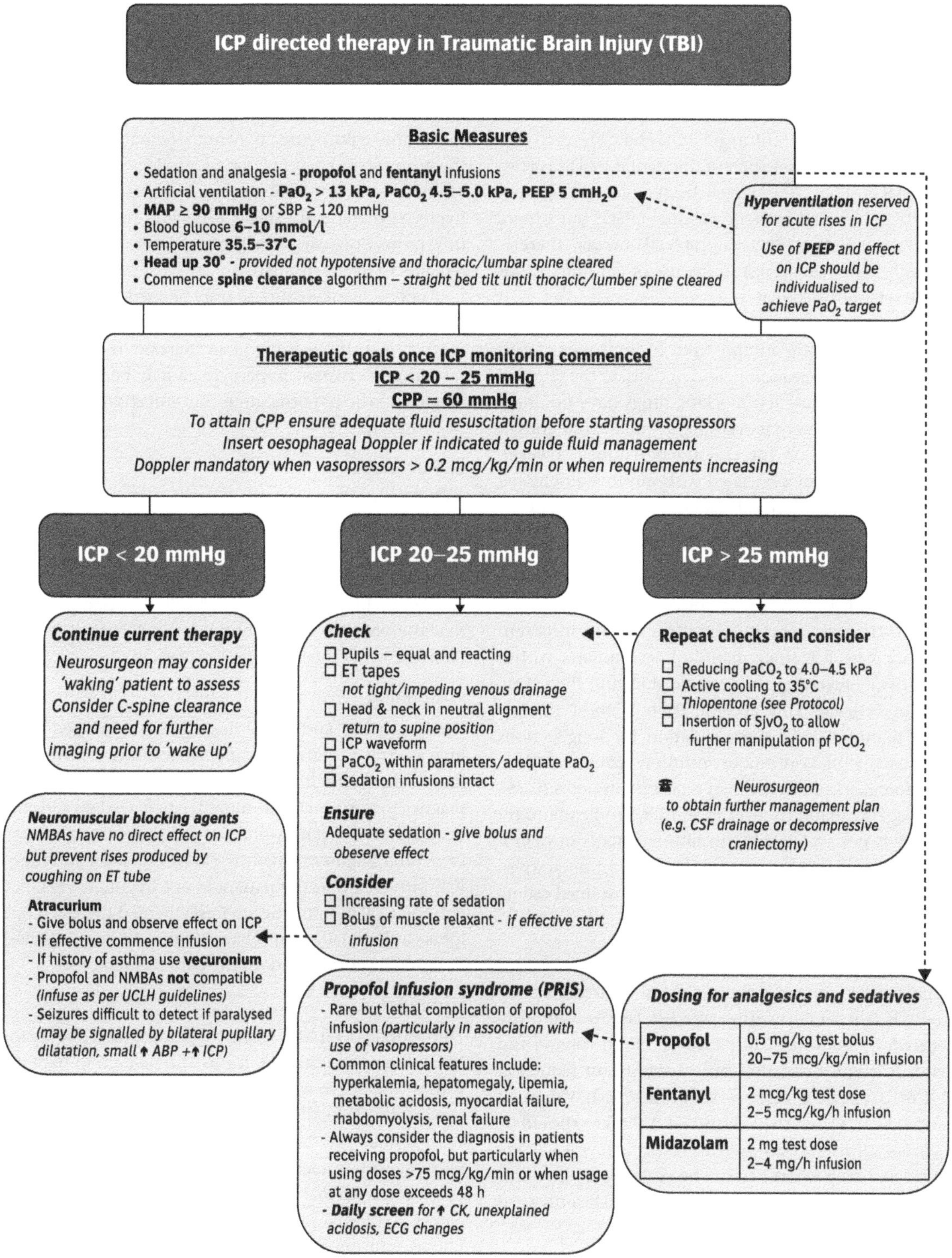

ICP directed therapy in Traumatic Brain Injury (TBI)

Basic Measures

- Sedation and analgesia - **propofol** and **fentanyl** infusions
- Artificial ventilation - **PaO_2 > 13 kPa, $PaCO_2$ 4.5–5.0 kPa, PEEP 5 cmH_2O**
- **MAP ≥ 90 mmHg** or SBP ≥ 120 mmHg
- Blood glucose **6–10 mmol/l**
- Temperature **35.5–37°C**
- **Head up 30°** - *provided not hypotensive and thoracic/lumbar spine cleared*
- Commence **spine clearance** algorithm – *straight bed tilt until thoracic/lumber spine cleared*

***Hyperventilation** reserved for acute rises in ICP*

*Use of **PEEP** and effect on ICP should be individualised to achieve PaO_2 target*

Therapeutic goals once ICP monitoring commenced

ICP < 20 – 25 mmHg

CPP = 60 mmHg

To attain CPP ensure adequate fluid resuscitation before starting vasopressors

Insert oesophageal Doppler if indicated to guide fluid management

Doppler mandatory when vasopressors > 0.2 mcg/kg/min or when requirements increasing

ICP < 20 mmHg

Continue current therapy

Neurosurgeon may consider 'waking' patient to assess

Consider C-spine clearance and need for further imaging prior to 'wake up'

ICP 20–25 mmHg

Check

- ☐ Pupils – equal and reacting
- ☐ ET tapes
  not tight/impeding venous drainage
- ☐ Head & neck in neutral alignment
  return to supine position
- ☐ ICP waveform
- ☐ $PaCO_2$ within parameters/adequate PaO_2
- ☐ Sedation infusions intact

Ensure

Adequate sedation - *give bolus and obeserve effect*

Consider

- ☐ Increasing rate of sedation
- ☐ Bolus of muscle relaxant - *if effective start infusion*

ICP > 25 mmHg

Repeat checks and consider

- ☐ Reducing $PaCO_2$ to 4.0–4.5 kPa
- ☐ Active cooling to 35°C
- ☐ *Thiopentone (see Protocol)*
- ☐ Insertion of $SjvO_2$ to allow further manipulation pf PCO_2

☎ *Neurosurgeon to obtain further management plan (e.g. CSF drainage or decompressive craniectomy)*

Neuromuscular blocking agents

NMBAs have no direct effect on ICP but prevent rises produced by coughing on ET tube

Atracurium

- Give bolus and observe effect on ICP
- If effective commence infusion
- If history of asthma use **vecuronium**
- Propofol and NMBAs **not** compatible *(infuse as per UCLH guidelines)*
- Seizures difficult to detect if paralysed *(may be signalled by bilateral pupillary dilatation, small ↑ ABP +↑ ICP)*

Propofol infusion syndrome (PRIS)

- Rare but lethal complication of propofol infusion *(particularly in association with use of vasopressors)*
- Common clinical features include: hyperkalemia, hepatomegaly, lipemia, metabolic acidosis, myocardial failure, rhabdomyolysis, renal failure
- Always consider the diagnosis in patients receiving propofol, but particularly when using doses >75 mcg/kg/min or when usage at any dose exceeds 48 h
- ***Daily screen** for ↑ CK, unexplained acidosis, ECG changes*

Dosing for analgesics and sedatives

Propofol	0.5 mg/kg test bolus 20–75 mcg/kg/min infusion
Fentanyl	2 mcg/kg test dose 2–5 mcg/kg/h infusion
Midazolam	2 mg test dose 2–4 mg/h infusion

Figure 8.9 ICP directed therapy.

routine use of sedatives, analgesics, and neuromuscular blocking agents to facilitate mechanical ventilation and treat intracranial hypertension.

Intravenous anaesthetic agents cause a dose-dependent reduction in cerebral metabolism, CBF, and ICP while maintaining pressure autoregulation and CO_2 reactivity. The use of barbiturates such as thiopental in TBI is controversial and they have largely been replaced by propofol, which has similar cerebrovascular effects but a more favourable pharmacological profile. However, there is currently renewed interest in the use of barbiturates for an intractably raised ICP.

Potent parenteral narcotics such as fentanyl and morphine are frequently administered to limit pain, facilitate mechanical ventilation, and potentiate the effect of sedation. Neuromuscular blocking drugs have no direct effect on ICP, but may prevent rises produced by coughing and straining on the endotracheal tube. However, such agents are not associated with improved outcome and their use is currently the subject of much debate.

Mannitol

Mannitol is an effective agent for reducing cerebral oedema and ICP in certain settings of intracranial hypertension. However, repetitive administration can potentially increase ICP since mannitol accumulates within brain tissue, reversing the osmotic shift and increasing cerebral oedema. This accumulation is most marked when mannitol is in the circulation for long periods as occurs with continuous infusion administration. Therefore it should be given in repeat bolus doses (0.25–1.0 g/kg 20% mannitol over 15 min). Chronic mannitol therapy is not associated with improvements in neurological outcome, so its use should be discontinued when it no longer produces a significant and sustained reduction in ICP.

Hyperventilation

Hyperventilation, once the mainstay of treatment to reduce ICP in patients with severe TBI, is now vigorously debated. Its aim is to reduce cerebral blood volume and hence ICP, but it can also cause a significant reduction in CBF. Current guidelines advocate P_aCO_2 values of 4.5–5.0 kPa. Further reductions to 4.0–4.5 kPa should be used only if ICP is >20 mmHg. Levels below 4 kPa are considered only when ICP has been shown to be sensitive to changing the P_aCO_2 level and should be only used in conjunction with $S_{jv}O_2$ monitoring.

Therapeutic hypothermia

Elevations in temperature worsen outcomes after TBI so pyrexia should be avoided. Brain temperature tends to be higher than core temperature, and the brain's oxygen consumption increases by 6–9% for every degree Celsius elsius rise in temperature. Moderate reductions in brain temperature reduce the release of excitatory amino acids. Moderate hypothermia (to 33–35°C) has been shown to be beneficial in animal models. There is some evidence that while hypothermia may not attenuate damage from the primary injury, it may provide a degree of protection against secondary brain injury from hypotension and hypoxia in the early stages following injury. Whether this protection can be sustained over longer periods remains to be determined.

Cooling blankets should only be used in sedated and paralysed patients to avoid a shivering response which may cause a rise in ICP and an increase in oxygen consumption. Persistent hyperpyrexia may be the result of damage to the hypothalamus, but infection should also be considered.

CSF drainage

CSF drainage by insertion of an external ventricular drain is frequently employed to treat intracranial hypertension in severe TBI. While it is established as a first-line treatment, there are no consensus guidelines for its use. Some advocate continuous CSF drainage provided that the ventricle size is normal, and intermittent CSF drainage when the ventricle size is small.

Positioning

Head rotation and neck flexion are associated with increased ICP, decreased jugular venous return, and localized changes in cerebral blood flow. It is traditional practice to position head-injured patients in bed with the head elevated to a maximum of 30° above the heart and in neutral alignment with the trunk in order to reduce ICP, provided that the patient is not hypotensive. Once ICP and CPP monitoring are implemented there is scope for an individualized approach (within these guidelines) to head elevation based on the patient's response.

Barbiturates

Thiopental is a rapidly acting barbiturate used mainly for induction of anaesthesia. It can also be used in patients with severe TBI to control intractable intracranial hypertension by decreasing the brain's metabolic demands. The use of barbiturates for ICP control is usually reserved for refractory intracranial hypertension unresponsive to other conventional medical and simple surgical treatments. An initial loading dose will indicate whether or not an infusion should be commenced. A loading dose of 250 mg is given intravenously and repeated until a reduction in ICP is observed (up to a maximum of three bolus doses). A bolus dose acts within one arm–brain circulation time (i.e. 1 min), with the effect lasting for 5–15 min, and is cumulative after repeated administration. If there is no reduction in ICP after three doses then a high dose infusion should not be commenced. However, if the bolus doses are effective, an infusion running at 3–8 mg/kg/h should be commenced and titrated to achieve the target ICP (<25 mmHg). Other sedation should be reduced, but the thiopental infusion should be reviewed after 48 hours.

Decompressive craniectomy

Patients who do not have an operable mass lesion but who have progressive intracranial hypertension that is unresponsive to standard medical management should be considered for decompressive craniectomy to lower ICP. However, while early decompression can lower ICP, evidence of improved outcome is less certain.

Neuroprotective drugs

Corticosteroids have been used for treating certain neurological conditions since the 1950s. While producing rapid improvement in patients with brain tumours associated with oedema, there is also some evidence of benefit from early administration of high dose methylprednisolone in spinal cord injury. However, several prospective randomized clinical trials failed to show that steroid therapy reduced ICP or improved outcomes in patients with severe TBI. Indeed, the CRASH trial (Corticosteroid Randomization after Significant Head Injury) had to be stopped prematurely because of an increased risk of death in the corticosteroid-treated group.

Evidence from experimental studies suggests that modification of neurochemical and cellular events with targeted pharmacotherapy can promote functional recovery following TBI. Moreover, it is likely that there is a therapeutic window following injury during which such pharmacological intervention must be initiated in order to be effective. Such drugs (e.g. antioxidants, ion-channel blockers, and membrane stabilizers) aim to protect brain cells from secondary injury by interrupting one or more of the mediating factors that cause tissue damage. However, while animal studies show good effect, there is little clinical evidence to date of brain protection with new drugs.

Respiratory management

A large proportion of patients with severe TBI are hypoxaemic without ventilatory support or added oxygen, and many require advanced ventilatory support within a short period of time. Acute lung injury (ALI) (see Chapter 4) is common in patients with isolated head injury, particularly those with a post-resuscitative GCS ≤8. It is an additional marker of the severity of brain injury and is associated with an increased risk of morbidity and mortality.

Neurogenic pulmonary oedema (NPE) represents the most severe form of ALI and is seen in cases of fatal or near-fatal head injury and after abrupt elevations in ICP. The exact mechanisms responsible for this acute condition are unclear. Primary treatment consists of methods to reduce ICP and appropriate ventilation management, increasing inspired oxygen concentration, controlling carbon dioxide levels, and increasing PEEP to maximize oxygenation with minimal effect on ICP and cardiac output.

The development of the acute respiratory distress syndrome (ARDS) complicates the management of severe TBI as many of the therapies used to protect the lungs can raise ICP or decrease CPP. Furthermore, the initial catecholamine storm following injury leads to changes in pulmonary pressures and capillary leak. The ventilatory strategies used to protect the lungs, such as reduced tidal volume, permissive hypoxaemia and hypercarbia, increased levels of PEEP, and prone positioning, pose problems for these patients not only during the acute course of head injury when ICP may be high, but also in terms of delaying the early rehabilitation therapy which is essential to maximize recovery. The management of fluid balance, BP, and CPP can also be difficult issues. While aggressive CPP management (maintaining CPP >70 mmHg) decreases the risk of brain ischaemia, it has been shown to increase the incidence of ARDS.

Following head injury, respiratory function may be depressed. A period of apnoea may have occurred at the accident, resulting in atelectasis. Aspiration of gastric contents may also have occurred due to a decreased level of consciousness. Coma, prolonged bed rest, mechanical ventilation and sedation, and a diminished cough reflex make these patients extremely susceptible to pulmonary complications which could further compound their neurological status. Chest physiotherapy is essential in severe TBI patients. However, the care needed to prevent and treat these complications is often associated with significant increases in ICP. Provided that the patient's head and neck are kept in alignment, side-turning is advocated for chest management. How long and how often they should remain on their side is determined by intracranial and cardiovascular stability.

Increasing sedation or administering a bolus of sedation may lessen the adverse effects of treatment, but timing is vital if it is to be effective as an adjunct to treatment. During suctioning and chest physiotherapy, the aim is to prevent hypoxaemia (current guidelines recommend P_aO_2 >13 kPa in severe TBI) and hyper/hypocarbia, and to avoid excessive and prolonged increases in ICP.

Patients should be pre-oxygenated with 100% O_2 prior to suctioning and, provided that their carbon dioxide levels are not already at the minimum limit, may be mildly hyperventilated. In most cases, the rise in ICP is temporary and returns to baseline in 30–60 sec. Suction should be limited to a maximum of two or three passes of the catheter in one session to avoid a cumulative effect on ICP.

Cardiovascular management

High levels of sympathetic activity and circulating catecholamines after severe TBI can have an adverse effect on cardiac function. There is myocardial damage (evidenced by raised troponin, creatine kinase MB isoform) and also electrocardiographic abnormalities including atrial and ventricular arrhythmias, abnormalities of the QRS complex, T wave, and ST segment, and QT prolongation. These are most common in patients with diffuse injury, oedema, and contusions. Life-threatening arrhythmias require prompt treatment; however, most cardiac arrhythmias in acute CNS disorders do not require therapeutic intervention.

An inotrope (usually norepinephrine) is required in most patients to counteract the hypotensive effects of sedation and facilitate CPP management.

Fluid management

Several factors must be considered in the fluid management of patients following severe TBI, including clinical and laboratory assessment of volume status, the effects of different fluids on CPP and cerebral oedema, osmotic therapy, and water and electrolyte disturbances.

Following TBI, the BBB is likely to be disrupted and different fluids can have an effect on cerebral oedema. If the serum osmolarity falls, water moves across the BBB along the altered osmotic gradient, causing cerebral oedema, increased ICP, and decreased CPP. Therefore hypotonic fluids should be avoided. Glucose-containing solutions should not be used unless specifically indicated to correct hypoglycaemia. There are still questions regarding the optimal target for glucose control after severe brain injury, but evidence suggests that the aim for blood glucose levels should be 6–10 mmol/L.

Disturbances of sodium and water balance are common following severe TBI, and accurate diagnosis and treatment are essential (see section on 'Management of sodium and water balance').

Nutrition

TBI patients are often hypermetabolic and hypercatabolic, resulting in increased energy and protein requirements. Early feeding, within hours of injury, is associated with improved clinical outcomes so nutritional support should begin within 24 hours following injury. Enteral nutrition is the method of choice for nourishing this group of patients.

Several problems can affect successful delivery of enteral nutrition to TBI patients. In the early stages, delayed gastric emptying/gastroparesis may affect the patient's ability to tolerate feeds and is often more prolonged than found in patients suffering other types of trauma. In most cases this will improve after 3 weeks. The exact mechanism for gastroparesis in TBI is unclear, but is thought to be related to either the head injury itself, the host of mediators released following cerebral injury, or raised ICP. In many circumstances, the sudden development of intolerance after a period of successful enteral feeding is probably due to a change in clinical status, such as deterioration in neurology or sepsis. In such cases, parenteral feeding may be necessary.

Posture and tone

Patients with neurological dysfunction resulting in abnormal posture and movement are at great risk of developing structural deformity. Treatment must be initiated at the onset of neurological damage and continued as long as the risk of secondary complications exists. The role of the physiotherapist in preventing long-term physical disability is crucial. Passive movements are regularly performed on patients who are unconscious in order to maintain muscle and joint range, as ICP allows. In addition, splinting of limbs may be required. Different postures and positions and their influence on tone and movement should be considered. For these patients rehabilitation starts from the moment of admission to the critical care unit, as this is a crucial factor in the rehabilitation process.

Protection of the cervical spine

All severe TBI patients are at risk of having sustained a cervical spine injury (Figure 8.10). In unconscious or sedated patients clinical assessment cannot exclude cervical injury and therefore early diagnostic imaging is essential. This also prevents prolonged unnecessary immobilization, with its associated complications. If a fracture or dislocation is diagnosed, management is dictated by the precise nature of the injury and its stability. However, routine radiological examination cannot reliably exclude ligament injury; in the unconscious patient a cervical collar is often kept in place until such injury can be ruled out. This may mean waiting until the patient has regained consciousness and can describe signs and symptoms.

Level of spine involved	Number of people required	Role of each person	Positioning
Multilevel - Cervico-thoracic and Thoraco-lumbar	Unstable – 5 Stable and fixed—moving and handling as for non-spinal patient	1- Head—Team leader 2- Upper body 3- Pelvis, upper thigh 4- Lower leg 5- Skin check, pillow person	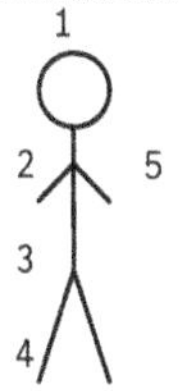 1, 2, 5, 3, 4
C1 to T4	Unstable – 3 Stable and fixed—moving and handling as for non-spinal patient	1- Head—Team leader 2- Upper body 3- Skin check, pillow person (cross patient's legs for turning)	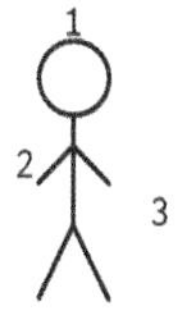 1, 2, 3
T4 to L5	Unstable – 4 Stable and fixed—moving and handling as for non-spinal patient	1- Upper body—Team leader 2- Pelvis, upper thigh 3- Lower leg 4- Skin check, pillow person	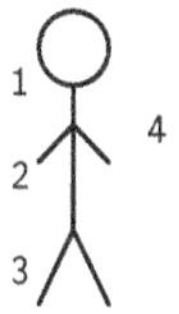 1, 4, 2, 3

Figure 8.10 Spinal clearance.

Collars can cause chin and occipital pressure sores from prolonged tight application and can occlude skin capillary blood flow. They can also cause significant elevations in ICP by obstructing venous drainage. Once bony injury has been excluded, and provided that the patient is adequately sedated, the collar can be removed and replaced briefly for turning and repositioning. The collar should be applied when sedation is being weaned and the patient 'woken'.

Subarachnoid haemorrhage

Subarachnoid haemorrhage (SAH) is defined as bleeding into the subarachnoid space and therefore into the CSF (Figure 8.11). Cerebral arteries lie in the subarachnoid space and give off small perforating branches to the brain tissue. Bleeding from these vessels or from an associated aneurysm occurs primarily into this space. Some intracranial aneurysms are embedded within the brain tissue and their rupture causes intracerebral bleeding with or without subarachnoid haemorrhage. Occasionally, the arachnoid layer is disrupted and a subdural haematoma results. Following subarachnoid haemorrhage, blood within the CSF can disrupt the reabsorption of CSF and lead to secondary hydrocephalus.

The leading cause of SAH, accounting for about 60% of cases, is rupture of an intracranial saccular aneurysm. This is a dilatation in the wall of an artery, and usually occurs at the junction or bifurcation of arteries. Other causes include arteriovenous malformations, hypertension, tumours, bleeding diathesis, anticoagulants, and idiopathic causes.

The incidence of SAH increases with age, with the peak occurrence between 40 and 60 years and a female to male ratio of 3:1. The aetiology of cerebral aneurysms remains unclear, but several factors (congenital defects, degenerative change, and hypertension) are implicated. Hypertension is not only a risk factor for bleeding but is also an unfavourable prognostic factor, increasing the likelihood of a poor outcome from 5% to 32%. The cardinal symptom of SAH is the sudden onset of severe headache, present in up to 97% of patients, often accompanied by vomiting.

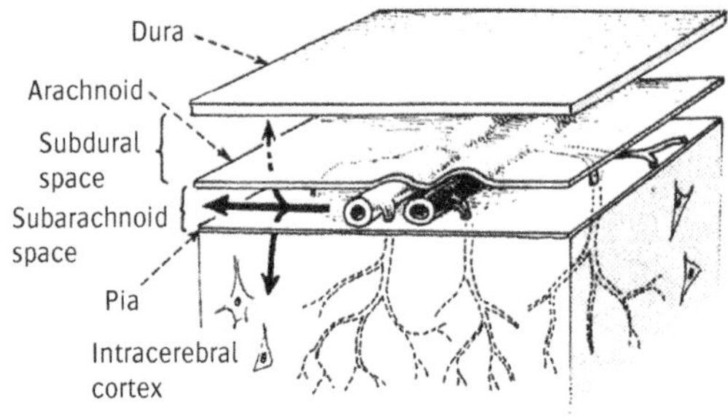

Figure 8.11 Subarachnoid space.

This figure was published in *Neurology and Neurosurgery Illustrated*, Lindsay, K.W. and Bone, I. Copyright Elsevier (2004).

Despite advances in subarachnoid haemorrhage management, the associated mortality and morbidity remain high. Nearly half the patients die within 60 days of the initial bleed. Since management varies depending on the cause, for the purposes of this chapter the management of patients with aneurysmal subarachnoid haemorrhage only will be discussed.

Grading of SAH

The single most important independent predictor of outcome after aneurysmal rupture is the clinical status of the patient on admission after initial resuscitation and stabilization. Several clinical grading systems have been proposed to guide treatment or prognosticate. The World Federation of Neurological Surgeons (WFNS) Scale, with grading from I to V, uses the GCS to assess the level of consciousness and the presence or absence of a major focal deficit to distinguish between grades II and III (Table 8.8). Therefore a grade I SAH with a GCS of 15 is the best score while grade V with a GCS of 3–6 is the worst.

Table 8.8 World Federation of Neurological Surgeons SAH Grading Scale

WFNS grade	GCS score	Motor deficit absent or present
I	15	Absent or present
II	14–13	Absent
III	14–13	Present
IV	12–7	Present or absent
V	6–3	Present or absent

Reproduced from *Journal of Neurosurgery*, Report of World Federation of Neurological Surgeons Committee on a Universal Subarachnoid Hemorrhage Grading Scale, Volume 68, Issue 6, pp. 985–986. Copyright (1988) American Association of Neurological Surgeons, http://thejns.org/toc/jns/68/6.

Complications of SAH

Rebleeding

The commonest cause of early death after SAH is an immediate rebleed. Rebleeding can occur at any time but most frequently from day 3 to day 11, with a peak incidence around day 7 after the original bleed. The mortality rate for patients who have a rebleed from an aneurysm is 80%.

Cerebral vasospasm

Cerebral vasospasm is a leading cause of death and disability, and is present in 20–30% of patients with aneurysmal SAH. The presence of blood products around the large arteries at the base of the brain is the most likely cause of vasospasm. It typically occurs 3–5 days following the initial bleed, but onset may be delayed up to 21 days, with the highest risk period between days 3 and 14. The risk of vasospasm is related to the amount of blood seen on CT, the patient's condition (20% and 75% risk for WFNS Grades I and V, respectively) and the location of the aneurysm (more common with anterior communicating artery aneurysm than with middle cerebral artery aneurysm).

Hydrocephalus

Hydrocephalus occurs when blood impairs either the reabsorption of CSF (communicating) or the intraventricular flow of CSF (non-communicating). It can develop either acutely (within the first few days) or chronically (in the second week) following SAH. Acute hydrocephalus carries a poor prognosis; when it causes an acute deterioration in conscious level it requires urgent CSF drainage with an external ventricular drain.

Seizures

The highest risk of seizures is within the first 24 hours following SAH, but they may occur at any stage, especially if a haematoma has caused cortical damage. Seizures may be generalized or focal. Anti-epileptic medication is not normally prescribed for a first seizure.

Diagnosis of SAH

- **Computed tomography** (CT) is the first-line investigation to confirm the diagnosis of SAH. It can also show associated problems such as hydrocephalus and intracerebral haematoma, and may help identify the site of an aneurysm.

- **Lumbar puncture** is only used when CT imaging is negative but the patient has a history suggestive of SAH. Lumbar puncture commonly reveals an elevated opening pressure with release of blood-stained CSF that does not clear with sequential samples. Xanthochromia (yellow coloration) may take 24–48 hours to develop, but can be present within 6 hours of the bleed.
- **Digital subtraction angiography (DSA)** is the definitive investigation for identification of aneurysms and for treatment planning. A normal angiogram is seen in 15–20% of cases so the aetiology in these cases is unclear, but may be due to a venous haemorrhage.
- **CT angiography** is useful in the unstable patient requiring craniotomy for aneurysmal intracerebral haemorrhage before a cerebral angiogram can be performed.

Cerebral angiography (ideally four-vessel) should be performed within 24 hours of admission and a treatment plan made. The treatment plan would broadly fall into one of three categories: (i) early treatment (clipping/coiling), (ii) late treatment (clipping/coiling)< or (iii) no treatment (conservative management).

Treatment

The neurosurgeon, in consultation with the neuroradiologist, will determine which therapeutic option, either surgery (clipping of the aneurysm) or endovascular (coiling of the aneurysm), is most appropriate. Factors influencing their decision include the site, size, and shape of the aneurysm and the patient's condition.

Surgical treatment

The ideal goal is to place a clip across the neck of the aneurysm to exclude it from the circulation. Timing of surgery remains the most controversial aspect of treatment and depends on both surgeon and patient. The surgeon has to decide whether to operate early (days 0–3) or to delay until after day 10; both options avoid the highest risk period for vasospasm. Early surgery eliminates the risk of rebleeding and also enables intensive management of vasospasm without danger of aneurysm rupture.

Endovascular treatment

Endovascular coiling (using Gugliemi detachable coils) is increasingly being used as an alternative to surgical clipping. This procedure is minimally invasive and can be carried out at the same time as diagnostic angiography. The approach is via the femoral artery from where a microcatheter is navigated to the aneurysm site. Coils are then deposited within the aneurysm sac, sufficient to obliterate it. These coils cause thrombosis by inducing flow stagnation within the aneurysm.

Intensive care management

Recent consensus guidelines address key issues faced by the multidisciplinary team in managing such patients. The main aim in early management is stabilization of the patient with optimization of their condition for aneurysm obliteration, together with prevention of secondary cerebral insults. Initial priorities include adequate ventilation and oxygenation, haemodynamic stability, and control of raised ICP.

Neurology

Early detection and treatment of a developing neurological deficit may prevent progression from ischaemia to infarction. The significance of changes, however small, should never be overlookedfor example, mild weakness, arm drift, dysphasia. Therefore, wherever possible, the patient should be clinically assessable. If not (i.e. when sedation is required to facilitate ventilation), ICP monitoring may be indicated, with a target range of 20–25 mmHg and a CPP of 60 mmHg (although evidence for this is taken from studies in TBI). In most instances there is no need for an ICP bolt to be inserted if an external ventricular drain is required to treat secondary hydrocephalus. However, ICP monitoring may be indicated in some SAH patients with massive intraventricular bleeding where drain function is difficult to assess.

Neurological deterioration, such as a drop in GCS or a new focal deficit, in a patient with an untreated aneurysm may be the result of rebleeding, an expanding intracerebral haematoma, vasospasm, or evolving hydrocephalus. Once the aneurysm has been treated, such neurological deterioration is likely to be due to either vasospasm or hydrocephalus.

Nimodipine

This calcium antagonist significantly lowers the incidence of death caused by delayed cerebral ischaemia and the occurrence of cerebral infarcts in patients with aneurysmal SAH. It has become standard therapy in the prophylactic treatment of cerebral vasospasm in these patients (Table 8.9).

Respiratory management

Respiratory problems following SAH are a common complication. Neurogenic pulmonary oedema occurs particularly in patients in coma and in those with fatal SAH.

Table 8.9 Nimodipine in subarachnoid haemorrhage

	Oral/NG	IV (only administered IV if patient not absorbing NG)
Dose	60 mg	Initial rate of 1mg/hour for first hour Increased to 2 mg/hour if BP adequate
Timing	Four-hourly from diagnosis for 21 days	Continuous infusion

Side effects: hypotension can occur. It can be an irritant to blood vessels. If so, it should be given into a central line and run in divided doses of 30 mg two-hourly. This should be run concurrently with 40 ml/h normal saline via a dedicated lumen

As in TBI, these patients often need advanced respiratory support in the acute stage. However, there are important differences in their respiratory management. Ventilation should be adjusted to maintain a PaO_2 >13 kPa and a normal P_aCO_2 (not less than 4.5 kPa). Patients with SAH should not be hyperventilated because of the added risk of ischaemia from vasospasm. If sedation is required to facilitate ventilation, any hypotensive side effects should be avoided with adequate volume expansion and inotropes, if necessary. Sedation or neuromuscular blockade should be adequate to prevent an intubated patient with an untreated aneurysm from coughing on the ET tube because of the hypertension and raised ICP that this can induce.

A patient with an untreated aneurysm often needs to be awakened and extubated quickly. If extubation is not possible, an early tracheostomy may be needed to stop/reduce sedation to enable clinical assessment and determination of future management.

Cardiovascular management

Cardiac changes in the acute stage following SAH are common and can range from asymptomatic ECG changes to significant life-threatening arrhythmias. These changes are attributed to high levels of circulating catecholamines, injury to the posterior hypothalamus, and blood in the CSF affecting brainstem centres, and do not necessarily mean that myocardial function is impaired.

ECG abnormalities are common following SAH and are particularly prevalent in the more severe grades. These include SVT, VT, bundle branch block, and sinus arrhythmias. Such arrhythmias usually occur within 48 hours of the onset of SAH but can be delayed for 1–2 weeks and can persist for up to 6 weeks post-bleed. In the acute phase, pharmacological management should be implemented with care since many of the arrhythmias are brief; aggressive management may lead to a prolonged opposite effect or reduce blood pressure to undesirable levels.

Reactive arterial hypertension for 24–48 hours following SAH is common, most likely due to catecholamine release. Extremes of blood pressure should be avoided, but the normal BP for each individual patient should be taken into account. A high BP in a patient with an untreated aneurysm is more likely to cause a rebleed, while a low BP will exacerbate hypoxic or ischaemic cerebral damage from vasospasm.

For patients with an untreated aneurysm, the patient's normal BP should be maintained as far as possible, treating hypotension initially with fluids. Inotropes (usually norepinephrine) are used only if their circulation or urine output cannot be maintained by fluid replacement alone. Care should be taken to avoid hypertension and the sudden drop or surge in BP that can occur during pump changes. Gross hypertension should be treated using a short-acting agent (e.g. labetalol). This should preferably be administered intravenously to allow careful titration, since patients on antihypertensive agents have a significantly higher risk of cerebral infarction.

For patients with a treated (clipped or coiled) aneurysm, BP management should be guided primarily by the neurological status of the patient, aiming for a 'high normal' BP. Following SAH, cerebral autoregulation can be impaired, making CBF more dependent upon CPP and blood viscosity. Historically, Triple H therapy (Hypertensive Hypervolaemic Haemodilution) has been used as a therapeutic approach to prevent a delayed ischaemic deficit (DID) by improving CBF using fluids and inotropes to increase MAP, increasing circulating volume, and reducing blood viscosity. Recent controlled studies have concluded that there is no good evidence that Triple H therapy (or each separate component) improves CBF in these patients. However, some uncontrolled studies show that, of the three components of Triple H, hypertension seems to be the most effective in improving CBF. The general management of SAH patients is outlined in Figure 8.12. Monitoring the patient for signs of vasospasm and taking prompt action when it occurs is crucial (Figure 8.13).

Pain management

Headache experienced at the time of SAH is often described as explosive. It may continue to be intense for the first 48 hours owing to meningeal irritation and raised ICP. The distress it causes often increases BP to dangerous levels and increases the risk of rebleeding. Effective

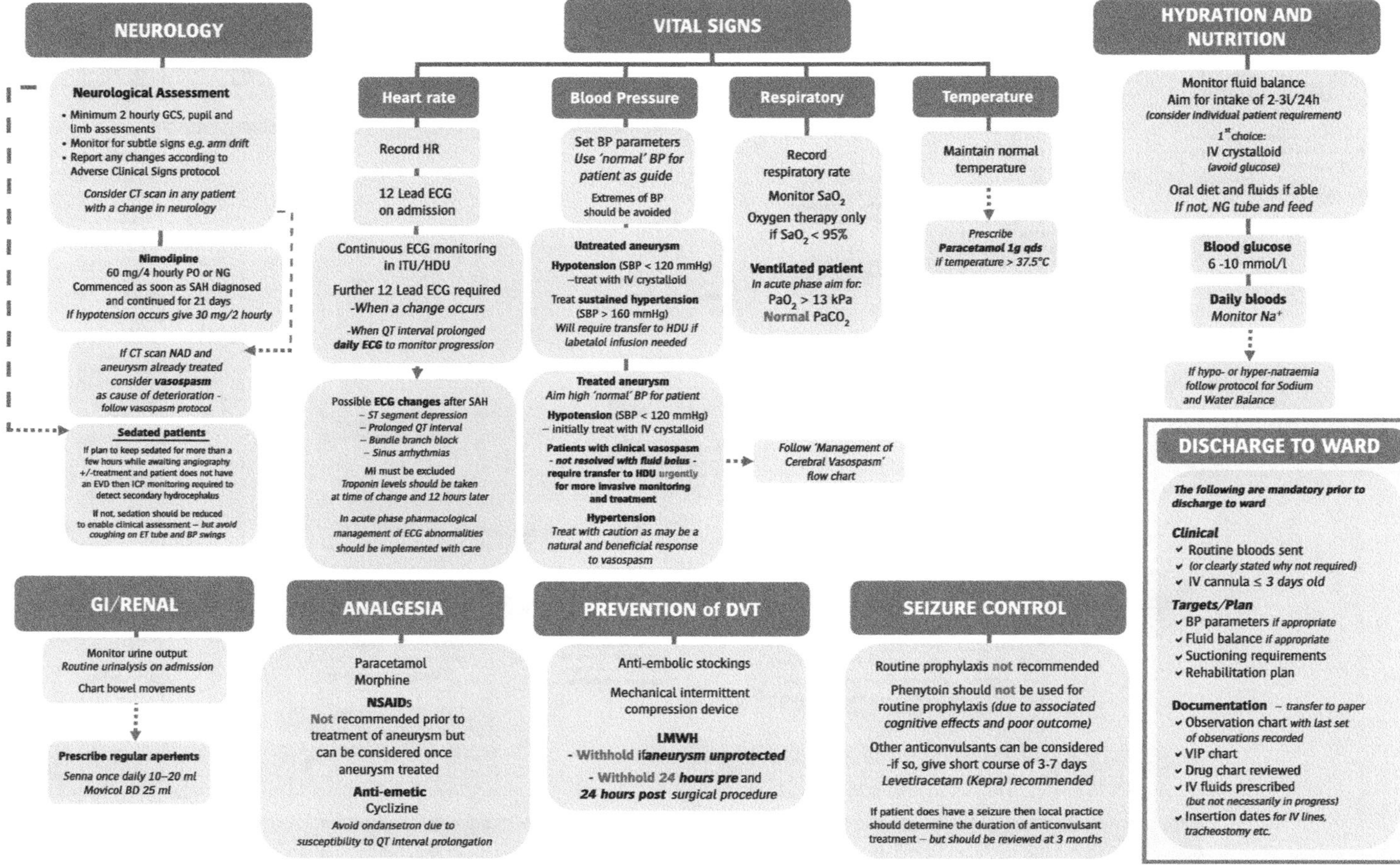

Figure 8.12 Management of SAH.

Subarachnoid Haemorrhage (SAH)
Management of Cerebral Vasospasm

MONITORING AND DIAGNOSIS

MONITORING

Observations
GCS, pupil and limb assessment
Vital signs - set BP target

*Neurocritical care patients will have daily **Transcranial Dopplers** during risk period*

Ventilated patients

BP 'high normal' for patient

<u>Blood gas targets</u>
PaO_2 > 13 kPa
Normal $PaCO_2$
Do not hyperventilate due to added risk of ischaemia from vasospasm

Daily Transcranial Dopplers

If there is good evidence of vasospasm from angiography or direct observation of blood vessels at operation a period of prophylactic hypertensive therapy may be specified if the patient is not clinically assessable

DIAGNOSIS

Detected clinically:
Reduction in conscious level
Focal neurological deficit
- Dysphasia
- Limb weakness
(May be subtle sign e.g. arm drift)

Diagnosis of exclusion
∴ Patient needs CT scan to exclude hydrocephalus or established stroke

Clinical signs of vasospasm?
- YES → BP
- NO → **Continue monitoring and preventive measures**

PREVENTION AND TREATMENT

Nimodipine
60 mg/4 hourly PO or NG
Commenced as soon as SAH diagnosed and continued for 21 days
If hypotension observed after administration give 30mg/2 hourly
If patient not absorbing give IV (1–2 mg/hr) via dedicated central line lumen (run concurrently with 0.9% saline 40 ml/hr)

BP

BP 'high normal' for patient

Euvolaemia
2-3 litres in 24 hours will be target for most patients but consider individual requirements

Clinical signs of vasospasm?
- NO → **Continue monitoring and preventive measures**
- YES → Give fluid bolus; Patient may require transfer to HDU for more invasive monitoring and treatment

FLUID THERAPY

Monitor fluid balance

1st choice: IV crystalloid

Give fluid bolus

Clinical signs of vasospasm?
- NO → **Continue monitoring and preventive measures**
- YES → Induced hypertension

VASOPRESSORS

Secured aneurysm

Induced hypertension
Patient requires HDU bed
1. Metaraminol infusion
(see Protocol)
If still required after 24 hours insert central line and start noradrenaline
2. Noradrenaline infusion
Make stepwise increases and titrate to neurology to determine BP target

↑ Systolic BP to reverse neurological deficit
(may be up to 180 mmHg)
BP target set by ICU Consultant *after d/w Interventional Neuroradiologist and Neurosurgeon*
Adjust target based on patient response to initial elevation of BP

Clinical signs of vasospasm?
- NO → **Continue monitoring and preventive measures**
- YES → *If no reversal of neurological deficit seen after 1 hour of hypertensive therapy discuss with Interventional Neuroradiologist*
  1. Transcranial Dopplers (TCD)
  2. CT perfusion – after d/w Interventional Neuroradiologist
  3. Proceed to angiography after d/w Interventional Neuroradiologist

Endovascular options
- Angioplasty
- Direct intra-arterial injection with vasodilators

Duration of induced hypertension
- Review every 24 hours
- Review TCD results
- Consider trial of lowering BP targets to determine continued need for induced hypertension
- Stepwise reduction in vasopressor based on neurology
- Set new BP target
- Consider rescan to rule out established infarct contra-indication to induced hypertension

Unsecured aneurysm

*If aneurysm thought to have ruptured is unsecured **cautious BP elevation** may be attempted*

Unsecured aneurysm not thought responsible for acute SAH should not influence haemodynamic management

<u>CEREBRAL VASOSPASM</u>

With current emphasis on early protection of a ruptured aneurysm, cerebral vasospasm leading to delayed ischaemic neurologic deficit (DIND) is the most common cause of late morbidity and mortality

Vasospasm is angiographically demonstrable in about two thirds of patients and one third will go on to develop clinical symptoms of cerebral ischaemia

Vasospasm occurs in a delayed fashion and may be reversible with aggressive preventive and treatment strategies in intensive care

<u>PATHOPHYSIOLOGY</u>

Peaks at 4–10 days after ictus and persists for several days but can occur up to 1 month after ictus

Exact cause remains obscure but its development is directly correlated with blood load in basal cisterns

Constituents of oxyhaemoglobin are likely spasmogenic factors

Most significant consequence of vasospasm is development of DIND secondary to reduced regional cerebral perfusion

Figure 8.13 Management of cerebral vasospasm.

management of pain and nausea is essential, and may calm an otherwise agitated patient. Paracetamol and dihydrocodeine are most commonly used and should be prescribed regularly. Morphine should also be prescribed, ideally by patient-controlled infusion (PCA) in suitable patients. The use of non-steroidal anti-inflammatory drugs (NSAIDs) is not recommended for patients with an untreated aneurysm as their antiplatelet effects can increase the risk of rebleeding. However, once the aneurysm has been treated NSAIDs may be considered.

Fluid and electrolyte balance

SAH patients are normally maintained on 3 L of fluid in 24 hours (2 L normal saline and 1 L colloid). As in TBI patients, dextrose-containing solutions are avoided and blood glucose is controlled between 6 and 10 mmol/L. Depleted volume states require close monitoring and treatment in view of the risk of cerebral vasospasm following SAH; treatment should aim for a normal to high CVP.

As with TBI patients, disturbances of water and electrolyte balance can occur following SAH. Hyponatraemia (serum sodium <135 mmol/L) has an associated morbidity and mortality if left untreated. Cerebral salt wasting (CSW) and the syndrome of inappropriate antidiuretic hormone (SIADH) are the two commonest causes; their distinction is important since CSW has an associated depleted circulating volume making spasm a great risk. Diabetes insipidus (DI) is particularly associated with anterior circulation aneurysms. It can also present post-operatively in these patients (see section on 'Management of sodium and water balance').

Nutrition

As in TBI, nutritional support should be commenced as soon as possible.

Positioning

Forced bed rest is a traditional part of SAH management, with patients nursed flat or with a head elevation of 15° if there are respiratory complications. Since subcutaneous heparin is not recommended in SAH patients, DVT prophylaxis consists of graduated elastic stockings and mechanical calf compression. Once the aneurysm has been treated, there are no restrictions on mobilizing the patient as their condition allows, except in the case of patients who have been fully anticoagulated following endovascular treatment when some restrictions may apply.

Stroke

Developments in acute stroke management, with improved pre-hospital recognition of stroke and early access to a specialist hyperacute stroke unit (HASU), have resulted in patients with acute severe stroke now being admitted to intensive care for more aggressive treatments. Such treatments include invasive blood pressure management, decompressive surgery, thrombectomy, treatment of hydrocephalus, and management of raised intracranial pressure. The complexities of management require a robust transfer pathway for patients at high risk of clinical deterioration who require on-site neurosurgical facilities (e.g. large middle cerebral artery/cerebellar infarct) and those who require time-critical interventional neuroradiology.

Differences in the treatment of ischaemic stroke and haemorrhagic stroke make a protocol-based approach essential, importantly in managing blood pressure and anticoagulation. Figure 8.14 details important aspects of care for these patients.

Status epilepticus

Epilepsy is a condition characterized by periodic disturbances of brain electrical activity that can lead to seizures, loss of consciousness, and sensory disturbances. Any of the classified seizure types can progress to status epilepticus. However, since generalized convulsive seizures are most commonly seen in critical care units, this section will focus on its management.

Status epilepticus (SE) is a clinical term referring to a series of generalized seizures without recovery of consciousness between attacks lasting for at least 30 min. Status epilepticus is usually easily diagnosed by observation, with seizures characterized by loss of consciousness, tonic (ongoing) and/or clonic (rhythmic) muscle activity, tongue biting, and urinary

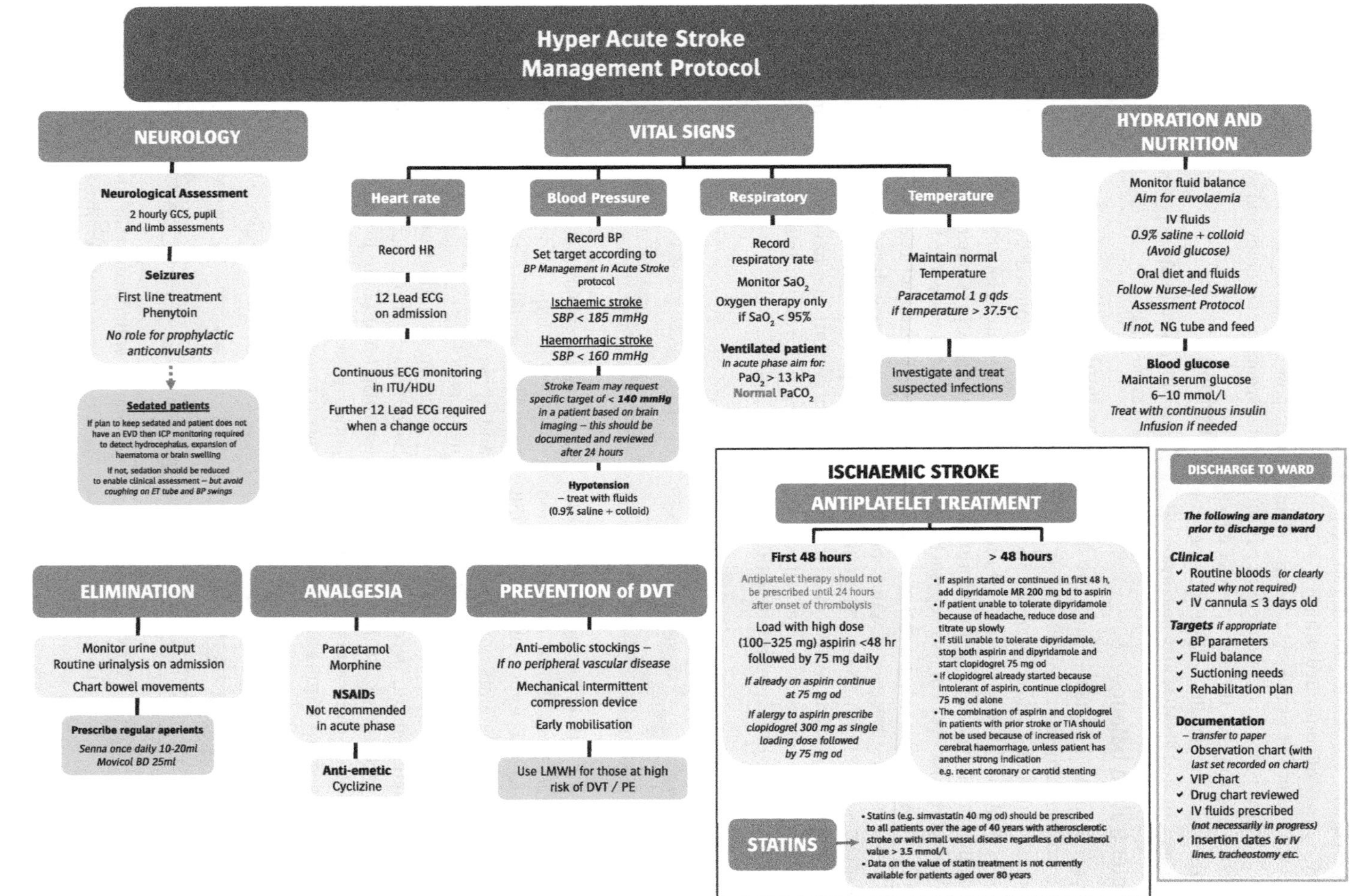

Figure 8.14 Management of acute stroke.

incontinence. However, as the duration of seizures increases, convulsive activity may become less obvious as depleted cerebral oxygen supplies are unable to meet demand (electromechanical dissociation). Only subtle twitching may remain as an outward sign that seizures are persisting.

Causes of status epilepticus include:

- metabolic abnormalities
- CNS infection (e.g. encephalitis, meningitis)
- vascular brain injury
- traumatic brain injury
- drug toxicity (e.g. cocaine, alcohol)
- cerebral anoxic/hypoxic damage
- pre-existing epilepsy
- non-compliance with or withdrawal of anticonvulsant drug therapy
- chronic alcoholism
- cerebral tumours/space-occupying lesions.

Management

Status epilepticus carries a high risk of mortality and morbidity, and therefore is a medical emergency requiring prompt action. Management should be directed at terminating the seizures, preventing recurrence of seizures once status is controlled, investigating and managing the precipitating causes of status epilepticus, and managing the potentially serious and cumulative complications of status epilepticus.

Many patients will respond to first-line treatment with benzodiazepines. However, note that all anti-epileptic medication is sedative in nature; therefore these patients will need nursing in a high dependency environment that has access to resuscitation equipment. In addition, these patients should be nursed in the recovery position, given oxygen therapy, and have continuous ECG, BP, and pulse oximetry monitoring. Steps should be taken to reduce the risk of self-harm/injury occurring during the seizures by removing all unnecessary equipment from the immediate vicinity of the patient.

Figure 8.15 is an algorithm showing the suggested treatment cycle of anti-epileptic drugs that should be considered. If the patient fails to respond to this treatment plan they should be considered to be in refractory status and transferred to a critical care unit. During prolonged status (60–90 min) the outward signs of motor activity diminish despite the presence of continued electroencephalographic (EEG) seizure activity. Here, the patient will require sedation with general anaesthetic agents, requiring that they be intubated and ventilated. Management is ideally aimed at suppressing this activity by titrating anaesthetic agents to the neurophysiological monitoring, usually recorded on a portable EEG monitor, until burst suppression of such activity is achieved. Full supportive treatment of the intubated patient is needed until the seizures stop and they regain consciousness.

Myasthenia gravis

Myasthenia gravis (MG), derived from the Greek for 'severe muscle weakness', is an autoimmune disease of varying severity characterized by relapses and spontaneous remissions. Its incidence is about 1 in 20,000 of the adult population, and is more prominent among women in their second to third decade and among men in their sixth to seventh decade. Without treatment, 20–30% of myasthenics will die from the disease, 39–50% improve spontaneously, and the remainder continue to worsen or remain symptomatic. Its cause is unknown, but the thymus gland may play some role in the autoimmune process since 80% of MG patients have thymic hyperplasia and 15% have thymic tumours.

Pathophysiology

MG affects the neuromuscular junction (Figure 8.16), specifically the acetylcholine (ACh) receptor site. Neurotransmission relies on release of ACh into the neuromuscular junction with subsequent binding to receptors on the post-synaptic membrane, triggering muscle contraction. The enzyme acetylcholinesterase (AchE) rapidly breaks down ACh allowing the muscle to relax. In MG the immune system generates antibodies that bind to these receptor sites and interfere with normal transmission, making it less effective or causing it to fail completely.

Signs and symptoms

The disorder is characterized by weakness and fatiguability of voluntary muscles; it typically involves muscles of the eye, face, and mouth. Skeletal muscles can also be affected, and in severe cases weakness of the muscles of swallowing and respiration can be life-threatening. The severity of muscle weakness fluctuates, typically worsening with repeated or sustained exertion or towards the end of the day, and is relieved by rest.

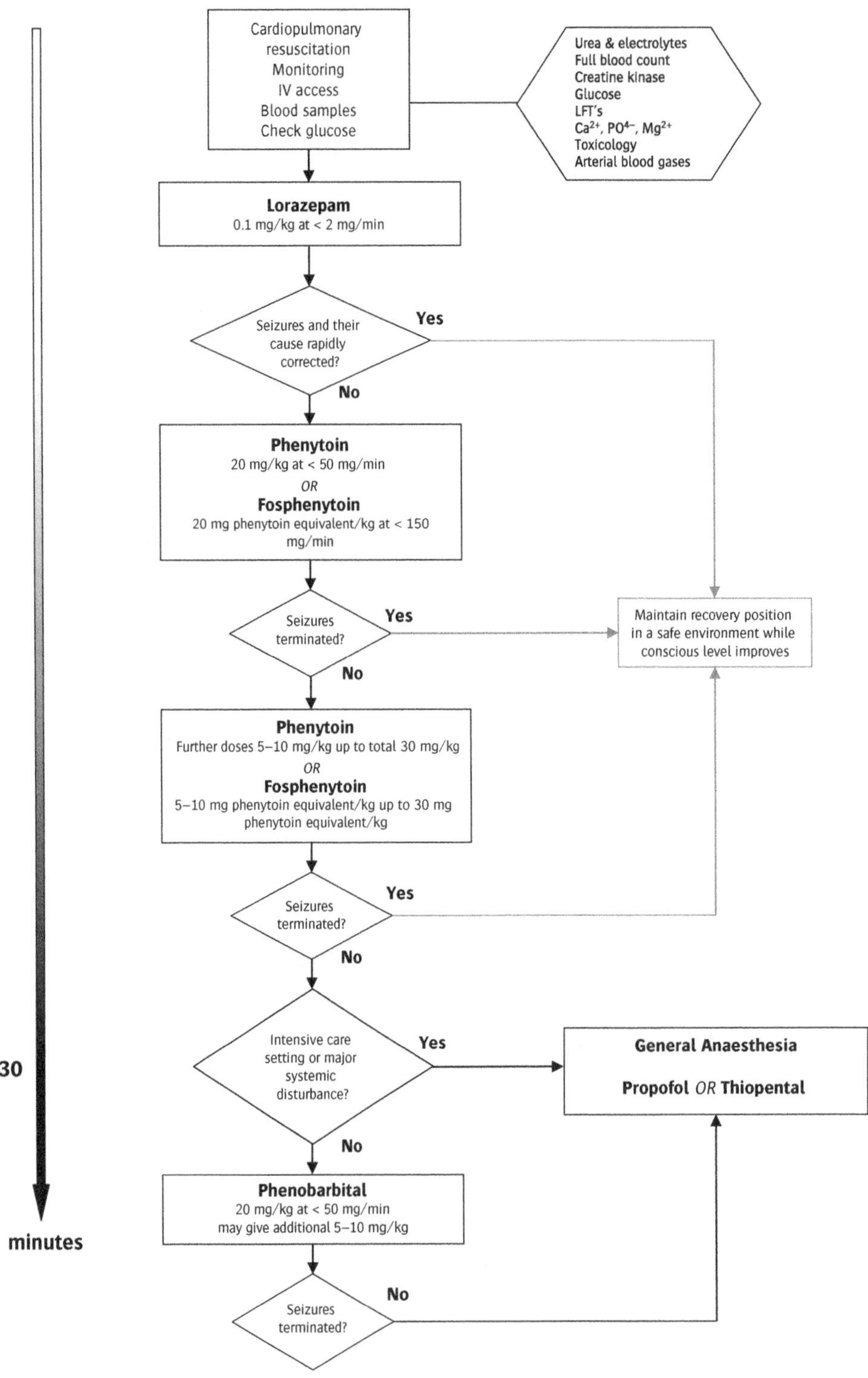

Figure 8.15 Algorithm for the treatment of status epilepticus.

Reproduced with permission from Chapman, M.G. *et al.*, Status epilepticus, *Anaesthesia*, Volume 56, Issue 7, pp.648–659, Copyright © 2001 The Association of Anaesthetists of Great Britain and Ireland

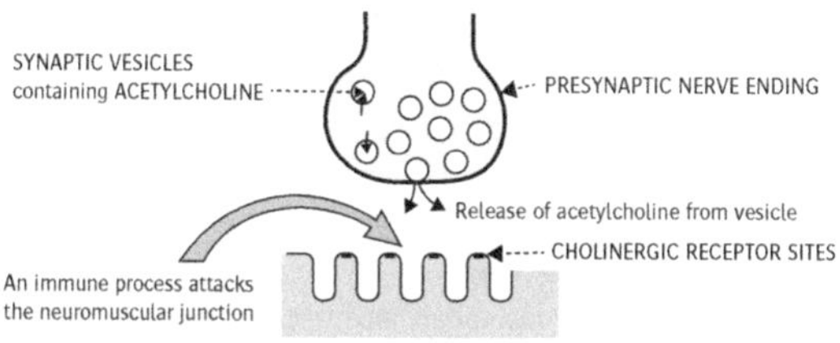

Figure 8.16 The neuromuscular junction

This figure was published in *Neurology and Neurosurgery Illustrated*, Lindsay, K.W. and Bone, I. Copyright Elsevier (2004).

Classic signs and symptoms include:

- ocular problems of ptosis and diplopia
- facial weakness
- bulbar weakness—difficulty swallowing and managing saliva
- dysarthria—voice nasal and weak and fades when talking
- weakness and fatiguability of skeletal muscle exacerbated by exercise and worsening as the day goes on
- loss of strength in limbs—arms more affected than legs, and proximal muscles more affected than distal muscles
- neck muscle weakness with head falling forward
- respiratory muscle weakness (not usually affected in isolation).

Diagnosis

Diagnosis is based on history, physical examination, electromyography (EMG), which may include diaphragmatic EMG, and confirmatory laboratory testing which should include detection of the anti-ACh receptor antibodies. An MRI/CT scan is carried out to determine if the thymus gland is enlarged.The Tensilon (edrophonium) test involves injection of the cholinesterase inhibitor edrophonium chloride, which produces rapid, but brief, return of muscular power. By decreasing the amount of cholinesterase, edrophonium makes more ACh available to their receptors, thus improving muscle strength. In addition to being used to diagnose MG, it is also used to distinguish between myasthenic crisis, where there is ACh deficiency, and cholinergic crisis, where there is an excess of ACh due to overdose with anticholinesterase drugs. As with any cholinergic drug, edrophonium can have adverse cardiac effects, such as bradycardia and arrhythmias, and adverse respiratory effects, such as respiratory muscle weakness, brochospasm, laryngospasm, and increased bronchial secretions. Atropine, the antidote to the muscarinic side effects of edrophonium, should be available during testing.

Treatment

There is no single therapy that works best for all patients; therefore treatment is based on the individual's response to specific therapies.

1. Symptomatic therapy with anticholinesterase agents:
   - pyridostigmine (Mestinon)
   - neostigmine (rarely used).
2. Disease-modifying approaches:
   - immunosuppressant drugs—corticosteroids (e.g. prednisolone), azathioprine
   - thymectomy
   - plasma exchange
   - intravenous immunoglobulin (IVIg).

Cholinesterase inhibitors delay the breakdown of ACh at cholinergic synapses allowing ACh to accumulate at the neuromuscular junction with prolonged effect. While they produce dramatic improvement in some patients, treatment with these drugs alone rarely produces normal strength. Pyridostigmine is the drug of choice since it has a long half-life and fewer gastrointestinal side effects. Prednisolone is given until sustained improvement is seen (usually within 3–4 weeks) and then weaned to the lowest level necessary to maintain improvement. Worsening of symptoms occurs in 50% of patients after commencing prednisolone, and this may result in severe bulbar and respiratory muscle weakness, sometimes requiring tracheal intubation and ventilation.

Azathioprine produces improvement in most patients after 4 months but may not show significantly until up to 12 months of treatment. Improvement persists for as long as the drug is given, but weakness may return after the drug is stopped or the dose is reduced.

Thymectomy produces best results in young patients with a short history of MG and in the absence of a thymoma. This should always be an elective procedure with the patient's MG well stabilized prior to surgery. Response to thymectomy may take up to 2 years, with the ultimate aim of maintaining the patient on lower doses of immunosuppressive medication.

Plasma exchange and intravenous immunoglobulin (IVIg) therapy may produce a rapid, albeit short-term, improvement of severe symptoms. Almost all patients will improve after plasma exchange. Improvement may begin after the first exchange and is seen within 48 hours in most patients, continuing for weeks or months after a single course.

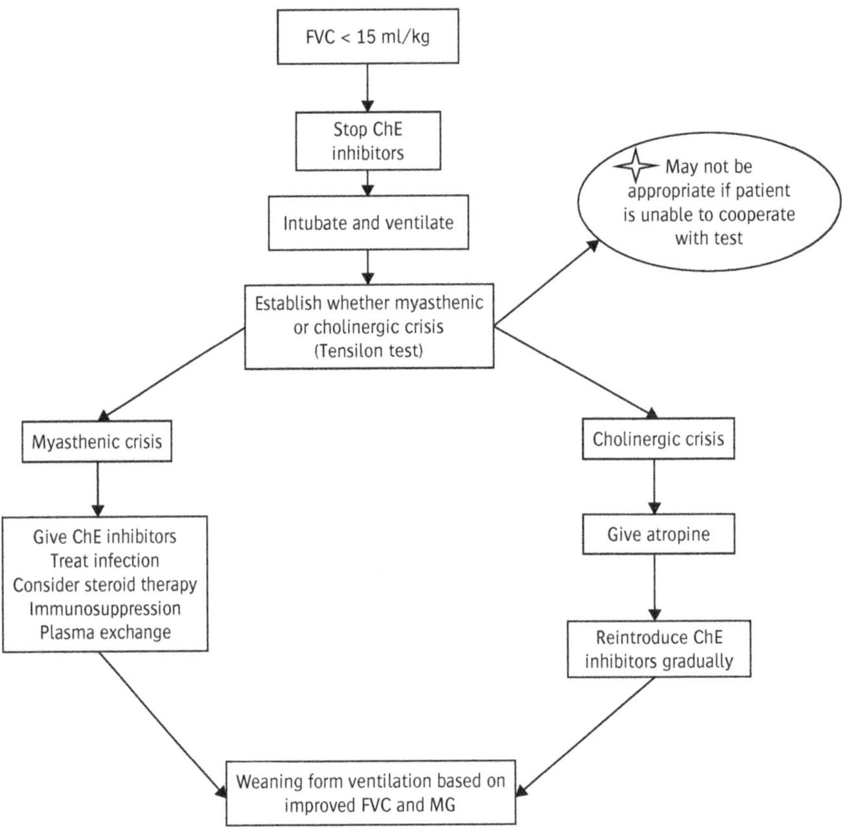

Figure 8.17 Myasthenic or cholinergic crisis?

Management in intensive care

Management will vary depending on whether admission is the result of an acute deterioration in a patient with known MG, or new onset in a previously undiagnosed MG patient. In severely ill patients the first priority is to maintain adequate ventilation and protection of the airway.

The development of respiratory insufficiency in MG is due to respiratory muscle weakness as a result of neuromuscular dysfunction and may be complicated by aspiration pneumonia secondary to bulbar weakness. Hypoxaemia, decreased tidal volume, dyspnoea, and abnormal arterial blood gases are all late findings in neuromuscular respiratory failure and are poor indicators of the need for ventilatory support. A more sensitive indicator of progressive respiratory failure is the forced vital capacity (FVC). As the FVC falls, spontaneous coughing weakens and there is greater difficulty in clearing secretions. Tracheal intubation is generally performed if FVC drops below 15 ml/kg but may be undertaken at a higher FVC if the patient also has bulbar weakness.

When there is an acute deterioration in a known myasthenic, it is vital to distinguish between *myasthenic crisis* and *cholinergic crisis* (Figure 8.17). The usual cause of myasthenic crisis is infection, and the signs and symptoms are those of myasthenia. Cholinergic crisis is caused by over-medication with anticholinesterase drugs, and symptoms include abdominal cramping and diarrhoea (muscarinic effects), profound generalized weakness, excessive pulmonary secretions, and impaired respiratory function (nicotinic effects). Both are medical emergencies that may require prompt tracheal intubation and assisted ventilation. The Tensilon test may reveal whether the patient is over- or under-dosed with anticholinesterase drugs, but its use in crisis may not be appropriate since the patient may not be able to cooperate with the test procedure. Delay in intubation may prove life-threatening. All ChE inhibitors should be disconitued and any underlying cause, such as infection or electrolyte abnormalities (in particular hypokalaemia, hypocalcaemia, and hypermagnesemia), treated. ChE inhibitors should be resumed at a dose lower than before the crisis and gradually increased.

Drug reactions and myasthenia gravis

Several drugs (including some aminoglycoside antibiotics such as gentamicin) exacerbate blockade at the neuromuscular junction, so use of any drug must be carefully considered. Some drugs, such as anti-spasmodics, carry a warning against their use in MG. The decision to extubate a patient with MG after an anaesthetic should be taken with caution.

Guillain–Barré syndrome

Guillain–Barré syndrome (GBS) is the commonest cause of acute neuromuscular paralysis in the UK with an annual incidence of 1–2 per 100,000 population. Despite advances in treatment and intensive care management, 3–8% die as a result of potentially avoidable complications including respiratory failure, respiratory or cardiac arrest, sepsis, pulmonary embolism, or the general medical complications of critical care. A further 10% remain severely disabled up to a year later.

Pathophysiology

GBS is an acute inflammatory neuropathy affecting peripheral nerves. The underlying pathology is usually demyelination of the nerves, with secondary axonal degeneration in the most severely affected cases. Two-thirds of patients describe an infectious illness in the 4 weeks prior to onset of symptoms, suggesting an immune basis for the inflammatory process. Bacterial and viral agents implicated include *Campylobacter jejuni, Mycoplasma pneumoniae*, Epstein–Barr virus, human immunodeficiency virus (HIV), and cytomegalovirus.

Signs and symptoms

GBS patients usually present with weakness and mild sensory symptoms (usually glove and stocking paraesthesiae). Typically, weakness starts from the feet up and, depending on severity, can gradually involve the rest of the body. Cranial nerves (in particular facial and bulbar) are commonly affected. Areflexia (loss of tendon jerks) is an early sign. In most cases weakness is maximal 3 weeks after the onset of neurological symptoms. Recovery usually begins 2–4 weeks after progression of weakness stops but, depending on severity, may be delayed for months. Respiratory muscle weakness requiring positive pressure ventilation occurs in 25–30% of patients. Bulbar dysfunction occurs in a similar proportion of GBS patients and may require tracheal intubation for airway protection. Autonomic dysfunction (dysautonomia) is extremely common and occurs in some form in 65% of patients. Sympathetic overactivity resulting in persistent tachycardia and hypertension is the most commonly seen manifestation, although severe parasympathetic manifestations may occur.

Diagnosis

The criteria for diagnosis include a history of presenting symptoms (progressive weakness of more than one limb with the duration of progression less than 4 weeks), clinical assessment (areflexia), laboratory studies of CSF (increased protein concentration with normal or only slightly raised white cell count) and blood (may reveal PCR positivity or rising titres to specific viruses), and nerve conduction studies (electromyography shows slowed nerve conduction, suggesting demyelination).

Treatment

1. **Supportive measures**: good general medical and nursing care, critical care management, rehabilitation.
2. **Specific therapy**: plasma exchange, intravenous immunoglobulin (IVIg).

Plasma exchange and IVIg therapy have been found to be equally effective in promoting recovery from GBS. They are most effective within a week of symptom onset or when there has been rapid deterioration in limb power. Owing to the ease of administration, IVIg is now the treatment of choice.

Management in intensive care

Up to 28% of all GBS cases present with a mild course of the disease, and are able to walk unaided throughout. Three factors determine whether the remainder will require critical care—respiratory failure, bulbar involvement, and autonomic dysfunction.

Close monitoring of respiratory function is essential to predict the respiratory needs of this group of patients and is usually done by monitoring the FVC. When the FVC falls to 15–20 ml/kg elective intubation should be considered. Likewise, when the recovering FVC reaches

20 ml/kg weaning is usually commenced. Intubation is often difficult in GBS patients because of autonomic instability. Bulbar dysfunction may require early intubation for airway protection even if the FVC remains adequate. Early tracheostomy should be considered if it is obvious that a prolonged period of artificial ventilation will be required. Autonomic dysfunction is usually benign and does not require any specific therapeutic intervention. However, close monitoring in a critical care unit is usually required to detect any life-threatening instability. Autonomic instability can cause extreme sensitivity to the effects of drugs, in particular sedatives, analgesics, and inotropes. Postural hypotension and bradycardia induced by vagal stimulation on suctioning are common. A persistent tachycardia (>120 bpm) is usually treated with short-acting drugs. Severe swings in BP should be treated symptomatically, though cautiously, with fluid and pressors for hypotension and cautious anti-hypertensive therapy for persistent elevations in BP. Delivery of nursing and therapy care should be observed for effects on the autonomic status of the patient, especially stimulatory interventions such as tracheal suction and chest physiotherapy.

Pain

Pain, arising from immobility, inflamed nerves, and denervated muscles, is a common problem and is often refractory to simple analgesics. It is often severe, usually neurogenic, and worse with remyelination of the nerves. Types of pain include paraesthesia (tingling, stinging, pins and needles), dysaesthesia (burning), backache and sciatica, meningism (meningeal irritation from swollen nerve roots), joint pain, and occasionally visceral pain (related to autonomic dysfunction). This can be compounded by problems of proprioception in some patients, making symptom relief difficult. Management requires thoughtful use of several types of analgesic. Simple analgesics and NSAIDs may be effective in relieving musculoskeletal symptoms, and paracetamol and NSAIDs should be prescribed routinely. Anticonvulsant agents such as gabapentin are effective for paraesthesia and dysaesthesia, while tricyclic antidepressants such as amitriptyline are effective for neurogenic pain. Opioids (e.g. meptazinol) may be required if pain persists.

Sleep

Pain is exacerbated by the poor sleep patterns and disorientation that can be experienced in the intensive care environment. Many patients describe periods of vivid and disturbing dreams, occurring during both day and night, during the rehabilitation period. Reorientating the patient and giving reassurance can help reduce anxiety and promote relaxation prior to sleep. GBS patients often benefit from regular night sedation and access to 'breakthrough' analgesia.

Positioning/rehabilitation

Careful positioning and passive full-range joint movements can prevent contractures; physiotherapy input is crucial to address these issues. Intermittent splinting of limbs (wrists, fingers, and ankles) may be needed. A graduated programme, which involves sitting the patient up in bed and on a tilt table to ensure that postural changes can be tolerated, is usually required before the patient can sit out of bed. Positioning can be compromised by the need for head and trunk support, and a fully supportive semi-reclining wheelchair with pressure-relieving cushions is essential.

Communication

The GBS patient presents a challenge in achieving effective communication. Acute GBS, where the patient is paralysed and requires mechanical ventilation, and is totally dependent on others, gives rise to understandable fear and anxiety. Sedation is usually given for the first 24–48 hours following intubation, but is generally not appropriate afterwards. Early intervention from a speech and language therapist will help identify the most appropriate aids to communication for individual patients. Patients with intact bulbar function can be taught to use a speaking valve with tracheostomy cuff deflation, while patients with impaired bulbar function will need to rely on a blink response to an alphabet board or picture cards in the early stages. If is seems likely that the disease process will be lengthy, early tracheostomy will aid lip reading (see Chapter 3).

Acute infection and inflammation of the central nervous system

Any CNS infection can have potentially devastating consequences and requires immediate medical attention. Patients often need admission to critical care for urgent airway protection, mechanical ventilation, and control of raised ICP. They may also require critical care management for seizure control or because agitation makes them difficult to manage, necessitating sedation and respiratory monitoring.

The infection can be regional (i.e. meningitis), diffuse (i.e. encephalitis), or focal (i.e. brain abscess). Clinical presentation will vary depending on which part of the CNS is affected. Meningitis is characterized by fever, headache, and neck stiffness, encephalitis is primarily characterized by altered mental status, and brain abscess gives rise to focal deficits. Meningitis is more common than either encephalitis or brain abscess. In meningitis and encephalitis, either syndrome can be accompanied by some features of the other; most cases of meningitis are complicated by some degree of inflammation of the brain tissue (sometimes termed meningoencephalitis).

Meningitis

Meningitis is an inflammation of the meninges, usually the arachnoid and pia mater, and the intervening subarachnoid space. There are three main types of meningitis: viral (e.g. herpes simplex virus), bacterial (e.g. *Neisseria meningitides, Streptococcus pneumoniae, Haemophilus influenzae*), and others (e.g. tuberculous, fungal). Most viral causes are usually self-limiting, resolving spontaneously with only supportive treatment, and the patient makes a full recovery. Other forms, in particular bacterial meningitis, constitute a serious and life-threatening illness. Even with modern treatment, there is a significant mortality, while many survivors will have complications of hydrocephalus, blindness, deafness, cognitive deficits, or epilepsy.

Signs and symptoms

Certain features are common to all types of meningitis, but the speed at which they develop and their intensity varies depending on the causative organism. Meningitis is not always obvious; some cases may not show the preceding 'typical' signs. Bacterial meningitis may strike suddenly, with the patient lapsing into coma within hours before other symptoms are established. Others may present with a seizure. If infection is confined to the spinal meninges, the CSF may be purulent without either disturbance of consciousness or even headache. Tuberculous and cryptococcal meningitis are insidious in onset, and their presenting symptoms may not arouse suspicion of meningitis.

More typically, the illness is preceded by a respiratory infection, otitis media, or pneumonia, or by a few days of pyrexia and a flu-like illness. This is followed by severe frontal/occipital headache, photophobia and drowsiness, and neck stiffness, which is the vital sign of meningeal irritation. This is demonstrated by attempting to bend the head forward so that the chin rests on the chest—neck rigidity will prevent this. In addition, attempting to straighten the knee when the hip is flexed will be painful and restricted (positive Kernig's sign) (Figure 8.18). On examination, a non-blanching petechial or purpuric rash is suggestive of meningococcal infection.

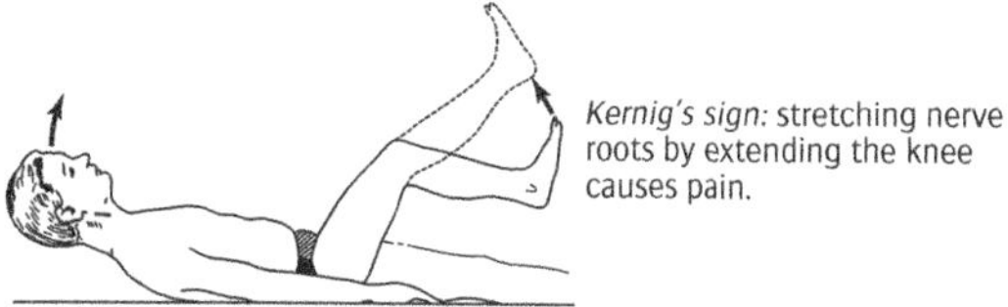

Figure 8.18 Signs of meningism

This figure was published in *Neurology and Neurosurgery Illustrated*, Lindsay, K.W. and Bone, I. Copyright Elsevier (2004).

Diagnosis

Diagnosis includes patient history and examination, throat swabs, blood culture, blood and urinary antigen testing, and CSF analysis. Microbiology samples should be taken from purpuric lesions by injecting small amounts of sterile normal saline into a lesion and then aspirating it. This is an effective means of isolating meningococci, even after antibiotics have been commenced. Lumbar puncture is usually needed to establish the diagnosis, though is not necessary if the patient has an obvious meningococcal rash. Patients in coma with focal neurological signs or papilloedema must first undergo CT scanning to exclude a mass lesion or significantly raised intracranial pressure prior to lumbar puncture. However, a normal CT scan does not fully exclude raised intracranial pressure, so a risk of coning remains. Regardless, it is essential to commence antibiotics promptly after taking blood samples for culture rather than waiting until a lumbar puncture is performed, unless this is done immediately. CSF results from lumbar puncture may show moderate increases in pressure, raised white cell count (neutrophils or lymphocytes), raised protein, and a normal or low glucose level depending on the infecting organisms. The organism may be seen in the CSF on Gram stain (bacteria) or other special stains (e.g. India Ink for *Cryptococcus*). Electron microscopy may identify a viral aetiology. Increasingly, molecular diagnostics (e.g. polymerase chain reaction(PCR)) is being used to facilitate prompt diagnosis, as traditional culture may take days to weeks to identify an organism.

Viral meningitis

Viral meningitis is caused by a number of different viruses, the commonest being enteroviruses, spread by the faecal–oral route (common in summer/autumn), and arboviruses (arthropod-borne viruses), transmitted by mosquito bite or tick bite (common in summer/autumn). Often the organism responsible remains unknown. With international travel, tropical viral diseases cannot be excluded, and a good history will establish if this is relevant or not. The onset and symptoms of viral meningitis are similar to bacterial forms but are usually less severe.

Aciclovir is active against herpes simplex virus and should be started immediately. Following this, management is purely supportive. Antibacterial agents are not appropriate unless there is a concurrent bacterial infection. The course of the illness is self-limiting and recovery usually begins within 7–14 days.

Tuberculous meningitis

Tuberculous meningitis is caused by the tubercle bacillus. It may be a primary meningitis but often is a secondary manifestation of tuberculosis elsewhere in the body, most commonly the lungs The primary lesion may have gone unrecognized, and the patient may have been unwell for weeks with gradually increasing headache and listlessness. Untreated tuberculous meningitis may progress over weeks to months from the non-specific symptoms of fever and lethargy to coma and death.

Tuberculous meningitis is treated with a cocktail of thre or four anti-tuberculous drugs such as rifampicin, isoniazid, and pyrazinamide. Treatment is normally for 6 months or longer. Steroids may be given in addition.

Bacterial meningitis

Bacterial meningitis results from invasion of bacteria, the commonest in adults being meningococci, pneumococci, and *Haemophilus*. The onset is acute, with bacteria invading the subarachnoid space either directly from adjoining structures, such as the sinuses, or indirectly from the bloodstream. Bacterial meningitis can be fatal, or may leave the patient with a severe handicap such as deafness or brain injury.

In the UK, *Haemophilus influenzae* type B meningitis (Hib) has been largely eliminated by vaccination of infants. Meningococcal meningitis (caused by *Neisseria meningitidis*) is the most common bacterial form in the UK, accounting for more than half the cases. Its incidence is also decreasing due to childhood vaccination against the *Meningococcus* C strain. It is spread by droplet infection, and the organism lodges and multiplies in the nasopharynx. It may also spread systemically, giving rise to generalized sepsis with organ dysfunction in approximately 55% of cases. Pneumococcal meningitis (caused by *Streptococcus pneumoniae*) is indicative of a secondary invasion of the meninges from an adjacent infected site or the result of a bacteraemia. Recent pneumonia, sepsis in the middle ear or sinuses, and a fractured base of skull are frequent causes. It is associated with a higher risk of death and permanent neurological damage compared with meningococcal infection.

The bacteria which cause both meningococcal and pneumococcal meningitis are very common. They live naturally in the back of the nose and throat or upper respiratory tract, and 10–25% of the population are carriers. However, only rarely do they overcome the body's natural defences and spread via the bloodstream to the subarachnoid space to cause meningitis. The incubation period is 2–10 days.

Treatment includes the urgent administration of antibiotics, at first empirical and then, if needed, adapted to the pathogen and antibiotic susceptibilities recovered from the CSF, suppression or removal of the initial infectious focus, steroids, and symptomatic and adjunctive therapy. Though studies suggest shorter courses are effective, treatment is often given for 10 days. For meningococcal and pneumococcal meningitis national guidelines advise treatment with ceftriaxone or cefotaxime. If the patient has a clear history of anaphylaxis to penicillin or cephalosporins, chloramphenicol and vancomycin or rifampicin should be given. Benzylpenicillin can be the initial therapy for meningococcal meningitis, provided that the patient has not recently visitied an area of high resistance such as Spain or the USA.

With meningococcal meningitis, close contacts of the patient (family, room-mates, nursery school contacts) are at increased risk of cross-infection. All such contacts should be offered antibiotics (e.g. one dose of ciprofloxacin to adults, or rifampicin to children) to eliminate the organism from the nasopharynx. Healthcare workers are not routinely offered prophylaxis unless they come into direct contact (e.g. the patient coughs into the carer's eyes). Protective goggles/hood and masks should be worn for the first few days, and the patient should be kept in isolation.

Steroid therapy (dexamethasone 10 mg four times daily for 4 days) has been shown to be effective for pneumococcal or haemophilus meningitis, but only if the first dose is given at the time of administration of the first dose of antibiotics.

Encephalitis

Encephalitis is an acute inflammatory process that affects brain tissue and, in some cases, will be accompanied by inflammation of the meninges (meningoencephalitis). Most cases are caused by viral infection and can manifest as either primary encephalitis, when the virus directly infects the brain, or secondary (post-infectious) encephalitis, where an often innocuous infection is thought to precipitate an autoimmune attack on the brain leading to inflammation. Some types of encephalitis are caused by parasitic or protozoal organisms including malaria, toxoplasma, or amoebae. Like meningitis, the seriousness of the disease depends upon the organism responsible. While some types of viral encephalitis are self-limiting and patients recover fully, others constitute a severe and life-threatening illness.

Signs and symptoms

Onset of encephalitis is usually acute, but signs and symptoms of CNS involvement are often preceded or accompanied by a non-specific acute febrile illness. The classic triad of features of encephalitis are confusion/reduced level of consciousness, fever, and seizures. Seizures may be frequent, and may involve increasing areas of the body as the cerebral inflammation extends. In secondary encephalitis symptoms usually appear within 1–2 weeks of the original infection and typically include fever, headache, behavioural changes, and impaired conscious level; seizures are less common than in primary encephalitis. Unless the meninges are also infected, there is relatively little neck stiffness and Kernig's sign is negative.

Diagnosis

History-taking and physical examination can provide clues to the cause, but the diagnosis is usually established on the basis of CSF analysis (including microscopy, culture, PCR, and electron microscopy), neurodiagnostic studies (CT scan, MRI scan, EEG), and brain biopsy if indicated. Serum and CSF antibody studies are useful in some instances such as arboviral encephalitis. When recording the history particular attention should be paid to recent illnesses, recent vaccinations, travel, contacts with pets or wild animals, or tick exposure, long-term immunosuppression or possible exposure to HIV, and a recent acquired immunodeficiency syndrome (AIDS) illness.

As in meningitis, lumbar puncture should be performed only after CT scan has excluded a space-occupying lesion in patients in coma or with focal neurological deficits, or the likelihood of a significantly raised intracranial pressure. In viral encephalitis CSF analysis will typically show a normal or moderately elevated opening pressure, a moderate increase in lymphocyte count, a normal or mildly elevated protein level, and a normal glucose level. Confirmation of diagnosis depends on identification of the virus within the CSF, or within brain tissue following biopsy. EEG is important to exclude non-convulsive status epilepticus.

Bacterial encephalitis

Bacterial pathogens invariably involve inflammation of the meninges out of proportion to their encephalitic components. The exception is *Listeria monocytogenes* which most commonly affects the elderly and pregnant women. Unlike the more common forms of bacterial meningitis, which are mostly restricted to the meninges, *Listeria* also has a propensity to infect the brain tissue itself, in particular the brainstem. *Listeria* encephalitis is treated with amoxicillin and gentamicin, or co-trimaxazole in the penicillin-allergic patient.

Viral encephalitis

More than 100 different viruses are known to cause acute viral encephalitis; the most frequently reported are seasonal enteroviruses, arboviruses, and herpes simplex virus (HSV).

Entry into the CNS depends on the virus. Some are spread through person-to-person contact (e.g. HSV, varicella zoster virus (VZV) associated with chickenpox, measles, mumps, and rubella virus). Important animal carriers are mosquitoes and ticks (arbovirus) and warm-blooded mammals (rabies virus). Some viruses will target specific areas of the CNS; for example, HSV selectively affects the inferior frontal and medial temporal lobes. Immunologically compromised patients are particularly susceptible to VZV and cytomegalovirus (CMV).

With a few exceptions, notably aciclovir for herpes simplex encephalitis (HSE), no specific therapy is available for most forms of viral encephalitis, so management consists of symptomatic and supportive care. However, since the early administration of antiviral therapy for HSE has been shown to reduce mortality and morbidity (note that evidence is only for HSV, but VZV is also sensitive), empirical therapy with intravenous aciclovir should be given in all cases of suspected HSE and varicella zoster encephalitis (VZE) until a definitive diagnosis is made. Similarly, until a bacterial cause can be excluded, parenteral antibiotics (ceftriaxone or cefotaxime) should be commenced. Treatment should continue until such time as a causative organism is identified or until medically directed otherwise. Secondary or post-infectious encephalitis is treated by immunosuppression, usually with steroids.

The time course for recovery from viral encephalitis can be protracted. However, supportive care should be given for as long as necessary since, even when recovery takes a long time, outcome can still be very good.

Behavioural changes can be dramatic and may continue for many months into the recovery stage.

Cerebral malaria

Malaria should always be suspected as the cause of any neurological symptoms in a patient who has returned from an endemic area within the previous 2 months. Cerebral malaria frequently presents with non-specific influenza-type symptoms but can progress to coma and death and therefore requires urgent treatment. Cerebral malaria is treated with intravenous quinine or, increasingly, with artesunate.

Intracranial abscess

Intracranial abscess may develop due to direct spread from adjacent infections in the ear or sinuses following trauma (either penetrating head injury or closed head injury with base of skull fracture) or, alternatively, infection can spread through the bloodstream from a distant source or from an infected epidural/spinal anaesthesia. It can also occur as a complication of craniocerebral surgery or in immunologically compromised patients. The two main types are intracerebral abscess and subdural abscess (empyema). Chronic otitis media should be suspected in temporal lobe and cerebellar abscess, while frontal lobe abscess should raise suspicions of local sinus infection. While any organism is capable of producing a cerebral abscess, common organisms are *Streptococcus milleri*, anaerobic *Bacteroides* species, *Proteus*, and *Escherichia coli*.

The brain usually goes through a stage of cerebritis before the abscess forms. A capsule, which eventually becomes quite tough and thick, then begins to form around the infected area, a defence mechanism which prevents the infection from spreading through the brain. The abscess then acts as a space-occupying lesion, resulting in raised ICP and focal neurological deficits.

Signs and symptoms

Headaches are a common feature, becoming increasingly severe and leading to confusion and drowsiness. Focal signs and symptoms will usually reflect the site involved. With subdural empyema the spread of infection within the subdural space gives rise to more acute signs of increased ICP. Seizures are also a common feature of intracranial abscess.

Diagnosis

Plain X-rays of the skull may show abnormalities in the frontal sinuses or mastoid air cells, indicating a possible source of infection, but CT scan with contrast is the definitive investigation. A full blood count and blood cultures should also be taken.

Treatment

Treatment consists of surgical drainage via either craniotomy or burr-hole aspiration of the abscess, identifying the organism responsible and treating with appropriate antibiotics, plus therapeutic and supportive measures to reduce ICP in severe cases. In addition, the primary source of infection should be investigated and treated.

The algorithm in Figure 8.19 summarizes the treatment of a patient with a presumed CNS infection.

Brainstem death and organ donation

Brainstem death

Determining death by neurological criteria is accepted practice in many countries throughout the world and many religions accept the concept of brain death. However, there are some differences in practice between countries regarding the number of physicians required, the additional confirmatory tests recommended, and the time period for testing. Although the same principles apply to adults and children, testing in neonates and infants is more difficult because of size and developmental stage. The time course for maintaining the brain-dead patient is limited, and prolonged intervention cannot prevent cardiac arrest from haemodynamic instability (despite increasing levels of inotropic support) for more than a few days in most cases. Accounts of the preservation of brain dead patients for longer periods have been documented, but such cases are very rare, and in some cases the evidence is unclear.

The UK Code of Practice for the Diagnosis and Confirmation of Death (2008) recommends that the definition of brainstem death should be regarded as 'irreversible loss of the capacity for consciousness, combined with irreversible loss of the capacity to breathe'. It states that brainstem death, irrespective of its cause, produces irreversible cessation of brainstem function and therefore brainstem death equates to death of the brain and of the individual. In the UK there are three stages in

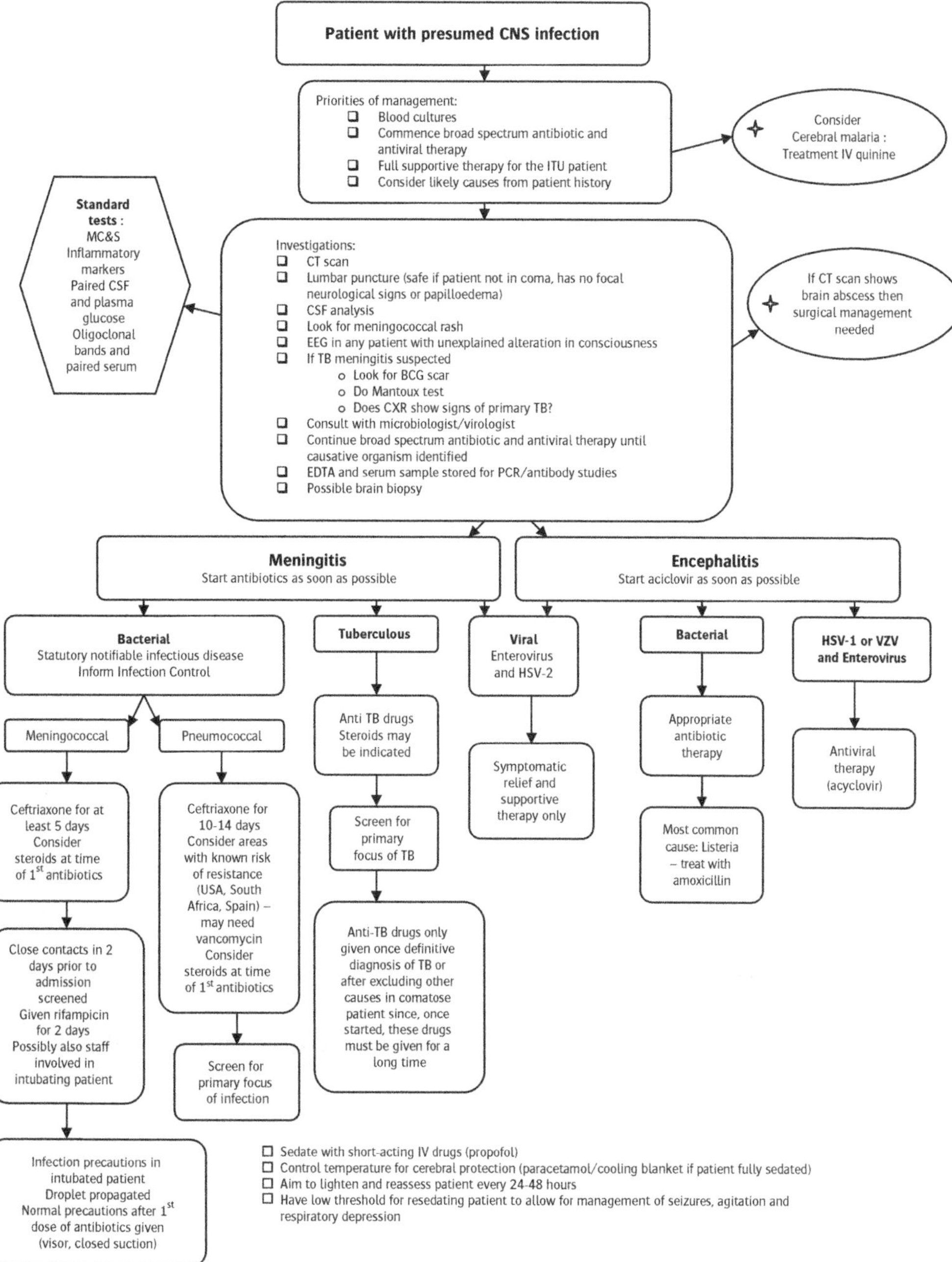

Figure 8.19 Algorithm summarizing the treatment of a patient with a presumed CNS infection.

the diagnosis of brain death—preconditions, exclusions, and clinical tests (Table 8.10).

Timing of brainstem death tests

The time before testing should equal the time taken to meet the essential preconditions and the necessary exclusions, and patient management should focus on specific preparation for the tests (Table 8.11).

Test procedure

The UK Code of Practice requires two doctors with expertise in the field to make the diagnosis of brain

Table 8.10 Stages in the diagnosis of brainstem death

Preconditions	Diagnosis compatible with brainstem death and evidence of irreversible structural brain damage Apnoeic coma dependent on mechanical ventilation
Exclusions	Causes of reversible coma and factors causing central depression excluded Absence of effects of sedative, hypnotic, analgesic, and muscle relaxant drugs confirmed Primary hypothermia excluded Metabolic disorders considered, with particular emphasis on the correction of abnormal sodium, glucose, and pH levels
Clinical tests	Tests to confirm the absence of brainstem reflexes and the presence of persistent apnoea

Table 8.11 Observation and management of the patient for brainstem death tests

Neurology	No cranial nerve function
Respiratory	No spontaneous respiration Absence of gag reflex on oral suction and absence of cough on tracheal suction Normal pH and acid–base balance Normalize CO_2 prior to testing
Cardiovascular*	Maintain: • MAP ≥60 mmHg (use vasopressors if required) • Temperature >35°C • Na^+ 135–155 mmol/L • K^+ 3.5–4.5 mmol/L • Glucose 4–9 mmol/L
Sedation	Sedatives, analgesics, and muscle relaxant drugs discontinued for >6 hours prior to testing: reversing drugs (e.g. naloxone, flumazenil) and a peripheral nerve stimulator can be used
Hydration	IV fluids to maintain BP and CVP Continue nasogastric feeding Insulin infusion if required to keep blood glucose at 4–9 mmol/L 5% glucose if required to keep Na^+ below 155 mmol/L
Elimination	DDAVP 0.4 mg if evidence of diabetes insipidus to control electrolyte balance and volume status

* It is recognized that circulatory, metabolic, and endocrine disturbances (e.g. hypernatraemia, diabetes insipidus) are probable accompaniments of brainstem death, but these are effect rather than cause. Provided that potentially reversible causes of unconsciousness are excluded, these do not preclude diagnosis of brainstem death.

DDAVP, l-deamino-8-d-arginine vasopressin (desmopressin).

death (Table 8.12). These will usually be senior clinicians (registered for more than 5 years) with an interest in intensive care medicine and anaesthesia. One should be a consultant and the other a consultant or senior registrar. The preconditions and exclusions must have been satisfied before the tests are carried out, and the two doctors must carry out the tests independently of each other. In adults, there is no formal requirement in the UK for a specified time interval between the two sets of tests. However, it is common practice to allow an interval of 2–4 hours between the first and second tests to allow time for relatives to come to terms with the diagnosis. It is during this period that the subject of organ donation may be broached. If hypoxic injury has occurred (e.g. following cardiac arrest), it is usual to allow at least 24 hours to elapse before brainstem tests are carried out. Although not specifically mentioned in the UK Code of Practice, the 'doll's eyes' response should be tested initially in every case. If this response is present, the patient is clearly not brainstem dead.

Limb and trunk movements

Reflex movements of the limbs and trunk may occur in brainstem-dead patients due to spinal reflexes. Their significance should be explained to relatives and staff to enable them to understand that they do not involve conscious voluntary movements (i.e. they do not originate in the cerebral cortex).

Documentation

Documented time of death is the time of the first set of brainstem tests when the diagnosis of brain death is confirmed, and not when mechanical ventilation is discontinued. Legally, the time of death is recognized when the first set of tests indicates brainstem death, but death cannot be pronounced and certified until after completion of the second set of tests.

Table 8.12 Tests for the absence of brainstem function and apnoea

Diagnostic test	Cranial nerve	Area of brainstem tested
Fixed diameter pupil, unreactive either directly or consensually to sharp changes in light intensity	Optic (II) Oculomotor (III)	Midbrain
Absent corneal reflex—no blink occurs when cornea is brushed with gauze	Trigeminal (V) Facial (VII)	Midbrain
Absent vestibulo-ocular reflex—no eye movement occurs during or following slow injection of at least 50 ml of ice-cold water into each external auditory meatus (clear access to the tympanic membrane must be established by direct inspection and the head should be flexed at 30°)	Acoustic (VIII) Abducens (VI)	Pons
No motor response within the cranial nerve distribution in response to stimuli and no limb response to supraorbital nerve pressure Absent grimacing to pain No head movement	Facial (VII) Accessory (XI)	Midbrain, medulla
No gag reflex in response to suction catheter passed down the trachea No slowing of heart rate	Glossopharyngeal (IX) Vagus (X)	Medulla
No respiratory movements occur when disconnection from ventilator allows P_aCO_2 to rise above the threshold for respiratory stimulation (6.65 kPa)		Respiratory centre in medulla
Testing for apnoea • Reduce SIMV rate to allow P_aCO_2 to rise to 6.0 kPa prior to testing • Pre-oxygenate with 100% oxygen for 10 min • Disconnect from ventilator • Insufflate oxygen at 6 L/min via suction catheter placed in endotracheal tube to maintain adequate oxygenation during testing • Allow P_aCO_2 to rise to 6.65 kPa • Confirm no spontaneous respiration • Reconnect ventilator		

SIMV, synchronized intermittent mandatory ventilation.

Turning off the ventilator

If the patient is not to be an organ donor, when appropriate time has been given to relatives, the ventilator should be switched off and all infusions discontinued. There should be no 'weaning' process since the patient has been certified dead.

Care of the family

It is well documented that caring for the relatives of a critically ill patient can be extremely stressful. When the patient has had a catastrophic brain injury and is awaiting brainstem tests the degree of stress can be very high. These patients are often young, previously fit individuals and the circumstances leading to their admission sudden and tragic. Initial intensive nursing and medical management suddenly changes to supportive care for the patient whose diagnosis is irreversible and often difficult to comprehend. There may be little time for the intensive care team to build up a rapport with the family and for the family to come to terms with imminent loss. These factors alone can make the task of explaining the already complex concept of brainstem death difficult for all those involved.

The nurse's role in preparing the family for the diagnosis of brainstem death and supporting them through the process is crucial. Some relatives may request to be at the bedside when the tests are carried out and will need the support of an experienced and knowledgeable nurse.

Despite confirmation of the diagnosis of brainstem death, the patient remains warm to touch and continues to display physiological signs of life (heart rate and blood pressure) until the ventilator is switched off. This can make acceptance of the diagnosis difficult. Relatives should be given appropriate time at the bedside and given the choice to be there when ventilation is discontinued. If they do choose to be at the bedside when the ventilator is switched off, some explanation should be given of possible reflex movements that the patient may make. Some families may want the patient be an organ donor, and once brainstem death has been confirmed the focus of care will be to fulfil the family's wish.

Approaching the family of a potential organ donor

Broaching the subject of organ donation with a bereaved family is often seen as one of the most difficult stages in the organ donation process and many factors have been identified as potential obstacles to organ donation: dislike of adding to relatives' distress, lack of training in how to approach families, adverse media publicity, fear of being blamed, and fear of saying or doing the wrong thing.

Who can ask?

There are no set rules about who should ask. However, the person asking should be comfortable with the concept of brainstem death and the idea of organ donation. This should be a collaborative approach. The intensive care team who have been involved in the care of the patient and family since admission can provide support and guidance. Involving the specialist nurse for organ donation (SNOD) in the initial stages ensures expert advice from someone who can answer all questions regarding the donor process.

When to ask

Some families may spontaneously raise the issue of organ donation prior to brainstem testing and information should be provided as required. The SNOD might be contacted at this point to answer questions about the donor process. However, if the option of donation needs to be broached by the intensive care team, ideally this should be done in the interval between the two sets of brainstem tests. It is important that within this process the family is given sufficient time to accept the diagnosis of brainstem death.

Donation after brainstem death (DBD)

Once a family has decided that their relative should be an organ donor, the aim of management is to support the patient's organs for transplantation (Table 8.13). Brain death affects nearly every organ system, and there are many complications that can make donor management difficult. These complications include hypotension, diabetes insipidus, hypothermia, electrolyte abnormalities, coagulopathy, hypoxia, and cardiac arrhythmias. At the present time, the only absolute contraindication to organ donation is Creutzfeldt–Jakob disease (CJD) or a family history of CJD.

Table 8.13 Maintenance of the organ donor

Respiratory support	P_aO_2 >10 mmHg with the lowest possible FiO_2 (<0.6) Normal pH (7.35–7.45) PEEP <7.5 cm
Cardiovascular support	Maintain intravascular volume (CVP 10 mmHg) Treat CVP <6 mmHg with fluid bolus Systolic BP 90–100 mmHg (mean 65 mmHg) Vasopressors if required HR 100 bpm SVR <1000 dyn sec/cm^5 Urine output 100 ml/hour (DDAVP for diabetes insipidus)
Endocrine support	Hormone replacement therapy for severe cardiovascular instability or high inotrope requirement (T_3, pitressin, methylprednisolone) Glucose 6–11 mmol/L
Haematological support	Fresh frozen plasma (FFP) Platelets
Temperature support	Core temperature >35°C Warming blankets Warmed IV fluids Heated and humidified inspired gases

DDAVP, l-deamino-8-d-arginine vasopressin (desmopressin).

Donation after cardiac death (DCD)

Unlike in DBD, where the patient will be transferred to theatre ventilated with a heartbeat, donation after cardiac death only proceeds once the patient has become asystolic. DCD should be considered after the decision has been made that withdrawal of treatment is in the patient's best interests. As a result of improvements in surgical techniques, immunosuppression, and organ preservation, it is now possible for these patients to donate lungs, liver, kidneys, and pancreas. As good organ function is necessary, most potential DCD donors will have suffered a neurological insult but will not satisfy brainstem death criteria. DCD can also be offered to those families who would otherwise refuse DBD donation because they wish to remain with their relative until their heart stops beating. For DCD to proceed< cardiac death must occur within 4 hours of extubation. Regardless of the outcome, the focus in these patients is good end-of-life care.

Management of sodium and water balance

Disturbances of sodium and water balance are common following brain injury and accurate diagnosis and treatment is essential.

Hyponatraemia

Hyponatraemia is defined as a plasma sodium concentration <130 mmol/L. Patients with no primary cerebral disease will develop symptoms of hyponatraemia (nausea, anorexia, emesis, confusion, seizures, and impairment of consciousness) when sodium levels fall below 120–125 mmol/L. In contrast, patients with CNS lesions may demonstrate symptoms at much higher sodium levels. Accurate diagnosis and treatment is essential because of the high risk of seizures if the plasma sodium falls below 120 mmol/L.

In hospital settings iatrogenic hyponatraemia is often due to inadequate sodium replacement (and/or loss) or dilution from excessive infusion of water (e.g. 5% glucose). Psychogenic polydipsia, where the patient drinks excessive amounts of water, may also result in hyponatraemia. Two pathological syndromes leading to hyponatraemia, namely the syndrome of inappropriate antidiuretic hormone secretion (SIADH) and cerebral salt wasting syndrome (CSW), are most commonly seen in patients with severe TBI and poor grade SAH. Although the serum electrolyte profile of the two syndromes is similar, it is important to distinguish between them because the management is markedly different. SIADH is characterized by increased intravascular volume, water retention, and dilutional hyponatraemia and is treated with volume restriction, while CSW is a state of decreased intravascular volume, increased urine output, and hyponatraemia and is treated by re-establishing normovolaemia.

Antidiuretic hormone (ADH) is produced in the supra-optic and paraventricular nuclei in the hypothalamus and stored in the posterior lobe of the pituitary gland, from where it is secreted into the blood depending largely on the plasma osmolality. Its major function is to regulate body fluid tonicity. Without the action of ADH, the kidney would generate 20–30 L of free water per day. SIADH may develop due to persistent release of ADH resulting in increased intravascular volume, water retention, and dilutional hyponatraemia. SIADH is usually self-limiting with brain injury and resolves as brain tissue recovers; hypertonic saline (± furosemide) is rarely required.

Cerebral salt wasting (CSW), on the other hand, is thought to be due to increased release of atrial natriuretic factor (ANF) from the brain and is characterized by water loss with hypovolaemia. Hyponatraemia may be associated not only with a progressive naturesis but also with a tendency to diuresis, leading to a significant contraction of circulating and extracellular volumes. In CSW, fluid restriction will not correct the hyponatraemia and

Table 8.14 Diagnosis of disorders of sodium and water balance

Disorder	CVP	Urine output	Specific gravity	Serum Na^+ (mmol/L)	Urinary Na^+ (mmol/L)	Serum osmolality (mOsmol/kg)	Urine osmolality (mOsmol/kg)
SIADH	High	Low (no evidence of volume depletion)	Normal	Low (<135)	Normal	Low	High (compare with serum osmolality)
CSW	Low	High	Normal	Low (<135)	High	High/normal	Variable
DI	Low	High (>1000 ml/4 h)	Low (1.005)	High (>148)	Normal	High	Low

SIADH,syndrome of inappropriate ADH secretion; CSW, cerebral salt wasting syndrome; DI, diabetes insipidus.

Table 8.15 Treatment of disorders of sodium and water balance

SIADH	Restrict water intake to 500–1000 ml per day Check urine and serum sodium and osmolality
CSW	Re-establish normovolaemia with the administration of sodium-containing isotonic solutions Check urine and serum sodium and osmolality In severe cases hypertonic saline should be given over 24–48 hours at a rate to increase sodium concentration by <12 mmol/L/24 h
DI	If urine output >1000 ml in 4 hours and specific gravity <1.005 give 0.4 mg DDAVP IV If urine output remains high after 30 min give further 0.4 mg DDAVP IV Accurate fluid balance, aiming for even balance, is essential (urine output should not be chased) If sodium >148 mmol/L give 5% glucose, with insulin infusion if needed to keep blood glucose 4–9 mmol/L In addition, water can be given via a nasogastric or orogastric tube

DDAVP, l-deamino-8-d-arginine vasopressin (desmopressin).

may be harmful, as it will reduce intravascular volume further. This may lead to hypotension and an increased risk of cerebral infarction.

Hypernatraemia

Hypernatraemia may result from fluid restriction or from the osmotic diuretic agents used for ICP control. This can easily be corrected by the administration of isotonic fluids. Urine output is usually reduced and the urine specific gravity is elevated (>1.020). Hypernatraemia can also be iatrogenically induced through excessive use of sodium-containing fluids.

Diabetes insipidus (DI)

Diabetes insipidus may develop after brain injury, surgery, or tumours when there has been damage to the hypothalamus or pituitary gland. It occurs when over 80% of neurons synthesizing vasopressin are destroyed or become temporarily non-functional. It is characterized by a high urine output (>200 ml/h) and low urine specific gravity (<1.005).

Diagnosis and treatment of disturbances of sodium and water balance are outlined in Tables 8.14 and 8.15.

Bibliography

Academy of the Medical Royal Colleges (2008) *A Code of Practice for the Diagnosis and Confirmation of Death.* London: PPG Design and Print Ltd.

Alderson, P., Roberts, I. (1997). Corticosteroids in acute traumatic brain injury: systematic review of randomised controlled trials. *British Medical Journal*, **314**, 1855–9.

Association of Anaesthetists of Great Britain and Ireland. *Recommendations for the Transfer of Patients with Acute Head Injuries to Neurosurgical Units*. London: AAGBI, 1996.

Barker, R.A., Barasi, S., Neal, M.J. (1999). *Neuroscience at a Glance.* Oxford: Blackwell Science.

Bear, M.F., Connors, B.W., Paradiso, M.A. (1996). *Neuroscience: Exploring the Brain.* Baltimore, MD: Williams & Wilkins.

Bouma, G.J., Muizelaar, J.P. (1992). Cerebral blood flow, cerebral blood volume and cerebrovascular reactivity after severe head injury. *Journal of Neurotrauma*, **9**(Suppl 1), 333–48.

Brain Trauma Foundation (2007) *Guidelines for the Management Of Severe Traumatic Brain Injury* (3rd edn). New York: Mary Ann Liebert.

Bratton, S.L., Davis, R.L. (1997). Acute lung injury in isolated traumatic brain injury. *Neurosurgery*, **40**, 707–12.

Bullock, R., Povlishock, J.T. (1996). Guidelines for the management of severe head injury. *Journal of Neurotrauma*, **264**, 1085–8.

Carter, P., Edwards, S. (1997). General principles of treatment. In *Neurological Physiotherapy: A Problem Solving Approach* (ed. S. Edwards), pp. 87–113. London; Churchill Livingstone.

Chalela, J.A. (2001). Pearls and pitfalls in the intensive care management of Guillain–Barré syndrome. *Seminars in Neurology*, **21**, 399–405.

Chapman, M.G., Smith, M., Hirsch, N.P. (2001). Status epilepticus. *Anaesthesia*, **56**, 648–59.

Chesnut, R.M. (1995). Secondary brain insults after injury: clinical perspectives. *New Horizons*, **3**, 366–75.

Clifton, G.L., Robertson, C.S., Kyper, K., *et al.* (1983). Cardiovascular response to severe head injury. *Journal of Neurosurgery*, **3**, 447–54.

Contant, C.F., Valadka, A.B., Shankar, M.D., *et al.* (2001). Adult respiratory distress syndrome: a complication of induced hypertension after severe head injury. *Journal of Neurosurgery*, **95**, 560–8.

Crossman, A.R., Neary, D. (1995). *Neuroanatomy: an Illustrated Colour Text*. Edinburgh: Churchill Livingstone.

Cunning, S., Haudek, D.L. (1999). Preventing secondary brain injuries. *Dimensions of Critical Care Nursing*, **18**, 20–2.

Dankbaar, J.W., Slooter, A.J., *et al.* (2010). Effect of different components of triple-H therapy on cerebral perfusion in patients with aneurysmalsubarachnoid haemorrhage: a systematic review. *Critical Care*, **14**, R23.

Dearden, N.M. (1998). Mechanisms and prevention of secondary brain damage during intensive care. *Clinical Neuropathology*, **17**, 221–8.

Drake, G.C. (1988). Report of the World Federation of Neurological Surgeons Committee on a universal subarachnoid haemorrhage rading scale. *Journal of Neurosurgery*, **68**, 985–6.

European Brain Injury Consortium (1997). Guidelines for the management of severe head injury in adults. *Acta Neurochirurgica*, **139**, 286–94.

Feldman, Z., Kanter, M.J., Robertson, C.S., *et al.* (1992). Effect of head elevation on intracranial pressure, cerebral perfusion pressure and cerebral blood flow in head injured patients. *Journal of Neurosurgery*, **76**, 201–11.

George, M.R. (1988). Neuromuscular respiratory failure: what the nurse knows may make the difference. *Journal of Neuroscience Nursing*, **20**, 110–17.

Graham, D.I., Hume Adams, J., Nicoll, J.A.R., *et al.* (1995). The nature, distribution and causes of traumatic brain injury. *Brain Pathology*, **5**, 397–406.

Greenberg, M.S. (1994). Subarachnoid haemorrhage and aneurysms. In *Handbook of Neurosurgery* (ed. M.S. Greenberg) (3rd edn), pp. 711–52. Lakeland, FL: Greenberg Graphics.

Gupta, A.K., Summors, A. (eds) (2001). *Notes in Neuroanaesthesia and Critical Care*. London: Greenwich Medical Media.

Hartung, H.P., Willison, H.J, Kieseier, B.C. (2002). Acute immunoinflammatory neuropathy: update on Guillaine–Barré syndrome. *Current Opinion in Neurology*, **15**, 571–7.

Holly, L.T., Kelly, D.F., Counelis, G.J., *et al.* (2002). Cervical spine trauma associated with moderate and severe head injury: incidence, risk factors and injury characteristics. *Journal of Neurosurgery. Spine*, **96**, 285–91.

Jennett, B. (1991). Diagnosis and management of head trauma. *Journal of Neurotrauma* **8**(Suppl. 1), S15–18.

Jennett, B., Lindsay, K.W. (1994). *An Introduction to Neurosurgery* (5th edn). Oxford: Butterworth-Heinemann.

Lawn, N.D., Wijdicks, E.F.M. (2002). Status epilepticus: a critical review of management options. *Canadian Journal of Neurological Science*, **29**, 206–15.

Lindsay, K.W., Bone, I., Fuller, G. (2010). *Neurology and Neurosurgery Illustrated* (5th edn). Edinburgh: Churchill Livingstone.

McLeod, A.A., Neil-Dwyer, G., Meyer, C.H.A., *et al.* (1982). Cardiac sequelae of acute head injury. *British Heart Journal*, **47**, 221–6.

Maas, A.I.R., Dearden, M., Teasdale, G.M., *et al.* (1997). EBIC guidelines for management of severe head injury in adults. *Acta Neurochirurgica*, **139**, 286–94.

Martin, N.A., Patwardhan, R.V., Alexander, M.J., *et al.* (1997). Characterisation of cerebral haemodynamic phases following severe head trauma: hypoperfusion, hyperaemia and vasospasm. *Journal of Neurosurgery*, **87**, 9–19.

Miller, J.D., Becker, D.P. (1982). Secondary insults to the injured brain. *Journal of the Royal College of Surgeons of Edinburgh*, **27**, 292–8.

Morris, C.G.T., McCoy, E. (2004). Clearing the cervical spine in unconscious polytrauma victims, balancing risks and effective screening. *Anaesthesia*, **59**, 464–82.

Ng, K.K.P., Howard, R.S., Fish, D.R. *et al.* (1995). Management and outcome of severe Guillain-Barré syndrome. *Quarterly Journal of Medicine*, **88**, 243–50.

Oppenheimer, S.M., Cochetto, D.F., Hachinski, V.C. (1990). Cerebrogenic cardiac arrhythmias. *Acta Neurologica*, **47**, 513–19.

O'Riordan, J.I., Miller, D.H., Mottorshead, J.P., *et al.* (1998). The management and outcome of patients with myasthenia gravis treated acutely in a neurological intensive care unit. *European Journal of Neurology*, **5**, 137–42.

Palace, J., Vincent, A., Beeson, D. (2001). Myasthenia gravis: diagnostic and management dilemmas. *Current Opinion in Neurology*, **14**, 583–9.

Palmer, J.D. (ed.) (1996). *Manual of Neurosurgery*. London: Churchill Livingstone.

Parsons, I.C., Wilson, M.M. (1984). Cerebrovascular status of severe closed head injured patients following passive position changes. *Nursing Research*, **33**, 68–75.

Piek, J., Chesnut, R.M., Marshall, L.F., *et al.* (1992). Extracranial complications of severe head injury. *Journal of Neurosurgery*, **77**, 901–7.

Poulter, A. (1998). The patient with Guillaine–Barré syndrome: implications for critical care nursing practice. *Nursing in Critical Care*, **3**, 182–9.

Rabinstein, A.A., Wijdicks, E.F.M. (2003). Hyponatraemia in critically ill neurological patients. *Neurologist*, **9**, 290–300.

Rappaport, Z.V., Vajda, J. (2002). Intracranial abscess: current concepts in management. *Neurosurgery Quarterly*, **12**, 238–50.

Rees, G., Shah, S., Hanley, C., *et al.* (2002). Subarachnoid haemorrhage: a clinical overview. *Nursing Standard*, **16**, 47–56.

Robertson, C.S. (2001). Management of cerebral perfusion pressure after traumatic brain injury. *Anaesthesiology*, **95**, 1513–17.

Robertson, C.S., Valadka, A.B., Hannay, H.J., *et al.* (1999). Prevention of secondary insults after severe head injury. *Critical Care Medicine*, **27**, 2086–95.

Ropper, A.H. (ed.) (1993). *Neurological and Neurosurgical Intensive Care* (3rd edn). New York: Raven Press.

Rosner, M.J., Rosner, S.D., Johnson, A.H. (1995). Cerebral perfusion pressure—management protocol and clinical results. *Journal of Neurosurgery*, **83**, 949–62.

Scherer, P. (1986). Coma assessment. *Journal of Nursing*, May, 542–55.

Scottish Intercollegiate Guidelines Network (2009). *Early Management of Patients with a Head Injury: A National Clinical Guideline*. Report, SIGN, Edinburgh. http://www.sign.ac.uk/pdf/sign110.pdf.

Seelig, J.M., Becker, D.P., Miller, J.D. *et al.* (1981). Traumatic acute subdural haematoma: major mortality reduction in comatose patients treated within four hours. *New England Journal of Medicine*, **304**, 1511–18.

Shafer, P.O. (1999). New therapies in the management of acute cluster seizures and seizure emergencies. *Journal of Neuroscience Nursing*, **31**, 224–9.

Shorvon, S. (1994). *Status Epilepticus: Its Clinical Features and Treatment in Children and Adults*. Cambridge: Cambridge University Press.

Slade, J., Kerr, M.E., Marion, D. (1999). The effect of therapeutic hypothermia on the incidence and treatment of intracranial hypertension. *Journal of Neuroscience Nursing*, **31**, 264–9.

Smith, M. (1998). Management of the multiple organ donor. *Surgery* **16**, 180–3.

Stone, J.D., Sperry, R.J., Johnson, J., *et al.* (eds) (1996). *The Neuroanaesthesia Handbook*. St Louis, MO: Mosby.

Sullivan, J. (2000). Positioning of patients with severe traumatic brain injury: research based practice. *Journal of Neuroscience Nursing*, **32**, 204–9.

Sutcliffe, A. (2001). Hypothermia (or not) for the management of head injury. *Care of the Critically Ill*, **17**: 162–5.

Teasdale, G., Jennett, B. (1974). Assessment of coma and impaired consciousness: a practical scale. *Lancet*, **2**(7872), 81–4.

Teasdale, G., Jennett, B. (1976). Assessment and prognosis of coma after head injury. *Acta Neurochirurgica*, **34**, 45–55.

Teasdale, G., Maas A., Lecky, F., *et al* (2014) The Glasgow Coma Scale at 40 years: standing the test of time. *Lancet Neurology*, **13**, 844–54.

Twyman, D. (1997). Nutritional management of the critically ill neurologic patient. *Critical Care Clinics*, **13**, 39.

Valadka, A.B., and Andrews, B.T. (2005) *Neurotrauma: Evidence-based Answers to Common Questions*. New York: Thieme Medical Publishers.

Walker, M. (1998). Protection of the cervical spine in the unconscious patient. *Care of the Critically Ill*, **14**, 4–7.

Watkins, L.D. (2000). Head injuries: general principles and management. *Surgery*, 219–24.

Wijdicks, E.F.M. (2001). *Brain Death*. Philadelphia, PA: Lippincott–Williams & Wilkins.

Wijdicks, E.F.M. (2003). *The Clinical Practice of Critical Care Neurology* (2nd edn). New York: Oxford University Press.

CHAPTER 9

Gastrointestinal problems and nutrition

Introduction

The gastrointestinal (GI) tract has not always been considered an area of vital importance in the care of the critically ill. However, its effectiveness as a defence system and in delivering essential resources for other organs makes support of this organ system as important as any other. Protection of these functions is now considered an essential part of optimal care of the critically ill. A survey of critical care units in England (Sharifi *et al.* 2011) showed that 66% of patients in critical care were receiving nutritional support, and 83% of these patients received it via the enteral route. The proportion of patients with malnutrition in intensive care is as high as 43% (Giner *et al.* 1996), and this group have an increased incidence of complications. A more recent study from Newcastle using the MUST (Malnutrition Universal Screening Tool) (Lamb *et al.* 2009) identified that 77% were at risk of malnutrition. Early intensive care focused on the use of parenteral nutrition as the delivery method of choice (Jeejeebhoy 2012), often with an unnecessarily high level of nutrient delivery, with detrimental results. The gradual move to enteral nutrition delivery ameliorated some of this and reduced the negative impact of overfeeding, but difficulties in tolerance meant that some patients were receiving less than their requirements. The compromise of feeding enterally where possible and supplementing or subsitituting parenterally where necessary is the current approach.

Nutrition forms a vital part of the comprehensive and proactive care of the patient. A significant responsibility for the delivery of nutrition falls on the nurse caring for the patient, not only in ensuring that what is prescribed gets delivered, but also in monitoring and evaluating the patient's ability to tolerate the mode of nutritional delivery. Both under- and overfeeding are associated with worse outcomes in specific ICU patient groups (Jeejeebhoy 2012; Krishnan *et al.* 2003; Rapp *et al.* 1983).

Anatomy and physiology

The anatomy and physiology of the GI tract will be described briefly, with particular reference to those aspects relevant to the critically ill. The GI tract acts as both a point of access and a protective barrier to the external environment. Its major functions are:

- breakdown of complex nutrients
- absorption of predigested molecules
- movement of food through the digestive tract
- elimination of waste matter
- recycling of materials used in digestion
- protection of vulnerable internal organs from ingested organisms.

The GI tract is mostly under the control of the autonomic nervous system. The oropharyngeal cavity, upper oesophagus, and external anal sphincter are under voluntary control via somatic motor fibres. Most of the GI tract is supplied by both sympathetic and parasympathetic nerves. Parasympathetic innervation is mainly via the vagus and pelvic nerves, and sympathetic innervation is via nerves from the spinal cord and pre-vertebral ganglia, and from these ganglia to the gut.

Sympathetic stimulation decreases gut motility, increases sphincter tone, and decreases exocrine secretions (i.e. substances locally discharged from a gland via a duct). Norepinephrine (noradrenaline) is the transmitter most commonly found in the post-ganglionic efferent nerves and neurons of the symapthetic system. Parasympathetic stimulation has the opposite effects, with acetylcholine being the most common parasympathetic transmitter. Sympathetic and parasympathetic responses can be altered by psycho-emotional stimuli mediated by the brain. Thus, fear may increase the viscosity and decrease the amount of saliva secreted, producing the characteristic dry mouth, while any strong emotion may increase gut motility.

Gut function

The gut functions of secretion, absorption, and motility are controlled by interaction between the autonomic nervous system and the endocrine and paracrine systems. Function is highly organized and integrated within the GI tract, allowing movement, digestion, and absorption of food to take place.

Oropharyngeal cavity

The functions of the oropharyngeal cavity are:

- mechanical breakdown of food
- swallowing of food bolus (voluntary)
- saliva production.

Saliva is a complex substance consisting mainly of water, but it also contains (Johnson 2007):

- mucus
- salivary amylase (ptyalin), a starch-digesting enzyme
- lingual lipase, a hydrolysing enzyme for lipids
- lysozyme, an enzyme which attacks bacterial cell walls
- lactoferrin, an iron-chelating agent preventing the growth of organisms that require iron
- secretory IgA, an immunoglobulin active against viruses and bacteria.

The mucus lubricates and binds food while the enzymes break down carbohydrate and lipids. The other agents protect both the mouth and the upper GI tract from ingestion of pathological organisms. The amount of saliva produced is increased by parasympathetic stimulation and decreased by sympathetic stimulation. Saliva is produced by the parotid, submandibular, and sublingual glands.

Swallowing

The swallowing centre in the medulla is responsible for the coordination of the highly complex muscle activation associated with swallowing. The tongue, oropharynx, soft palate, laryngeal muscles, glottis, and epiglottis work together to protect the respiratory tract and to ensure that the food bolus is propelled through the pharynx into the upper oesophageal sphincter. A swallow can be initiated voluntarily, but then becomes an involuntary reflex. The upper oesophageal sphincter relaxes to allow food to move into the oesophagus.

Swallowing can be affected by a number of neurological diseases or events such as cerebrovascular accidents. In critical care, endotracheal intubation for more than 48 hours can result in disturbances of swallowing in up to 50% of patients after the tube has been removed. This usually corrects itself after 4 days (Barquist *et al.* 2001).

Oesophagus

The oesophagus secretes mucus (for lubrication and protection) and propels food (by peristalsis). The speed of transition through the oesophagus depends on the size and consistency of the food bolus.

Lower oesophageal sphincter

The lower oesophageal sphincter is the last centimetre or so of the oesophagus. It prevents reflux of gastric contents by continuous smooth muscle contraction, but relaxes in response to peristalsis to allow food to pass through to the stomach.

Stomach

The stomach has a primary digestive function but its highly acidic environment also acts as an effective barrier to foreign organisms. Specialized cells within the gastric mucosa secrete the constituents of gastric juice: pepsin, intrinsic factor, hydrogen ions, and mucus. The functions of the stomach are:

- breakdown of food by pepsin and gastric acid (hydrochloric acid (HCl))
- production of intrinsic factor (facilitates absorption of vitamin B_{12} by the small intestine)
- production of gastrin (promotes growth and repair of gastric mucosa and stimulates secretion of pepsinogen and HCl).

Gastric acid secretion is regulated by gastrin and the parasympathetic mediator acetylcholine (ACh); their effect is potentiated by histamine via H_2 histamine receptors in the gastric mucosa. The basal rate of acid secretion has a diurnal rhythm which is higher in the evening and lower in the morning (Johnson 2007). Other factors which affect secretion include:

- conditioned reflexes such as smell, taste, chewing, swallowing
- alcohol and caffeine acting on gastric chemoreceptors and nerve plexuses within the stomach wall
- hypoglycaemia via the brainstem and vagal fibres.

Distension of the stomach and the presence of digested protein in the intestine will also stimulate gastric acid release. The human stomach secretes 1–2 L of gastric juice per day. This is an important point when considering the volumes associated with aspirating gastric contents to check tolerance of enteral feeding. Protection of the gastric epithelium from gastric acid is vital, as the gastric luminal pH is maintained at a potentially damaging value of 2–3. This protection is achieved by the following mechanisms.

1. Tight fitting of the gastric mucosal cells, forming a barrier against HCl damage. As this barrier is impermeable to hydrogen ions, it maintains a pH gradient between stomach wall and lumen. It can be disrupted by bile salts, alcohol, aspirin and steroids. Mucosal blood flow, and thus oxygenation, is an important factor in maintaining mucosal integrity.
2. Secretion of a mucus–bicarbonate gel by mucosal cells to cover the mucosal epithelium. This gel is capable of maintaining a pH gradient from approximately 2 on the gastric luminal side to approximately 7.3 on the epithelial side.

Endogenous prostaglandins play an important role in maintaining gastric mucosal integrity by influencing mucosal blood flow, stabilizing the mucosal barrier, and stimulating mucus–bicarbonate secretion. Inhibition of prostaglandins by non-steroidal anti-inflammatory drugs (NSAIDs) may result in gastric erosions or deeper ulceration. Enteral nutrition, or the presence of any food in the stomach, is also important in maintaining mucosal integrity (see Box 9.1).

Pancreas

The pancreas secretes both exocrine substances (assisting digestion and absorption of nutrients) and endocrine substances (e.g. insulin, glucagon, pancreatic polypeptide). Stimulation of the water and bicarbonate component of the exocrine secretions occurs in response to acid entering the duodenum, while the principal stimulant of enzyme secretion is cholecystokinin (CCK) which is released in response to amino acids, peptides,

Box 9.1 Factors affecting movement of nutrients through the gut

1. Gastric to duodenal delivery of nutrients: antral peristalsis and fundal tone are reduced by the arrival of nutrients and hyperosmolar solutions in the duodenum, maintaining a constant delivery of 1–2 kcal/min.
2. Malabsorbed nutrients (particularly fat) are detected by sensors in the ileum which exert a further inhibitory effect on gastric emptying and small intestinal motility.
3. Additional fibre may reduce glucose absorption, thus inhibiting total transit time.

Data from Scott, A., Skerratt, S., Adam, S., *Nutrition for the Critically Ill: A Practical Handbook*, p. 67. 1998, CRC Press.

and fatty acids in the small intestine. Secretin is released in response to a drop in pH in the proximal duodenum and stimulates water and bicarbonate release. There are also vasovagal-mediated responses.

Exocrine function consists of the following:

- Secretion of water to dilute chyme (a mixture of semi-digested food and gastric enzymes) and increase nutrient absorption.
- Secretion of bicarbonate to neutralize post-gastric chyme and prevent damage to the duodenal mucosa.
- Secretion of inactive forms of enzymes including protein-digesting trypsin, chymotrypsin, elastase, and carboxypeptidase; and nucleic-acid-digesting nuclease. Once in the duodenum, trypsin is activated by the intestinal mucosal enzyme enterokinase, and this in turn activates other pancreatic enzymes.
- Secretion of active forms of enzymes including fat-digesting lipase and esterase, and starch-digesting amylase.

Endocrine secretions from the islets of Langerhans, such as insulin and glucagon, are discussed in Chapter 14.

Gall bladder

The gall bladder holds and concentrates bile, a complex mixture of organic components such as bile acids, phospholipids, cholesterol, and bile pigments, and inorganic ions including sodium, potassium, calcium, chloride, and bicarbonate. Many of these components (e.g. bile acids) are synthesized and secreted by hepatocytes. Bilirubin is the primary bile pigment; this is derived from the breakdown of haemoglobin from ageing red blood cells by the reticuloendothelial system. The hepatocytes extract bilirubin from the blood, conjugate it with glucuronic acid, and secrete the conjugated molecule into the bile.

Bile plays an essential part in the digestion and absorpion of lipids by:

- emulsifiying fat into small droplets for degradation by lipase and esterase into micelles (particles with a fatty core and water-soluble coat) which are then transported across the intestinal lumen, leaving the bile behind.
- ionizing fat-soluble vitamins into absorbable forms.
- suspending cholesterol, triglycerides, and medium-density lipoproteins within the blood, preventing their precipitation and deposition.

When digestion is not occurring, the gall bladder collects and stores bile, distending to do so. Once food passes into the duodenum, CCK release stimulates gall bladder contraction, releasing bile into the duodenum.

Duodenum and jejunum

The duodenum and jejunum constitute the sections of the small intestine where absorption of food primarily takes place. Digestion occurs intraluminally under enzymatic initiation. However, further denaturing of chemical bonds also takes place in the brush border of the small intestine, as this contains hydrolytic enzymes which produce even smaller fragments of nutrient substrate.

A number of other highly complex mechanisms are associated with this part of the gut.

- Secretion of water to further dilute chyme in the proximal part of the small intestine.
- Secretion of bicarbonate to neutralize post-gastric acidic chyme.
- Mucus secretion to protect the duodenal lumen.
- Secretion of enterokinase to convert trypsinogen (inactive form) to trypsin (active form).
- Secretion of secretin and CCK in response to acidity and proteins. These stimulate pancreatic secretion and the release of the contents from the gall bladder.
- Secretion of maltase, lactase, and sucrase to convert carbohydrates to simple sugars.
- Mixing of chyme to allow exposure of all molecules to the absorptive surface.
- Peristalsis to propel chyme along the small intestine.
- Absorption of carbohydrates by active and passive transport across the intestinal lumen into the bloodstream.

- Absorption of protein as amino acids and protein fragments by active diffusion (assisted movement across a concentration gradient) and passive diffusion (movement from high to low concentration).
- Absorption of fats in the form of fatty acids and monoglycerides by passive transport in the duodenum and the first half of the jejunum.
- Reabsorption of water and electrolytes (Na^+, Cl^-) following an osmotic gradient occurs through the rest of the small intestine. This is enhanced by opiates. but other agents such as serotonin and dopamine increase secretion into the gut. The high volume diarrhoea seen in diseases such as cholera is caused principally by a greatly increased secretion of fluid into the gut.
- Reabsorption of iron, usually in the form of heme, but also as inorganic iron bound to transferrin, an iron-binding protein released by enterocytes in the small bowel.

Colon

Between 7 and 10 L of water enter the small intestine over a 24-hour period. Because of highly efficient reabsorption mechanisms, only 600 ml or so reaches the colon, where up to 500 ml are then reabsorbed along with sodium, potassium, chloride, and bicarbonate. The colon is capable of reabsorbing up to 6 L of fluid per day (Johnson 2007). Other functions of the colon include:

- secretion of mucus to lubricate faecal material and protect mucosa
- mixing of contents to allow exposure to the absorptive surface and peristalsis to propel contents
- mass movement to propel faecal matter rapidly into the rectum from the sigmoid and descending colon
- absorption of water, potassium, and chloride
- absorption of folic acid
- absorption of ammonia.

Delayed movement of faecal material through the colon leads to constipation. Most of this is diet-related as there is a strong relationship between volume of dietary fibre, increased material bulk, and rate of movement through the colon. However, some disorders, such as irritable bowel syndrome, which can result in constipation are associated with altered contraction of the sigmoid colon, known as segmentation contraction. These forms of contraction are resistant to movement of faecal material. Segmentation contractions are also seen following opiate administration, thereby contributing to the constipation associated with their use.

Rectum

The rectum is usually almost empty. It fills intermittently and when distended with faecal material the internal sphincter relaxes unless voluntarily over-ridden. If defecation is appropriate, rectal propulsion moves contents into the anal canal and both internal and external rectal sphincters relax to allow passage of the faecal bolus.

Effect of tonicity of gastrointestinal contents

Tonicity is defined as the effective osmotic pressure of a fluid in relation to plasma.The GI tract is highly permeable to water in both directions. Water is absorbed passively throughout the stomach and small and large intestines and is also secreted into chyme. If the gastrointestinal contents are hypertonic, osmosis (the movement of water from an area of low solute concentration to an area of high solute concentration across a semi-permeable membrane) into the lumen will occur. If the contents are hypotonic, water moves from the gastrointestinal contents into the bloodstream. Such movements can obviously affect the fluid and electrolyte balance of the body as a whole, but they will also affect the amount of fluid within the gut contents. Thus a hypertonic enteral feed could produce diarrhoea due to the movement of water into the gut lumen via osmosis.

The immune function of the gut

The dual functions of connection with, and protection from, the external environment require both accessibility for absorption of required substances and complex defences against external harmful organisms. Protection is achieved by the following.

1. The gut mucous layer protecting the gastric and duodenal epithelium by acting as a physical barrier against systemic invasion by bacteria that colonize the gut. This layer is a continuous viscous adherent mucous coating produced by mucus-producing cells to protect the epithelium.
2. The gut epithelial cells preventing migration of organisms.
3. The bowel wall containing large numbers of lymphocytes and macrophages.
4. The mesentery containing regional lymph nodes.
5. Secretory immunoglobulin A (IgA) produced intraluminally by specialized cells (Peyer's patches). This prevents adherence of bacteria to mucosal cells and is the principal component of the gut mucosal defence system.

6. Fixed tissue macrophages in the liver (Kupffer cells) and the spleen that trap and phagocytose bacteria and toxic products if penetration does occur.

In the healthy person this protection is highly organized and effective. However, when the patient becomes critically ill several factors may compromise this system and allow migration of gut organisms into the circulation (bacterial translocation).

1. Altered permeability or loss of integrity of the intestinal mucosa as a result of ischaemia, sepsis, or other inflammatory insult (see Chapter 10).
2. Decreased host defence mechanisms (e.g. immunosuppression).
3. Increased bacterial numbers within the intestine caused by either overgrowth or intestinal stasis. The normal gut maintains a balance of commensal bacteria which restricts the numbers of any one type. This balance can be disturbed by antibiotics preventing the growth of one organism and thus allowing overgrowth of another.
4. Other drugs and treatments affecting gut blood flow (e.g. catecholamines), acid production (e.g proton pump inhibitors (PPIs)), and immune function (e.g. corticosteroids).
5. Protein malnutrition may also affect the integrity of the gut mucosa or the immunocompetence of the gut and contribute to an increased risk of bacterial translocation. Early enteral feeding is thought to protect against loss of mucosal integrity possibly through the action of intestinal alkaline phosphatase (Lalles 2013; Hamarneh *et al.* 2014; Berger *et al.* 2007; Marik and Zaloga 2001).

Colonization by *Helicobacter pylori (H.pylori)* also causes disruption of the integrity of the mucous barrier and altered inflammatory responses in susceptible patients, resulting in development of peptic ulceration (Bi and Kaunitz 2003).

Absorption and storage of digested food

Absorption primarily takes place through the brush border of the intestine. Within villi (finger-like projections that protrude from the epithelium) there are many microvilli which contain enzymes needed for the large stages of absorption.

Carbohydrate

Digestion reduces carbohydrate polymers to monosaccharides (mainly glucose). The intestinal epithelial cells (brush border) contain glucoamylase and sucrase which split polysaccharides into monosaccharides. These are then absorbed in the small intestine via the sodium active transport mechanism which allows absorption to occur against a concentration gradient. Glucose is carried by the bloodstream to the individual cells where it is transported through the cell membrane by a process known as facilitated diffusion (see Figure 9.1). Glucose is stored as glycogen either in the liver or in muscle cells. This is usually sufficient to maintain blood glucose levels for about 18-24 hours under normal fasting conditions.

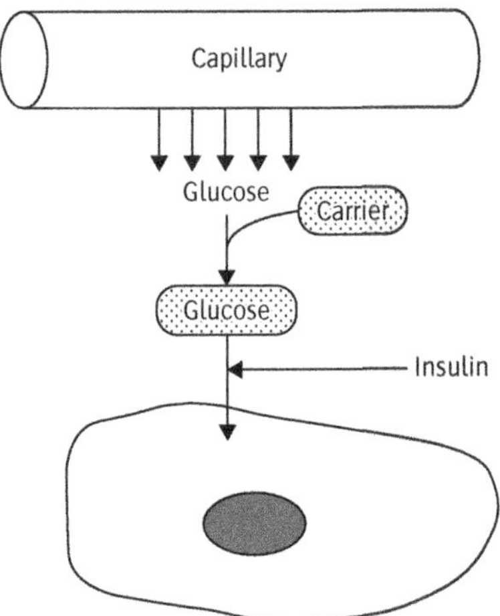

Figure 9.1 The mechanism of facilitated diffusion of glucose through the cell membrane.

Fat

Digestion of fat is by hydrolysis catalysed by the enzyme lipase. The end-products are fatty acids, glycerol, and glycerides. These molecules are highly soluble within the brush border of the epithelial cells and diffuse readily from the intestinal lumen. The molecules are then re-synthesized and expelled into the lymph system as small globules of fat called chylomicrons. The chylomicrons are transported via the thoracic lymph duct to empty into the bloodstream at the junction of the left internal jugular and subclavian veins. Fat is stored in modified connective tissue cells as triglycerides (see Figure 9.2). These are broken down and re-synthesized continuously with net breakdown or synthesis being controlled by blood levels of glucose, insulin, catecholamines, and glucagon. High levels of glucose and insulin increase synthesis, while high levels of catecholamines or glucagon stimulate breakdown.

Protein

Protein is digested by pepsin in the stomach to form small protein molecules (proteoses, polypeptides,

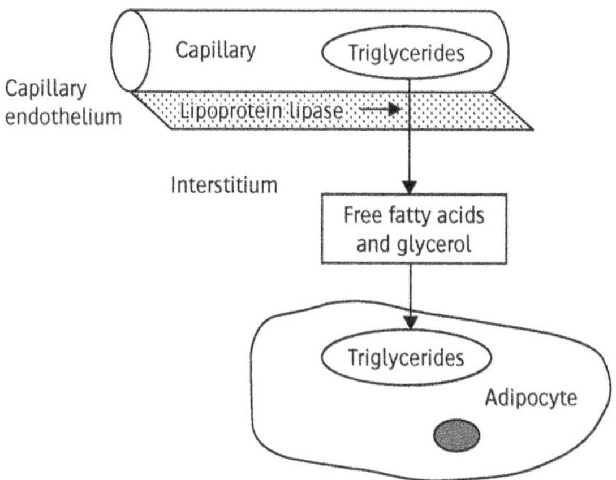

Figure 9.2 The mechanism of triglyceride (fat) storage in adipocytes.

peptones). Pepsin activity is neutralized when the pH becomes alkaline. These small proteins are further split by trypsin and other enzymes into amino acids and dipeptides, and are then absorbed by active transport into the brush border cells and then the bloodstream. Many organs, including the liver, can store amino acids and release them into the bloodstream when levels fall (Figure 9.3).

The liver

A wide variety of metabolic functions are performed by hepatocytes (liver cells). The liver has both an arterial and a venous blood supply, with approximately three-quarters of the blood flow to the liver coming from the portal vein which drains the gut. Arterial blood is supplied via the hepatic artery. The portal vein drains blood from the gut containing nutrients for storage and synthesis plus debris, including bacteria, for filtration and phagocytosis. The healthy liver has the ability to regenerate itself after injury.

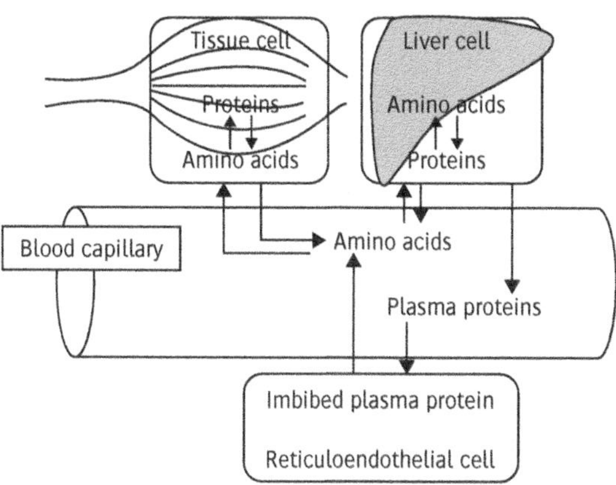

Figure 9.3 The mechanism of the storage and breakdown of amino acids (proteins).

Function of hepatocytes

Carbohydrate metabolism

The liver is a key component of the management of glucose availability to tissues. It is the only organ that both stores and releases glycogen (a complex of thousands of glucose molecules) into the circulation. Other sites of glycogen storage, such as myocytes, can only utilize the glycogen within the cell itself. Glucose homeostasis is maintained by the liver through glycogen storage and release, gluconeogenesis (production of glucose from non-carbohydrate sources, such as lactate, and some amino acids and fatty acids), and release of glucose into plasma.

When exogenous carbohydrate is not available the blood glucose concentration is maintained by endogenous glucose production, 90% of which is derived from the liver by glycogenolysis (breakdown of glycogen) or gluconeogenesis (see Box 9.2). This response is affected by levels of circulating insulin, cortisol, glucagon, epinephrine (adrenaline), and thyroxine.

Degradation of drugs (including alcohol, benzodiazepines, tranquillizers, phenobarbital, phenytoin, warfarin) and toxins

The liver protects the body from a wide range of potentially harmful substances by transforming them into a more water-soluble form that can be excreted safely.

> **Box 9.2 Breakdown and storage of glucose**
>
> **Gluconeogenesis**
>
> Formation of glucose from lactate, pyruvate, amino acids, and glycerol through a series of chemical reactions in the liver cells.
>
> **Glycogenolysis**
>
> Breakdown of glycogen stored in the muscle and liver cells to glucose by enzymes in the liver cells.
>
> **Glycogenesis**
>
> Excess glucose, fructose, and lactose molecules are converted to glycogen and stored in the liver cells.

Most drugs when metabolized are fat soluble, and their conversion by the liver into water-soluble substances facilitates their excretion into bile or urine.

Drugs are principally metabolized by hepatic enzymes in a process known as biotransformation which has two phases.

1. Cytochrome P450 enzymes expose functional groups such as –OH or –COOH in the molecule by oxidation, reduction, or hydrolysis.
2. Biotransformative enzymes attach other substances, such as glucuronic acid, acetate, and sulphate, to the functional groups to increase their water solubility.

The pharmacological consequences of drug metabolism vary according to the drug and the reaction it undergoes. Conjugation almost always causes loss of activity (e.g. salicylates, paracetamol, and morphine). Acetylation of sulphonamides makes drugs less soluble and potentially more harmful. When two drugs are metabolized by the same microsomal enzymes there may be prolongation of drug action. Drug metabolism may be impaired in liver disease. The extent to which individual drugs are metabolized in an altered manner is highly variable and care must be taken to avoid overdosage, particularly with sedative drugs.

Elimination of bilirubin

Eighty per cent of bilirubin is derived from heme following the breakdown of haemoglobin in the liver, spleen, and bone marrow. Bilirubin is not water soluble and is carried in the plasma bound to albumin. In the liver it is transported into the hepatocytes, conjugated with glucuronic acid, which makes it water soluble, and excreted by active transport into the bile. In the terminal ileum and colon, bacteria reduce bilirubin to stercobilinogen which is excreted in the stool. A small amount is reabsorbed and excreted in the urine as urobilinogen.

Fat metabolism

The liver receives fats in a range of sizes: chylomicron remnants (the products of brush border processing of fats in the duodenum, which are 98% lipid and 2% protein), very low density lipoproteins (VLDLs) (90% lipid 10% protein), low density lipoproteins (LDLs) (70% lipid, 30% protein), high density lipoproteins (HDLs) (50% lipid and 50% protein), and fatty acids.

Large lipoprotein molecules are split into smaller units by lipoprotein lipase (LPL) which is expressed on the endothelium of blood vessels. Circulating lipoproteins that are small enough attach to receptors on the hepatocyte, and LDL receptors transfer the lipoprotein fragments into the hepatocyte by endocytosis.

In a constant process of breakdown and synthesis, the liver will also:

(i) synthesize lipoprotein from cholesterol, phospholipid, and triglycerides combined with apoproteins

(ii) synthesize cholesterol and other lipid molecules

(iii) convert excess protein and carbohydrate to fat.

Mineral and vitamin storage

Hepatocytes store minerals (up to 60% of excess iron), vitamins (including A, D, K, and B_{12}), and folate.

Production of bile

The primary bile acids (cholic and chenodeoxycholic acid) are produced from cholesterol. They are secreted into bile with water-soluble bilirubin and then reabsorbed into the portal blood at specific sites in the terminal ileum.

Protein metabolism

Protein is transported to the liver as amino acids which are further broken down to form ketoacids, ammonia, and then urea. Oxidative deamination can be an important energy source for the liver. The liver has the following roles:

- synthesis of plasma proteins including albumin, globulins (other than gamma-globulins), transferrin, caeruloplasmin, and components of the complement system.
- deamination (breakdown) of proteins and conversion of ammonia to urea, with the production of energy (ATP).
- transamination (movement of amino acids from one molecule to another).

Steroid catabolism

The liver is responsible for the catabolism of some hormones, including insulin, glucagon, cortisol, and oestrogens.

Synthesis of coagulation factors

The following coagulation factors are synthesized by hepatocytes: factor I, fibrinogen; factor II, prothrombin; factor V, proaccelerin; factor VII, proconvertin; factor IX, plasma thromoplastin component; factor X, Stuart factor.

Mononuclear phagocytic function

The mononuclear phagocytic process for clearing the body's own debris, and for killing and digesting bacteria, is carried out by the Kupffer cells. These are fixed tissue macrophages located in the walls of blood sinuses that can filter particles and foreign bodies/antibody-coated cells.

Assessment of the patient's gastrointestinal function

Assessment of gastrointestinal function should assess both potential or actual GI dysfunction, and the patient's overall nutritional status.

Physical examination

As with all acute situations, assessment should follow an ABCDE structure to ensure the safety of the patient.

Airway

Airway compromise can be associated with vomiting, acute GI bleeding, altered conscious level from hepatic encephalopathy, and misplacement of nasoenteral tubes.

Breathing

Breathing can be compromised by a range of GI dysfunction including intra-abdominal hypertension from ascites or ileus (increasing the work of breathing), protein malnutrition and muscle wasting (affecting respiratory muscles), and altered conscious level related to hepatic encephalopathy.

Circulation

Altered circulating blood volume and blood pressure can be affected by various GI disorders, for example acute bleeding from peptic ulceration or oesophageal varices, increased capillary leak and vasodilatation from inflammatory conditions such as severe acute pancreatitis, intraluminal fluid accumulation with bowel obtruction and ileus, and increased fluid losses following diarrhoea and vomiting.

Disability (neurological care)

Conscious level can be affected by a wide range of pathological states associated with GI dysfunction, including:

- metabolic (e.g. hypoglycaemia in acute liver failure)
- circulatory (e.g. hypovolaemia from excess vomiting)
- organ failure (e.g. liver failure)
- acid–base and/or electrolyte disturbance (e.g. from excess vomiting)
- drugs and poisons (e.g opiates, carbon monoxide)
- hypo/hyperthermia (e.g. acute liver failure)
- intracranial dysfunction (e.g. cerebral oedema).

Everything else

A full physical examination allows evaluation of muscle wasting, breakdown in skin integrity, and generalized and focal areas of oedema and ascites. Specific elements related to disease pathology, such as the Grey–Turner sign (flank bruising) for retroperitoneal haemorrhage following pancreatitis or spider naevi for hepatic disease, can also be sought.

The patient's general appearance can only give a limited evaluation of nutritional state. Obvious signs of obesity and emaciation are easily discernible, but muscle wasting (suggesting protein deficiency) may be obscured in the obese patient. Generalized oedema may also mask recognition of muscle wasting, and only in the resolution stage of the illness may the degree of loss become apparent. Features of individual vitamin and trace element deficiency, such as dryness, reddening, and petechial haemorrhage of the skin in vitamin C, K, or A deficiencies, may be attributed to other causes such as coagulation disorders.

Jaundice and the almost green tinge associated with bile duct obstruction may be indicators of hepatic dysfunction, although there may be few overt signs until hepatic dysfunction is quite severe.

Examination of the oral cavity

This should assess the condition of the mucosa, teeth (or dentures), and lips. Signs of inflammation, fungal infection such as *Candida albicans*, aphthous ulcers, and herpetic lesions should be noted and swabs taken for culture if necessary. Medical staff should be informed.

Teeth need to be examined for blackening, dental caries, loose sockets, and plaque or debris. The gums should be assessed for signs of inflammation, recession, bleeding, and overgrowth. Bleeding may be related to poor dental hygiene or to coagulation disorders, and should be considered in context with the patient's underlying condition. Medical staff should be informed of loose teeth, bleeding gums, and very severe tooth decay, as a dental referral may be necessary.

The patient's breath should also be assessed and any unusual odour, such as hepatic fetor (a sweet musty odour) or ketones (a sweet smell of acetone), should be noted and reported.

Abdominal assessment

The abdomen should be examined for symmetry, size, evidence of distension (taut, swollen skin often with an everted umbilicus), and signs of pulsation (usually visible epigastrically). Dilated veins may be visible and any rashes, bruising, scars, or lumps (such as hernias) should be noted. Palpation should assess tenderness, muscle resistance, masses, and a fluid thrill (present in ascites). Auscultation with the diaphragm of the stethoscope should assess the presence and character of bowel sounds. 'Tinkling' high-pitched sounds may be heard with mechanical obstruction. The absence of bowel sounds cannot be confirmed unless auscultation continues for at least 3 min. Rectal examination may be necessary if the patient complains of constipation or has diarrhoea that may constitute faecal overflow.

History

Useful information can be obtained from the patient, family, and friends concerning nutritional status immediately prior to admission. In particular, recent weight loss, change in eating habits, and appetite should be noted. Other areas which should be explored are bowel function, dental hygiene, and previous GI problems. A history of drug and/or alcohol abuse will also have an impact on nutritional status.

Specific problems associated with the gastrointestinal tract

Acute gastrointestinal bleeding

Acute GI bleeding can be the reason for admission to critical care or can occur as a secondary complication. Causes of acute GI bleeding include oesophageal varices, peptic ulcers, vascular lesions, and neoplastic lesions (Bordas *et al.* 2006). A review of the incidence of GI bleeding in 1034 patients from 97 ICUs (Krag *et al.* 2015) found that clinically significant bleeding was rare (2.6%) and was not associated with increased adjusted mortality. Protection from the risk of bleeding is part of standard intensive care and the use of acid suppressants (such as PPIs or H_2 receptor antagonists) is widespread.

Acute GI bleeding may be manifested by either:

- haematemesis—usually related to a bleeding point above the duodenojejunal junction, or
- melaena—altered blood appearing black and tarry from passage through the upper GI tract lipoprotein lipase. Lower GI bleeding usually looks fresh and bright red (haematochezia). If upper GI bleeding is copious and current, the patient may pass virtually unaltered blood per rectum.

If bleeding is severe, the patient will appear shocked, pale, and distressed. This is an emergency situation and should be dealt with as such with immediate fluid resuscitation, oxygen and, if necessary, urgent blood and blood product transfusion.

Assessment of the bleeding patient

Initial assessment of the patient should follow the ABCDE (Airway, Breathing, Circulation, Disability, Everything else) approach.

1. Airway—check that the airway is not compromised (see Chapter 1). Blood aspirated during episodes of haematemesis or a decrease in conscious level can affect the ability to maintain an adequate airway.
2. Breathing—assess respiratory rate and effort, oxygen saturation, and arterial blood gases.
3. Circulation—assess markers such as heart rate, blood pressure, peripheral perfusion, and capillary refill time. If devices are in situ, measure CVP, cardiac output, and central venous oxygen saturation. If a urinary catheter is in place, measure urine output. Ensure that there is adequate venous access to enable rapid high volume fluid replacement.
4. Disability—assess level of consciousness, mental state, and degree of weakness.
5. Everything else—assess colour, volume and rapidity of blood loss, skin colour, and evidence of sweating.

If the patient is able to give a history, details of the frequency and volume of haematemesis or melaena should be determined. See Table 9.1 for causes of GI bleeding.

Priorities of management

1. Airway management and protection—if necessary, clear the airway using suction. If the patient cannot maintain an adequate and protected airway, they should be intubated and mechanically ventilated.
2. Breathing—supplemental oxygen should be given to maintain an acceptable oxygen saturation. Intubation and mechanical ventilation may be required if gas exchange is impaired, or to facilitate endoscopy or surgery.
3. Circulation—fluid resuscitation should be given via large bore IV access. Multiple cannulae may be needed for profuse bleeding. Central venous access is useful to assess CVP. Fluid should be replaced as rapidly as necessary to maintain an adequate circulation. In the first instance, clear fluid (colloid or crystalloid)

Table 9.1 Causes of gastrointestinal bleeding

Problem	Area affected by problem			
	Upper GI bleeding		Lower GI bleeding	
	Oesophagus	Stomach	Small intestine	Large bowel and rectum
Varices	✓	✓(less common)	✓(less common)	
Inflammation	✓	✓(gastritis)		✓(ulcerative colitis)
Ulcers	✓	✓	✓	
Tumours	✓	✓		✓
Mallory–Weiss tear	✓			
Angiodysplasia		✓(less common)	✓	✓(less common)
Crohn's disease			✓	✓
Diverticula			✓(Meckel's diverticulum)	
Haemorrhoids				✓
Rectal fissures				✓

should be given urgently while blood is being cross-matched. If the haemoglobin is very low (<5 g/dl) and the patient is compromised, group-specific or O-negative blood should be used.

4. Disability—conscious level should be monitored closely using either GCS or AVPU scores (see Chapter 8). Reduced mental alertness is an early indicator of decreased cerebral blood flow. Reduce anxiety levels by maintaining calm, explaining and informing about what is happening, and building confidence and reassurance in responding to and managing the situation. Check and correct abnormal levels of blood glucose and electrolytes.
5. Everything else—fresh frozen plasma and platelets ± cryoprecipitate should also be requested if bleeding is severe or the patient has an underlying coagulopathy. Calcium chloride may be needed if the patient becomes hypocalcaemic.

Further management

1. If the patient remains hypotensive, despite continued fluid resuscitation, investigation of uncontrolled bleeding should be instigated as soon as possible. Ideally, the patient should be resuscitated and stabilized before endoscopy or surgery. If the patient does respond to fluid resuscitation and transfusion, the procedure may be delayed until the patient's condition has stabilized. Investigation of bleeding may require endoscopy for upper GI bleeding, and sigmoidoscopy/colonoscopy for lower GI bleeding. A variety of endoscopic treatments are available to stop bleeding (e.g. injection of sclerosants and/or epinephrine, banding of varices, electrocoagulation, laser therapy). Angiography is increasingly performed in patients with massive or recurrent bleeding, particularly where the source of bleeding is unknown, and to enable therapeutic embolization as a preference over laparotomy. Open surgery may be required for persistent or recurrent severe undiagnosed bleeding, or where embolization has proved unsuccessful or cannot be performed (Bordas *et al.* 2006).
2. A large bore nasogastric tube should be inserted to allow drainage and assessment of upper GI bleeding, prevent gastric dilatation, and allow administration of medication. The patient should remain nil by mouth initially in case surgery is required. If the patient has known, or suspected, varices as the source of bleeding, an endoscopy should first be performed.
3. A proton pump inhibitor (e.g. pantoprazole, omeprazole) or H_2 receptor antagonist (e.g. ranitidine) should be given for bleeding due to known or suspected peptic ulceration and oesophagitis. For severe bleeding, a continuous IV infusion is generally preferred. Best results are achieved if the gastric pH is >4; this should be checked four-hourly. Antacids may have to be administered as well in order to achieve this.

Oesophageal varices

Aetiology

Oesophageal varices occur when obstruction to the portal vein produces portal hypertension. Development of varices starts once the hepatic venous pressure gradient (HPVG) rises above 10 mmHg and bleeding can occur at pressures >12 mmHg (Villanueva and Balanzo 2008). Portal hypertension may be due to destruction of the hepatic vasculature, as in cirrhosis, or obstruction of the portal vein itself. The back pressure produced is transmitted throughout the portal system and has the effect of producing dilatation of the surface blood vessels in the lower oesophagus or the fundus of the stomach and the duodenum (Figure 9.4). The protruding veins can become eroded and bleed. Varices should be suspected in patients with acute GI bleeding, particularly with a history/physical examination suggestive of chronic liver damage. Some evidence now exists that concurrent infection may precipitate a variceal bleed. The most effective current therapy to prevent bleeding is the use of non-selective beta-blockers and regular endoscopic band ligation (O'Brien *et al.* 2013).

Priorities of management

1. As before, resuscitation of the patient with fluid and blood/blood product transfusion is of paramount importance.
2. An infusion of vasopressin (antidiuretic hormone) or terlipressin (a synthetic vasopressin analogue) may control variceal bleeding in 60% of cases. These drugs constrict splanchnic arterioles, increasing their resistance to flow. This reduces the amount of blood entering the portal venous system, reducing portal pressure and, to some extent, variceal pressure. Its side effects are systemic hypertension and intestinal colic, and it may cause severe ischaemia in gut, skin, and heart. Simultaneous infusion of glyceryl trinitrate is often used to reduce coronary and splanchnic vasoconstriction side effects. Somatostatin or octreotide (a somatostatin analogue) are also commonly used as splanchnic vasoconstrictors. They are more expensive, though no more effective than vasopressin or terlipressin.
3. If bleeding is severe, a Sengstaken–Blakemore or modified Sengstaken (four-lumen Minnesota) tube can be inserted to apply balloon tamponade (Figure 9.5). This tube is inserted through the nose or mouth and fed into the stomach. It has two balloons which can be used to apply local pressure to the cardia and

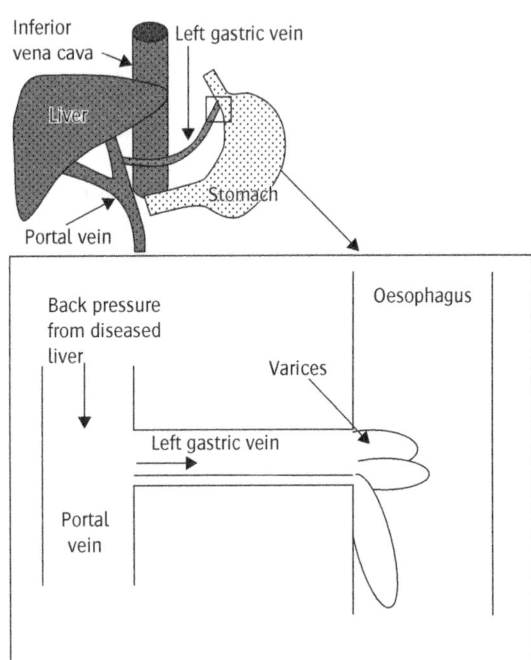

Figure 9.4 Diagrammatic representation of oesophageal varices.

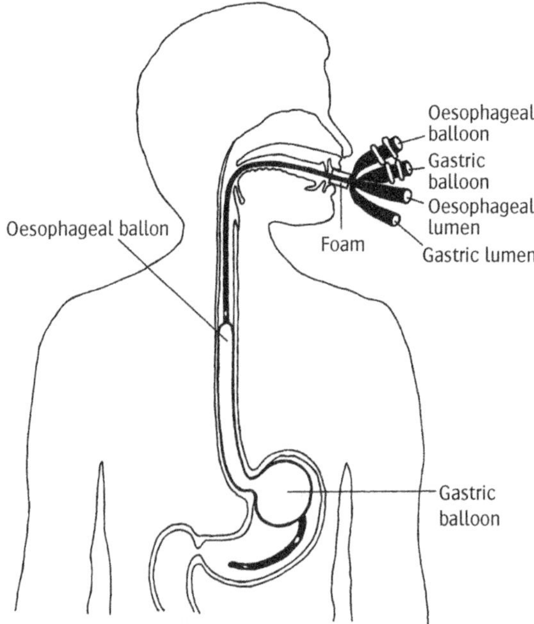

Figure 9.5 The Sengstaken (modified) tube

(very occasionally) the oesophagus. The Sengstaken tube has a lumen for gastric aspiration while the Minnesota tube has an extra lumen for oesophageal aspiration. It is used as a temporary bridge to other treatment in situations where massive bleeding is not controlled by initial drug or endoscopic interventions (Bordas *et al.* 2006).

4. If the patient is not protecting their airway, they should be intubated and ventilated.
5. A broad spectrum antibiotic that covers Gram-negative bacteria (e.g. ciprofloxacin) should be prescribed (O'Brien *et al.* 2013).

Insertion and care of the Sengstaken tube (balloon tamponade)

This is a difficult manoeuvre which is usually complicated by patient agitation and persistent haematemesis. It is easier and probably safer to perform with the patient sedated, intubated, and mechanically ventilated. Particular care should be taken by staff to prevent contamination by blood splashes. All staff involved in the procedure should wear full-face visors, gloves, and plastic aprons. See Box 9.3 for further equipment required.

- The patient requires explanation and preparation for the procedure (see later). They are likely to be considerably distressed and may also have hepatic encephalopathy with alterations of perception and behaviour. Explanations should include the sensations the patient may experience (fullness of stomach, tube in the mouth and back of the throat, not able to swallow saliva easily) and the likelihood of success (around 90%).

Box 9.3 Sengstaken (modified) tube: equipment required for insertion

- Sengstaken or equivalent tube (red rubber or latex tubes should be made firmer by placing in the freezing compartment of a refrigerator for at least 15 min prior to the procedure)
- Laryngoscope
- Tongue depressor
- Magill's forceps
- Anaesthetic spray
- Lubricating jelly
- Tape to fix the tube
- Piece of sponge, weight, or splint to apply traction
- 50 ml syringe

- Prior to insertion, the balloons should be checked for leaks and patency. The oesophageal balloon should not generally be used.
- The tube is inserted per-orally with the patient sitting at an angle of about 30° or in the left lateral position. The choice of position will depend on the patient's conscious level and ability to cooperate.
- Confirmation of correct placement is important, as inflation of the gastric balloon whilst still in the oesophagus can result in oesophageal rupture. Checking placement is best carried out by X-ray or possibly by ultrasound scan (Lin *et al.* 2006).
- When the tube is in position the gastric balloon is inflated with 150–200 ml of air (or water) and drawn back until it sits firmly against the cardia of the stomach.
- The tube should be secured with tape and splints or foam applied at the exit point from the mouth in order to maintain traction. Alternatively, firm traction can be maintained using a 500–1000 mg weight (e.g. a bag of fluid).
- The oesophageal balloon is not usually inflated unless bleeding continues despite the gastric tamponade. If it has to be inflated a manometer should be used to ensure that pressures are <30–40 mmHg (4.5–5.4 kPa). It should not be left inflated for longer than 24 hours as the risk of oesophageal wall ischaemia and rupture is high.
- If the tube has an oesophageal aspiration lumen this should be aspirated frequently or placed on continuous suction to prevent build up of secretions and the risk of aspiration.
- The patient will be unable to swallow and saliva will require removal by suction if they is unable to spit. Mouth care is essential, although difficult to achieve.

The balloon is usually deflated at 24-hour intervals; once bleeding has ceased the tube can be removed. The patient will then undergo sclerotherapy, endoscopic variceal band ligation (VBL), or transjugular intrahepatic portal systemic shunt (TIPS). TIPS is associated with a reduced incidence of rebleeding from varices, although survival is similar to band ligation and encephalopathy may be a problem (Pomier-Layrargues *et al.* 2001).

Removal of the Sengstaken tube

- The procedure should be explained to the patient.
- If not intubated, the patient should be sitting upright. If there is any concern over the patient's ability to protect their airway, the anaesthetic staff should be consulted to ensure that adequate back-up is present to prevent aspiration of any gastric contents.

- The balloon(s) should be deflated and a period of time allowed before removal to ensure that bleeding does not recur. If the oesophageal balloon has been used, it should always be deflated first.
- Immediately prior to removing the tube the gastric (and oesophageal, if present) lumen(s) should be aspirated to clear any gastric contents.

Stress ulceration

The incidence of stress ulceration in ICU patients may remain relatively high, but the clinical impact of these lesions has reduced significantly, with studies suggesting that between 1% and 2.6% of patients suffer clinically important bleeding as a result (Marik *et al.* 2010; Krag *et al.* 2015). This is probably related to increased use of early enteral nutrition, gastric acid suppressants and protectants, and better maintenance of organ perfusion (see Box 9.4).

Pathogenesis

Decreased mucosal blood flow

Mucosal blood flow is vital in maintaining the gastric mucosal barrier; even a short period of ischaemia may be enough to disrupt the protective function of the mucosa.

Breakdown of the mucosal barrier

The viscoelastic mucus layer acts as a physical barrier to protect the gastric epithelium. Disruption of the mucus-producing cells and reduction in mucus and bicarbonate production and secretion allows back-diffusion of H^+ ions into the mucosa. Factors affecting mucosal breakdown are:

- bile salts and urea damage the epithelial cells
- salicylates and local prostaglandin production inhibit active ion transport and bicarbonate secretion, thus reducing the pH gradient between mucosa and gastric lumen
- ethanol decreases the thickness of mucus and stimulates histamine release which increases acid secretion
- corticosteroids alter the composition, decrease the production of mucus and cause an increase in acid secretion.

Increased intraluminal acidity

The level of intraluminal pH is not necessarily a causative factor in itself. Stress ulceration seems to be related to other factors such as the integrity of the mucosal defence mechanisms.

Decreased epithelial regeneration

Decreased cellular proliferation and deoxyribonucleic acid (DNA) synthesis in the gastric mucosa occur during stress. Thus regeneration of the mucosal barrier for protection against intraluminal acid is compromised and may lead to ulceration.

While the pathogenesis of stress ulceration remains complex and, as yet, incompletely explained, some interventions have clearly helped to prevent bleeding from stress ulcers. Probably the most important is maintaining adequate blood flow to the gastric mucosa by early and appropriate resuscitation. An acidic intraluminal environment and the loss of the protective mucosal barrier are also thought to be important contributory features (Johnson 2007, p.81). The use of early enteral nutrition to maintain the integrity of the mucosa and, where this is not possible, the use of PPIs or H_2 receptor antagonists has greatly contributed to the reduction of clinically significant bleeding from the GI tract (Marik *et al.* 2010).

Box 9.4 Risk factors associated with stress ulceration

- Hypoperfusion and ischaemia
- Sepsis
- Head injury
- Renal failure
- Multiple trauma
- Respiratory failure and prolonged mechanical ventilation
- Severe burn injuries
- Major surgical procedures
- Fulminant hepatic failure or severe hepatic dysfunction
- Drugs (e.g. NSAIDs)

Neutralizing the acidic intraluminal environment

Antacids

Antacids are suspensions of magnesium and aluminium hydroxides. They act as a base, combining with H^+ ions to neutralize gastric acid. They are effective in reducing the incidence of bleeding provided that pH is kept >4. Side effects include diarrhoea, hypermagnesaemia, increased plasma aluminium levels, and alkalosis. An increased incidence of aspiration pneumonia has been associated with their use, possibly as a result of bacterial overgrowth (Brett 2005). The requirement of hourly to four-hourly monitoring of gastric pH and administration of antacid is time-consuming (Brett 2005). There may be difficulty aspirating a representative sample of gastric contents if a fine bore feeding tube is used. The use of enteral nutrition is likely to be more effective in maintaining gastric pH >4.

Histamine (H_2) receptor antagonists (e.g. ranitidine)

Increased gastric acid secretion is stimulated by histamine release acting via the H_2 receptors on acid-secreting cells in the stomach. Ranitidine is an H_2 receptor antagonist that decreases the incidence of bleeding in selected groups of patients. However, there is no evidence that its use improves overall survival of critical care patients, or that it is effective in clinically important bleeding (Messori *et al.* 2000).

Side effects of H_2 receptor antagonists include drug interactions, suppression of ADH release, and reports of mental confusion. The increase in intraluminal pH associated with H_2 receptor antagonist use may also result in bacterial overgrowth and an increased incidence of pneumonia (Messori *et al.* 2000) and *Clostridium difficile* diarrhoea.

Proton pump inhibitors

Omeprazole or pantoprazole are intravenous proton pump inhibitors. These drugs act by binding to and inhibiting the potassium-dependent ATPase proton pump of the gastric parietal cell. They do not appear to cause tolerance, and are used extensively to prevent rebleeding following endoscopic management of the various causes of upper GI bleeding. In patients with severe bleeding, they are best administered as continuous IV infusions (following an initial IV bolus) to maintain gastric pH >4–6 (Morgan 2002). As PPIs are more potent in raising intraluminal pH than H_2 receptor antagonists, the risk of pneumonia and *C.difficile* diarrhoea is higher.

Improving the protective mucosal barrier

Sucralfate (the basic aluminium salt of sucrose octasulphate) forms a protective barrier over the gastric mucosa and facilitates healing of ulcers while gastric pH is maintained. It is effective in the treatment of duodenal ulcers and in the prevention of gastric ulcers (Tryba 1991); however, evidence is conflicting with regard to stress ulceration. Complications associated with its use include constipation, feeding tube occlusion, bezoars, aluminium accumulation, and hypophosphataemia (Brett 2005). There may be less risk of nosocomial pneumonia, probably because of the maintenance of gastric pH (Messori *et al.* 2000).

Enteral feeding

Enteral feeding protects the gastric mucosa, and this protection may be as effective as the use of gastric acid blockers (Marik *et al.* 2010). However, this has not been tested in the prevention of rebleeding following primary haemostasis by endoscopic intervention—see following section.

The liver

Acute-on-chronic liver failure is the commonest reason for admission to intensive care. In the USA there are only 2000 cases of acute liver failure per year.

Acute liver failure

The incidence and aetiology of acute liver failure varies by country and custom, with paracetamol (acetaminophen) induced liver failure being more common in the UK, although changes in the law restricting dispensed packs to a maximum of 32 tablets may have reduced this (Hawkins *et al.* 2007; Pettie and Dow 2013). Worldwide, viral hepatitis is the commonest cause. *Amanita phalloides* (mushroom) poisoning is particularly prevalent in France and parts of North America. Causes can broadly be grouped into drugs, infection, poisoning, immune/metabolic, and a range of relatively rare causes such as heatstroke or the Budd–Chiari syndrome.

Defining types of acute liver failure depends on the interval between onset of jaundice and onset of encephalopathy (see Box 9.5). The Acute Liver Failure Study Group (Stravitz *et al.* 2007) defined acute liver failure as the onset of hepatic encephalopathy and coagulopathy within 26 weeks of jaundice in a patient without pre-existing liver disease. Cross *et al.* (2006) outlined a subclassification of hyperacute (jaundice to encephalopathy <7 days), acute (jaundice to encephalopathy in 7–28 days), and subacute (jaundice to encephalopathy from 28 days to 3 months). Prognosis is better in the hyperacute group than in the acute or subacute groups.

Box 9.5 Definitions of acute liver failure

1. O'Grady *et al.* (1993)
   - Hyperacute liver failure (0–7 days)
   - Acute liver failure (8–28 days)
   - Subacute liver failure (29–72 days)
2. The Acute Liver Failure Study Group (Stravitz *et al.* 2007)
   - Onset of hepatic encephalopathy and coagulopathy within 26 weeks of jaundice in a patient without pre-existing liver disease

Hyperacute (fulminant) hepatic failure

Common causes include viral hepatitis (A, B, C, E) and paracetamol (acetaminophen) overdose. Other causes include idiosyncratic drug reactions, ingestion of other toxins (e.g. *Amanita phalloides*), acute fatty liver of pregnancy, inhalation of carbon tetrachloride or halothane, and Wilson's disease. Prognosis is poor, and mortality remains between 40–80% without liver transplantation (Gill and Sterling 2001). However, liver transplantation has improved the outcome of acute liver failure dramatically with 1 and 5 year survival rates of 65% and 59%, respectively (Cross *et al.* 2006). In general, management of such patients is best carried out in regional specialist centres. Early transfer based on criteria for poor prognosis is recommended.

Acute and subacute (subfulminant) hepatic failure

The onset of encephalopathy is delayed and can occur several months after the initial insult. The most frequent causes are viral infections and idiosyncratic drug reactions. Prognosis is also very poor, and mortality without liver transplantation is >80% (Gill and Sterling 2001) although more recent survival (Lee 2012) is thought to be around 60–70% with changing aetiology associated with liver failure.

Acute-on-chronic hepatic failure

This is defined as an acute exacerbation of existing liver disease precipitated by a specific cause such as infection, GI haemorrhage (varices, peptic ulcer), administration of sedatives, surgery, a high protein load, or any other cause of hepatic decompensation. Short-term survival is better than for fulminant hepatic failure.

See Table 9.2 for the classifcation of liver failure according to the Child–Pugh score.

Table 9.2 Classification of liver failure according to Child–Pugh score

	1 point	2 points	3 points
Bilirubin (µmol/L))	<34.2	34.2–51.3	>51.3
Albumin (g/100ml)	>3.5	2.8–3.5	<2.8
Prothrombin time INR	<1.7	1.8–2.3	>2.3
Presence of ascites	No	Mild	Moderate to severe
Hepatic encephalopathy (grade)	No	1–2	3–4
Total points	5–6	7–9	10–15
Child–Pugh class	A	B	C
3 year predicted survival*	73%	59%	46%

*Angermayr *et al.* 2003.

Reproduced with permission from R.N.H. Pugh, M.M. Lyon, J.L. Dawson, *et al.*, Transection of the oesophagus for bleeding oesophageal varices, *British Journal of Surgery*, Volume 60, Issue 8, pp.646–9, Copyright © 1973 John Wiley & Sons.

Problems associated with acute/acute-on-chronic hepatic failure

Hepatic encephalopathy

Encephalopathy (see Table 9.3) describes a range of changes in cerebral function associated with liver failure (Felipo 2013). The cognitive and behavioural changes

Table 9.3 Grades of encephalopathy

Grade	
0	Normal awareness.
I	Mood change, slow mentation, disturbed sleep, restless, forgetful, mild confusion, tremor, apraxia
II	Lethargy, drowsiness, disorientation, inappropriate behaviour, arousable and conversant, dysarthria, ataxia, asterixis (liver flap)
III	Marked confusion and disorientation, aggression, agitation, stuporose but rousable, hyper-reflexia, muscle rigidity, clonus
IV	Unrousable to noxious stimuli, decerebrate, or decorticate posturing

This article was published in *Gastroenterology*, Volume 72, Conn, H.O., Leevy, C.M., Vlahcevic, Z.R., Rodgers, J.B., Maddrey, W.C., Seeff, L., Levy, L.L., Comparison of lactulose and neomycin in the treat- ment of chronic portal-systemic encephalopathy. A double blind con- trolled trial, pp. 573–83, Copyright Elsevier (1977).

associated with acute-on-chronic hepatic failure are relatively unusual in acute hepatic failure. Encephalopathy is associated with hyperammonaemia. Ammonia levels >150 µmol/L greatly increase the risk of cerebral oedema and death. It is not clear what exactly causes encephalopathy. Many factors have been implicated, including free fatty acids, mercaptans, phenols, bilirubin, and bile acids. Gamma-aminobutyric acid (GABA) and aromatic amino acids have also been associated with encephalopathy. EEG findings typically show diffuse slowing of cortical activity and a high amplitude waveform of 5–7 Hz. Subclinical seizure activity can be seen on an EEG in encephalopathy grades III and IV; this often responds to phenytoin, resulting in a reduction in cerebral oedema.

Cerebral oedema

Cerebral oedema is common in grade III–IV encephalopathy, affecting >80% of patients with grade IV coma. It is related to disruption of the blood–brain barrier with increased flux of water, and loss of autoregulation of blood flow. Prognosis worsens as the grade of encephalopathy increases. Diagnosis and management may be facilitated by intracranial pressure (ICP) monitoring (see Chapter 8), though no studies have shown outcome benefit through its use.

Coagulopathy

Liver synthesis of fibrinogen and factors V, VII, IX, and X is impaired in liver failure. This is evidenced by prolongation of the prothrombin time (PT) and international normalized ratio (INR) which is used as a prognostic index—the greater the prolongation the worse the likely outcome. Alterations in platelet count (thrombocytopaenia) and function are also seen during hepatic failure.

Renal failure

This occurs in approximately 50% of cases, and in up to 75% of those with grade IV coma. Causes include hypovolaemia, hepatorenal syndrome, sepsis, and direct nephrotoxicity from drugs such as paracetamol (Cross *et al.* 2006). The blood urea is often low, and does not reflect renal function as urea is produced by the liver and its production is affected by hepatic failure. Hepatorenal syndrome refers to a functional renal failure probably due in the majority of cases to generalized intense renal vasoconstriction, the exact mechanism of which remains unknown. There are specific criteria associated with the syndrome, including a low glomerular filtration rate, and the absence of other causes such as sepsis or nephrotoxicity, proteinuria <500 mg/day, and no sustained improvement in renal function following diuretic withdrawal and volume expansion.

Hypoglycaemia

This is related to failure of hepatic gluconeogenesis and reduced glycogen stores, and can develop rapidly in the early stages. Hypoglycaemia is frequently seen in acute liver failure and requires close monitoring and management (Whitehouse and Wendon 2013). Provision of enteral nutrition will support blood glucose levels, but acute drops in blood glucose will require immediate treatment with high concentration glucose solutions intravenously.

Acid–base and electrolyte imbalance

Hypokalaemia due to inadequate potassium intake, vomiting, and secondary hyperaldosteronism occurs in the early stages of failure. It may be replaced later by hyperkalaemia if renal failure occurs. Hypomagnesaemia, hyponatraemia, hypophosphataemia, and hypocalcaemia can all develop and may exacerbate neurological complications.

Metabolic alkalosis may occur as a response to hypokalaemia and gastric acid loss through vomiting or aspiration. It can also be due to an inability to deal with amino acids in the urea cycle, i.e. removal of the amino radical ($-NH_2$) by conversion into ammonia which combines with carbon dioxide to form urea which is excreted renally.

Metabolic acidosis can occur with paracetamol (acetaminophen) overdose and is also possible as a result of lactic acidosis due to tissue hypoxia.

Respiratory problems

The patient's airway may be compromised due to a decreased conscious level, and the ventilatory response to hypoxaemia is decreased. Patients can develop pulmonary oedema which is thought to be related to alterations in membrane permeability and is associated with cerebral oedema. They may have intrapulmonary shunting (either anatomical and/or functional) leading to ventilation/perfusion mismatch and hypoxaemia.

Cardiovascular problems

Hypotension due to vasodilatation and relative hypovolaemia, with a high cardiac output and low systemic vascular resistance are commonly seen. Arrhythmias related to electrolyte disturbances are common, necessitating continuous monitoring.

Sepsis

The patient is immunocompromised, and sepsis due to bacteraemia or fungaemia is common. This is related to reduced reticulo-endothelial clearance, impaired leucocyte function, and deficient complement activity, as well as the impact of liver dysfunction on the production of immune system components such as acute phase proteins and complement. In addition, the portal filtering of bacteria is compromised. Up to 80% of liver failure patients develop bacterial infections (Whitehouse and Wendon 2013).

Management of patients with acute hepatic failure

Owing to the high risk nature of some of the causes of acute hepatic failure, source isolation barrier nursing precautions should be followed initially when caring for these patients. Blood tests for all hepatitis-causing viruses should also be performed.

Management is composed of both general interventions and cause-specific interventions (e.g. *N*-acetylcysteine for paracetamol overdose). General management is discussed first and cause-specific management at the end of the section (Patton *et al.* 2012).

Encephalopathy

The aims of management in the early stages of encephalopathy are to limit the production of ammonia and avoid precipitating factors such as benzodiazepines or other potentially hepatotoxic drugs. Most ammonia comes from 'ammonia- forming' intestinal bacteria and the breakdown of dietary proteins (Riordan and Williams 1997). At encephalopathy grades 3–4, the aims of management focus on the prevention or reduction of cerebral oedema and intracranial hypertension.

Encephalopathy grade 1–2

- A high carbohydrate diet to prevent endogenous protein breakdown may help; however, low protein diets are no longer recommended.
- Lactulose (a non-absorbable disaccharide) is used to empty the bowel and reduce reabsorption of protein. The aim is to produce two to four soft stools daily.
- Sedation should be avoided unless essential. Use of opiates and benzodiazepines should be minimized.
- Continuous assessment of the patient's mental state is important so that alterations in conscious level are quickly detected. Patients in the early stages of encephalopathy may be confused and difficult to manage. Considerable nursing time and expertise may be needed to avoid using sedation unless absolutely necessary and to prevent the patient coming to harm. Tranquilizers may be needed to control agitation.
- Reduce sensory load by ensuring a quiet environment with minimal handling, and providing reassuring and calming speech and touch (see Chapter 8).

Encephalopathy grade 3–4

- Elective sedation, intubation, and ventilation are commonly required to reduce cerebral metabolic demands and thus cerebral blood flow (CBF), thereby reducing the risk of cerebral oedema and intracranial hypertension. The aim is to maintain normal values of PCO_2 and pH (Felipo 2013).
- Maintaining normal blood electrolyte and glucose levels is also key owing to the impact of hyponatremia and hypoglycaemia on osmotic balance within the brain and the highly increased likelihood of developing cerebral oedema (Patton *et al.* 2012).

Cerebral oedema

- All patients with grade 3–4 encephalopathy are at high risk of developing intracranial hypertension and cerebral oedema.
- Elective sedation, intubation, and ventilation are commonly initiated to reduce cerebral metabolic demand and thus cerebral blood flow (CBF). Some specialist centres will place a reverse internal jugular venous catheter to monitor jugular bulb venous saturation (SjO_2) to monitor the adequacey of CBF. SjO_2 should be between 60% and 80% (Cross *et al.* 2006).
- Although there is no evidence of an impact on outcome, monitoring of ICP may be used to manage cerebral oedema (Stravitz *et al.* 2007). The aim is to reduce ICP to <20 mmHg and to maintain cerebral perfusion pressure >50–60 mmHg.
- The importance of nursing measures such as maintaining head elevation >30° and avoiding prolonged coughing or suctioning must be emphasized (full details of these are given in Chapter 8).
- Hypotension, hypoxaemia, and hypercapnia should be avoided as these all cause cerebral vasodilatation and thereby increase ICP (Patton *et al.* 2012).
- Maintaining body temperature between 35 and 36.5°C may avoid exacerbating intracranial hypertension (Whitehouse and Wendon 2013).
- As an immediate response to raised ICP, a rapid intravenous dose of mannitol (0.25–0.5 g/kg) is used to rapidly reduce the ICP (Patton *et al.* 2012). Serum osmolality is monitored, and excess fluid volumes associated with its administration should be removed from the circulation by either spontaneous diuresis or haemofiltration.
- Other interventions used in the treatment of raised ICP include bolus hypertonic saline, thiopental, indomethacin, and short-term hyperventilation. However, evidence of their impact on outcome is limited.

Coagulopathy

- Avoid procedures likely to cause bleeding (e.g. prolonged or excessive suction, vigorous mouth care, IM injections).
- Vitamin K (10 mg IV) is usually prescribed on a daily basis for 2–3 days.
- Bear in mind the increased risk of bleeding and observe the patient closely for early indications of covert bleeding.
- Administer H_2 antagonists or proton pump inhibitors, with or without antacids, to maintain gastric pH >4.
- Administer fresh frozen plasma (FFP), whole blood, and platelets as necessary. This is generally only needed if spontaneous bleeding occurs or prior to an invasive procedure. The aim is to keep the haemoglobin above 7 g/dl and to treat bleeding problems.

Renal failure

The development of renal failure is associated with a worse outcome, so prevention is the most important aspect of management. The most effective interventions are:

- correction of hypovolaemia and maintenance of renal perfusion pressure
- avoidance of nephrotoxic drugs including high dose furosemide.

Continuous renal replacement therapy is preferred to intermittent dialysis because of the reduced fluid shifts involved and their effect on cerebral perfusion (Whitehouse and Wendon 2013).

Hypoglycaemia and nutrition

Hypoglycaemia occurs frequently in the advanced stages of liver failure.

- Monitor blood glucose levels regularly (hourly until stable). If blood glucose is <3.5 mmol/L, 10–20% glucose should be infused to maintain normoglycaemia.
- Nutrition should be commenced as soon as possible and consist of a normal protein, high carbohydrate feed.
- Vitamin supplementation is usually given (e.g. parentrovite).
- Enteral feeding is possible provided that the patient has not recently bled and the GI tract is functioning. A nasogastric tube can be safely placed if done cautiously and as atraumatically as possible.
- There is no evidence that use of high branched chain, low aromatic amino acid feed formulae improves the level of encephalopathy.

Acid–base and electrolyte management

Acid–base and electrolyte disturbances are commonplace and should be monitored/managed carefully. Hyponatraemia, hypokalaemia, hypophosphataemia, alkalosis, and acidosis may all occur. Avoidance of hyponatraemia is particularly important as it will precipitate cerebral oedema.

- Monitor electrolyte levels frequently (once or twice daily as a minimum) and correct as necessary.
- Metabolic alkalosis may be corrected by correcting any potassium deficiency.
- Respiratory alkalosis associated with hyperventilation and metabolic acidosis does not usually require treatment.

Respiratory problems

The patient may need to be intubated to protect the airway. If grade III or IV encephalopathy is present, elective ventilation is recommended (Cross *et al.* 2006). If severe hypoxaemia, hypoventilation, or fitting occurs, the patient should also be ventilated. Airway pressures should be kept as low as possible and the use of PEEP minimized.

Cardiovascular problems

- A hyperdyanamic circulatory state occurs in acute liver failure with vasodilatation, hypotension, and a high cardiac output. Optimal intravascular volumes should be maintained by appropriate fluid challenges against CVP or stroke volume.
- Treat any causes of hypotension, such as hypovolaemia and arrhythmias. If necessary, maintain mean arterial pressure with vasopressors (norepinephrine or vasopressin/terlipressin) and/or inotropes if cardiac output is low (cardiomyopathy may be present, e.g. in alcoholics).
- Relative adrenal insufficiency may be a cause of persistent hypotension which can be treated with hydrocortisone (Stravitz *et al.* 2007).

Risk of infection

- Scrupulous attention should be paid to infection control measures. Infective complications occur in 20–35% of liver failure patients due to their impaired immune function.
- Regular cultures should be taken and appropriate antibiotics prescribed if organisms are found.
- Note that there is a high incidence of fungal infection in such patients, and this needs to be recognized and treated early.

Management of cause-specific acute liver failure

Paracetamol overdose

Administration of *N*-acetylcysteine (NAC) should be started immediately. Efficacy reduces as time passes though it is still effective for up to 72 hours. It is given intravenously with a loading dose followed by continuous infusion.

Acute fatty liver of pregnancy (AFLP) and the haemolysis, elevated liver enzymes, low platelet (HELLP) syndrome

Immediate delivery of the fetus usually reverses the condition. Otherwise management is supportive.

Amanita phalloides poisoning

Although evidence in support is limited, some experts recommend the use of high dose penicillin G and *N*-acetylcysteine (Stravitz *et al.* 2007).

Viral hepatitis

Viral hepatitis may respond to the use of antivirals (Patton *et al.* 2012).

Acute-on-chronic hepatic failure

Acute-on-chronic hepatic failure is characterized by jaundice, ascites, and encephalopathy. The two main causes of chronic hepatic failure are viral hepatitis (especially B and C) and alcohol (see Box 9.6). It is most likely that patients with chronic hepatic failure admitted to critical care unit will have suffered an acute decompensation, most commonly due to GI bleeding or infection.

Problems associated with chronic hepatic failure

Encephalopathy

The mechanisms underlying encephalopathy are presumed to be similar to those for acute hepatic failure, but development is slower and cerebral oedema is rare. It is usually known as porto-systemic encephalopathy because of the development of a porto-systemic collateral circulation caused by portal hypertension. This allows bypassing of the liver by the blood supply of the GI tract. Encephalopathy is often precipitated by an increased protein load in the gut, particularly following GI haemorrhage.

Box 9.6 Causes of liver cirrhosis

- Alcohol
- Infection
- Metabolic disorders (fibrocystic disease, Wilson's disease, glycogen storage diseases)
- Drugs (e.g. methotrexate, methyldopa)
- Cholestasis
- Immune factors
- Congestion (hepatic venous outflow obstruction)

Ascites

This is not solely due to portal hypertension in cirrhosis. Sodium and water retention are increased due to a fall in renal blood flow and hyper-reninaemia leading to secondary aldosteronism. This secondary aldosteronism is intensified by failure of the liver to metabolize aldosterone and vasopressin. Hypoalbuminaemia due to liver failure also lowers colloid osmotic pressure, further encouraging the formation of ascites. Treatment is as follows:

- sodium restriction of <40 mmol/24 hours
- fluid restriction of 1500 ml/24 hours
- diuretic therapy
- paracentesis (drainage of ascites via an indwelling catheter), with or without infusion of salt-poor 20% albumin.

Oesophageal varices

The pathogenesis of oesophageal varices and their management is discussed earlier in this chapter. Treatment of the precipitating factor is an important aspect of management. Blood cultures and diagnostic paracentesis should be taken to rule out infected ascites, and active measures should be carried out to prevent further GI bleeding.

Jaundice

This word 'jaundice' refers to the yellow appearance of the skin and mucous membranes seen with an increased bilirubin concentration in the body fluids. It is detectable when the serum bilirubin concentration exceeds 50 μmol/L. Causes of jaundice are haemolytic, obstructive, or hepatocellular.

Haemolytic jaundice

An increased rate of destruction of red blood cells produces an increased amount of bilirubin which is excreted by the liver until its capacity is overwhelmed. The jaundice is usually mild, as the healthy liver can excrete up to six times the normal bilirubin load. Causes of haemolytic jaundice include drugs, erythrocyte abnormalities (e.g. sickle cell disease), and malaria.

Obstructive jaundice

Jaundice occurs due to obstruction of the excretion of bilirubin anywhere between the biliary canaliculi and the ampulla of Vater. Causes of large duct obstruction include gallstones in the common bile duct, biliary duct strictures, sclerosing cholangitis, carcinoma of the head of the pancreas, and other tumours. Causes of small duct obstruction include drugs and alcohol, which damage liver cells and bile ducts, sepsis, viral hepatitis, Hodgkin's disease, primary biliary cirrhosis, and cholangitis. Jaundice can be prolonged and severe, and the patient will pass pale or clay-coloured stools due to the lack of bilirubin entering the gut. Urine will be dark due to renal excretion of conjugated bilirubin.

Hepatocellular jaundice

Jaundice results from the inability of the liver to transport bilirubin into the bile as a result of liver cell damage. Common causes are alcohol, drugs, sepsis, and viral hepatitis. Various drugs can interfere with bilirubin metabolism by:

- displacing bilirubin from protein binding in the blood (e.g. salicylates)
- impairing bilirubin uptake and transport (e.g. rifampicin)
- blocking excretion into the canaliculi (e.g. oral contraceptives).

Liver dysfunction

Critically ill patients may develop liver dysfunction as part of multiple organ failure. This can be either a result of circulatory disturbance or a reaction to one or more of the drugs used in treatment. Factors involved are numerous and may produce both hepatocellular damage and intrahepatic cholestasis. Decreased hepatic perfusion with tissue hypoxia is a common cause although cholestasis due to extrahepatic bile duct obstruction may also occur. Importantly, drug metabolism is impaired, so dosages should be carefully reviewed by the CCU pharmacist.

Management depends on the precipitating cause, but is usually dependent on treating the underlying disease. If drugs are suspected as a cause, they should be discontinued and alternatives used.

Liver support systems

Liver transplantation is considered the only fully effective treatment for acute liver failure which does not respond to supportive management. However, the growing disparity between donor availability and demand has meant that many patients do not receive a donor organ in time. Therefore research has been concentrated on alternative liver assist devices to allow support until either a donor can be found or liver function is recovered. These support systems are of two types.

1. **Extracorporeal blood purification** This technique involves use of a double-sided albumin-impregnated hollow-fibre dialysis membrane (which adsorbs molecules onto its surface). Blood travels through one side of the membrane, allowing adsorption of protein-bound toxins onto the membrane, and albumin is then run through the other side of the membrane and removes the toxins via the concentration gradient (in a similar manner to haemodiafiltration—see Chapter 7). The albumin is then run through a charcoal filter, an ion exchange resin, and another dialyser run against ordinary dialysate. This clears all the toxins picked up by the albumin which is then returned to the patient circuit in a closed loop. This is known as the Molecular Adsorption Recycling System (MARS).
2. **Biological liver support** This technique combines the use of artificially generated hepatocytes in a system again based on a dialyser. The hepatocytes are either grown in the dialyser plates themselves or attached to a matrix within the dialyser.

There are several forms of this type of purification. Trials to date have not yet demonstrated significant improvements in outcome across all types of liver failure, although a systematic review and meta-analysis of use in acute liver failure (Stutchfield *et al.* 2011) found a significant improvement in survival rates ($P = 0.05$).

Liver transplantation

This procedure is necessary in patients who have severe acute liver failure or chronic, irreversible, and progressive liver disease that does not respond to alternative medical and surgical interventions (see Box 9.7). A review of the last 20 years of liver transplantation reported in the European Liver Transplant Registry (Germani *et al.* 2012) showed survival rates for patients at 1, 5, and 10 years of 74%, 68%, and 63%, respectively. This was despite a rise in the age of both donors and recipients, and an increased likelihood of graft failure in the first year in recipients aged over 50 years with donors aged over 60 years.

Major contraindications are extrahepatic malignancy, severe sepsis, and active alcoholism. Relative contraindications are portal vein thrombosis, severe cardiopulmonary or renal disease, age over 55 years, past multiple abdominal operations, psychological instability, and a positive hepatitis B e-antigen.

Box 9.7 Conditions in which liver transplant may be appropriate

- Biliary atresia
- Inborn errors of metabolism
- Chronic active cirrhosis
- Primary biliary cirrhosis
- Sclerosing cholangitis
- Primary hepatic malignancy
- Acute liver failure
- Subacute hepatic necrosis (Sibulesky *et al.* 2013)

More recently. auxiliary liver transplantation has been undertaken where a remnant part of the recipient liver is left in situ and a partial graft transplanted from the donor. The advantage of this technique is that the native liver can potentially regenerate, regaining function and allowing immunosuppressive therapy to be withdrawn, thus allowing the transplanted liver to atrophy.

Donors

Live donor liver transplantation (LDLT)

Development of techniques in splitting livers to produce firstly reduced size grafts from adult donors for children and then split-liver transplants, where two recipients could be transplanted with one donor liver, have resulted in the technique of live organ donation of livers in adults, first performed in 1996. This is possible because of the segmental structure of the liver, which allows surgical division with vascular and biliary access, and the regenerative capacity of the liver itself. Although a success rate of >85% survival at 1 year has been cited (Tat Fan 2006), there is a risk to the donor as well as the recipient because of the large volume of liver tissue required in adults. Donor mortality rate is 0.08–0.5% (Tat Fan 2006). Over 1500 live donor transplants have already taken place.

Cadaveric organ donation

The same criteria for approach to donation are required as for any other organ (see Chapter 8).

Transplantation

Orthotopic (replacement of the recipient's liver with that of the donor) transplantation is the usual method. Donor livers can be maintained for 8–20 hours using a perfusion solution. Blood loss can be high and transfusion requirements may range from 10 to 100 units. Large quantities of FFP and platelets are also required.

Post-operative management

Haemodynamic problems

- Monitoring and maintenance of an adequate (but not excessive) intravascular volume with appropriate monitoring is vital.
- Hypotension not related to low intravascular volume is corrected using inotropes or pressors, as indicated by systemic vascular resistance and cardiac output (see Chapter 5).
- Hypertension occasionally occurs and should be controlled to protect the integrity of the vascular anastomoses. Treatment is usually related to the underlying cause, such as inadequate sedation or continuing cerebral oedema, in patients with previous acute hepatic failure. Occasionally, antihypertensive agents are required.
- Hypothermia is common due to the length of operation and the use of bypass. Gradual warming is instituted using temperature management systems.

Respiratory problems

The majority of patients are ventilated post-operatively to allow optimal respiratory support. PEEP at moderate levels is used to minimize basal atelectasis. Deep breathing and postural changes should be encouraged. Pleural effusions are common and the majority resolve spontaneously or with diuretic therapy. Development of ARDS is associated with intra-abdominal sepsis, allograft rejection, and hepatic artery thrombosis.

Metabolic disturbances

- Hypokalaemia can be severe due to absorption of potassium into the reperfused hepatocytes. Potassium supplements are given routinely unless serum levels are high.
- Insulin may be needed to maintain normal blood glucose levels.
- Metabolic alkalosis is related to the large amounts of citrate in transfused blood, as well as to hypokalaemia.

Bleeding and coagulopathy

Continuous bleeding is usually surgical in origin and may necessitate a return to theatre. Coagulopathy can usually be controlled using FFP and platelet infusions.

Immunosuppression

The exact programme and timing of immunosuppression varies, but the primary agents used are prednisolone, azathioprine, and ciclosporin. Newer agents, such as polyclonal and monoclonal antilymphocyte globulin preparations, are used in some centres as initial immunosuppression, which is then followed by long-term ciclosporin. Ciclosporin is a highly effective immunosuppressant but its use carries the risk of a number of side effects (e.g. nephrotoxicity), some of which can be severe.

Infection

- The patient will be susceptible to infection because of their state of chronic ill health and decreased immune function due to the liver failure. This will then be compounded by the introduction of immunosuppressive drugs.
- Bacterial infections frequently occur post-operatively and are treated with the appropriate antibiotics. Fungal infections (especially Candida species and Aspergillus) are treated with appropriate antifungals. Viral infections can also occur and aciclovir or ganciclovir may be needed.
- Patients should be nursed in side rooms with protective isolation. Scrupulous care is required for all clean and aseptic procedures.

Renal dysfunction

Renal dysfunction occurs in up to two-thirds of transplant patients post-operatively. It may result from continued bleeding and poor renal perfusion, sepsis, and poor allograft function. Drugs used for immunosuppression and to treat infection can be highly nephrotoxic. Management consists of maintaining intravascular volume and blood pressures. The aim is to produce 0.5 ml/kg/h urine.

Neurological dysfunction

Patients who have undergone transplant for acute liver failure may receive continual ICP monitoring throughout the post- operative period. Neurological assessment is regularly carried out to monitor status in all liver transplant patients. Complications, such as fitting, can occur and these are usually associated with ciclosporin neurotoxicity or hypomagnesaemia. Other neurological problems may occur as a result of intracerebral haemorrhage, hepatic or metabolic encephalopathy, and opportunistic infection.

Pain

An opiate, such as morphine, is usually given as an infusion or IV bolus. Some centres also use sedatives, such as midazolam, to reduce the patient's awareness of discomfort and to facilitate ventilation.

Psychological problems

Numerous psychological problems are associated with adjusting to transplantation (see Box 9.8). The nearness of death will have caused fear and anxiety to transplant recipients, and a necessity to confront their own mortality. The adjustment to accepting the presence of another person's organ within their own body may also take considerable support and rationalization. Forsberg *et al.* (2000) identified a range of profound emotions experienced by transplant recipients. Patients require trained counselling and support which is an important part of any transplant programme.

Box 9.8 The patient experience of transplant

Categories of experience include:

1. Facing the inevitable
2. Recapturing the body
3. Emotional chaos
4. Leaving the experts
5. Family and friends
6. The threat of graft rejection
7. Honouring the donor

Forsberg *et al.* (2000)

Nutritional deficit

Because of prolonged liver disease patients are often severely malnourished pre-operatively. Energy expenditure is significantly raised by the stresses associated with transplantation and patients are hypercatabolic in the post-operative phase. Therefore nutrition is required and can be given either enterally or parenterally.

Liver dysfunction

Liver function usually returns to normal soon after transplantation, but up to two-thirds of patients suffer some degree of liver dysfunction. In the extreme situation the graft fails to function immediately due to ischaemic injury, and there may be total hepatic failure. Retransplantation is the only possible course, although prognosis is poor. There may be some lesser degree of failure related to technical complications, such as bleeding, and these may be repaired on return to theatre. Rejection is the commonest cause of graft dysfunction and occurs to some extent in most patients, usually at 2–3 weeks. Rejection can occur slowly and progressively, or acutely. Treatment consists of increasing levels of steroids and use of antilymphocyte globulin or monoclonal antilymphocyte antibody (OKT3).

Survival following liver transplant is around 63% at 10 years. It is an accepted form of treatment in both end-stage liver disease and acute liver failure.

Acute pancreatitis

The incidence of acute pancreatitis has been rising over the past three decades and now affects 22.4 per 100,000 population per year in the UK (Pavlidis *et al.* 2013). It is associated with alcohol abuse or gall bladder disease in 75% of cases. Severe acute pancreatitis occurs in 25% of cases and is associated with a significant hospital mortality.

The exact aetiology is unknown, but its pathogenesis involves the activation of pancreatic enzymes within the pancreas rather than in the duodenum, or their retrograde diffusion in the activated state from the duodenum. This leads to autodigestion and an acute inflammatory response. Alcohol may cause irritation and protein precipitation which obstructs the acinar ductules and traps enzymes within the pancreas. The irritant factor in gall bladder disease is thought to be bile. Blockage of the pancreatic duct by gallstones may also precipitate pancreatitis. Many of the multisystem problems associated with pancreatitis (respiratory complications, cardiac abnormalities, impaired renal function, disseminated intravascular coagulation, etc.) are related to both the local inflammatory response and transfer of enzymes and products of pancreatic tissue destruction to the circulation, This is thought to happen via the lymphatic drainage of the pancreas to the thoracic lymph duct. Overall mortality associated with acute pancreatitis has steadily reduced over the past 20 years to between 4% and 8% (Bank *et al.* 2002). The vast majority of deaths occur in those with the most severe form, where mortality is approximately 20% (Pavlidis *et al.* 2013). Ideally, this high risk group should be treated in specialized referral centres.

Diagnosis of pancreatitis is difficult and is usually based on a number of differential diagnoses as well as the interpretation of laboratory data (see Boxes 9.9 and 9.10). The use of CT scans is considered an effective method of assessment of acute pancreatitis and associated complications.

Various scoring systems, such as the Ranson score (see Box 9.11), allow early recognition of the severity of the disease and prognostication.

Strategies for management

Correction of hypovoloemia and fluid volume imbalances

The release of vasoactive substances following autodigestion of pancreatic tissue causes alterations in the permeability of the capillary membrane. This leads to large losses of fluid into the extravascular space, and into the peritoneal space in particular. Fluid losses lead to a low circulating blood volume with reactive constriction of the splanchnic (abdominal organ) blood vessels, resulting in poor perfusion of the pancreas, further damage to the pancreatic tissue, and a continuing downward spiral in the patient's condition. Further fluid losses related to nasogastric aspiration and vomiting must also be taken into account.

- Adequate volume loading is essential in the management of these patients and should be given with pressure ± cardiac output monitoring.

Box 9.9 Signs and symptoms of acute pancreatitis

- Acute epigastric and peri-umbilical pain
- Nausea and vomiting
- Abdominal distension associated with a small bowel ileus, or pseudocyst in severe disease
- Low grade pyrexia, occasionally hypothermia
- Shock: ↑ pulse, ↓BP, etc.
- Retroperitoneal haemorrhage showing as either the Grey–Turner sign (grey discoloration (bruising) over the flanks) or Cullen's sign (bruising in and around the umbilicus)

Box 9.10 Laboratory indicators of acute pancreatitis

- Serum amylase is high (usually >1000 IU/L)
- Serum lipase is high in 75% of cases
- Total calcium levels are decreased (due to hypoalbuminaemia or extravascular precipitation)
- Ionized calcium levels decrease due to intraperitoneal combination with free fatty acids
- Hyperglycaemia is common (related to hyperglucagonaemia, insulin deficiency, or insulin resistance)
- Hyperbilirubinaemia and raised transaminase and alkaline phosphatase levels may be seen
- Hypoalbuminaemia

> **Box 9.11 Ranson score for prognostic factors in acute pancreatitis**
>
> **On admission**
>
> - Age >55 years
> - White cell count >16,000/mm^3
> - Glucose >11 mmol/L
> - LDH >400 IU/L
> - AST >250 IU/L
>
> **Within 48 hours of hospitalization**
>
> - Decrease in haematocrit >10%
> - Increase in blood urea >1.8 mmol/L
> - Calcium <2 mmol/L
> - P_aO_2 <8 kPa
> - Base deficit >4 mmol/L
> - Fluid deficit >6 L
>
> **Mortality rates**
>
> - 0–2 risk factors: mortality rate <1%
> - 3–4 risk factors: mortality rate 15% (approx.)
> - 5–6 risk factors: mortality rate 40% (approx.)
> - >6 risk factors: mortality rate 100% (approx.)
>
> Reprinted from *Surgery, Gynecology & Obstetrics*, J.H Ranson, K.M Rifkind, D.F Roses, *et al*, Prognostic signs and the role of operative management in acute pancreatitis, Volume 139, Issue 1, pp.69–81, 1974. Reprinted with permission from the *Journal of the American College of Surgeons*, formerly *Surgery Gynecology & Obstetrics*.

> **Box 9.12 Signs of hypocalcaemia**
>
> - *Chvostek's sign*: twitching of the lip and cheek in response to tapping of the side of the face over the facial nerve in the parotid gland.
> - *Trousseau's sign*: carpopedal spasm with wrist and metacarpophalangeal joints flexed and interphalangeal joints extended when a blood pressure cuff placed on the same arm is inflated to just above systolic pressure. (The response should occur within 2 min.)

- Crystalloid fluid replacement should continue at a rate suitable for the patient's normal fluid requirements. The aim is to preserve organ perfusion and maintain renal function with a urine output >0.5 ml/kg/h.

Correction of electrolyte imbalances

Imbalances in calcium, magnesium, phosphate, and potassium are also related to alterations in capillary permeability, nasogastric losses, vomiting, and diarrhoea. Calcium levels are reduced as a result of intraperitoneal saponification (combination to form a soap-like compound) with free fatty acids released during fat necrosis. Alcohol abusers may also suffer from diet-related decreases in these levels.

- Electrolyte and calcium levels should be monitored regularly, and corrected as required.
- The patient should also be observed for signs of hypocalcaemia (see Box 9.12).

Compromised circulatory function

Haemodynamic disturbances are related to the acute inflammatory process as well as to hypovolaemia, hypocalcaemia, hypokalaemia, and possible myocardial depressant factors released as part of the inflammatory response.

- There is a need for continuous monitoring of blood pressure, ECG, filling pressures (CVP), and cardiac output if myocardial depression is suspected.
- Ideally, the patient should be catheterized to monitor urine output.
- Intravascular volume should be optimized and electrolyte levels corrected. If cardiac output remains low, inotropes will be required, or vasopressors if in high output shock.

Compromised respiratory function

Hyperventilation may occur as a response to the acute pain associated with pancreatitis. Pain relief is important in limiting this response. Respiratory complications occur in 30–50% of patients, and up to 70% are hypoxaemic. There are several possible contributory factors.

- Increased likelihood of developing ARDS (see Chapter 4). Non-cardiogenic pulmonary oedema occurs in 10–30% of patients.
- Pleural effusions may form from the passage of pancreatic exudate via lymph channels into the chest, or extravasation of exudate through the diaphragm.
- Pseudocysts or abscesses may form a fistula into the chest cavity.
- Atelectasis may occur as a result of hypoventilation due to pain-related splinting of the abdominal wall.

Management consists of supporting respiratory function with appropriate oxygen therapy, and mechanical ventilation when necessary. Monitoring should include pulse oximetry and frequent arterial blood gases.

Pain

The epigastric and peri-umbilical pain in acute pancreatitis is caused by extravasation of inflammatory exudate and enzymes into the retroperitoneum. This may lead to digestion of the fat in the pancreatic bed and surrounding tissue. Another cause may be distension of pancreatic ducts and obstruction of the ampulla of Vater or swelling of the head of the pancreas, producing duodenal obstruction.

- Analgesia is essential, usually by opiate infusion. Pethidine is the traditional opiate of choice. While morphine was avoided due to its potential ability to cause spasm of the sphincter of Oddi, this does not appear to be a common problem.
- Localized analgesia, such as nerve blocks or ganglion blocks, may be useful, although epidurals should be used with caution.
- Other methods of pain relief, such as warmth, positioning, and relaxation, may have a minimizing effect but are unlikely to remove the pain completely.
- Continuous nasogastric aspiration and keeping the patient nil by mouth may sometimes help to limit pancreatic stimulus to release enzymes.

Hyperglycaemia

This can occur secondary to hyperglucagonaemia, insulin deficiency, or insulin resistance related to the critical illness. An insulin infusion, titrated to blood glucose levels, should be administered.

Nutrition

There is now clear evidence of the benefit of enteral nutrition in pancreatitis. A Cochrane review (Al-Omran *et al.* 2010) found that enteral nutrition significantly reduced mortality, multiple organ failure, systemic infections, and the need for operative interventions compared with parenteral nutrition. Marik and Zaloga (2004) also found a significant reduction in length of hospital stay ($P < 0.001$) in a meta-analysis of six randomized controlled trials comparing enteral with parenteral nutrition in pancreatitis. Recent studies (Wereszczynska-Siemiatkowska *et al.* 2013; Pavlidis *et al.* 2013) have shown that early enteral nutrition is beneficial in the management of severe acute pancreatitis, with commencement within 48 hours of admission being associated with reduced mortality ($P < 0.05$) and infection ($P < 0.05$) (Wereszczynska-Siemiatkowska *et al.* 2013).

In mild uncomplicated pancreatitis nutritional support may not be necessary initially. However, in moderate to severe pancreatitis nutritional support should be instituted early, ideally with placement of a jejunal tube. Gastric feeding can be attempted if a jejunal tube cannot be inserted. Parenteral nutrition should be considered if enteral nutrition is not feasible.

Secondary infection

Use of prophylactic antibiotics is not supported by evidence (Bai *et al.* 2008). Due to the risks of resistance and superinfection, antibiotics should only be initiated for confirmed infection.

Surgery or drainage of abscesses/necrosis/pseudocyst

Radiologically guided drainage with siting of a percutaneous drain or surgical debridement may be indicated, particularly if the general state of the patient deteriorates and there are concerns about super-infection of necrosis or a pseudocyst.

Intra-abdominal hypertension

Fluid movement into the interstitium as a result of capillary endothelial damage causes the abdominal wall to expand. As the volume of fluid increases and the distension reaches the stretch end-point, the pressure within the abdominal cavity starts to rise. Causes are varied and include direct peritoneal and retroperitoneal injury as well as a more system-wide inflammatory response (for full details see Chapter 11). Abdominal compartment syndrome, reduced renal perfusion, and renal failure can result if intra-abdominal hypertension is not controlled (Cheatham *et al.* 2007)

Normal intra-abdominal pressure (IAP) is 0–5 mmHg and can be monitored via a Foley bladder catheter. Intra-abdominal hypertension (IAH) is present if IAP exceeds 12–15 mmHg. The degree of IAH is graded, as shown in Table 9.4.

Table 9.4 Intra-abdominal hypertension grading

Grade	Intra-abdominal pressure (mmHg)
I	12–15
II	16–20
III	21–25
IV	>25

Reproduced from *Intensive Care Medicine*, Cheatham, M.L., Malbrain, M.L., Kirkpatrick, A., *et al.*, Results from the International Conference of Experts on Intra-abdominal Hypertension and Abdominal Compartment Syndrome. II. Recommendations, Volume 33, pp. 951–62, Copyright © 2007 with permission of Springer.

Endoscopy

Oesophagogastroduodenoscopy (OGD) is the examination of the upper GI tract using a flexible fibreoptic instrument which is passed via the mouth and then through the oesophagus, stomach, and duodenum to allow direct visualization of the mucosal surface. Procedures such as sclerosis of varices or biopsies of lesions such as ulcers can be performed via an instrument channel within the scope.

The critically ill patient is most likely to require endoscopy for investigation of GI haemorrhage, severe epigastric pain, unexplained anaemia, and attempted correction of upper gastrointestinal bleeding (see Box 9.13).

Preparation of the patient for endoscopy

The patient should be adequately resuscitated prior to endoscopy, though resuscitation may be ongoing for a massive bleed. An explanation of the procedure, the reasons for it, and the probable sensations/discomfort should be given to the patient and their family. Routine gastric lavage prior to the procedure is unnecessary. Increased levels of sedation are usually required for the procedure. However, if there are concerns about the airway, the patient should be electively ventilated. Endoscopy can cause hypoxaemia and cardiorespiratory compromise, so close monitoring should continue throughout and following the procedure. The inspired oxygen concentration may have to be increased. Following the procedure, the patient should be observed for signs of further bleeding and/or perforation (see Table 9.5 for haemostasis).

Box 9.13 Indications for endoscopy

- Acute gastrointestinal haemorrhage (identification of site and haemostasis)
- Biopsy of lesions such as tumours and ulcers
- Placement of duodenal and jejunal feeding tubes
- Sclerosis of oesophageal varices
- Removal of ingested foreign objects
- Studies of biliary and pancreatic ducts

Table 9.5 Haemostasis of bleeding points

Method	Procedures	Use and efficacy
Chemical	Injection of sclerosants, such as epinephrine and alcohol, directly into the base of an ulcer	Can control arterial bleeding in >90% of cases
Thermal	Electrocoagulation: monopolar and bipolar diathermy Heater probe Laser photocoagulation	Haemostasis of most vessels apart from brisk arterial bleeding Can control arterial bleeding from peptic ulcers Effective in 80–90% of ulcer bleeds Can reduce the incidence of arterial rebleeding from ulcers

Delivery of nutritional support

Most critically ill patients cannot meet their own nutritional requirements. This may be related to increased or altered nutritional requirements associated with their illness, and/or limitations associated with other supports such as sedation, intubation, and mechanical ventilation. Nutritional needs should be carefully assessed, leading to the most appropriate type of support. Patients who do not receive their nutritional needs over a long period (several days) have a reduced likelihood of survival (Villet *et al.* 2005; Weijs *et al.* 2012).

Assessment of the patient's nutritional status and requirements

This is difficult to assess accurately in the critically ill patient because of alterations in metabolic function, associated particularly with sepsis and trauma, but also because of other stressors (for details see Chapter 3). Methods of assessing nutritional requirements are approximate at best. Improved patient outcome is associated with neither over- nor underfeeding. Moderate levels of nutrition or those matched to individual needs appear to work best. Krishnan *et al.* (2003) found that improved outcomes for medical ICU patients was associated with moderate levels of nutritional intake (approximately 9–18 kcal/kg per day or 33–65% of targets associated with American College of Chest Physicians recommended levels). However, current ESPEN guidelines and expert consensus (Singer *et al.* 2014; Kreymann *et al.* 2006) suggest 20–25 kcal/kg/day in the acute phase and 25–30 kcal/kg/day in the recovery phase.

Most of the methods used to assess nutritional status and requirements were produced for relatively well patient populations and may not apply to the critically ill. Some of these methods, together with details of their application in intensive care, are described in the following sections.

Anthropometry

Daily weight is not a reliable measure of nutritional status in the critically ill. Fluctuations in fluid balance associated with the illness or therapy may produce considerable changes in weight which are unrelated to nutrition. Patients may be 10 L, or even more, positive. Weight loss itself also gives little indication of the composition of that loss. Thus a 2 kg weight loss in starvation may have a ratio of fat to protein of 2:1, but in the hypercatabolic patient the ratio may be 1:4 with much graver consequences.

Measurements of skinfold thickness and midarm muscle circumference have also been used to gauge muscle mass, but this too has problems in the critically ill patient. Oedema may seriously alter the measurement, changes develop slowly, and there can be considerable inter-operator variation.

Measurements of hand-grip muscle strength by dynamometry and respiratory muscle strength using maximal inspiratory force have been used but are affected by other variables such as patient cooperation and respiratory muscle fatigue.

Assessment of nitrogen balance (as an indicator for loss of lean body mass)

Loss of protein stores can be profound in acute illness. Maintenance of lean body mass is associated with improved outcomes in critically ill patients (van Schijndel *et al.* 2009). Finn *et al.* (1996) found that up to 17% of body stores were lost in 21 days in multiple trauma patients, two-thirds of which was skeletal muscle mass. Thus muscle wasting in these patients can be severe.

Nitrogen balance, as the end-product of amino acid breakdown, can provide an insight into whether protein (and therefore lean body mass) is being gained or lost. Intake of nitrogen (usually in the form of protein) is compared with nitrogen losses as urinary urea in a 24-hour urine collection as approximately 90–95% of nitrogen losses are excreted via the urine (see Box 9.14).

Urinary nitrogen losses can range from <10g/70 kg body weight in patients following surgery to >25g/70 kg in patients with burns (Chiolero *et al.* 2006) The difference between nitrogen intake and loss is termed

Box 9.14 Calculation of nitrogen balance

Nitrogen balance = (intake − loss / 24 h)

Intake (g / 24 h) = protein / 6.25 (g / 24 h)

Loss (g / 24 h) = urinary urea (mmol / L) × urinary volume / 24 h (L) × 0.028

'nitrogen balance', and this is rarely positive in the critically ill patient.

An estimate of faecal losses of 4 g/day of nitrogen has been suggested. However, this will overestimate losses in the parenterally fed patient with minimal or absent stools, and vice versa in the patient with diarrhoea. Therefore it must be added to the nitrogen balance calculation with caution.

The usefulness of nitrogen balance in assessing the patient's nutritional state is debatable. Assumptions are made that a steady state exists within the body pool of nitrogen, but this may not be the case. For instance, a rising blood urea in acute renal failure will affect the amount of urinary urea lost, giving a falsely low level of nitrogen loss. Therefore correct interpretation of nitrogen balance is important, and assessment of the patient's overall nutritional status must be made in order to evaluate the results correctly.

Levels of serum proteins as nutritional indicators

Most investigators have concluded that levels of plasma proteins do not accurately assess whole-body nutritional status in individual patients during the critical illness phase. Various factors in the critically ill patient alter plasma protein levels without affecting nutritional status (see Box 9.15). The most commonly used indicator has been albumin. However, albumin levels are frequently low due to:

- fluid shifts producing dilution
- movement of proteins into extravascular spaces through leaky capillary membranes
- dilution by infusion of artificial colloids
- decreased liver production of albumin due to liver dysfunction associated with the catabolic state of critical illness.

Thus, despite the absence of significant malnutrition, low albumin levels are often found. Hypoalbuminaemia is considered to be a non-specific indicator of illness. However, in the *pre-disease* state, low albumin levels (<30 g/L) are an indicator of malnutrition (Chiolero *et al.* 2006).

Box 9.15 Plasma proteins used to assess nutritional state

Serum albumin

May fall precipitately in the critically ill without significant nutritional deficit

Rises slowly in repletion

Serum transferrin

Can also be raised in iron deficiency

Frequently underestimates nutritional status in the critically ill

Rises earlier than albumin in repletion

Indirect calorimetry

Indirect calorimetry is able to provide a more accurate assessment of the individual patient's energy requirements (Martindale *et al.* 2009) than energy expenditure formulae. It is a technique whereby the patient's energy expenditure is calculated from the inspired and expired gases (i.e. the amount of oxygen consumed and the amount of carbon dioxide produced by the patient). These gases are consumed and produced during the oxidation of food substances, and the amount of oxygen and carbon dioxide can be directly related to the amount of food oxidized to produce energy:

$$C_6H_{12}O_6(\text{carbohydrate}) + 6O_2 = 6H_2O + 6CO_2 + \text{energy (kCal)}.$$

Indirect calorimetry requires a stand-alone metabolic monitor (such as the MedGraphics system) or a ventilator that incorporates metabolic monitoring. Mass spectrometry, whereby different constituents of a gas are detected by passing them through an electron beam which ionizes them and then a magnetic field which separates the ionized molecules by their mass and electric charge, is a very expensive alternative that is rarely available clinically.

The advantages of indirect calorimetry for assessment of energy expenditure are as follows

1. It is more accurate for the individual patient than formulae and tables which are created for populations of patients.
2. If continuous measurements are performed, changes in metabolic rate (for instance, as a result of activity or drugs) can be measured (McClave *et al.* 2003).
3. It gives an immediate answer to the patient's energy requirements rather than waiting for any laboratory analysis.

Other information can be gained from indirect calorimetry, such as an indirect measure of the work of breathing. If the patient is being weaned from the ventilator and support is decreased, and provided that no other changes in the patient's condition are occurring, the increase in oxygen consumption will reflect the increased work required from the patient to compensate for the decrease in ventilatory support.

The disadvantages of indirect calorimetry for assessment of energy expenditure are as follows.

1. Accuracy decreases with increasing inspired oxygen concentrations; an error >5% exists with an FiO_2 >0.6. Therefore it is more inaccurate in those critically ill patients least able to tolerate the consequences of over- or underfeeding.
2. Other sources of error during mechanical ventilation relate to leaks in the ventilator circuit and use of flow-by ventilation and humidication.
3. The assumption that steady state conditions exist may not always apply. In particular, body carbon dioxide pools are likely to change if there are pH imbalances.
4. If the patient is on haemofiltration, there may be carbon dioxide loss across the filter membrane in solution in the ultrafiltrate, and as bicarbonate. This results in potential underestimation of carbon dioxide production by the indirect calorimeter.
5. Hypoventilation and hyperventilation will also affect the measurement of expired gases as carbon dioxide accumulates or is blown off. This results in over- or underestimation of energy expenditure.
6. The equipment is expensive.

If used correctly, indirect calorimetry is the most accurate way of assessing an individual patient's energy needs (Martindale *et al.* 2009).

Markers of gut function

While various markers have been proposed for assessment of gut function, some are more useful than others (Table 9.6).

Presence or absence of bowel sounds

While traditionally used as an absolute indicator of gut function, the presence or absence of bowel sounds should be interpreted with caution and should not be a deciding factor in the initiation of enteral feeding (Martindale *et al.* 2009). Bowel sounds are produced by disruption of the gas–fluid interface of the intestinal and gastric lumen by peristaltic waves. The largest areas of gas–fluid interface are in the stomach and the colon, i.e. the two areas of bowel most sensitive to loss of function. In some circumstances, gastric and colonic function may be affected following an insult but small bowel function may continue or return more quickly. Bowel sounds may thus be absent although only parts of the gut are non-functioning. As the small bowel is the major site for absorption of nutrients, it may still be possible to feed the patient enterally using a nasoduodenal tube or jejunostomy tube placed directly into the small bowel. Therefore bowel sounds should be interpreted in context with other indicators of bowel function such as pain, distension, vomiting, gastric aspirate, and diarrhoea. See Box 9.16 for indications for parenteral nutrition.

High volumes of nasogastric aspirate

There is no definitive level at which the amount of aspirate clearly indicates absence of gut function. Volumes

Table 9.6 Factors involved in deciding the mode of nutritional support

Gut function	Oral/oesophageal route	Mastication and swallowing	Mode of nutritional support
Gut is fully functioning and is patent	Oral/oesophageal route is patent	Patient is able to masticate and swallow	Patient can eat a normal diet
Gut is functioning, although tolerance of certain foods may be affected	Oral/oesophageal route is patent	Patient may have difficulty with mastication but can swallow	Patient can eat a modified diet
Gut is functioning, although tolerance of certain foods may be affected	Oral/oesophageal route has some degree of restriction or damage so that whole foods are not tolerated	Patient may have difficulty with mastication but can swallow	Patient can take nourishing fluids
Gut is functioning, although tolerance of certain foods may be affected or parts of the gut, such as the stomach, may not function	Oral/oesophageal route may be restricted or damaged or gastric function may be absent	Patient has difficulty masticating or swallowing	Patient requires enteral feed via nasoenteric or percutaneous gastrostomy/ jejunostomy tube
Gut is not functioning or requires rest from stimulation			Patient requires parenteral nutrition

Box 9.16 Indications for parenteral nutrition

- GI tract obstruction (adhesions, hernia, carcinoma of the oesophagus or colon, intussusception, volvulus, and diverticular disease)
- Prolonged paralytic ileus (post-surgery, peritonitis, post-spinal injury)
- Enterocutaneous fistulae
- Malabsorption and short-bowel syndromes (<100cm)
- Inflammatory intestinal disease (some patients with Crohn's disease or ulcerative colitis)
- Severe pancreatitis and cholecystitis
- Repeated failure to establish enteral feed

used as a cut-off point should reflect the amount of feed being given and the likely amount of gastric secretions. Gastric secretions are approximately 2 L/day in the healthy person but can be increased by stimulation, such as the presence of a nasogastric tube (Johnson 2007). The amount of aspirate used in most ICUs as a cut-off point for continuing or commencing enteral feed is 200–250 ml after a 4-hour period without aspiration, occurring on two occasions in a 24-hour period (Metheny *et al.* 2012; McClave and Snider 2002). Again, this must be considered in context with other factors.

Vomiting/regurgitation of feed

This is a dangerous situation if the patient cannot protect their airway, as the risk of aspiration is considerable. Endotracheal intubation should not be considered totally protective as aspiration of feed is not uncommon in intubated patients despite a fully inflated endotracheal tube cuff. Patients should be nursed in the semi-recumbent position (45° to the horizontal) to reduce the risk of regurgitation (Williams and Leslie 2004). However, this concept has recently been challenged, as early animal studies suggest that a head-down position may actually offer more protection (Zanella *et al.* 2011; Li Bassi 2008); further work is needed on this. Enteral feeding should always be stopped and the patient assessed for other signs of intolerance such as abdominal distension, pain, and diarrhoea if vomiting or regurgitation is evident. If there is no evidence of an abdominal disorder, drugs that increase gastric motility and emptying, such as metoclopramide, may be used to improve gastric emptying and feed restarted cautiously at a low rate. See Box 9.17 for factors associated with increased risk of regurgitation of feed and nosocomial pneumonia.

Box 9.17 Factors associated with increased risk of regurgitation of feed and nosocomial pneumonia

- Presence of enteral feeding tube (Kearns *et al.* 2000; Tejada Artigas *et al.* 2001)
- Size of enteral feeding tube (NB: not supported by evidence) (Metheny *et al.* 1986; Ferrer *et al.* 1999).
- Placement of enteral feeding tube (NB: not supported by evidence) (Strong *et al.* 1992; Kearns *et al.* 2000)
- Position of patient (Zanella *et al.* 2011; Drakulovic *et al.* 1999)
- Increased delay in gastric emptying (Mentec *et al.* 2001)

Assessment of nasogastric aspirate or vomit

The colour, amount, pH, and consistency of nasogastric aspirate or vomit can provide useful information. It should be observed and recorded, and any significant change reported. Gastric or duodenal bleeding will either appear as a normal red colour if it has spent little time in the stomach itself, or will be altered to so-called 'coffee grounds' (brownish-black particles) following denaturation by gastric acid. Normal biliary secretions are dark-green to yellow-brown.

Diarrhoea

Up to half of critically ill patients develop diarrhoea (DeLegge 2013; Mentec *et al.* 2001; Montejo 1999; McClave *et al.* 1999). Many of the causes are not simply related to intolerance of enteral feed (see Box 9.18), although this may aggravate the situation. The patient should be investigated and treated for likely causes prior to discontinuing enteral feeding. For further details see the section on 'Care of the enterally fed patient'.

Box 9.18 Factors implicated in diarrhoea

- Lactose intolerance
- Antibiotic therapy
- Other drug therapy (e.g. digoxin)
- Zinc deficiency
- Feed osmolality
- Low serum albumin levels
- Bacterial contamination of feeds
- Infection such as *Clostridium difficile* (Bliss *et al.* 2000)
- Fat malabsorption

Table 9.7 Types of diarrhoea

Frequency	Colour	Texture	Cause
Occasional	Black	Tarry	Old bleeding—upper GI tract: melaena
Frequent depending on the rate of bleeding	Dark red	Viscous but liquid	Fresh bleeding: melaena
Constant	Brighter red	Liquid	Rectal bleeding: haemorrhoids
Frequent	Green/khaki	Soft stool or liquid	Infective: *Clostridium difficile*, Salmonella
Frequent	Pale brown/clay coloured	Loose, bulky, may float or be frothy	Malabsorption, obstruction of the biliary duct
Frequent	Bloody	Loose with obvious blood	Ischaemic or infarcted bowel
Frequent	Flecks of blood and mucus	Loose with mucus	Ulcerative colitis, Crohn's disease

Assessment of bowel movements and constipation

There is a considerable variation in the normal frequency of bowel movements between individuals. The patient's normal frequency should be ascertained before deciding whether there is a problem with constipation or diarrhoea. Patients are as likely to become constipated in critical care as they are to experience diarrhoea because of the use of opioids, low-residue feeds, etc. (Btaiche *et al.* 2010). Montejo *et al.* (1999) reported a 15.7% incidence of constipation and a 14.7% incidence of diarrhoea in 400 ICU patients studied in a prospective survey.

Valuable information about gastrointestinal dysfunction can be obtained from a thorough assessment of the patient's stools and an accurate record of frequency, consistency, and texture (see Table 9.7). Many units now use a monitoring chart such as the Bristol Stool Chart which allows common understanding of description of the consistency of bowel movements (Lewis and Heaton 1997).

The Bristol Stool Chart categorizes consistency into seven types:

1. separate hard lumps, like nuts
2. sausage shaped but lumpy
3. like a sausage or snake, but with cracks on its surface
4. like a sausage or snake, smooth and soft
5. soft blobs with clear cut edges
6. fluffy pieces with ragged edges, a mushy stool
7. water, no solid pieces[1]

[1] Reproduced with permission from S.J. Lewis, K.W. Heaton, Stool form scale as a useful guide to intestinal transit time, *Scandinavian Journal of Gastroenterology*, Volume 32, Issue 9, pp.920–4, Copyright © 1997 Taylor & Francis.

Box 9.19 Conditions producing abdominal pain/tenderness

Intra-abdominal causes

- (Perforated) peptic ulcer
- Oesophagitis
- Trauma
- Dissecting or ruptured aneurysm
- Pancreatitis
- Cholecystitis
- Cholangitis
- Acute renal tract infection
- Crohn's disease
- Pelvic inflammatory disease
- Ulcerative colitis
- Hepatitis
- Ruptured ectopic pregnancy
- Diverticulitis
- Occlusion of mesenteric artery
- Appendicitis
- Ileus
- Bowel obstruction
- Peritonitis

Extra-abdominal causes

- Myocardial disease
- Respiratory disease including pneumonia
- Diabetic or thyroid crisis
- Spinal cord lesion
- Acute intermittent porphyria
- Lead poisoning
- Endometriosis
- Sickle-cell disease

Pain

Acute abdominal pain is frequently associated with gut dysfunction and should always be taken seriously (see Box 9.19). It is an important sign in ileus, peritonitis, obstruction, and ischaemia. If accompanied by other signs, such as abdominal distension and vomiting, feed should be stopped immediately and medical staff informed.

Distension

The abdomen may be distended for various reasons (see Box 9.20). When associated with pain, vomiting, or diarrhoea, enteral feeding may need to be discontinued; senior medical staff should be informed.

Box 9.20 Causes of abdominal distension

- Intestinal obstruction
- Malabsorption
- Peritonitis
- Abdominal haemorrhage (see Chapter 11)
- Ascites
- Gas
- Paralytic ileus
- Gut wall oedema

Priorities of care

Priorites of care for the GI tract are (Martindale *et al.* 2009):

- Prevention of further complications associated with the GI tract.
- Maintenance of nutritional intake in order to preserve lean body mass, avert metabolic complications, and maintain immune function.

Prevention of further complications associated with the gastrointestinal tract

Problem 1—Pulmonary aspiration of stomach contents

The incidence is difficult to establish, as much of it may occur unnoticed (McClave *et al.* 2002). Overt aspiration has been quoted to be as high as 38% (Winterbauer *et al.* 1981), though this figure is probably lower in modern practice. It is a potentially lethal complication leading to pneumonia or ARDS, and it is important to avoid any potentiating factors. Even intubated patients or those with tracheostomies can aspirate gastric contents despite an inflated cuff (see Box 9.21).

Strategies to avoid aspiration include (Williams and Leslie 2004; Drakulovic 1999; Martindale *et al.* 2009; Kreymann *et al.* 2006):

- monitoring gastric residual volumes (the amount of gastric aspirate in the stomach) four-hourly when feeding is being established and eight-hourly once it is established (NB: some individual critical care feeding protocols may differ)
- checking gastric residual volumes prior to any vigorous head-down procedures such as postural drainage and, if necessary, aspirate gastric contents
- nursing the patient in a 30–45° upright position to reduce the risk of reflux, provided that cardiovascular status allows this
- monitoring the tube position externally by marking the entry site with tape or ink on the tube and checking that this has not migrated outwards
- monitoring the tube position internally by performing gastric aspiration, checking pH, and confirming a satisfactory position on chest X-ray.

Problem 2—Hospital-acquired (nosocomial) pneumonia

Transfer of bacteria from the stomach to the oropharynx and trachea is recognized as a major factor in the development of nosocomial pneumonia in ventilated patients—ventilator-associated pneumonia (VAP) (Tejada Artigas *et al.* 2001). Increased growth of organisms

Box 9.21 Increased risk of aspiration is associated with

- reduced level of consciousness
- diminished or absent cough or gag reflexes
- incompetent oesophageal sphincters
- delayed gastric emptying (such as that associated with diabetes or malnutrition)
- paralytic ileus
- displacement of enteral feeding tube into either the oesophagus or the pharynx (can be associated with vigorous coughing or retching)
- presence of an enteral feeding tube

in the stomach is associated with an increase in gastric pH. This can be due to the common use of gastric acid inhibitors or antacids, as well as enteral feeding. Tejada Artigas *et al.* (2001) reported a 54% incidence of VAP in patients who were continuously enterally fed.

The use of selective decontamination of the digestive tract (SDD) or selective oropharyngeal decontamination (SOD) has been successful in reducing the incidence of nosocomial pneumonia and improving outcomes in critical care populations (de Smet *et al.* 2009). However, equipoise still remains in many ICU practitioners about its worth.

Strategies to reduce the incidence of nosocomial pneumonia include:

- elimination/reduction of the factors contributing to the incidence of aspiration (see above)
- avoidance of exogenous bacterial contamination (see Chapter 3)
- avoidance of use of antacids or gastric acid inhibitors, if possible.
- SDD or SOD.

Problem 3—Stress ulceration and acute bleeds

This is discussed in the section on 'Acute gastrointestinal bleeding'.

Maintenance of nutritional intake

Nutritional support does not constitute a first-line life-saving intervention, but it does carry a significant impact on recovery of the critically ill patient. Progressive weight loss adds to debility, while patient mortality and morbidity correlate closely with loss of body weight. Loss of >30% of body weight is usually fatal. Weijs *et al.* (2012) showed that those patients who achieved their protein and calorie targets had an improved outcome. However, recent studies (Hermans *et al.* 2013; Puthucheary *et al.* 2013) suggest that provision of additional parenteral nutrition and increased levels of protein in early critical illness may actually delay recovery of muscle atrophy and weakness.

In a study of 129 patients admitted to critical care, Giner *et al.* (1996) identified 43% as malnourished. This group had a significantly higher incidence of complications. Thus it is important both to identify patients likely to be at risk and to ensure that nutritional support meets their needs.

The goal of nutritional therapy in the acute phase of critical illness is to provide sufficient calories and protein to maintain lean body mass, reduce nitrogen loss, and supply the range of nutrients required to support cellular function. It is not generally possible to replenish body stores until the recovery phase of critical illness because of the degree of catabolism associated with the severely stressed state.

Provision of optimum protein and energy requirements

The debate around the optimal levels of protein and energy for critically ill patients continues. The amount of calories required varies hugely. The accepted rule of thumb is to supply 20–25 kcal/kg/day to females and 25–30 kcal/kg/day to males (Singer *et al.* 2014). However, some recent studies support 'permissive underfeeding' of calories (Arabi *et al.* 2012; Needham *et al.* 2013). Permissive underfeeding is based on animal research which shows a reduction in metabolic rate and oxidative stress, an improvement in insulin sensitivity, and lowered mitochondrial free-radical production associated with delivering <70% of energy requirements. Permissive underfeeding aims to provide around 60–70% of accepted calorie targets in order to initiate a similar response in the critically ill patient.

Protein requirements are also complex. Recommendations from different guidelines give varying ranges from 1.3–1.5 g/kg/day to 1.2–2.0 g/kg/day. A recent meta-analysis of studies which measured protein requirements with 24-hour urinary nitrogen excretion and energy requirements with indirect calorimetry showed that protein needs varied from 1.2 to 3.2 g/kg/day (Kreymann *et al.* 2012). The difficulty of monitoring lean body mass means that the provision of protein requirements will remain a best estimate for now. As mentioned earlier, there is a suggestion that increased protein feed may be deleterious (Hermans *et al.* 2013; Puthucheary *et al.* 2013).

Management of blood glucose levels

Hyperglycaemia is associated with poor outcome in the critically ill. Using an intensive insulin regimen van den Berghe *et al.* (2001) showed significantly reduced mortality rates associated with maintenance of 'tight' blood glucose control with levels between 4.5 and 6 mmol/L (81–108 mg/dl) (see Chapter 10 for details). However, subsequent large multi-centre randomized controlled trials could not reproduce this benefit. A large study (NICE-SUGAR Study 2009) found that outcomes were better when blood glucose levels were kept between 7.8 and 10 mmol/L (140–180 mg/dl). Current recommendations are to maintain sugar levels below 180 mg/dl (10 mmol/L) but not to aim for very tight control.

Immunonutrition

A number of nutrients have specific effects on the immune response in critically ill patients (see Box 9.22). As nosocomial infection is associated with an increased risk of both morbidity and mortality in the critically ill, it would be extremely advantageous if immune function could be manipulated by the addition of one or more of these nutrients. There have been over 60 studies of feeds combining various immune-enhancing nutrients (usually three or more in each feed), with a variety of results and recommendations. A systematic review of studies in over 1900 high risk surgical patients (Marik and Zaloga 2010) suggested that immune-enhancing feeds significantly reduced the risk of acquired infections, wound complications, and length of stay, but this required the use of both arginine and fish oil. A large prospective multi-centre trial (Heyland *et al.* 2013) examining glutamine and/or antioxidants (selenium, zinc, beta-carotene, and vitamins C and E) found harm from glutamine and no benefit from the antioxidant cocktail. At present, there is no overall view that any specific immunonutrient should be given to critically ill patients.

Modes of nutrition

Provision of nutritional support can be accomplished either enterally and/or parenterally. There are pros and cons associated with each method, but all have a place depending on the needs of the patient. For an individual patient the decision must be made on the basis of their GI tract function, metabolic problems, and knowledge of the potential risks and advantages of each route. One method may have to be substituted for another as the patient's condition changes. It is generally accepted that if the patient is unable to take food orally but the GI tract is otherwise functioning, enteral nutrition is the first choice for nutritional support (Martindale *et al.* 2009).

The advantages of enteral nutrition are:

- more physiological, using the normal route for absorption and subject to the checks and balances associated with the uptake of oral nutrition
- cheaper (an important aspect in view of limited resources)
- does not require central venous access with the associated risks of catheter insertion, infection, etc.
- preserves gut mucosal integrity
- possible role in modifying the immune response to stress.

The disadvantages of enteral nutrition are as follows.

- An association with diarrhoea (14.7% (Montejo 1999)) which can cause dehydration, electrolyte imbalance, skin excoriation, and discomfort, as well as increasing nursing workload considerably.
- In many cases, patients do not receive the amount of feed prescribed; in some cases these may not even satisfy basic metabolic requirements (McClave *et al.* 1999; De Jonghe *et al.* 2001). This shortfall is related to non-patient factors including (i) stopping feeds for an hour each time gut absorption is checked, (ii) keeping patients nil by mouth for excessive periods prior to procedures, and (iii) poor systems for checking that the amount prescribed is actually being delivered.
- a possible increased risk of nosoomial pneumonia associated with continuous enteral feeding. may be related to an increase in gastric pH, allowing bacterial colonization of the stomach and retrograde migration of the organisms via the oesophagus to the respiratory tract.
- not all patients will be capable of absorbing enteral feed. However, it is possible to feed a high percentage of critically ill patients enterally, but this requires commitment and a willingness to tackle associated problems.

See Table 9.8 for further complications of enteral feeding.

Box 9.22 Nutrients associated with altering inflammatory response

- **Glutamine**: major fuel source for activated immune cells and enterocytes (cells that line the intestine). Also acts as a precursor for glutathione (extracellular antioxidant).
- **Arginine**: precursor to nitric oxide with immunoregulatory properties. Essential for wound healing and lymphocyte response.
- **Omega-3 polyunsaturated fatty acids**: associated with downregulation of inflammatory response by altering the arachidonic acid pathway (see Chapter 10).
- **Nucleotides**: important for lymphocyte reproduction.

Differences in metabolism between parenteral and enteral feeding

Assimilation of digested enteral feed occurs via the portal system and liver, while parenteral feed passes directly into the circulation. Amino acids, with the exception of branched-chain amino acids, are extracted by the liver from the enteral route. Branched-chain amino acids pass directly into the systemic circulation and are taken up

Table 9.8 Complications of enteral feeding

Type of complication	Causes and manifestations of complication
Mechanical	• Knotting of the tube • Clogging or blockage of the tube due to (i) fragments of inadequately crushed tablets, (ii) adherence of feed residue, and (iii) incompatibilities between feed and medication given (e.g. phenytoin) • Incorrect placement (usually in the bronchial tree) (See Figure 9.6) • Nasopharyngeal erosions and discomfort • Sinusitis and otitis • Oesophageal reflux and oesophagitis • Tracheo-oesophageal fistula • Ruptured oesophageal varices • Pyloric or intestinal obstruction by gastrostomy or jejunostomy tubes
Nausea and vomiting	• High infusion rates • Large gastric volumes • Fat or lactose intolerance • Hyperosmolality • Delayed gastric emptying
Aspiration	See section on priorities of care
Diarrhoea (see also section on markers of gut function)	• Osmotic load associated with hypertonic medication)e.g sorbitol-containing elixirs) • Medication-induced (e.g. magnesium and phosphate salts) • Infection and antibiotic-related overgrowth(e.g. *C.difficile*) • Low fibre feed formula • Feeding contamination • Lactose intolerance • Diarrhoea has been particularly associated with enteral feeding in the critically ill. It does not necessarily indicate that the gut is unable to function, and the patient should be assessed for precipitating factors which can be dealt with before feed is discontinued.
Abdominal distension/ delayed gastric emptying	• Critical illness • Formula (associated with high density, high lipid content) • Medication (opiates) • Ileus • Gastric atony • Medical conditions such as pancreatitis, diabetes, and malnutrition, or post-vagotomy
Cramping	• Lactose intolerance • High fat content formulae • Malnutrition-related malabsorption
Constipation	• Opiate infusions • Previous laxative abuse • Long-term feeding regimens (particularly low fibre formulae)
Hyperglycaemia	• Associated with sepsis, age, renal insufficiency, diabetes, steroid therapy, and high caloric density formulae • High rates of infusion, or inadequate endogenous insulin production and inadequate exogenous insulin supplementation can also induce hyperglycaemia • Prolonged hyperglycaemia may develop into hyperosmolar hyperglycaemic non-ketotic states, although this is unlikely to develop in the critical care area because of close monitoring and management

(continued)

Table 9.8 **Continued**

Type of complication	Causes and manifestations of complication
Hypercapnia	• High levels of carbohydrate can produce large amounts of CO_2 that require increased minute volumes and respiratory rate to be excreted • May precipitate ventilatory failure in the patient with compromised respiratory function or in the weaning patient
Electrolyte and trace element abnormality	• Hypernatraemia due to high sodium intake and dehydration • Hyponatraemia due to overhydration and GI water loss (diarrhoea, drains, etc.) as well as insufficient sodium intake • Hyperkalaemia, usually associated with renal insufficiency and metabolic acidosis • Hypokalaemia, usually associated with diarrhoea, high dose insulin, or diuretics, but can also be due to insufficient intake or replacement • Hyperphosphataemia, usually caused by renal dysfunction in tube-fed patients • Hypophosphataemia occurs in the same way as hypokalaemia but may also be seen in malnourished patients when feeding is restarted (refeeding syndrome) along with low serum levels of zinc, copper, and magnesium

primarily by muscle. However, in parenteral feeding all amino acids enter the systemic circulation, though the same pattern of uptake is then followed. Carbohydrate normally passes directly from intestine to liver, but with parenteral feeding it first passes into the circulation; this may have an effect upon levels of insulin-mediated uptake by the liver. Fat metabolism may also be affected by parenteral administration as hepatic steatosis (fatty liver) is a complication not seen in the enterally fed. The mechanism is not known but is related to high levels of glucose feeding.

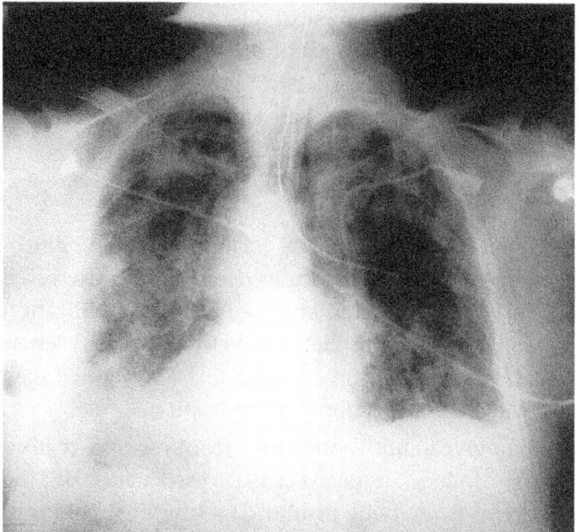

Figure 9.6 Incorrect placement of nasogastric tube.

These differences have led to the assumption that enteral nutrition is better controlled by the body as it more closely mimics the normal oral diet. It is subject to physiological feedback mechanisms which dictate hormone release and support the balance between anabolism/catabolism and the maintenance of plasma nutrient levels.

Complications associated with parenteral feeding

Complications include the risks associated with intravascular catheter placement, as well as the metabolic and infectious complications of parenteral delivery itself.

Vascular problems

Problems associated with central venous catheterization include pneumothorax, arterial puncture, and catheter misplacement during insertion, and line-related infections subsequently. Most infections are thought to be due to poor insertion technique or failure to observe infection control protocols (see Chapter 3). Repeated cannulation can lead to thrombosis of central veins.

While peripheral cannulae can be used to administer specific formulations of parenteral feed, these are prone to infection, thrombosis, and cellulitis, and thus should be viewed as a short-term measure only.

PICC (peripherally inserted central catheter) lines are increasingly being used for long-term delivery of parenteral feed. Some lines can be in place for up to 12 months. PICCs are long narrow lines made from either silicone or polyurethane (see Figure 9.7). They are inserted percutaneously into the antecubital veins or the basilic/cephalic veins in the forearm, usually under

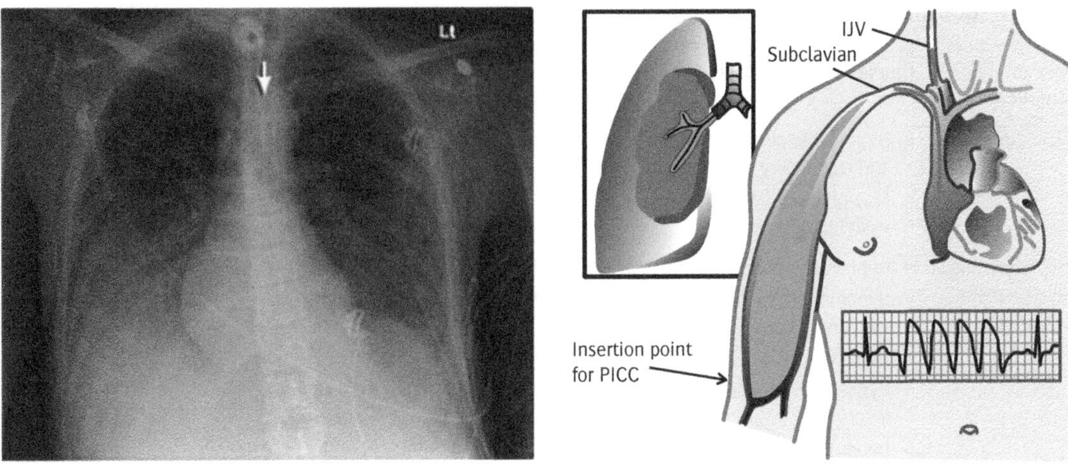

Figure 9.7 PICC line.

Reproduced with permission from Wijdicks, E.F. Management of Complications Associated with Venous Access, In Wijdicks E.F., *The Practice of Emergency and Critical Care Neurology*. Copyright (2010) with permission from Oxford University Press

ultrasound guidance. From this position, the catheter is advanced into the central circulation with the tip lying either in the superior vena cava or at the caval–atrial junction. Multi-lumen devices are available allowing a dedicated lumen for delivery of parenteral nutrition. PICC line insertion is less risky than central line insertion, and rates of infection are similar (Al Raiy *et al.* 2010), but evidence suggests that they are associated with increased risk of thromboembolism (Bonizzoli *et al.* 2011; Johansson *et al.* 2013).

Care of PICC lines

Preventing infection

PICC lines require the same scrupulous care as central lines to prevent infection and should be secured with a catheter fixation device as well as a transparent semi-permeable dressing over the entry site. The PICC line site should be viewed daily for signs of inflammation and dressings changed every 7 days, or sooner if wet, soiled, or no longer intact. The use of 2% chlohexidine in alcohol is recommended for cleaning the site and a chlorhexidine-impregnated patch should be placed over the entry point to reduce the likelihood of infection.

Preventing occlusion

Flushing of lines with normal saline should be carried out following delivery of medication or changing of infusions. If the line is unused, it should be flushed every 12–24 hours. Heparinized saline is no longer used for routine flushing because of the limited evidence of advantage (Guthrie *et al.* 2007).

If occlusion occurs the cause can be thrombotic, mechanical (due to kinks or malpositioning), precipitate from medication incompatibility, or fat emulsion build-up. Initial checks for obvious causes, such as kinking or in-line filter clogging, should be carried out and flushing re-tried. Never force flush against resistance. Use of fibrinolytic agents may be necessary to clear the line.

Removal of PICC lines

The procedure is similar to the removal of central lines. The patient should be supine and be asked to carry out a Valsalva manoeuvre as the line exits the insertion site. The line should be removed using slow intermittent traction and a clean dressing should be available to apply pressure to the exit site once the line is out. Examination of the length of the line and the integrity of the tip should be carried out post-removal to ensure that there is no fragmented element which has broken off and remains within the patient.

Metabolic complications

1. **Hyperglycaemia** Causes include persistent gluconeogenesis, blunted insulin release and/or decreased sensitivity to insulin, impaired peripheral utilization of glucose or phosphate, and chromium deficiency. Late development in a previously stable patient may signal a new infection or complication.
2. **Hypoglycaemia** A sudden discontinuation of feed may induce hypoglycaemia, particularly if the patient is receiving insulin. The insulin should usually be discontinued or reduced prior to stopping the feed. If this is not possible 10–20% glucose may

be commenced. Blood glucose should be frequently monitored.

3. **Hyperlipidaemia** Lipid clearance may be impaired in liver disease. Rapid infusion of lipid may also result in transient hyperlipidaemia.
4. **Hepatic dysfunction** Abnormal liver function tests (LFTs) and fatty infiltration of the liver can develop in carbohydrate-based parenteral nutrition. This is treated by reducing the number of calories or increasing the proportion of fat.
5. **Acid–base disturbances** Hyperchloraemia can develop from amino acid metabolism, but the resulting acidosis is usually mild. Most amino acid preparations contain acetate as a buffer. Metabolic alkalosis can be seen with diuretic use, continuous nasogastric drainage, or corticosteroid therapy if concomitant replacement of sodium, potassium, and/or chloride ions is inadequate.
6. **Electrolyte imbalance** Generally, electrolytes are monitored and corrected before problems occur. However, significant body deficiencies may not be reflected by plasma levels due to the effect of pH and serum albumin levels or hormonal influences such as aldosterone or ADH, which are often altered in the critically ill. Occasionally, magnesium, calcium, and phosphate may become imbalanced. Hypophosphataemia is often seen when parenteral nutrition is first started following a period of semi-starvation. This is due to poor prior intake of phosphate, increased glucose phosphorylation, and augmented intracellular transport of phosphates once feeding is restarted. Plasma phosphate levels below 0.3–0.5 mmol/L can potentially cause haemolysis, rhabdomyolysis, and respiratory failure, and hamper weaning attempts though the evidence base for this is weak. Low levels may persist for several days after adequate replacement. Other effects of electrolyte imbalance include arrhythmias, decreased myocardial contractility, seizures, diminished tissue sensitivity to insulin, abnormal calcium and magnesium metabolism, and decreased sensitivity to vasoactive drugs.

Other complications associated with parenteral feeding

1. Precipitation of respiratory failure and failure of weaning due to excessive carbohydrate administration.
2. Hyperosmolar states with an excessive osmotic diuresis.
3. Abnormal platelet function and hypercoagulability states.
4. Anaemia after prolonged use of IV lipids.

Many of the potentially serious complications associated with parenteral feeding can be avoided or controlled by rigorous monitoring and observation of the patient. A high index of suspicion for complications should also be maintained.

Nutritional requirements

It is only possible to give an approximate guide to the amount of nutrients required by the individual patient (see Tables 9.9–9.13). Factors such as age, weight, sex, severity of illness, use of catecholamines, body temperature, and injury will all affect nutrient and energy needs. Electrolyte and fluid balance are also important factors in deciding the composition of feeds.

The exact requirements for trace elements in the critically ill have not been determined, but deficiency can have significant effects on a number of metabolic processes. Most enteral feeds contain stated amounts of most essential trace elements. Multiple additives for parenteral feeding may be supplemented as necessary.

Insertion of nasogastric and duodenal feeding tubes

Enteral feeding tubes are normally inserted blind by appropriately experienced nursing staff. However, the presence of an endotracheal tube cuff increases the difficulty of entry to the oesophagus by pressing on its soft walls and decreasing its size. The risk of misplacement in the bronchial tree is increased in ventilated patients. A review of 9931 blindly placed nasoenteral tubes found that 60% of misplacements occurred in ventilated patients, 74% in the critically ill, and 96% in patients with altered conscious level (Sparks *et al.* 2011). Therefore it may be necessary to insert the tube under direct visualization of the pharynx. This is usually carried out by experienced medical staff. The ET tube cuff does not provide complete protection against inadvertent tracheal intubation with the nasogastric tube. Thus it is always essential to confirm accuracy of tube placement before starting the feed. If there is any doubt about the position, the tube should be removed and reinserted.

The technique for insertion will differ slightly according to the type of tube but the principles are the same.

Principles of insertion

1. Explanation to the patient is required whether they are sedated or awake. This should include the need for the tube, where the tube will be placed, probable sensations/discomfort that the patient may feel, and how long the tube is likely to be in place.

Table 9.9 Monitoring nutritional support

Variable to be monitored	Enteral nutrition	Parenteral nutrition
Electrolytes	Daily	Daily
Serum magnesium, calcium, phosphate	Twice weekly	Twice weekly
Acid–base status	Daily	Daily
Gastric residuals (aspirate)	Four-hourly when starting feeding; eight-hourly when established	As required by pathology
Abdominal function (distension, vomiting, nausea, diarrhoea, constipation)	Continuously	As required
Flow rate and volume infused	Hourly	Hourly
Blood glucose	Eight-hourly	Hourly to two-hourly at first; when stable four- to six-hourly
Urinalysis for glucose and ketones	Daily	Daily
Urea and creatinine (plasma)	Daily	Daily
Urea and creatinine clearance (urinary)	24-hour urine collection weekly	24-hour urine collection weekly
Weight (if mobile or on a weigh bed)	For fluid status: daily For nutritional status: weekly	For fluid status: daily For nutritional status: weekly
Haematological and coagulation screens	Every 1–2 days	Every 1–2 days
Serum albumin, proteins, LFTs, trace elements (e.g. copper, zinc, etc.)	Weekly	Weekly

Table 9.10 Daily nutritional requirement during enteral and parental nutrition

Nutrient	Amount per day	Influencing factors
Protein (nitrogen)	1.2–2.0 g/kg/day (0.19–0.32 g/kg/day)	Hypermetabolism can increase protein requirements
Carbohydrate	Need will depend on the patient's energy requirements, two-thirds of which are usually provided by carbohydrate, and one-third by fat. A useful quick estimate of Energy requirements is: Male: 25–30 kcal/kg/day Female: 20–25 kcal/kg/day	Patients with respiratory insufficiency or those who are weaning after long-term ventilation may not cope with the high CO_2 levels associated with high intakes of carbohydrate. Energy requirement can then be supplied as half fat and half carbohydrate.
Fat	The minimum amount of fat necessary to prevent fatty acid deficiency is 1 L of 10% fat emulsion (e.g. Intralipid) weekly. However, the amount of fat delivered is usually aimed at providing energy rather than preventing deficiency and is adjusted to between a third and half of total calories required. A safe quantity to deliver is thought to be 0.7–1.5 g/kg/day (Kreymann *et al.* 2006).	Tolerance of intravenous fat can be limited (see parenteral nutrition complications), and the amount delivered may need to be adjusted if this is the case

Note: this table represents only a rough guide, and each patient should be assessed individually.

Table 9.11 Electrolyte requirements during enteral or parenteral nutrition

Typical daily requirement	Additional factors
Sodium: 70–100 mmol	More may be needed with loop diuretic therapy or increased GI losses such as diarrhoea, fistulae. etc. Less may be needed in oedema and hypernatraemia.
Potassium: 70–100 mmol	More may be needed during early repletion, post-obstructive diuresis, loop diuretic therapy and increased GI losses. Less may be required in renal failure.
Magnesium: 7.5–10 mmol	As above.
Calcium: 5–10 mmol	
Phosphate: 20–30 mmol	More may be needed in early nutritional repletion when there may be dramatic falls in serum phosphate (see refeeding syndrome). Less may be required in renal failure.

2. Insertion is treated as a clean rather than aseptic technique, with handwashing prior to commencement and non-sterile gloves worn for the protection of the operator.
3. Measurement of the length of tube is required to ensure placement within the stomach or duodenum. This can be fairly accurately measured using the formula shown in Figure 9.8 for 91% of tubes placed within the stomach (Hanson 1979). However, in practice the simpler method of measuring nose to ear to xiphisternum is a reasonable approximation of length. Most tubes are marked at 10 cm intervals and the stomach should be reached by the time the 40 cm mark is at the nares, except in tall people.
4. Placement in the duodenum requires insertion of at least 85 cm of feeding tube to allow direct passage, or to allow a coil of tube in the stomach which may then migrate spontaneously through the pylorus into the duodenum.
5. Lubrication is necessary to promote atraumatic insertion. Some tubes are pre-lubricated and require placing in water to activate the lubricant, while others require lubricant jelly.
6. The tube is inserted along the floor of the nose; this avoids the sensitive conchae and will provide a guide

Table 9.12 Trace element requirements during enteral and parenteral nutrition (recommendations for parenteral amounts from the American Society of Parenteral and Enteral Nutrition)

Trace element	Recommended daily dietary allowance		Effects of deficiency
	Enteral nutrition(mmol/L)	Parenteral nutrition	
Zinc	110–145	2.5–5.0 mg	Impaired cellular immunity, poor wound healing, diarrhoea
Chromium	0.5–1.0	10–15 mcg	Insulin-resistant glucose intolerance, elevated serum lipids
Copper	16–20	0.3–0.5 mg	Hypochromic microcytic anaemia, neutropenia, arrhythmias, pseudo scurvy
Iodine	1–1.2	1.0 mmol/L	
Selenium	0.8–0.9	20–60 mcg	Cardiomyopathy
Molybdenum	0.5–4.0	0.2–1.2 mmol/L	
Manganese	30–60	60–100 mcg	CNS dysfunction
Fluoride	95–150	50 mmol/L	

Data from American Society of Parental and Enteral nutrition for parenteral amounts: Mirtallo, J., Canada,T., Johnson, D., *et al.*, Safe practices for parenteral nutrition. *Journal of Parenteral and Enteral Nutrition*, Volume 28, S39–69, 2004, American Society for Parenteral and Enteral Nutrition; Singer, P., Berger, M., van den Berghe, G. *et al.*, ESPEN Guidelines on Parenteral Nutrition: intensive care. *Clinical Nutrition*, Volume 28, 387–400, 2009, European Society for Clinical Nutrition and Metabolism.

Table 9.13 Vitamin requirements during enteral or parenteral nutrition

Vitamin	Recommended daily dietary allowance	
	Enteral nutrition	Parenteral nutrition
A (retinol) 5000 (µg)	600–1200 µg	800–2500 µg
B_1 (thiamine) (mg)	0.8–1.1	6*
B_2 (riboflavin) (mg)	1.1–1.3	3.6*
Niacin (mg)	2–18	40
B_6 (pyridoxine) (mg)	1.2–2.0	6.0*
B_{12} (cyanocobalamine) (µg)	1.5–3.0	5*
C (ascorbic acid) (mg)	40–60	200*
D (cholecalciferol) (µg)	5	5*
E (δ- and α-tocopherol) (mg)	10	10
Folic acid (µg)	400	600
K (phytomenadione) (µg/kg)	1	0.03–1.5
Pantothenic acid (mg)	3–7	15*
Biotin (µg)	10–200	60*

Data from the Parenteral and Enteral Group of the British Dietetic Association, 1997. For more recent guidance see *A Pocket Guide To Clinical Nutrition*, 4th edition, 2014.

* Jeejeebhoy, K.N., Parenteral nutrition in the intensive care unit, *Nutrition Reviews*, Volume 70, pp. 623–30, 2012, John Wiley & Sons, Inc.

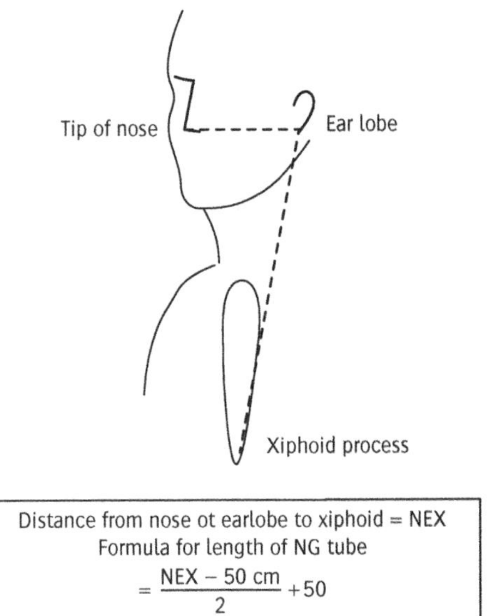

Distance from nose ot earlobe to xiphoid = NEX
Formula for length of NG tube

$$= \frac{\text{NEX} - 50 \text{ cm}}{2} + 50$$

Figure 9.8 Calculation of the length of the nasogastric tube

through the nasal cavity to the nasopharynx. If the patient is conscious they may assist insertion by swallowing once the tube is felt at the back of the nasopharynx.

7. Once the tube has been inserted, the position should be checked using specific recommended methods (Taylor 2013). Insufflation of air with auscultation (the 'whoosh' test) is no longer considered a safe or effective test. A range of methods are available, although none on their own are considered absolutely certain of correct placement.
   - Aspiration of gastric contents and testing of the pH of fluid withdrawn. This should be done with an appropriate pH indicator paper and not standard litmus paper. A pH <4 indicates gastric placement. Care must be taken with critically ill patients and those receiving gastric acid inhibitors or antacids, as the gastric pH may be as high as 5–6. It is also possible to withdraw tracheobronchial secretions in certain conditions with a low pH (Metheny and Clouse 1997): for example, pH 7.0–7.29 (malignancy), pH 6 (oesophageal rupture), and pH 5.5 (empyema).
   - Capnography will detect pulmonary placement and can be used to rule out tracheobronchial placement in high risk patients. It has a high level of success in detecting pulmonary placement during tube insertion and to check placement once the tube is in situ (Meyer *et al.* 2009). It can be used in combination with pH testing to determine gastric placement.
   - Electromagnetic tracing—a magnetic tracer incorporated into the enteral tube is tracked using a tracer placed on the patient's xiphisternum. This allows both depth and position to be monitored. However, this is still open to interpretation and requires experience and trained operators (Taylor 2013).
   - Chest X-ray was traditionally used as the 'gold standard' to locate placement of enteral tubes, particularly in high risk patients. However, this method depends on the quality of imaging, the opacity of the tube, and the training and experience of the interpreter. Incorrectly placed tubes in the left lung have been misinterpreted as being in the stomach. According to the National Patient Safety Agency (2011), misinterpreted X-rays are now the largest

cause of undetected lung placement, occurring in 45% of cases of misplacement.

8. If the tube has a guidewire it should be removed after the tube has been confirmed as being in the correct position. The tube should not be flushed until there is confirmation of placement. If there is difficulty withdrawing the guidewire, 1–2 ml water inserted into the tube may assist in facilitating its removal.

Care of the enterally fed patient with a nasogastric tube

Checking gastric residual volumes (aspirate)

These checks are used to confirm the gastric placement of the tube and to determine the level of tolerance for the volume of feed.

- Residual volumes should be checked four-hourly when feeding is first commenced, and then eight-hourly once the feed has been running without large amounts of residual volumes. This may differ according to unit protocols and various expert practice recommendations (Williams *et al.* 2014; Williams and Leslie 2004).
- It is unnecessary to stop feeds for an hour in order to check residual volumes. The minimal time necessary to demonstrate reduced absorption has not yet been determined, but it is probably less than 30 min even with reduced gastric motility.
- If all is well following a check for residual volumes, the rate of feed delivery should be increased to cover delivery of the feed volume missed prior to the check.
- It is possible to aspirate fine bore nasogastric tubes of internal diameter 1.5–2.0 mm. Using a 50 ml syringe exerts less pressure and therefore is less likely to cause the tube to collapse.
- In practice, gastric residual volumes <200 ml are an acceptable cut-off limit. There is little published research in this area, with recommendations ranging from '>1.5 times the previous hour's input of feed' (Koruda *et al.* 1987) to '400 ml' (Metheny *et al.* 2012) A systematic review by McClave and Snider (2002) suggested that monitoring gastric residual volumes gives little real indication of the risk of aspiration or clinical deterioration and does not relate to the ability of the patient to continue to tolerate feed. However, at present it remains difficult to continue to feed patients if there are very high volumes of gastric residual aspirates, and it remains sensible to use this as a signal to either monitor more frequently or review the rate of feeding.
- If residual volumes ≥200 ml are obtained, the feed is either held at the current level if feeding is just building up, or reduced to a lower rate if it has been in progress for some time. Volumes are then checked again 4 hours later and the manoeuvre repeated. If this occurs three times in succession, or is accompanied by vomiting and abdominal pain or distension, medical staff should be informed and the feed stopped. There is little evidence to support either returning residual volumes to the patient or discarding them. In a small study, Booker *et al.* (2000) found no significant difference in weight, electrolyte levels, or CO_2 levels between patients randomized to have either discarded or returned gastric residual aspirates.
- Stimulants of intestinal motility (prokinetic agents), including metoclopramide and erythromycin, may be used if the patient has no acute signs of feed intolerance but continues to have high volumes of gastric residuals. Although they have not been shown to improve outcomes, they have been recommended as a first-line response to improving poor gastric motility and increasing tolerance of enteral feed (Booth *et al.* 2002; Doherty and Winter 2003). However, these drugs do carry potential side effects, for example related to dopamine antagonism and prolactin stimulation with metoclopramide, or antibiotic resistance and overgrowth with erythromycin.
- Feeding into the duodenum may still be possible and should be tried if there is no evidence of general gut dysfunction (pain, distension, vomiting). Care should be taken when feeding into the duodenum, and this may require assessment of gastric contents regularly by aspiration either using a double-lumen tube with a gastric outlet or inserting a nasoduodenal/nasojejunal tube.

Prevention of tube obstruction

Tube obstruction can be common with fine bore enteral tubes, particularly if feed is stopped or medication is given via the tube (Williams and Leslie 2005). The following recommendations can be made, albeit on the basis of limited evidence.

- Avoid giving crushed tablets down the enteral tube. Any drugs given in the nasogastric tube should be either soluble or in the form of linctus. A 20–30 ml flush of water should be given after administration of drugs; more may be required if crushed tablets are given.
- Some recommend flushing the tube with at least 30 ml of water every 4 hours during continuous feeding (Kohn and Keithley 1989).

- Water is the most appropriate fluid for flushing tubes (Metheny *et al.* 1988).
- Use a continuous delivery method of feeding (drying and encrustation between feeds may obstruct the tube).
- Use a polyurethane or PVC material tube as these have a larger internal diameter and better flow rates than silastic tubes (Metheny *et al.* 1988).

Prevention of tube displacement

- Use a firm but easily removable tape to attach the tube to the nose or face.
- The point of entry into the nose should be marked on the tube with fine tape once correct placement has been established. This can then be checked to ensure that it remains in the same place. This does not guarantee that the tube has remained in the stomach. The tube may be brought up by vigorous coughing or retching and sit coiled in the mouth or oropharynx, particularly when the patient is unconscious.

Current advice and evidence support checking tube placement in the following circumstances (Curtis 2013):

- before administering every feed
- at least once a day during continuous feeding
- before administering medication
- following episodes of vomiting, retching, and coughing
- following oropharyngeal suction
- following any signs or suspicion of tube movement
- following any change in the patient's respiratory status.

PEG (percutaneous endoscopic gastrostomy) and PEJ (percutaneous endoscopic jejunostomy) tubes

Feeding via a PEG or PEJ tube should be considered if the patient is likely to require enteral nutritional support for a period exceeding 2–3 weeks.

Placement of PEG or PEJ tubes

Placement is simple and safe in the hands of a skilled endoscopist, although the added complications of critical illness can increase the complexity of the procedure (see Figure 9.9). Increased likelihood of complications is associated with a high BMI (>30 kg/m^2) and a serum albumin <2.5g/dl (Shah *et al.* 2009). PEG and PEJ tubes can also be placed directly during bowel surgery or under radiographic guidance.

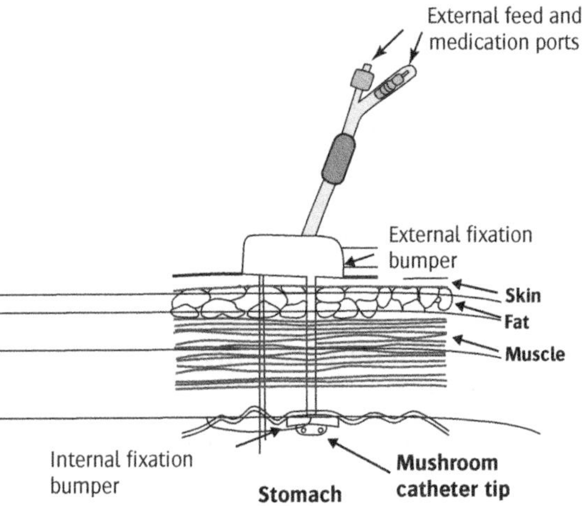

Figure 9.9 PEG tube placement

Prior to placement of a PEG or PEJ, a full diagnostic endoscopy is carried out to ensure that there are no local contraindications such as erosive gastritis, ulcer, or extensive tumour infiltration around the site. Contraindications to carrying out a PEG/PEJ placement include INR >1.5, thromboplastin time <50%, partial thromboplastin time >50 sec, and platelet count <50 000/mm^3.

The patient should be nil by mouth for 8 hours prior to the procedure with functioning intravenous access. Routine antibiotic prophylaxis is no longer thought necessary, but should be considered where there is a high risk of infection for the patient (Löser *et al.* 2005).

A tube larger than 15Ch is recommended as smaller diameter tubes are associated with higher rates of clogging.

There are several placement techniques, the most common being the 'pull' technique, where a suture thread or guidewire is passed through the cannula sheath of a puncture needle into the stomach and drawn up through the oesophagus using the biopsy forceps of the endoscope. The thread is fastened to the PEG tube, which is then pulled down to the stomach and out through the puncture site until the internal fixation bumper is fast against the anterior stomach wall. A second external fixation bumper ensures that the PEG is retained against the abdominal wall. A low level of traction is maintained on the tube for several hours post-insertion and then a sterile Y-compress is applied under the external fixation bumper and a small amount of free movement (approximately 5 mm) is maintained to prevent tension on the abdomen or stomach wall causing ischaemia.

Placement of a PEJ tube involves threading a jejunal catheter through the PEG and along the small intestine past the flexure of Treitz into the jejunum. Jejunal placement decreases the likelihood of oesophageal reflux and is of benefit where there is impaired gastric motility. An increased risk associated with jejunal placement is the possibility of tube migration, which can result in either gastric or distal intestinal displacement. Symptoms include vomiting, abdominal distension, and pain.

Complications of tube placement

Complications include aspiration, haemorrhage, and inadvertent bowel perforation, all of which are relatively rare (Stayner *et al.* 2012). Subclinical pneumoperitoneum is common, but not clinically significant, and does not generally indicate perforation.

Complications of PEG/PEG tubes

Development of gastric mucosal ulceration around the site of the tube, peristomal infection, peristomal leakage and irritation, gastric outlet obstruction, buried bumper syndrome. and inadvertent removal are the most common complications (Stayner *et al.* 2012). Fistulous tracts into other parts of the bowel, tumour seeding in patients with upper GI malignancy, and intramural displacement and feeding are rarer complications (Zerizer *et al.* 2005)

Care of PEG/PEJ tubes

If placement is uncomplicated, feeding through the tube can commence from an hour after placement, although many places wait for longer. A trial flush of 40 ml water is recommended to ensure that the lumen is clear (Simons and Remington 2013).

Prevention of infection

Initially, the PEG/PEJ site should be dressed daily, cleaned with sterile water, and covered with a dry dressing. Later, once the stoma has healed, dressing frequency can be reduced to every 2–3 days provided that the site is clean and dry (Löser *et al.* 2005).

- Maintaining patency of the tube—flushes of 30–50 ml of water should be carried out post enteral feeding or medication delivery. If the tube is not being used it should be flushed regularly
- Checking residual volumes—this should be carried out in the same way as for other enteral feeding routes.

Prevention of buried bumper syndrome

This occurs when the internal fixation bumper has been pulled in tight against the stomach wall resulting in overgrowth of gastric mucosa around the fixator. It is avoided by ensuring there is no tension on the tube and free movement away from the stomach wall of 5 mm or more.

Diarrhoea

Diarrhoea is defined as at least three or four liquid stools daily in adults. The causes of diarrhoea are frequently multifactorial in the critically ill patient. A full assessment of the patient should be undertaken to identify all relevant causal factors.

1. Drugs
   - The following drugs are particularly associated with diarrhoea:
     - antibiotics, as these alter the gut flora and increase the likelihood of *Clostridium difficile* infection
     - acid-suppressive medication (proton pump inhibitors, H_2 receptor antagonists) increases the likelihood of diarrhoea and *C.difficile* infection (Btaiche *et al.* 2010)
     - magnesium-containing antacids and electrolyte elixirs are known irritants to the gastrointenstinal mucosa
     - hypertonic sugary elixirs which, being hyperosmolar, increase the osmolality of GI secretions causing diarrhoea
     - laxatives (van der Spoel *et al.* 2006).
     - The patient's drugs should be reviewed. Any likely causative agent should ideally be stopped, with alternatives sought if necessary. Hypertonic elixirs can be diluted prior to administration.
   - Addition of a probiotic, prebiotic, or synbiotic have been suggested as a method of modifying gut flora (e.g. *Lactobacillus acidophilus* which is present in live yoghurt) (see Box 9.23). This remains a much debated area with some studies showing decreased diarrhoea with the addition of a probiotic, while

Box 9.23 Supporting gut microflora

Probiotics—live (non-pathogenic) micro-organisms (e.g. *Lactobacillus acidophilus*)

Prebiotics—dietary supplements and foods which in sufficient quantity may alter the normal microflora of the gut (e.g. nondigestible plant fibres)

Synbiotics—combinations of probiotics and synbiotics

others showed either no impact or, in one study (Besselink *et al.* 2008), increased harm.

- It may be appropriate to give antidiarrhoeal drugs, such as loperamide or codeine phosphate, for drug-related diarrhoea, with the exception of antibiotic-related diarrhoea. Cholestyramine (an insoluble ion exchange resin that binds bile acids in the gut) has been suggested for diarrhoea caused by *C.difficile* toxin as it binds the toxin to the resin. This is given in addition to treating the *C.difficile* infection with appropriate antibiotics such as metronidazole or vancomycin.

2. Bacterial contamination
   - Potential sources of contamination should be investigated and stool specimens sent for microscopy, culture, sensitivities, and *C.difficile* toxin screen.
   - Feed should not be hung at room temperature for >12 hours and feed bags should not be 'topped up'. Feed-giving sets should be changed every 24 hours.
   - Ready-made feed should be used wherever possible. If feed has to be reconstituted, or substances added, great care should be taken to maintain sterility.
3. Feed constituents
   - High-osmolality, high-fat-content, and high-lactose-content feeds have all been associated with diarrhoea. Most formulae no longer contain lactose and evidence of a link between high osmolality and diarrhoea is conflicting. Problems with fat tolerance are more likely with special feeds such as Pulmocare (50% of non-protein calorie content from fat, 50% from carbohydrate). If appropriate, an alternative feed with less fat or a lower osmolality may be tried instead.
   - Fibre—in same cases a bulking agent (fibre) such as methylcellulose or psyllium hydrophilic mucilloid or guar gum has been used to good effect. Insoluble fibres increase stool bulk and absorb water (Btaiche *et al.* 2010). The addition of soluble fibre which can be degraded to short-chain fatty acids in the colon and provide a fuel source for colonocytes may also mitigate diarrhoea by improving sodium and water reabsorption in the colon.
4. Albumin levels. Hypoalbuminaemia may cause an osmotic diarrhoea due to a lowering of colloid oncotic pressure (COP). If the COP is reduced, feed within the intestinal lumen creates an osmotic gradient with fluid moving into, rather than out of, the intestine, resulting in a loose watery stool. Artificial colloids may maintain an adequate COP despite a low albumin level. However, there is no evidence base that demonstrates improved diarrhoea through increasing COP levels.
5. Intestinal effects of malnutrition and parenteral nutrition.
   - Malnutrition is associated with a loss in the number and height of intestinal villi and decreased levels of brush border enzymes. This reduces the absorptive capability of the intestine. Similar effects can be seen following long periods of parenteral feeding (Koruda *et al.* 1987). Intestinal epithelial cells may benefit from direct uptake of glutamine from feed given via the intestinal tract as a source of energy for maintenance of the intestinal barrier and the gut's immune function.
   - Commencement of enteral feeding in a malnourished patient may require a very slow increase in delivery rates and use of a peptide-based formula which is more easily absorbed.
   - In same cases, it may be appropriate to feed both enterally and parenterally to encourage return of gut function and to maintain a suitably high level of nutritional intake.

Many critically ill patients with diarrhoea associated with enteral feed can be managed simply by altering the feed formula, reviewing implicated factors, and adjusting treatment accordingly. Frequently, enteral feeding can be continued at a reduced level until the appropriate treatment has been started. Diarrhoea should not prevent enteral feeding unless associated with severe absorptive disorders or infection such as *C.difficile*.

Evaluating delivery of feed

Patients frequently do not receive the amount of feed prescribed, and in some patients the amount received may be very low (Adam and Batson 1997; McClave *et al.* 1999). Daily evaluation should compare feed delivered to that prescribed. Otherwise the patient may become malnourished before the deficit is detected.

- Feed should be prescribed in *calories* per 24 hours rather than *millilitres* per hour.
- The total calorie intake over 24 hours should be calculated by the nurse. Any large deficit or excess, and underlying reasons, should be reported to the dietitian or medical staff.
- Nursing evaluation should include details of the patient's ability to absorb and tolerate enteral feed.

The most important aspects of feeding are that patients should receive what they require in the form best suited to their ability to absorb and utilize it.

Care of the parenterally fed patient

Insertion of the central venous catheter (CVC)

More details are given in Chapter 5. In some ICUs, a dedicated port of a triple-lumen line is considered adequate for short-term parenteral feeding. However, long-term feeding should be via either a tunnelled feeding line or a Hickman catheter. Debate continues as to whether the risk of inserting a tunnelled feeding line into a critically ill patient outweighs the (slightly increased) incidence of infection in triple-lumen lines. Many units are now using PICC lines for delivery of parenteral nutrition, and long-term venous access where central venous access is difficult. Insertion is less risky and can be carried out by highly trained nurse specialists. There is also some evidence supporting reduced infection rate. However, a systematic review (Johansson *et al.* 2013) could not find sufficient high quality evidence to provide a good comparison of risks versus benefits and only two medium quality studies which showed significantly increased rates of DVT but decreased rates of occlusion in PICC lines compared with tunnelled or central venous access. Infection rates in PICC lines are comparable to those in CVC lines and therefore considered to be safe (Al Raiy *et al.* 2010). Further high quality study is needed to determine the advantages and disadvantages of PICC lines

Infection of central venous catheters: mechanisms and management.

1. Organisms may migrate down the dermal tunnel. This is preceded by colonization of the skin surrounding the site of insertion. that occurs during insertion or redressing.
    - Management strategy:
        - Scrupulous aseptic technique (surgical gowns, sterile gloves, 2% chlorhexidine in alcohol skin preparation, removal of any blood from insertion site prior to dressing) when inserting or dressing the catheter.
        - Use of an occlusive dressing which should be re-dressed according to unit policy. Some centres also use an impregnated chlorhexidine patch at the site of insertion, although current evidence does not show any impact on reductions in infection or colonization (Schroeder *et al.* 2012).
2. Bacterial colonization of the tip—this is generally a result of bacteraemia from another source. The problem is then compounded by the formation of a fibrin sheath within 3 days of insertion which acts as a shield to bacteria against antibiotics.
    - Management strategy
        - Maintenance of a high index of suspicion for catheter infection.
        - Removal of the catheter if patient shows evidence of infection (without any other obvious cause) and send tip for culture—appropriate systemic antibiotics can then be prescribed if indicated.
        - Change non-tunnelled lines if there is evidence of infection at the site or systemically.
3. Colonization of the hub or intraluminal segment of the catheter—this is generally due to contamination during tubing changes or by the infusion of contaminated solutions.
    - Management strategy
        - Scrupulous aseptic technique (sterile field, surgical gloves, spray hub, and connections with isopropyl alcohol) during changes of administration set or infusions.
        - Change the administration set every 24 hours unless using pre-mixed 48-hour infusion bags when the administration set should be changed with the infusion bag.
4. Infected infusate—this is less likely than in many other IV infusions owing to the amino acid content of the feed, which decreases the pH. However, if lipid emulsion is present in the bag, bacterial and fungal growth will be supported. Lipid emulsion alone is almost as good a growth medium as that normally used to culture organisms.
    - Management strategy
        - Premixed bags prepared in sterile conditions should be used wherever possible. If not, scrupulous aseptic precautions should be taken in setting up individual bottles and bags for concurrent infusion.
        - Infection rates have been shown to be reduced to 1–2% by using specially trained personnel. This is probably due to both an increased understanding of the risks and a high level of competence in manipulating lines. The same standards should be expected of the critical care nurse in order to limit the likelihood of infection in the highly vulnerable patient.

Prevention of intolerance of glucose load

Hyperglycaemia associated with stress (see Chapter 3) is often exacerbated by infusing glucose. This is related to either a failure to release more insulin from the pancreas or a problem at the cell level (e.g. impaired sensitivity of the insulin receptor). The glucose infusion may also fail to suppress hepatic gluconeogenesis in the critically ill. The management strategy is as follows

- Regularly monitor blood glucose with measurements made every 15–30 min in the hour following commencement or discontinuation of parenteral nutrition, and following any sharp rise or fall (Krzywda *et al.* 1993).
- Intravenous insulin infusions should be titrated to maintain blood glucose <10 mmol/L but to avoid hypoglycaemia.
- Large changes in insulin infusion rates are not recommended because of the dangers of hypo- and hyperglycaemia. Insulin infusions should not be stopped abruptly even when the blood glucose is very low; it is better to infuse more glucose in order to maintain blood levels and reduce insulin as necessary to avoid rebound hyperglycaemia.
- Infusion rates of glucose should be kept within the limits of metabolic requirements; if tolerance limits the amount to below acceptable levels for nutrition, further calories should be given (e.g. as a lipid infusion).
- Consideration should be given to discontinuation of insulin infusions prior to stopping parenteral nutrition in order to avoid hypoglycaemia.

Prevention of problems from volumes of fluid infused

Owing to its hypertonicity, most parenteral feed requires a considerable amount of fluid volume to deliver the nutritional requirements of the patient. This may cause fluid overload in the patient in renal failure or in critically ill patients who have problems with oedema. Parenteral nutrition may have to be discontinued until either renal replacement therapy is commenced or the patient passes sufficient volumes of urine, and fluid overload is less of a problem.The managment strategy involves accurate calculation of fluid balance and hourly monitoring of intake and output.

Box 9.24 Psychosocial effects of parenteral nutrition

- Dependence on catheter and infusion pump
- Loss of potential comfort source
- Loss of taste and pleasure associated with eating
- Anxiety about whether it will ever be possible to eat again
- Anxiety about the effects of the feed itself and its ability to provide adequate nutrition
- Loss of the social aspects of eating (togetherness, communication, family relationships)

Psychological aspects

Many of the psychosocial problems associated with parenteral nutrition (see Box 9.24) do not apply to the critically ill as they may have little awareness of the need for food or the lack of it. It is also unlikely that their parenteral feeding will continue in the long term. However, during the convalescent phase the patient may become more aware, and the route for feeding, the reason for it, and the length of time it will continue should be carefully explained.

References and bibliography

Adam, S., Batson, S. (1997). A study of problems associated with the delivery of enteral feed in critically ill patients in five ICUs in the UK. *Intensive Care Medicine*, **23**, 261–6.

Al-Omran, M., Albalawi, Z.H., Tashkandi, M.F., Al-Ansary, L.A. (2010). Enteral versus parenteral nutrition for acute pancreatitis. *Cochrane Database of Systematic Reviews*, (1), CD002837.

Al Raiy, B., Fakih, M.G., Bryan-Nomides, N. *et al.* (2010). Peripherally inserted central venous catheters in the acute care setting: a safe alternative to high-risk short-term central venous catheters. *American Journal of Infection Control*, **38**, 149–53.

Angermayr, B., Cejna, M., Karnel, F., *et al.* (2003) Child–Pugh versus MELD score in predicting survival in patients undergoing transjugular intrahepatic portosystemic shunt. *Gut*, **52**, 879–85.

Arabi, Y., Tamim, H., Gousia, S., *et al.* (2011). Permissive underfeeding and intensive insulin therapy in critically ill patients: a randomized controlled trial. *American Journal of Clinical Nutrition*, **93**, 569–77.

Bai, Y., Gao, J., Zou, D.W., Li, Z. S. (2008). Prophylactic antibiotics cannot reduce infected pancreatic necrosis and mortality in acute necrotizing pancreatitis: evidence from a meta-analysis of randomized controlled trials. *American Journal of Gastroenterology*, **103**, 104–10.

Bank, S., Singh, P., Pooran, N., *et al.* (2002). Evaluation of factors that have reduced mortality from acute pancreatitis over the past 20 years. *Journal of Clinical Gastroenterology*, **35**, 50–60.

Barquist, E., Brown, M., Cohn, S., *et al.* (2001) Postextubation fiberoptic endoscopic evaluation of swallowing after prolonged endotracheal intubation: a randomized, prospective trial. *Critical Care Medicine*, **29**, 1710–13.

Belknap M.D., Davidson, L.J., Flournoy, D.J., *et al.* (1990). Contamination of enteral feedings and diarrhea in patients in intensive care units. *Heart & Lung & Lung*, **19**, 362–70.

Besselink, M.G.H., van Santvoort, H.C., Buskens, E., *et al.*(2008). Probiotic prophylaxis in predicted severe acute pancreatitis: a randomised,double-blind, placebo-controlled trial. *Lancet*, **371**, 651–9.

Bi, L.C., Kaunitz, J.C. (2003). Gastroduodenal mucosal defense: an integrated protective response. *Current Opinions in* Gastroenterology, **19**, 526–32.

Bliss, D.Z., Johnson, S., Savik, K., *et al.* (2000). Fecal incontinence in hospitalized patients who are acutely ill. *Nursing Research*, **49**, 101–8.

Bonizzoli, M., Batacchi, S., Cianchi, G., *et al.*(2011). Peripherally inserted central venous catheters and central venous catheters related thrombosis in post-critical patients. *Intensive Care Medicine*, **37**, 284–9.

Booker, K.J., Niedringhaus, L., Eden, B., *et al.* (2000). Comparison of 2 methods of managing gastric residual volumes from feeding tubes. *American Journal of Critical Care*, **9**, 318–24.

Booth, C.M., Heyland, D.K., Paterson, W.G. (2002) Gastrointestinal promotility drugs in the critical care setting: a systematic review of the evidence. *Critical Care Medicine*, **30**, 1429–35.

Bordas, J., Escorsell, A., Faust, F., Mas, A. (2006). Gastrointestinal bleeding. In *Clinical Critical Care Medicine* (eds R.K. Albert, A. Slutsky, M. Ranieri, *et al.*), pp 517–24. Philadelphia, PA: Mosby Elsevier.

Brett, S., (2005). The use of proton pump inhibitors for gastric acid suppression in critical illness. *Critical Care*, **9**, 45–50.

Brinson, R.R., Pitts, W.M. (1989). Enteral nutrition in the critically ill patient: role of hypoalbuminemia. *Critical Care Medicine*, **17**, 367–70.

Btaiche, I., Chan, L., Pleva, M., *et al.* (2010). Critical illness, gastrointestinal complications and medication therapy during enteral feeding in critically ill adult patients. *Nutrition in Clinical Practice*, **25**, 32–49.

Cheatham, M.L., Malbrain, M.L., Kirkpatrick, A., *et al.* (2007) Results from the International Conference of Experts on Intra-abdominal Hypertension and Abdominal Compartment Syndrome. II. Recommendations. *Intensive Care Medicine*, **33**, 951–62.

Chiolero, R., Soguel, L., Berger, M. (2006) Nutritional support. In *Clinical Critical Care Medicine*. (eds R.K. Albert, A. Slutsky, M. Ranier, *et al.*), pp. 205–16. Philadelphia, PA: Mosby Elsevier.

Cross, T., O'Beirne, J., Wendon, J. (2006). Acute liver failure. In *Clinical Critical Care Medicine* (eds R.K. Albert, A. Slutsky, M. Ranieri, *et al.*), pp 531–42. Philadelphia, PA: Mosby Elsevier.

Curtis,K. (2013). Caring for adult patients who require nasogastric feeding tubes. *Nursing Standard*, **27**, 38, 47–56.

De Jonghe, B., Appere-De-Vechi, C., Frounier, M., *et al.* (2001). A prospective survey of nutritional support practices in intensive care unit patients. What is prescribed? What is delivered? *Critical Care Medicine*, **29**, 8–12.

DeLegge, M.H. (2013). Nutrition support in the intensive care patient. *Journal of Infusion Nursing*, **36**, 262–8.

de Smet, A.M., Kluytmans, J.A., Cooper, B.S., *et al.* (2009) Decontamination of the digestive tract and oropharynx in ICU patients. *New England Journal of Medicine*, **360**, 20–31.

Doherty, W.L., Winter, B. (2003) Prokinetic agents in critical care. *Critical Care*, 7, 206–8.

Drakulovic, M., Torres, A., Bauer T., *et al.* (1999). Supine body position as a risk factor for nosocomial pneumonia in mechanically ventilated patients: a randomised trial. *Lancet*, **354**, 1851–8.

Felipo, V. (2013). Hepatic encephalopathy: effects of liver failure on brain function. *Nature Reviews Neuroscience*, **14**, 851–8.

Ferrer, M., Bauer, T.T., Torres, A., *et al.* (1999). Effect of nasogastric tube size on gastroesophageal reflux and microaspiration in intubated patients. *Annals of Internal Medicine*, **130**, 991–4.

Finn, P., Plank, L., Clark, M., *et al.* (1996) Assessment of involuntary muscle function in patients after critical injury or severe sepsis. *Journal of Parenteral & Enteral Nutrition*, **20**, 332–7.

Forsberg, A., Backman, L., Moller A. (2000). Experiencing liver transplantation: a phenomenological approach. *Journal of Advanced Nursing*, **32**, 327–34.

Germani, G., Theocharidou, E., Adam, R., *et al.* (2012). Liver transplantation for acute liver failure in Europe: outcomes over 20 years from the ELTR database. *Journal of Hepatology*, **57**, 288–96.

Gill, R.Q., Sterling, R.K. (2001). Acute liver failure. *Journal of Clinical Gastroenterology*, **33**, 191–8.

Giner, M., Laviano, A., Meguid, M.M., *et al.* (1996). In 1995, a correlation between malnutrition and poor outcome in critically ill patients still exists. *Nutrition*, **12**, 23–9.

Guthrie, D., Dreher, D., Munson, M. (2007) What you need to know about PICCs. Part 2. *Nursing*, 14 September, pp. 14–15.

Hanson, R.L. (1979). Criteria for length of nasogastric tube insertion for tube feeding. *Journal of Parenteral and Enteral Nutrition*, **3**, 160–3.

Hamarneh, S.R., Mohamed, M.M., Economopoulos, K., *et al.* (2014). A novel approach to maintain gut mucosal integrity using an oral enzyme supplement. *Annals of surgery*, **260**, 706.

Hawkins, L.C., Edwards, J.N., Dargan, P.I. (2007) Impact of restricting paracetamol pack sizes on paracetamol poisoning in the United Kingdom: a review of the literature. *Drug Safety*, **30**, 465–79.

Hermans, G., Casaer, M.P., Clerckx, B., *et al.* (2013). Effect of tolerating macronutrient deficit on the development of intensive-care unit acquired weakness: a subanalysis of the EPaNIC trial. *Lancet Respiratory Medicine*, **1**, 621–9.

Heyland, D., Muscedere, J., Wischmeyer, P., *et al.* (2013). A randomized trial of glutamine and antioxidants in critically ill patients. *New England Journal of Medicine*, **368**, 1489–97.

Jeejeebhoy, K.N. (2012). Parenteral nutrition in the intensive care unit. *Nutrition Reviews*, **70**, 623–30.

Johansson, E., Harrarskjöld, F., Lundberg, D., Arnlind, M. (2013). Advantages and disadvantages of peripherally inserted central venous catheters (PICC) compared to other central venous lines: a systematic review of the literature. *Acta Oncologica*, **52**, 886–92.

Johnson, L.R. (2007). *Gastrointestinal Physiology* (7th edn). St Louis, MO. Mosby–Yearbook.

Kearns, P.J., Chin, D., Mueller, L., *et al.* (2000). The incidence of ventilator-associated pneumonia and success in nutrient delivery with gastric versus small intestinal feeding: a randomized clinical trial. *Critical Care Medicine*, **28**, 1742–6.

Kohn, C.L., Keithley, J.K. (1989). Enteral nutrition: potential complications and patient monitoring. *Nursing Clinics of North America*, **24**, 339–51.

Koruda, M.J., Guenter, P., Rombeau, J.L. (1987). Enteral nutrition in the critically ill. *Critical Care Clinics* **3**,133–53.

Krag, M., Perner, A., Wettersley, J., *et al.* (2015). Prevalence and outcome of gastrointestinal bleeding and use of acid suppressants in acutely ill adult intensive care patients. *Intensive Care Medicine*, **41**, 833–45.

Kreymann, K.G., Bergerb, M.M., Deutzc, N.E.P., *et al.* (2006). ESPEN Guidelines on Enteral Nutrition: intensive care. *Clinical Nutrition*. **25**, 210–23.

Krishnan, J.A., Parce, P., Martinez, J.A., *et al.* (2003) Caloric intake in medical ICU patients: consistency of care with guidelines and relationship to clinical outcomes. *Chest*, **124**, 297–305.

Krzywda, E.A., Andris, D.A., Whipple, J.K., *et al.* (1993). Glucose response to abrupt initiation and discontinuation of total parenteral nutrition. *Journal of Parenteral and Enteral Nutrition*, **17**, 64–7.

Lalles, J.-P. (2013). Intestinal alkaline phosphatase: novel functions and protective effects. *Nutrition Reviews*, **72**, 82–94.

Lamb, C.A., Parr, J., Lamb,E.I., Warren, M.D. (2009). Adult malnutrition screening, prevalence and management in a United Kingdom hospital: cross-sectional study. *British Journal of Nutrition*, **102**, 571–5.

Lee, W.M. (2012). Recent developments in acute liver failure. *Best Practice & Research Clinical Gastroenterology*, **26**, 3–16.

Lewis, S.J., Heaton, K.W. (1997). Stool form scale as a useful guide to intestinal transit time. *Scandinavian Journal of Gastroenterology*, **32**, 920–4.

Li Bassi, G., Zanella, A., Cressoni, M., *et al.* (2008). Following tracheal intubation, mucus flow is reversed in the semirecumbent position: Possible role in the pathogenesis of ventilator-associated pneumonia. *Critical Care Medicine*, **36**, 518–25.

Lin, A. C-M., Hsu, Y-H., Wang, T-L., Chong, C-F. (2006) Placement confirmation of Sengstaken–Blakemore tube by ultrasound. *Emergency Medicine Journal*, **23**, 487.

Löser, C., Aschl, G.,Hebuterne, X., Mathus-Vliegen, E.M.H., *et al.* (2005). ESPEN guidelines on artificial enteral nutrition: percutaneous endoscopic gastrostomy (PEG). *Clinical Nutrition*, **24**, 848–61.

McClave S.A., Snider H.L. (2002). Clinical use of gastric residual volumes as a monitor for patients on enteral tube feeding. *Journal of Parenteral and Enteral Nutrition*, **26**(Suppl 6), 43–8.

McClave, S.A., Sexton, L.K., Spain, D.A. *et al.* (1999). Enteral tube feeding in the intensive care unit: factors impeding adequate delivery. *Critical Care Medicine* **27**, 1252–6.

McClave, S.A., McClain, C.J., Snider, H.L. (2001). Should indirect calorimetry be used as part of nutritional assessment? *Journal of Clinical Gastroenterology*, **33**, 14–19.

McClave, S.A., DeMeo, M.T., DeLegge, M.H. (2002). North American Summit on Aspiration in the Critically Ill Patient: consensus statement. *Journal of Parenteral and Enteral Nutrition*, **26**, S80–5.

McClave, S.A., Spain, D.A., Skolnick, J.L., *et al.* (2003). Achievement of steady state optimizes results when performing indirect calorimetry. *Journal of Parenteral and Enteral Nutrition*, **27**, 16–20.

Marik, P., Zaloga, G.P. (2004). Meta-analysis of parenteral nutrition versus enteral nutrition in patients with acute pancreatitis. *BMJ*, **328**, 1407.

Marik, P., Vasu, T., Hirani, A., Pachinburavan, M. (2010). Stress ulcer prophylaxis in the new millennium: a systematic review and meta-analysis.*Critical Care Medicine*, **38**, 2222–8.

Martindale, R.G., McClave, S.A., Vanek, V.W., *et al.* (2009). Guidelines for the provision and assessment of nutrition support therapy in the adult critically ill patient. Society of Critical Care Medicine and American Society for Parenteral and Enteral Nutrition: Executive Summary. *Critical Care Medicine*, **37**, 1757–61

Meijer, K., van Saene, H.K.F., Hill, J.C. (1990). Infection control in patients undergoing mechanical ventilation: traditional approach versus a new development—selective decontamination of the digestive tract. *Heart & Lung*, **19**, 11–20.

Mentec, H., Dupont, H., Bocchetti, M., *et al.* (2001). Upper digestive intolerance during enteral nutrition in critically ill patients: frequency, risk factors, and complications. *Critical Care Medicine*, **29**, 1955–61.

Messori, A., Trippoli, S., Vaiani, M., *et al.* (2000). Bleeding and pneumonia in intensive care patients given ranitidine and sucralfate for prevention of stress ulcer: meta-analysis of randomized controlled trials. *BMJ*, **321**, 1103–6.

Metheny, N.A., Clouse, R. (1997). Bedside methods of detecting aspiration in tube-fed patients. *Chest*, **111**, 724–31.

Metheny, N., Eisenberg, P., Spies, M. (1986). Aspiration pneumonia in patients fed through nasoenteral tubes. *Heart & Lung*, **15**, 256–61.

Metheny, N., Eisenberg, P., McSweeney, M. (1988). Effect of feeding tube properties and three irrigants on clogging rates. *Nursing Research*, **37**, 165–9.

Metheny, N., Dettenmeier, P., Hampton, K., *et al.* (1990). Detection of inadvertent respiratory placement of small-bore feeding tubes: a report of 10 cases. *Heart & Lung*, **19**, 631–8.

Metheny, N., Mills, A.C., Stewart, B.J. (2012) Monitoring for intolerance to gastric tube feedings: a national survey. *American Journal of Critical Care*, **21**, e33–40.

Meyer, P., Henry, M., Maury, E., *et al.* (2009) Colorimetric capnography to ensure correct nasogastric tube position. *Journal of Critical Care*, **24**, 231–5.

Mirtallo, J., Canada,T., Johnson, D., *et al.* (2004) Safe practices for parenteral nutrition. *Journal of Parenteral and Enteral Nutrition*, **28**, S39–69.

Montejo, J.C. (1999). Enteral nutrition-related gastrointestinal complications in critically ill patients: a multicentre study. *Critical Care Medicine*, **27**, 1447–53.

Morgan, D. (2002). Intravenous proton pump inhibitors in the critical care setting. *Critical Care Medicine*, **30**(Suppl), S369–72.

Naik, R.P., Joshipura, V.P., Patel, N.R., Haribhakti, S.P. (2009). Complications of PEG—prevention and management. *Tropical Gastroenterology*, **30**, 186–94.

National Patient Safety Agency (2011). *Patient Safety Alert NPSA/2011/PSA002: Reducing the Harm Caused by Misplaced Nasogastric Feeding Tubes in Adults, Children and Infants. Supporting Information*. http://www.nrls.npsa.nhs.uk/resources/type/alerts/?entryid45=129640

Needham, D., Davidson, J., Cohen, H. (2012) Improving long-term outcomes after discharge from intensive care unit: report from a stakeholders' conference. *Critical Care Medicine*, **40**, 502–9.

NICE-SUGAR Study Investigators (2009). Intensive versus conventional glucose control in critically ill patients. *New England Journal of Medicine*, **360**, 1283–97

O'Brien, J., Triantos, C., Burroughs, A. (2013). Management of varices in patients with cirrhosis. *Nature Reviews Gastroenterology and Hepatology*, **10**, 402–12.

O'Grady, J.G., Schalm, S.W., Williams, R. (1993). Acute liver failure: redefining the syndromes. *Lancet*, **342**, 273–5.

Patton, H., Misel, M., Gish, R.G. (2012). Acute liver failure in adults: an evidence-based management protocol for clinicians. *Gastroenterology & Hepatology*, **8**, 161–212.

Pavlidis, P., Crichton, S., Lemmic, H., *et al.*(2013) Improved outcome of severe acute pancreatitis in the intensive care unit. *Critical Care Research and Practice*, http://dx.doi.org/10.1155/2013/897107.

Pettie, J., Dow, M. (2013). Assessment and management of paracetamol poisoning in adults. *Nursing Standard*, **27**, 39–47.

Pomier-Layrargues, G., Villeneuve, J.-P., Deschênes, M., *et al.* (2001). Transjugular intrahepatic portosystemic shunt (TIPS) versus endoscopic variceal ligation in the prevention of variceal rebleeding in patients with cirrhosis: a randomised trial. *Gut*, **48**, 390–6.

Puthucheary, Z.A., Rawal, J., McPhail, M., *et al.* (2013). Acute skeletal muscle wasting in critical illness. *JAMA*, **310**, 1591–1600.

Rapp, R.P., Young, B., Twyman, D., *et al.* (1983). The favourable effect of early parenteral feeding on survival in head-injured patients. *Journal of Neurosurgery*, **58**, 906–12.

Riordan, S.M., Williams R. (1997). Current concepts: treatment of hepatic encephalopathy. *New England Journal of Medicine*, **337**, 473–9.

Scott, A., Skerratt, S., Adam, S. (1998). *Nutrition for the Critically Ill: A Practical Handbook*, p. 67. London Arnold.

Seaman, D.S. (2001). Adult living donor liver transplantation: current status. *Journal of Clinical Gastroenterology*, **33**, 97–106.

Schroeder, K.M., Jacobs, D.O., Guite, C., *et al.* (2012) Use of a chlorhexidine-impregnated patch does not decrease the incidence of bacterial colonization of femoral nerve catheters: a randomized trial. *Canadian Journal of Anesthesiology*, **59**, 950–7.

Shah, R. Tariq, N., Shanley, C., *et al.* (2009). Peritonitis from PEG tube insertion in surgical intensive care unit patients: identification of risk factors and clinical outcomes. *Surgical Endoscopy*, **23**, 2580–6.

Sharifi, M.N., Walton, A., Chakrabarty, G., *et al.* (2011). Nutrition support in intensive care units in England: a snapshot of present practice. *British Journal of Nutrition*, **106**, 1240–4.

Sibulesky, L., Heckman, M.G., Taner, C.B., *et al.* (2013). Outcomes following liver transplantation in intensive care unit patients. *World Journal of Hepatology*, **5**, 26–32.

Simons, S., Remington, R. (2013). The percutaneous endoscopic gastrostomy tube: a nurse's guide to PEG tubes. *MedSurg Nursing*, **22**, 77–83.

Singer, P., Berger, M., van den Berghe, G., *et al.* (2009) ESPEN Guidelines on Parenteral Nutrition: Intensive Care. *Clinical Nutrition*, **28**, 387–400.

Singer, P., Hiesmayr, M., Biolo, G., *et al.* (2014). Pragmatic approach to nutrition in the ICU: expert opinion regarding which calorie protein target. *Clinical Nutrition*, **33**, 246–51.

Sparks D.A., Chase, D.M., Coughlin, L.M., Perry E. (2011). Pulmonary complications of 9931 narrow-bore nasoenteric tubes during blind placement: a critical review. *Journal of Parenteral and Enteral Nutrition*, **35**, 625–9.

Stayner, J.L., Bhatnagar, A., McGinn, A. Fang J.C. (2012). Feeding tube placement: errors and complications. *Nutrition in Clinical Practice*, **27**, 738–48.

Stravitz, R.T., Kramer, A.H., Davern, T., *et al.* (2007) The Acute Liver Failure Study Group. Intensive care of patients with acute liver failure: recommendations of the US Acute Liver Failure Study Group. *Critical Care Medicine*, **35**, 2498–508.

Strong, R.M., Condon, S.C., Solinger, M.R., *et al.* (1992). Equal aspiration rates from postpylorus and intragastric-placed small-bore nasoenteric feeding tubes: a randomized, prospective study. *Journal of Parenteral and Enteral Nutrition*, **16**, 59–63.

Stutchfield, B.M., Simpson, K., Wigmore, S.J. (2011). Systematic review and meta-analysis of survival following extracorporeal liver support. *British Journal of Surgery*, **98**, 623–31.

Tat Fan, S., (2006) Live donor liver transplantation. *Transplantation*, **82**, 723–32.

Taylor,S. (2013). Confirming nasogastric feeding tube position versus the need to feed. *Intensive and Critical Care Nursing*, **29**, 59–69

Tejada Artigas, A., Bello Dronda, S., Chacun Valles, E., *et al.* (2001). Risk factors for nosocomial pneumonia in critically ill trauma patients. *Critical Care Medicine*, **29**, 304–9.

Tryba, M. (1991). Sucralfate versus antacids or H_2-antagonists for stress ulcer prophylaxis: a meta-analysis on efficacy and pneumonia rate. *Critical Care Medicine*, **19**, 942–9.

van den Berghe, G., Wouters, P., Weekers, F., *et al.* (2001). Intensive insulin therapy in critically ill patients. *New England Journal of Medicine*, **345**, 1359–67.

van der Spoel, J.L., Schultz, M.J., van der Voort, P.H.J., De Jonge, E. (2006). Influence of severity of illnes, medication and selective decontamination on defecation. *Intensive Care Medicine*, **32**, 875–80.

van Schijndel, S., Weijs, P., Koopmans, R., *et al.* (2009). Optimal nutrition during the period of mechanical ventilation decreases mortality in critically ill, long-term acute female patients: a prospective observational cohort study. *Critical Care*, **13**, R132.

Villanueva, C., Balanzo, J. (2008) Variceal bleeding: pharmacological treatment and prophylactic strategies. *Drugs*, **68**, 2303–24.

Villatoro, E., Bassi, C., Larvin, M. (2006). Antibiotic therapy for prophylaxis against infection of pancreatic necrosis in acute pancreatitis. *Cochrane Database of Systematic Reviews*, **4**, CD002941.

Villet, S., Chiolero, R.L., Bollman, M.D. (2005). Negative impact of hypocaloric feeding and energy balance on clinical outcome in ICU patients. *Clinical Nutrition*, **24**, 502–9.

Weijs, P.J., Stapel, S.N., de Groot, S.D., *et al.* (2012). Optimal protein and energy nutrition decreases mortality in mechanically ventilated, critically ill patients: a prospective observational cohort study. *Journal of Parenteral and Enteral Nutrition*, **36**, 60–8.

Wereszczynska-Siemiatkowska, U., Swidnicka-Siergiejko, A., Siemiatkowski, A., Dabrowski, A. (2013). Early enteral nutrition is superior to delayed enteral nutrition for the prevention of infected necrosis and mortality in acute pancreatitis. *Pancreas*, **42**, 640–6.

Whitehouse, T., Wendon, J. (2013) Acute liver failure. *Best Practice & Research Clinical Gastroenterology*, **27**, 757–69.

Williams, T.A., Leslie, G.D. (2004). A review of the nursing care of enteral feeding tubes in critically ill adults: Part I. *Intensive and Critical Care Nursing*, **20**, 330–343

Williams, T.A., Leslie, G.D. (2005). A review of the nursing care of enteral feeding tubes in critically ill adults: part II. *Intensive and Critical Care Nursing*, **21**, 5–15.

Williams, T.A., Leslie, G.D., Mills, L., *et al*. (2014). Frequency of aspirating gastric tubes for patients receiving enteral nutrition in the ICU: a randomised controlled trial. *Journal of Parenteral and Enteral Nutrition*, **38**, 809–16.

Winterbauer, R.H., Durning, R.B., Barron, E., *et al*. (1981). Aspirated nasogastric feeding solution detected by glucose strips. *Annals of Internal Medicine*, **95**, 67–8.

Zanella, A., Cressoni, M., Epp, M., *et al*. (2012). Effects of tracheal orientation on development of ventilator-associated pneumonia: an experimental study. *Intensive Care Medicine*, **38**, 677–85.

Zerizer, I., Chan, W.H., Singer M. (2005). Intramural feeding: a complication of percutaneous endoscopic gastrostomy feeding. *European Journal of Gastroenterology and Hepatology*, **17**, 131.

CHAPTER 10
Sepsis and multiple organ dysfunction

Introduction

Some of the greatest challenges in critical care are presented by patients suffering from multiple organ dysfunction syndrome (MODS). MODS is most often caused by sepsis (see Box 10.1), but is also associated with other conditions such as pancreatitis or trauma that trigger exaggerated, dysregulated systemic pro- and anti-inflammatory responses (see Box 10.2).

All body systems and organs can be affected to a greater or lesser extent in MODS. Brain, lung, cardiovascular, gut, and kidney dysfunctions are revealed by various abnormal clinical signs and symptoms. Raised plasma bilirubin is generally used as an indicator of liver dysfunction, even though hyperbilirubinaemia is a late and relatively insensitive marker and more

Box 10.1 Sepsis

- Sepsis is defined as one or more life-threatening organ dysfunctions caused by a dysregulated host response to infection.
- The infectious process may be triggered by a bacterium, virus, fungus, or parasite.
- Organ dysfunction in these cases is indicated by an increase in the Sepsis-related Organ Failure Assessment* (SOFA) score of two or more points. Specific organ dysfunctions are revealed by:
    - a reduced P_aO_2/FiO_2 ratio or a requirement for mechanical ventilation—indicating respiratory failure
    - hypotension or a requirement for inotropes or vasopressors—indicating cardiovascular failure
    - decreased Glasgow Coma Score—indicating neurological failure
    - increased creatinine or decreased urine output—indicating renal failure
    - increased bilirubin—indicating hepatic failure
    - decreased platelets—indicating haematological failure.
- At the bedside, if and when blood values are not available, organ dysfunction may be revealed by increased respiratory rate (22 breaths/min or more (in the non-ventilated patient)), hypotension (systolic blood pressure 100 mmHg or less), or altered mentation. Two or more of these indicators in the patient with infection mean that they are likely to have sepsis.
- Sepsis is the most common cause of MODS.
- Most deaths in septic patients occur in those who develop MODS, with the mortality risk correlating with the number of affected organs.

* The Sepsis-related Organ Failure Assessment is now termed the Sequential Organ Failure Assessment. The precise values for each level of failure of each organ were set-out by Vincent *et al.* (1996), so see this source for further information.

Box 10.2 Non-septic triggers of dysregulated systemic pro- and anti-inflammatory responses

- Trauma
- Pancreatitis
- Major burns
- Major surgical procedures
- Infection
- Haemorrhage/major blood transfusion
- Ischaemic tissue
- Periods of inadequate perfusion followed by reperfusion

sophisticated tests can show evidence of liver dysfunction at an earlier stage, for example by failure to clear drugs or injected dyes. Patients with MODS also suffer coagulation disturbances, although severe complications such as major bleeding or thrombosis are rarely seen.

Patients with MODS are prone to many complications and often require complex modes of organ support and other treatments. However, the severity of organ dysfunction and subsequent requirements for organ support vary considerably between individuals. This is due to genetic and other factors including comorbidities, immunosuppressant medications, malnutrition, and excessive alcohol use, all of which affect intrinsic immune and inflammatory responses.

Definitions

Different definitions of sepsis and organ dysfunction have been used over the years, although the terminology has often been imprecise with little or no reference to the underlying pathophysiology or the immunological or biochemical mechanisms involved (Vincent *et al.* 2011, 2013). Until recently, it was suggested that

Table 10.1 Definitions

Term	Definition
Bacteraemia	The presence of viable bacteria in the blood.
Septicaemia	An imprecise term still sometimes used in various ways, e.g. to describe the presence of micro-organisms or their toxins in the blood. Its use is no longer recommended.
Sepsis	Life-threatening organ dysfunction due to a dysregulated host response to infection.
Septic shock	Septic shock is a subset of sepsis with circulatory, cellular, and metabolic abnormalities that significantly increase the risk of mortality. It is identified by a requirement for vasopressors to maintain mean arterial pressure at 65 mmHg or more with a serum lactate >2 mmol/L in the absence of hypovolaemia.
Apoptosis	Genetically programmed cell death.
Anergy	A general loss of immune responsiveness indicating deficient T-cell function.

patients should be said to be septic when some infectious process led to physiological disturbances defined by abnormal vital signs or blood results known as the systemic inflammatory response syndrome criteria, with the term 'severe sepsis' used to describe cases when acute organ dysfunction was also present (see Table 10.1).

However, it is apparent that sepsis involves both pro- and anti-inflammatory mechanisms, and that the existing model of a systemic inflammatory response syndrome (SIRS) is too simplistic. Furthermore, it is known that many patients with mild infections satisfy the traditional criteria for sepsis but do not need treatment in hospital. As a consequence, the term systemic inflammatory response syndrome and the so-called SIRS criteria are not used in the latest definition of sepsis, and are in fact redundant. Instead, the term 'sepsis' will now be used to describe infected patients with impending or established organ dysfunction; so the term 'severe sepsis' will also be removed.

As sepsis is a syndrome rather than a distinct disease, there is no specific test that provides a definitive diagnosis at present. Infection is frequently presumed rather than confirmed and the clinical picture can be very variable. For example, patients with proven sepsis are very often febrile, but can be normothermic or even hypothermic. Diagnosis is also complicated by the presentation being confounded by other pathologies such as chronic obstructive pulmonary disease or cancer. The source of infection also makes a difference; for example, patients with sepsis arising from abdominal infection are more likely to develop acute kidney injury, clotting disorders, and shock than patients with sepsis due to respiratory infection (Volakli *et al.* 2010). These variations in the presentation and progression of sepsis can make early diagnosis difficult and lead to delays in treatment. On the other hand, some patients may be treated unnecessarily for infection that is not actually present; no organism is identified in approximately 30–50% of patients believed to be 'septic'. This may reflect the inability of the laboratory to identify a causative organism, or the fact that MODS is a common end-point for many systemic inflammatory conditions such as trauma (including surgery), non-infective pancreatitis, and drug and blood transfusion reactions. Uncertainty exists in many cases. The varied case mix also complicates research studies comparing the effects of different therapies.

Incidence and impact of sepsis

The imprecision of previous definitions and methods of identifying sepsis also means that many publications about sepsis may not always be describing the same phenomena. Reported incidences of sepsis are very variable. An analysis of four US population studies described an average 13% rise in the incidence of 'sepsis' between 2004 and 2009 based on hospital discharge coding, but, depending on the method of coding used, the incidence varied from 300 to 1031 per 100,000 population with in-hospital mortality varying from 14.7% to 29.9% (Gaieski *et al.* 2013). The annual costs of septic patients in US hospitals have been claimed to be $24.3 billion (Lagu *et al.* 2012). In the UK, a study of 170 critical care units found that 21% of patients satisfied the old criteria for severe sepsis on admission, and reported an in-hospital mortality of 40.6% (Shahin *et al.* 2012). Furthermore, patients admitted to critical care without sepsis are at high risk of developing sepsis at some later time due to the many lines, drains, and catheters used in this population and the degree of immunosuppression suffered by the critically ill. A large European study found that 37% of critical care patients had sepsis during the study period (Vincent *et al.* 2006). Even in patients who survive to hospital discharge, sepsis increases the risk of death and reduces quality of life in later years (Winters *et al.* 2010).

Bacterial sepsis

Most cases of what has previously been termed severe sepsis arise from bacterial infection, although the prevalence of different types of micro-organism varies. The EPIC II point prevalence study of 13,796 patients in 1265 critical care units from 75 countries collected on one day in 2007 showed that patients in Europe had more Gram-negative bacterial infections whereas Gram-positive infections predominated in North America (Vincent *et al.* 2009). A total of 7087 patients (51%) were considered infected, with specific infective organisms identified for 70% of these. The predominant Gram-positive organisms included staphylococci (e.g. *Staphylococcus aureus*), enterococci, and streptococci (e.g. *Streptococcus pneumoniae*). Such infections were commonly respiratory, blood, and skin/soft tissue based or catheter-related (see Figure 10.1). Gram-negative bacteria were commonly *Pseudomonas, Escherichia coli, Klebsiella, Acinetobacter*, and *Enterobacter* species. These infections were mainly sourced to the lungs, abdomen, blood, or urinary tract.

The inflammatory response to sepsis is due in part to the bacterium itself, in part to release of its constituents such as cell wall products (e.g., endotoxin), and in part to damage of the host's own tissues.

Endotoxins are an integral part of the Gram-negative bacterium cell wall that are released when the cell disintegrates (lyses). This can occur through natural immune defences but also with antibiotic treatment. Endotoxins consist of large lipopolysaccharides, and their toxicity is associated with the lipid A portion of the molecule. Exotoxins are proteins released outside the bacterium following their synthesis within the cytoplasm. They are predominantly associated with Gram-positive bacteria and may either cause a systemic illness (e.g. toxic shock syndrome produced by 'superantigens') or react with target tissues to cause specific types of damage (e.g. diphtheria with cardiac muscle, botulinism in nerve tissue, or *Clostridium difficile* and the gut wall). Bacteria also produce enzymes such as lipases, phosphatases, and proteases that destroy local tissue. Examples include streptokinase which dissolves fibrin clots, allowing infection to spread, hyaluronidase which digests hyaluronic acid in basement membranes permitting tissue penetration, and leukocidin which destroys leucocytes. The Panton–Valentine leukocidin in some strains of *Staphylococcus aureus* causes a particularly virulent and destructive form of pneumonia.

Endotoxin and the other distinctive molecules produced by invading micro-organisms are foreign

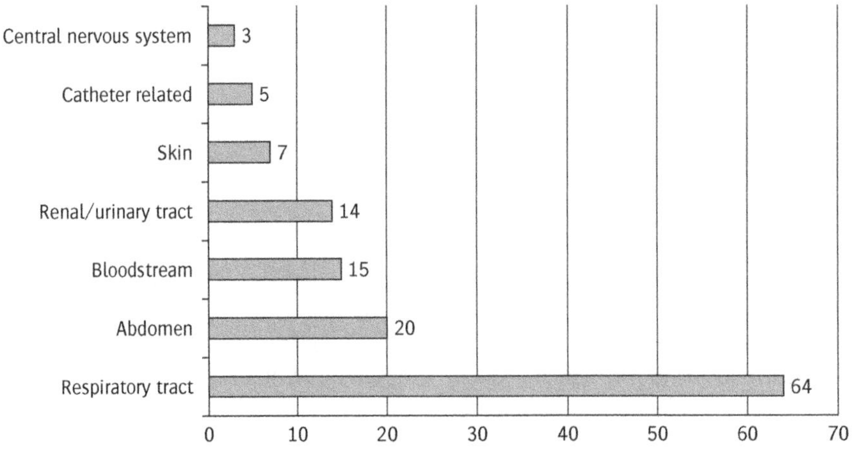

Figure 10.1 Percentage of ICU patients with confirmed infection at different sites.

Data from Vincent J.L., Rello J., Marshall J., *et al.*, International study of the prevalence and outcomes of infection in intensive care units, *JAMA*, Volume 302, Issue 21, pp. 2323–9. 2009, American Medical Association

to the body and are known as pathogen-associated molecular patterns (PAMPs). PAMPs are recognized by specialized pattern recognition receptors (PRRs) such as Toll-like receptors (TLRs) embedded in cell wall membranes and nucleotide oligomerization domain receptors (NOD-like receptors/NLRs) within the cytoplasm. These receptors trigger a cascade of immune and inflammatory responses that can lead to organ failure. Damage to tissues from infection and other insults like trauma or surgery also cause release of intracellular constituents such as mitochondria and proteins into the circulation. These damage-associated molecular patterns (DAMPs) are recognized by PRRs, again setting in train a series of immune and inflammatory responses similar to those induced by PAMPs (Cinel and Opal 2009).

Pathophysiology of sepsis and non-sepsis MODS

Rather than a particular insult simply triggering a pro-inflammatory response, it is evident that a complex series of overlapping processes occur with the overall effect varying over time (see Figure 10.2). Previously, several distinct stages were described. There was said to be an initial pro-inflammatory phase consisting of a 'cytokine storm', designed to eradicate invading pathogens and any damaged tissue but also potentially damaging the host itself, followed by an anti-inflammatory phase that would re-balance the body and restore homeostasis.

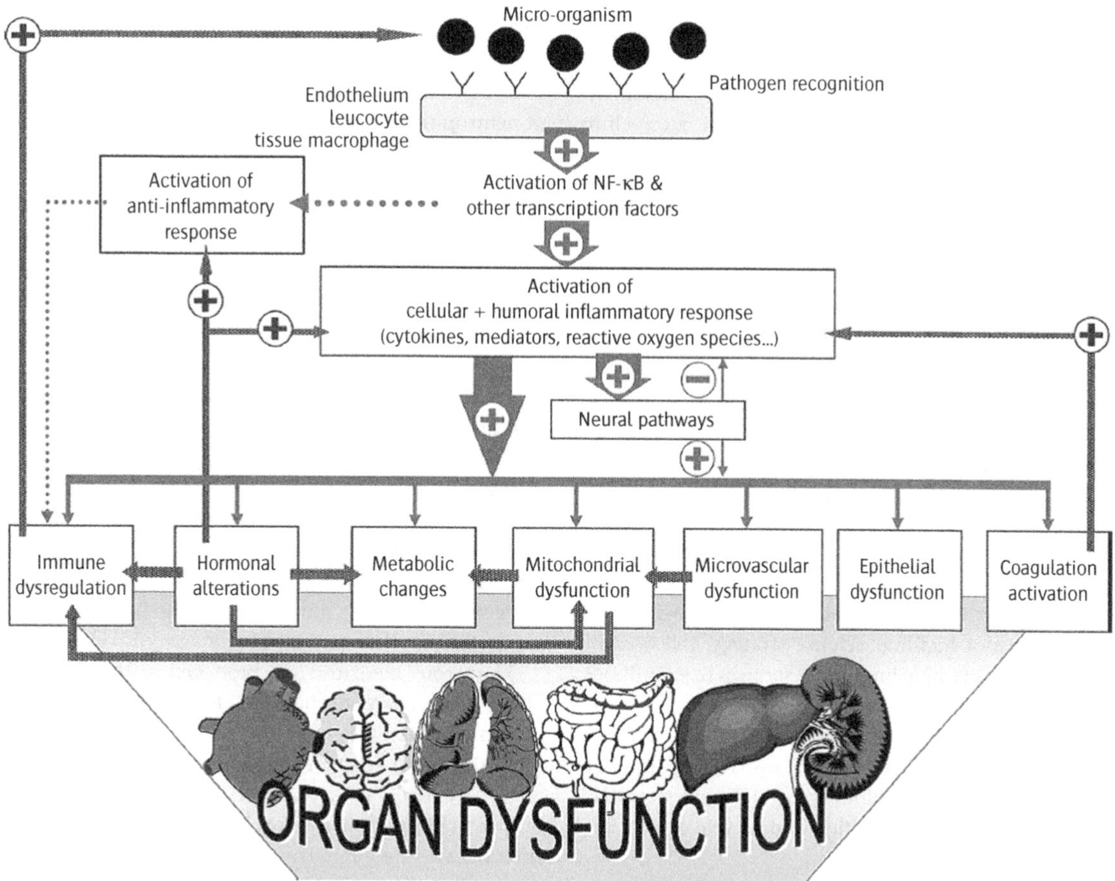

Figure 10.2 Mechanisms of sepsis-induced organ dysfunction.

Reproduced with permission from Edward Abraham and Mervyn Singer, Mechanisms of sepsis-induced organ dysfunction, *Critical Care Medicine*, Volume 35, Issue 10, pp.2408–16, Copyright © 2007 Wolters Kluwer Health, Inc.

(This relative immunosuppression may increase the risk of secondary infection.) It is now recognized that this model is over-simplistic and that, in reality, pro- and anti-inflammatory responses happen simultaneously, although one or other mechanism predominates at different times. Furthermore, the strength of different responses can be relatively mild or extremely excessive, with morbidity and mortality associated with higher levels of activation of both pro- and anti-inflammatory pathways. The duration of different responses also varies markedly between patients and over time, while different immune cell types (e.g. neutrophils and lymphocytes) show very different levels of activation or suppression at different times.

This complex picture highlights the difficulty in deciding which immunomodulatory treatments, if any, should be given to a patient at a particular time, at what dose, and for how long. For example, corticosteroids are anti-inflammatory agents that may be effective in dampening the effects of excessive pro-inflammatory processes, but could be counter-productive if the patient is already in an overall state of immunosuppression (Ward 2008). The naive approach until now has been to assume that there are relatively simple treatment protocols that can be used to manage the gross clinical features of sepsis; but the immunological/biological phenotype (characteristics) of individual patients at particular points in time were not taken into consideration. As a consequence, many therapeutic trials in sepsis have failed, even though a subset of treated patients could potentially benefit from more individually tailored approaches.

Processes occurring in sepsis are discussed in the following sections.

The immune/pro- and anti-inflammatory response

A series of interactive processes are activated via cellular and humoral (non-cellular) mediators. These involve both non-specific innate mechanisms (e.g. white cell activation) as a first-line defence strategy, followed by more specific adaptive immune responses (e.g. antibody formation). These are subject to considerable regulatory control in normal circumstances, including feedback loops and redundant pathways. However, in pathological conditions, these inhibitory regulatory systems fail to control prolonged activation and a cycle of continuous reactivation can occur.

The complement system is activated by antigen–antibody complexes or by specific micro-organisms. This is a complex cascade through a series of circulating proteins whose role is to initiate and enhance the immune response and to help destroy pathogens. These effects are protective if complement activation is localized to the site of injury, but more widespread activation causes gross vasodilatation, increased capillary permeability, and phagocytic activation with release of toxic by-products.

White blood cells include neutrophils, monocytes (circulating macrophages), and lymphocytes (see Figure 10.3). There are also fixed macrophages in tissues, for example Kupffer cells in the liver. The primary functions of the neutrophil are surveillance and phagocytosis of foreign pathogens and damaged tissue. They are drawn to the site of injury by chemotactic attraction to foreign organisms or the products of cell destruction. Neutrophils phagocytose ('eat up') pathogens by releasing proteases (cytotoxic enzymes such as elastase and catalase) and highly reactive oxygen-related molecules, collectively known as oxygen free radicals or reactive oxygen species (ROS). ROS attack pathogens in combination with proteases. These toxic substances can disperse into the extracellular environment, resulting in local tissue damage and, potentially, organ dysfunction. Binding to the endothelium is a key stage in the transfer of neutrophils out of the circulation and into the tissues, but excessive widespread activation can lead to generalized endothelial activation and damage.

Macrophages/monocytes also play an important role in the spread of inflammation. Their primary functions are to engulf and phagocytose foreign pathogens or antigens and process them for presentation to lymphocytes, and to produce inflammatory mediators (cytokines).

Lymphocytes form sensitized cells and antibodies that are highly specific to particular foreign pathogens. In cell-mediated immunity, T-lymphocytes proliferate in response to presentation of the antigen by the macrophage to T-cell lymphoid tissue. In humoral immunity, the B-lymphocytes recognize antigens and differentiate into antibody-producing cells. The antibodies bind with antigens, producing antigen–antibody immune complexes that are then removed by phagocytic cells.

Numerous mediators are produced in the pro- and anti-inflammatory mechanisms. It is beyond the scope of this chapter to describe the function and actions of all of these, but some of the more important mediators are briefly described here. Their relevance is underlined by the trialling of many novel therapies that modulate their release or antagonize their actions, for example by antibodies or receptor blockers. Such mediators are primarily produced by immune cells and the endothelium, but also by other cells (e.g. hepatocytes).

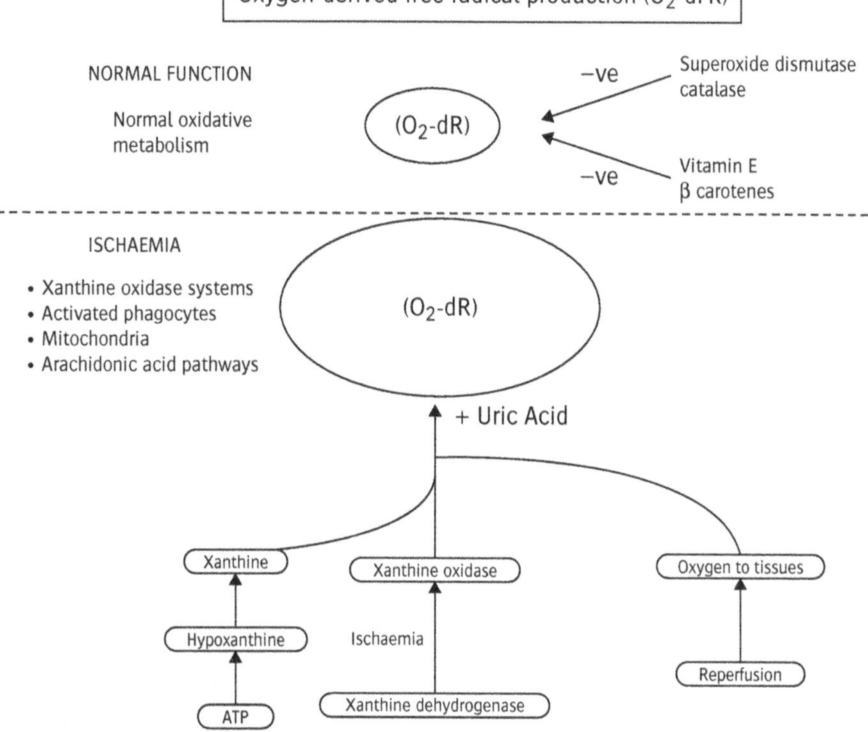

Figure 10.3 The generation of oxygen free radicals/reactive oxygen species.

Arachidonic acid metabolites

Arachidonic acid (AA) is a normal constituent of cell membranes released as a result of contact of the enzyme phospholipase A2 with injured cell walls. Arachidonic acid metabolism via cyclo-oxygenase and lipo-oxygenase pathways produces eicosanoids (prostaglandins, thromboxanes, and leukotrienes) that are essential for activation of macrophages as well as other roles including vasoconstriction *and* vasodilation, increased capillary leak, etc.

Tumour necrosis factor (TNF)

TNF is a polypeptide cytokine produced primarily by activated macrophages and T-lymphocytes. TNF release is stimulated by lipopolysaccharide (LPS), micro-organisms, ischaemic tissue, and tissue damage. It is an early release cytokine whose actions are central to the development of inflammatory responses, including neutrophil activation, platelet–neutrophil–endothelial interactions, endothelial activation, and adhesiveness, as well as mediation of both cell survival and cell death pathways (Bradley 2008). TNF stimulates secretion of other cytokines (e.g. interleukins 1 and 6), and acts on hepatocytes to stimulate the acute phase response, activate the coagulation system, and suppress division of bone marrow stem cells (Bradley 2008).

Interleukins (e.g. IL-1, IL-6, IL-8, IL-10, IL-18)

Interleukins are released by activated macrophages and other cells in inflammatory conditions, either locally and/or systemically. Some are associated with inducing pro-coagulant activity in the endothelium, mediating leucocyte adhesion, reducing vascular responsiveness to catecholamines, increasing muscle proteolysis, and causing a negative nitrogen balance. IL-1 also produces fever, enhanced activity and proliferation of various white cell populations, enhanced antibody production, and production of acute phase proteins. IL-6 works as a second-stage messenger released by macrophages, endothelium, and other cells in response to TNF or IL-1. Its most important actions are stimulation of acute phase protein production in the liver, antibody production, as a growth factor for B-cells, and maintenance of the metabolic response to stress. IL-8 is a chemokine, attracting neutrophils to regions of infected or injured tissue (chemotaxis). IL-10 on the other hand, is an anti-inflammatory cytokine.

Nitric oxide

Nitric oxide is a potent mediator released from many different cell types as well as from the endothelium. It has numerous effects, including vasodilation, myocardial depression, cytotoxicity (e.g. against bacteria), decreased platelet aggregation, mitochondrial inhibition, and neural transmission. Sepsis is associated with very high levels of NO caused, in large part, by increased expression of the inducible form of NO synthase.

Coagulopathy

Activation of the inflammatory response leads to concomitant activation of coagulation processes and alterations in haemostatic balance. Various circulating components, including tissue factor, the kallikrein–kinin cascade, complement, factor XII (Hageman factor), and platelets, play a role in both of these. Thrombin, generated by activation of the clotting cascade, is a potent inflammatory activator. However, while overt bleeding—disseminated intravascular coagulation (DIC)—is infrequently seen as a significant clinical problem, biochemical evidence of coagulopathy is present in most (if not all) patients with sepsis and organ dysfunction.

The contact system is activated at the same time as the coagulation system through factor XII (Hageman factor). The role of the contact system is not fully understood, but seems to include enhancement of the inflammatory response and fibrinolysis. Bradykinin is the major metabolite produced; this potent vasodilator increases capillary permeability and activates complement.

Fibrinolysis results in the breakdown of fibrin clot and is marked by increased levels of d-dimers in the plasma. Fibrinolysis is also enhanced in sepsis and other inflammatory conditions.

Disruption of the endothelium and exposure of the underlying collagen basement membrane causes the form of platelets to change from the normal disc shape to that of a swollen sphere with numerous projections called pseudopods. These expand the surface area available for adhesion and increase the likelihood of aggregation. During the shape change, adenosine diphosphate (ADP) is released which initiates platelet aggregation. Thromboxane A_2 (TXA_2) is also produced, causing vasoconstriction and further stimulation of platelet aggregation. The platelets release a platelet surface procoagulant that initiates formation of fibrin plugs and, eventually, clot. However, uncontrolled, excessive platelet activation may result in disruption of normal coagulation mechanisms and the development of DIC. Thrombocytopenia can occur due to increased consumption as well as decreased production from megakaryocytes.

Endothelial damage

The endothelium is highly susceptible to activation and damage, particularly by white blood cell–endothelial cell interactions. Effects of endothelial damage include:

- release of pro- and anti-inflammatory mediators including potent vasoactive substances such as prostaglandins, thromboxanes, nitric oxide, and endothelin
- potentiation of coagulation, as damaged endothelium may become the source of pro-coagulant substances such as tissue thromboplastin and tissue factor
- increased capillary permeability allowing increased movement of fluid and solute (and protein) from the vasculature, resulting in hypovolaemia and hypo-albuminaemia
- activation of coagulation pathways with consumption of clotting factors.

Neuroendocrine activation

Both sympathetic and parasympathetic mechanisms are activated in systemic inflammatory conditions, as is the hypothalamic–pituitary–adrenal system. An acute phase endocrine response occurs with release of adrenocorticotrophic hormone (ACTH), glucocorticoids, catecholamines (epinephrine (adrenaline)), and norepinephrine (noradrenaline)), endorphins, and prolactin. The net effect is increased cardiac output and blood flow to vital organs, with redistribution of blood flow away from secondary organs, increased capillary permeability, and increased blood glucose. These functions can be adaptive in the short term, but are damaging over extended periods, for example when excessive glucose damages protein structures through glycation, generates ROS, and promotes bacterial proliferation. This neuroendocrine activation also increases and perpetuates immune/inflammatory cascades; with prolonged activation over several days suppressing the immune response and thereby increasing the risk of secondary infection.

Many other endocrine changes occur in prolonged critical illness (e.g. with cortisol, thyroid hormones, sex hormones, and gut hormones/adipokines) (Langouche and van den Berghe 2006). There is a general loss of the diurnal rhythms of many hormones. Baseline cortisol levels may remain high, or be normal or low, possibly reflecting the degree of stress the patient experiences. ACTH stimulation tests show a variable response in septic shock patients, with those with high baseline cortisol levels and a poor increment to ACTH stimulation suffering higher mortality (Annane *et al.* 2000). Thyroid function is deranged with low levels of T_3 and T_4, the degree of which also relates to poor outcomes.

Cardiovascular effects

These effects include redistribution of circulating blood volume, increased capillary leak, overall vasodilation, and myocardial depression. While many mediators cause vasodilation, some cause vasoconstriction, affecting different vascular beds within the same organ. Digital ischaemia or infarction may be seen in particularly severe cases. The overall effect is vasodilation, and this is compounded by a decreased responsiveness of vascular smooth muscle to catecholamines. Hypotension results, and may progress to a shocked state.

Increased capillary vascular permeability causes intravascular fluid to move through the capillary membrane into the interstitial space (i.e. the 'third' fluid space). This results in tissue oedema and, in the lungs, acute respiratory distress syndrome (ARDS). Oedema compromises diffusion of oxygen and nutrients through to the cells. There may also be some obstruction to blood flow within the microvasculature caused by clumping or rolling of white cells and the development of microthrombi, although complete obstruction of blood vessels is relatively unusual.

Bioenergetic/metabolic effects

In healthy tissue, decreases in oxygen delivery do not necessarily reduce oxygen consumption, as tissue oxygen extraction is increased proportionately. Nonetheless, when oxygen delivery falls below a critical level, tissue oxygen extraction cannot increase enough to compensate and oxygen consumption reduces with further decreases in oxygen delivery. This is known as supply-dependent oxygen consumption. Furthermore, tissue oxygen extraction is often reduced in sepsis because of blood flow redistribution (shunting blood away from nutrient capillaries), cellular alterations related to decreased mitochondrial (aerobic) respiration (Brealey *et al.* 2002), and decreased metabolic rate. Oxygen is consumed by the body primarily for the production of ATP by the mitochondrial electron transport chain. This process is directly inhibited by mediators such as nitric oxide and other reactive oxygen species, downregulation of the genes encoding for mitochondrial proteins, and modifications in hormonal function (e.g. decreased thyroid activity). This model is supported by the finding that tissue oxygen tension is elevated in sepsis, i.e. oxygen is available to cells but utilization is still decreased. It has been proposed that organ dysfunction in sepsis and other critical illnesses may actually be adaptive, as the reduction in metabolism, and therefore reduced energy requirements, in the aftermath of a significant insult may protect the organs in a manner analogous to hibernation (Mongardon *et al.* 2009). Of note, metabolic rate increases in early sepsis but falls with increasing severity, so that patients in septic shock have a similar resting energy expenditure to healthy subjects. There is a rebound increase during the recovery phase as mobility increases and anabolism and healing occur (see Table 10.2).

Multiple organ dysfunction syndrome

The multi-centre SOAP study showed that 39% of ICU patients had multiple organ dysfunction syndrome (MODS) at some point during their stay, with most cases associated with sepsis (Sakr *et al.* 2012). MODS has been described as 'the final common pathway preceding death' and is the main cause of death in the critically ill, with mortality as high as 89% in those with sepsis and four or more failed organs (Sakr *et al.* 2012). Respiratory, renal, cardiovascular, central nervous, and coagulation systems are those most likely to fail during critical illness (Sakr *et al.* 2012).

Specific organ dysfunctions associated with septic and non-septic MODS are discussed in the following section.

Central nervous system dysfunction

CNS dysfunction is characterized by altered consciousness ranging from confusion/delirium to coma. Sepsis is a common cause of neurological dysfunction, although drug effects and structural and metabolic disorders should always be considered as possible factors as well. Up to 62% of septic patients develop 'septic encephalopathy' (Gofton and Young 2012) as well as complications such as seizures or stroke (usually following an intracerebral bleed or prolonged hypotension).

The precise mechanisms remain uncertain but include circulatory and microcirculatory perfusion

Table 10.2 Pathophysiological derangements associated with dysregulated systemic pro- and anti-inflammatory responses and the neuroendocrine response

1. Maldistribution of circulating blood volume	Systemic vasodilatation
	Increased microvascular permeability
	Vascular obstruction related to cellular aggregation, microthrombi, and tissue oedema
	Selective vasoconstriction
	Endothelial damage
	Coagulation/microvascular thrombi
	Loss of autoregulation
2. Imbalance of oxygen supply and demand	Maldistribution of circulating volume
	Microvascular abnormalities
	Increased oxygen demand due to pain, fever, tachycardia, restlessness, etc.
	Oxygen extraction defects
	V/Q mismatch
	Intrapulmonary shunt
	Excessive cellular activity
	Myocardial depression
3. Alterations in metabolism	Hypermetabolism
	Hyperglycaemia
	Protein catabolism and gluconeogenesis
	Resistance to insulin
	Excessive cellular activity
	Fatty acid mobilization and increased oxidation
	Hepatic dysfunction and lactate production

deficits, bioenergetic dysfunction, and reductions in cerebral metabolism. Excitatory neurotransmitters such as glutamine and aspartate may play a role in cerebral ischaemia. Reperfusion injury occurs, i.e. damage following restoration of the circulation after a period of ischaemia. This is predominantly related to local damage from the ROS produced in large quantities by mitochondria on resuscitation. There may also be post-ischaemic hypoperfusion where, after an episode of global ischaemia, there is a short period of hyperaemia (high blood flow) followed by more lengthy vasospasm-induced hypoperfusion. The no-reflow phenomenon is less common, but can occur for up to 3 days after an ischaemic insult. This is a continued decrease in cerebral blood flow despite normal mean arterial and cerebral perfusion pressures. Processes contributing to the no-reflow phenomenon include oedema, vasospasm, increased blood viscosity with red blood cell sludging, membrane damage, intracellular or mitochondrial calcium shifts, and increased production of ROS.

Assessment should include the following:

1. Level of consciousness—this is difficult to assess if sedation is required to maintain ventilation. However, a high degree of suspicion should be maintained if the patient remains unconscious when sedation is reduced, in which case it is usually appropriate to stop sedation, at least for a period, to give the patient the best possible opportunity to respond (see Chapter 8). Persistently low Glasgow Coma Scores are associated with the grade of encephalopathy, and with mortality.
2. Agitation and confusion—often apparent when the patient is first admitted. Other causes must be excluded (e.g. hypoxaemia). These can herald a further septic episode.
3. An EEG may exhibit evidence of changes consistent with metabolic or anoxic encephalopathy. Some will show evidence of profound abnormalities. Computed tomography (CT) and magnetic resonance imaging (MRI) may reveal both non-specific changes and distinct pathologies (e.g. intracerebral haemorrhage related to coagulopathy).

Critical illness polyneuropathy and myopathy

Critical illness polyneuropathy (CIP) and critical illness myopathy (CIM) are common accompaniments of critical illness, prolonging recovery time and increasing mortality (Hermans *et al.* 2008). Multiple mechanisms are implicated including ischaemia, cytokine–endothelial interactions leading to increased vascular permeability and oedema (which impairs the microcirculation), hyperglycaemia, mitochondrial dysfunction, and increased production of ROS. Primary axonal degeneration of motor and sensory fibres and denervation atrophy of limb and skeletal muscles follow. CIP usually presents as profound limb and chest wall weakness, although sensory deficits can occur alone or in combination. A primary CIM with protein catabolism and muscle degeneration that is not secondary to muscle denervation is also seen. Critical illness myopathy and neuropathy (CRIMYNE) is when myopathy and polyneuropathy coexist.

Profound weakness and muscle wasting may only become obvious as the patient begins to recover from MODS. It can be distinguished from simple weakness related to normal catabolic muscle wasting by electrophysiological studies showing signs of primary axonal degeneration of both sensory and motor fibres, or by myopathic changes (Bednarik *et al.* 2003). While the prognosis is generally good for CIM, recovery from CIP may take many months or may never be complete. Critical illness neuromyopathy delays weaning from mechanical ventilation and prolongs recovery.

Respiratory system involvement—ARDS

The most commonly recognized organ dysfunction in MODS is respiratory failure, formerly usually described as either 'acute lung injury' (ALI) or 'acute respiratory distress syndrome' (ARDS). ALI was defined in 1994 as a syndrome consisting of acute bilateral pulmonary infiltrates on chest X-ray, hypoxaemia (P_aO_2:FiO_2 ratio <40 kPa (<300 mm Hg)), the absence of heart failure or another cardiogenic cause of pulmonary infiltration, and a recognized predisposing condition (Bernard *et al.* 1994). ARDS had the same characteristics as ALI except that the hypoxaemia was worse, defined by a P_aO_2:FiO_2 ratio <26.7 kPa (<200 mmHg), indicating that ≥50% inspired oxygen was required to produce an acceptable P_aO_2. However, it became increasingly clear that these definitions of ALI and ARDS were flawed; the term 'acute' was not defined in terms of a specific timespan, different clinicians interpret X-rays in different ways, and standard treatments such as application of PEEP were not taken into consideration, even though these can have a significant impact on oxygenation.

Lung injury was redefined by an international expert group in 2012 ('the Berlin definition'). They proposed that the term 'acute lung injury' be discontinued and instead there should be descriptors of mild, moderate, or severe ARDS (ARDS Definition Task Force 2012). 'Acute' is now defined as development of the condition within a week of a likely causative event, and infiltrates should not be *wholly* explicable by heart failure or fluid overload, recognizing that patients with a degree of pulmonary hypertension may also have an ARDS pathology. Severe ARDS is indicated by a P_aO_2/FiO2 ratio ≤13.3 kPa (≤100 mmHg).

ARDS is essentially the pulmonary manifestation of organ dysfunction with inflammatory causes. Increased vascular permeability leads to fluid shifts from the pulmonary circulation into the interstitium and alveoli with ingress of inflammatory cells. These effects can be triggered by both infectious and non-infectious insults that may be either specific to the lungs (e.g. pneumonia or pulmonary aspiration) or result from distant conditions (e.g. abdominal sepsis). ARDS was traditionally said to be divided into periods of initial inflammation (an exudative phase) followed by proliferative and fibrotic phases, but these are now recognized to be overlapping rather than discreet. Fibrosis may even begin on the first day of development of ARDS. Fibrosis contributes to decreased lung compliance, as do decreased surfactant production, bleeding into the alveoli, and hyaline membrane formation (Dushianthan *et al.* 2011). These disease processes are compounded by other factors such as ventilator-induced lung injury (Matthay and Zemans 2012). The pulmonary fibrosis that develops in ARDS can take a long time to resolve and may lead to persistent respiratory problems both during weaning and after patients leave hospital. Recovery of lung function is slow; patients typically take up to 3 years to return to baseline performance (Herridge *et al.* 2011).

When assessing patients with ARDS, note their colour, the presence or otherwise of central cyanosis, the respiratory pattern, work of breathing/level of fatigue, mental state, and signs of sweating and distress. Auscultation of lung fields may sound fairly clear or reveal isolated or generalized crackles or wheezes. The volume, colour, and texture of pulmonary secretions should be assessed. There are usually minimal loose white secretions in the early stages of ARDS, but these tend to become more profuse and thicker over time, often due to secondary infection. Specimens should be sent for microbiological culture and serology for both primary pneumonia and secondary infection.

The chest X-ray may initially be relatively normal with clear lung fields or scant infiltrates in early ARDS. There may be unilateral lobar consolidation from a pneumonia, or diffuse lung involvement related to whichever precipitating factors are involved. Over time, interstitial oedema becomes more evident as the picture becomes one of diffuse alveolar infiltrates, sometimes termed a 'white-out'.

Patients are usually hypoxaemic from the early stages of ARDS with S_aO_2 often <90% when breathing room air. Oxygen therapy initially improves the S_aO_2, but non-invasive or invasive mechanical ventilation becomes necessary as gas exchange worsens. In the early stages of ARDS, the P_aCO_2 is generally either normal or low if the patient hyperventilates in response to hypoxaemia; therefore unless there is shock-induced metabolic acidosis and/or renal dysfunction the pH will usually be normal or even slightly raised if P_aCO_2 is reduced. Later on, as the patient tires and respiratory failure worsens,

Box 10.3 Definition of respiratory failure

Blood gases

- PO_2 <8.0 kPa, patient breathing air and at rest
- $\pm PCO_2$ >6.5 kPa in the absence of primary metabolic alkalosis
- ± pH <7.25 in the absence of primary metabolic acidosis.

Patient

- respiratory rate >40 or <6–8 breaths/min
- deteriorating vital capacity (<15 ml/kg).

P_aCO_2 rises and the pH will fall (see Box 10.3). The P_aO_2 remains low despite increased inspired oxygen, even up to an FiO_2 of 1.0.

Pulmonary compliance is reduced in ARDS, with a static compliance <40 ml/cmH_2O in severe cases (ARDS Definition Task Force 2012). Decreased pulmonary compliance increases airway pressures during positive pressure ventilation. Unless the ventilator is set up to limit such pressures, barotrauma and alveolar damage can result. The standard practice is to fix the ventilator so that airway pressures do not exceed 30 cmH_2O.

Pulmonary systolic and diastolic pressures are usually raised in ARDS. This can be measured using a pulmonary artery catheter or by echocardiography. Pulmonary hypertension places strain on the right ventricle (RV) and may bring about RV failure with subsequent haemodynamic deterioration. While well recognized, no studies have investigated the impact on outcomes of treating ARDS-induced pulmonary hypertension.

A retrospective analysis of 1256 patients found that those with mild, moderate, and severe ARDS had mortality rates of 27%, 32%, and 45%, respectively (ARDS Definition Task Force 2012). Of those who survive, pulmonary function may eventually return to normal, but a significant number have reduced exercise tolerance and quality of life five or more years after the original episode of ARDS (Herridge *et al.* 2011). Thus successful patient management requires respiratory support, identification and treatment of precipitating causes, and expert monitoring and prevention of further morbidity over the longer term. Management is covered in the Chapter 4. The aim of respiratory therapy is to reopen and stabilize collapsed but potentially functional alveolar units while minimizing barotrauma and over-distension of other lung areas.

Cardiovascular involvement

A major part of the cardiovascular dysfunction seen in MODS relates to the loss of peripheral vascular autoregulation with loss of vessel tone and vasodilation. There is redistribution of blood flow and decreased oxygen extraction. Fluid leak from the capillaries increases, leading to hypovolaemia, and there is also a depressant effect of inflammatory mediators on myocardial function (Zanotti-Cavazzoni and Hollenberg 2009). Sometimes even young, previously fit patients suffer sepsis-induced cardiogenic shock with very low cardiac output. Troponin levels can be markedly elevated in sepsis and may be considerably higher than those measured after acute myocardial infarction, but, while demonstrating cardiac involvement, this does not necessarily imply severe cardiac damage. Myocardial depression usually reverses within 7–10 days, and the development of chronic heart failure as a consequence is very unusual.

In general, the systemic vascular resistance (afterload) is decreased and cardiac output often increased with a concurrent tachycardia that persists despite adequate fluid resuscitation. Nevertheless, while cardiac output may remain normal or even increased, there is a decrease in ventricular ejection fraction, often with a degree of ventricular dilatation, particularly in the right ventricle (Vieillard-Baron 2011). There may also be an abnormal response to fluid volume loading, with relatively small increases in left ventricular end-diastolic volume and stroke work index for incremental increases in filling pressures (Vieillard-Baron 2011). Again, this is reversible as the patient recovers.

When assessing cardiovascular dysfunction, note the heart rate and rhythm. Tachycardia is commonplace, as are atrial and, occasionally, ventricular dysrhythmias. These rhythm abnormalities may reduce cardiac output and exacerbate hypotension. Blood pressure is a poor indicator of blood flow and the appropriate level for different patients will vary significantly; for example, a patient with chronic hypertension may need a relatively high mean arterial pressure (MAP), whereas a young fit adult may tolerate much lower values. A MAP of at least 60–65 mmHg is usually targeted to maintain the perfusion pressure of vital organs, but it may need to be higher (e.g. in cases of chronic hypertension).

Urine output may be affected as a consequence of decreased renal perfusion and/or direct renal injury. Catheterization and regular measurement of urine output provide a marker of renal perfusion in particular, and of other organs in general. Typically, the aim is to maintain a urine output >0.5 ml/kg/h. However, the quality of the urine produced may be poor and daily measurement of plasma urea and creatinine will be required for more complete assessment of renal function.

Patients with cardiovascular dysfunction undergo central venous catheterization for vascular access as well as for monitoring central venous pressures and central venous oxygen saturation ($S_{cv}O_2$). Rivers *et al.* (2001) found that many patients with what was then termed severe sepsis had subnormal $S_{cv}O_2$ values (<70%) which persisted even after what seemed to be adequate resuscitation, and that such patients had worse outcomes. Consequently, Rivers *et al.* (2001) used early goal-directed therapy to target normal $S_{cv}O_2$ values in a single-centre study, finding that this led to a major improvement in survival. However, three recent large multi-centre trials of this type of approach in the USA (ProCESS), Australasia (ARISE), and the UK (ProMISe) failed to reproduce the benefit, showing no advantage over standard practices (ProCESS Investigators 2014; ARISE Investigators 2014, Mouncey *et al.* 2015).

Echocardiography is increasingly being used to aid patient assessment, and many critical care units also monitor cardiac output either invasively or non-invasively. Cardiac output monitoring enables a more directed optimization of the circulation in terms of ventricular filling and use of vasoactive drugs such as inotropes and vasopressors. However, while intuitively sensible, no trial has yet been performed to definitively demonstrate improved outcomes in critically ill patients through more advanced haemodynamic monitoring.

Biochemical tests routinely used to monitor cardiovascular dysfunction include arterial base deficit and lactate. These are measured by blood gas analysis, using machines that are generally located in critical care areas. While base deficit and lactate are not specific markers of tissue hypoxia, rapidly increasing values are highly suggestive of worsening tissue ischaemia or infarction. However, a high lactate may be related to other causes, such as liver failure or drug side effects (e.g. from epinephrine), and base deficit may also be elevated for reasons other than circulatory failure (e.g. in renal failure or diabetic ketoacidosis). Conversely, a normal blood lactate does not always mean that all organs are adequately perfused; levels at the high end of the normal range have been associated with worse outcomes in critically ill patients presenting to emergency departments. In general, correction of metabolic acidosis should be achieved by treating the underlying cause, particularly by optimizing tissue perfusion if hypoperfusion is present.

Gastrointestinal involvement

Splanchnic hypoperfusion can occur as a consequence of the compensatory mechanisms associated with decreased cardiac output when there is blood flow diversion and local vasoconstriction. This may increase movement—'translocation'—of gut organisms and constituents such as endotoxin from the bowel lumen into the lymphatic system and thus the systemic circulation, and can, in itself, induce systemic inflammation. The importance of gut translocation as a pathological entity has been strongly debated over the years. Its role is still uncertain, but the frequent detection of increased levels of endotoxin in plasma, even in conditions unrelated to Gram-negative infection, does imply that translocation may be a significant process.

Apart from splanchnic hypoperfusion, the gut may be affected by autonomic dysfunction and the adverse effects of drug therapies such as opiates that can induce an ileus. The net effect is an inability to absorb nutrients from the gut with increased gastric aspirates, ileus leading to abdominal distension, and constipation. Diarrhoea is also common, although this is often a consequence of iatrogenic processes such as feed intolerance or overgrowth of pathogenic bacteria, such as *C.difficile*, following antibiotic therapy that eradicates normal gut flora as an unwanted side effect.

Specific areas of the gastrointestinal tract can also be affected. The stomach and upper duodenum may develop 'stress ulcers' that are usually superficial but may, on occasion, be extensive. These are again related to mucosal injury even though gastric acid production tends to be reduced in critical illness. Protective barriers are also lost and there may be concurrent mucosal hypoperfusion. Pancreatitis and acalculous cholecystitis (inflammation unrelated to gallstones) can also develop as stand-alone entities.

Assessing the abdomen should involve observation, palpation, and auscultation. Evidence of distension, discomfort and pain, and the presence of bowel sounds should be sought (see Chapter 9). The patient may feel nauseous or vomit, or have large volumes of aspirate (>200 ml) repeatedly obtained from the nasogastric tube. Note the colour, consistency, and frequency of stool and whether blood (fresh or old) is present in stool or gastric aspirate.

Ultrasound or CT scans can be used to diagnose specific abnormalities such as acalculous cholecystitis as well as to identify fluid collections within the abdomen, distended bowel, perforations, etc. Serum amylase or lipase may be measured to assess the presence of pancreatitis (see Chapter 9).

Liver involvement

Liver dysfunction (marked by hyperbilirubinaemia) is not usually identified using standard tests until several days after other organ dysfunctions are apparent (see Box 10.4). However, more sophisticated tests indicate that it develops much earlier than has been traditionally recognized. When the serum bilirubin exceeds 20 µmol/L there are usually other markers of hepatic dysfunction or injury such as increased hepatic enzymes (see Box 10.5), increased prothrombin time, ascites, or hepatic encephalopathy. The presence of any pre-existing liver disease is likely to lead to liver dysfunction in critical illness.

Underlying mechanisms include tissue hypoperfusion, the effects of inflammatory mediators causing direct injury, and down-regulation of genes encoding proteins involved in metabolism and elimination of waste products and drugs in bile. The mediators may be derived locally, particularly as Kupffer cells (tissue-based macrophages within the liver) are an important first-line defence against gut-derived organisms and bacterial products such as endotoxin translocating from the bowel. The synthetic function of the liver is also affected. e.g., with decreased manufacture of albumin and certain clotting products, although production of acute phase proteins involved in the inflammatory response will increase.

> **Box 10.4 Patient assessment for liver dysfunction**
>
> - Conscious level and neurological status
>   Assess for features of encephalopathy (see Chapter 9). This may be related to acute liver dysfunction, but other factors such as excessive sedation (particularly with reduced hepatic clearance) or a past history of liver disease should also be considered.
> - Conjunctival and skin colour
>   Observe for a yellow tinge indicating jaundice (see Chapter 9).
> - Skin, mucous membranes, and invasive line sites
>   Inspect these daily for evidence of coagulation abnormalities which give rise to bleeding from gums, purpura, bleeding from line sites, etc.
> - Urinalysis
>   Urinalysis may be done to check bilirubin levels.
> - Liver function tests
>   These should be performed at least every 2–3 days in the acute phase.
> - Clotting tests
>   These should be performed daily.

> **Box 10.5 Clinical markers of hepatic dysfunction**
>
> - Raised serum bilirubin (>20–30 µmol/L) (jaundice)
> - Raised AST and LDH (at least twice normal levels)
> - Abnormal prothrombin time or INR
> - Hepatic encephalopathy

Effects of liver dysfunction

The demands placed on the liver's metabolic functions (see Chapter 9) during the hypermetabolic phase are enormous. In conjunction with this, the combined effect of circulating inflammatory mediators and hypoperfusion on hepatic cell function is potentially highly damaging. The result is deranged carbohydrate, protein, and lipid metabolism, a dysfunctional immune response, reduced protein synthesis, and impaired detoxification processes (see Table 10.3).

Renal involvement

Renal dysfunction generally results from either circulatory failure and decreased renal perfusion, or a direct renal effect induced by toxins or inflammatory mediators. Notably, kidney histology (cell structure) usually remains remarkably normal. This suggests the possibility of a 'programmed metabolic shutdown' of kidney cells in response to a prolonged insult which then allows subsequent recovery of renal function once the sepsis or other disease process has resolved, i.e. the cells 'hibernate' as a response to ischaemia (Mongardon *et al.* 2009). Full details of the pathogenesis of acute kidney injury in critical illness are given in Chapter 7 (see Box 10.6 for assessments of renal involvement).

Typically, the clinical course of renal dysfunction has four phases.

1. Onset: a potentially reversible stage—if perfusion is restored, lasting hours to days depending on the cause. The disease course following ischaemic causes is generally shorter than for toxic causes.
2. Oliguric–anuric phase: lasts 1–6 weeks. The glomerular filtration rate is significantly reduced with a tendency to total body fluid overload, high blood urea and plasma creatinine levels, electrolyte abnormalities, and metabolic acidosis. Evidence of uraemic symptoms may be present.

Table 10.3 Effects of the dysregulated systemic inflammatory response/sepsis on liver function

Liver function	Effect of dysregulated systemic inflammatory response/sepsis
Protein metabolism	Increased rate of gluconeogenesis Concomitant rises in protein catabolism and urea production Increased urinary nitrogen excretion Decreased clearance of amino acids resulting in raised phenylalanine and tyrosine
Lipid metabolism	Lipolysis and lipogenesis may occur, resulting in: (a) high levels of serum lipids (b) decreased peripheral lipid clearance Reduced hepatocyte utilization of ketones produced from lipid conversion
Hepatic protein synthesis	Increased synthesis of acute-phase reactant proteins Decreased synthesis of albumin and transferrin Depletion of fibronectin (enhances phagocytosis) levels
Detoxification of drugs, toxins, and hormones	Increased levels of hormones normally detoxified by the liver (e.g. ADH, aldosterone) Higher serum levels, prolonged duration of action, and increased toxicity may occur with drugs normally metabolized by the liver
Clotting factors	Bleeding and DIC may be accentuated by limited removal of activated clotting factors Reduced clotting factor synthesis

3. Diuretic phase: an increased urine output is accompanied by a gradual improvement in renal function. Urine output may be more than 2–3 L/day in this period with little or no evidence of concentration or excretion. Gradually, the urinary urea increases and sodium falls. Acidosis and electrolyte imbalance begin to improve.
4. Recovery phase: glomerular filtration usually returns to at least 70–80% of normal within 1–2 years. Mild to moderate residual renal dysfunction may remain, though the need for long-term dialysis is rare if the kidneys were previously healthy.

Box 10.6 Patient assessment for renal involvement

The patient should be assessed for:

- oedema (peripheral and pulmonary), nausea, vomiting, pruritis, and other symptoms of uraemia
- urine output (the standard aim is > 0.5 ml/kg/h)
- urinalysis for specific gravity, protein, glucose, and blood ± urinary sodium and urea, ± urine and plasma osmolality
- blood urea
- plasma creatinine
- blood potassium
- blood pH
- intravascular fluid volume status.

Haematological involvement

The manifestations of coagulopathy most commonly seen in MODS are as follows.

1. Bleeding from line sites and wounds due to depletion of clotting factors.
2. Bleeding into the skin, ranging from petechiae to gross echymosis as well as bleeding from mucosa and gums.
3. Stress and peptic ulceration, and other causes of gastrointestinal bleeding (see Box 10.7).

Box 10.7 Patient assessment for haematological involvement

Observe/assess:

- skin for evidence of petechiae, purpura, bruising, and haematomas
- gums and mucous membranes for bleeding
- sclera and conjunctiva
- sites of any invasive devices or wounds for bleeding
- sputum during endotracheal suctioning for blood
- urinalysis for evidence of haematuria
- stools for evidence of melaena
- nasogastric aspirate for evidence of upper gastrointestinal bleeding
- blood tests including measurement of haemoglobin, platelet count, INR or prothrombin time, thrombin time, d-dimers, fibrinogen, partial thromboplastin time (PTT).

Disseminated intravascular coagulation (DIC) represents the severe end of a continuum of dysfunction of the haematological system. It arises from a pathological over-stimulation of normal coagulation that paradoxically causes both microvascular thrombi (thus depleting normal stores of clotting factors and activating the fibrinolytic system) and bleeding due to the resultant lack of clotting factors and overactive fibrinolysis (see Chapter 12). Although DIC occurs as a result of almost any severe disease process, there are a number of specific factors which predispose to its development in sepsis, namely arterial hypotension, inadequate tissue perfusion, and stasis of capillary blood flow.

Priorities and principles of management of sepsis

Internationally agreed guidelines for the management of what were then termed severe sepsis and septic shock were published by the Surviving Sepsis Campaign in 2013 (Dellinger *et al.* 2013). These still provide a useful overview of many of the key issues, although it should be stressed that the various recommendations have different levels of supportive evidence, depending on the quality of the available research. Furthermore, the guidelines will need to be revised following publication of the new Sepsis Definitions in 2016. Table 10.4 gives a summary of manifestations of organ failure associated with MODS.

Table 10.4 Summary of manifestations of organ failure in MODS

System	Manifestation
Neuromuscular	Encephalopathy Peripheral neuropathy Peripheral myopathy
Respiratory system	Acute respiratory distress syndrome (ARDS)
Renal system	Acute kidney injury
Gastrointestinal	Pancreatitis Gastric and intestinal stasis or hypokinesis Acalculous cholecystitis Stress ulceration and gastrointestinal bleeding
Hepatobiliary	Elevation in liver function enzymes to more than twice normal levels Serum bilirubin >20–30 times Prolonged INR or PT
Cardiovascular	Decreased response to catecholamines Loss of microvascular regulatory tone, peripheral vasodilatation Central myocardial depression
Coagulation	Thrombocytopenia Clinical evidence of bleeding Disseminated intravascular coagulation (DIC)
Neuroendocrine	Altered growth hormone release in prolonged critical illness Altered anterior pituitary function

Priorities

As with any critical illness initial resuscitation entails assessment and support of the airway, breathing, and circulation, aiming to avoid or minimize those insults capable of triggering the immune/inflammatory response, particularly hypoxaemia and organ hypoperfusion.

- **Airway** A patent airway is likely to be threatened in the patient who is comatose. Aspiration is also a high risk in the obtunded patient. In such cases, pre-emptive intubation should be considered earlier rather than later.
- **Breathing** Oxygen therapy and, if necessary, ventilatory support should be instituted to maintain oxygen saturation, ideally ≥94% in most patients. If ventilation is required, the aim is to minimize the risk of barotrauma with limitation of airway pressures (plateau pressures ≤30 cmH_2O) and relatively low tidal volumes (≤6–8 ml/kg of ideal body weight) (See Chapter 4). This approach may mean that some degree of respiratory acidosis is accepted rather than aggressively treated (permissive hypercapnia).
- **Circulation** The main aim is the rapid restoration of organ perfusion and perfusion pressure. Initially, the circulating volume should be optimized using fluid challenges (e.g. with aliquots of 200 ml, typically aiming to administer ≥30 ml/kg of fluid if there are signs of hypovolaemia and hypoperfusion (Dellinger *et al.* 2013)) with serial measurements of cardiac filling pressures and/or stroke volume. No clear benefit—and some suggestions of harm—has been found with synthetic colloids (particularly starch-based fluids), so current guidelines recommend crystalloid solutions (or human albumin). If adequate fluid loading does not restore perfusion pressure, vasopressor drugs are required (norepinephrine) to combat gross vasodilation, or inotropes (e.g. epinephrine, dobutamine, levosimendan) if there is severe myocardial depression.

Early interventions

Once airway, breathing, and circulation are stabilized, any injuries should be actively treated with particular attention to the removal of any necrotic tissue, debridement of eschar from burns or other insults, and stabilization of fractures if present. Drainage of any infected collections or abscesses is also a priority, as these can form a focus for further stimulation of the inflammatory/immune response. Further soft tissue damage and inflammation should be minimized, so scrupulous attention to skin integrity and avoidance of pressure damage is essential.

Blood, urine, and other cultures, such as cerebrospinal fluid (CSF), pleural fluid, or pus collections, should be sent to microbiology to attempt identification of any source of sepsis—ideally before the first doses of any antibiotics are given (although if antibiotics are indicated, there should be no significant delay in administration). Appropriate antibiotics should be prescribed and administered promptly, either as broad-spectrum cover prior to microbiological results being obtained, or according to culture sensitivities if these are available.

Ensuring adequate oxygenation

A crucial objective is the maintenance of tissue perfusion and oxygenation. As noted earlier, there are three distinct pathophysiological problems:

- maldistribution of circulating volume
- imbalance of oxygen supply and demand
- altered metabolism.

All can affect the ability of the cardiovascular system to respond to any increase in tissue oxygen requirements.

In addition, myocardial depressant factors associated with the inflammatory response may further reduce cardiac output.

Monitoring circulatory disturbances

Effective haemodynamic monitoring can establish the extent of cardiovascular derangement. Ideally, the patient should have some form of blood flow monitoring to allow measurement of cardiac output and other variables. The aim is to achieve an adequate mean arterial pressure (usually ≥65 mmHg but possibly lower in younger or previously very fit patients or higher in chronic hypertensives) to normalize blood lactate (<2.0 mmol/L) and, if possible, to maintain urine output ≥0.5 ml/kg/h and ensure effective cerebral perfusion. Markers of adequate renal perfusion also include measures of blood urea and creatinine. Markers of adequate cerebral perfusion are more difficult to obtain but levels of consciousness/alertness are useful indicators if the patient is not fully sedated and/or paralyzed with neuromuscular blockers. (See Chapter 5 for more details.)

Optimizing intravascular fluid volume

Early adequate resuscitation of the circulation can reduce the morbidity and mortality of sepsis. This concept is a central component of the Surviving Sepsis Campaign guidelines (Dellinger *et al.* 2013). Following the failure of Rivers' early goal-directed therapy strategy to show outcome benefit in two recently published trials, it is unclear what precise values should be targeted. However, it is reasonable to expect prompt restoration of adequate organ perfusion and an adequate blood pressure. Serial measurements of stroke volume/cardiac output can be used to assess the response to fluid resuscitation (see Chapter 5). The aim is to continue volume loading until the stroke volume shows no further improvement, i.e. so that the heart is adequately filled in order to pump an optimal volume of blood with least effort or additional support. An alternative dynamic challenge is to stop fluid loading when the central venous pressure has risen by >3 mmHg in response to a 200–250 ml fluid challenge. There are sometimes exceptions to this approach, for example in cases of severe ARDS when intravascular volume loading may be less aggressive in an effort to reduce extracapillary fluid shift and worsening pulmonary oedema.

Vasoactive drug support

If volume loading does not achieve the required goals, vasopressors or inotropes may be added. Vasopressors (e.g. norepinephrine) are used in high output states when there is low systemic vascular resistance (as is typically seen in sepsis). Inotropes (e.g. epinephrine, dobutamine, levosimendan) are given for low output states. There is no strong evidence base to support any of these therapies but it is generally advisable to use the lowest dose compatible with achieving the desired level of organ perfusion and blood pressure. Excessive sedation should be avoided, as these drugs have vasodilator and/or cardiac depressant effects. Vasopressin or its synthetic analogue terlipressin can be used to supplement norepinephrine in high output states. A side effect of these potent vasoconstrictors is ischaemia affecting digital, mesenteric, or myocardial vascular systems which may lead on to infarction. Such complications are more common in patients with low output states.

Ventilatory management

Physical measures supporting gas exchange and alternative modes of ventilation can be employed to achieve the aims of:

- maintaining oxygen saturations—usually ≥90%,
- minimizing the incidence of barotrauma by keeping airway plateau pressures below 30 cmH_2O.

See Chapter 4 for more details on the management of ARDS.

Metabolic management

Severe derangements should be corrected, although some degree of abnormality may be tolerated. Temperature control is contentious. Some relatively weak evidence suggests that hypothermia may be deleterious, and that a degree of fever may be beneficial as this is an intrinsic body mechanism that is both bacteriocidal and triggers production of protective heat shock proteins. On the other hand, very high temperatures may be harmful. A reasonable compromise is to aim to keep the core temperature between 36.5 and 39°C.

Blood glucose levels should be kept below 10 mmol/L, if necessary with a titrated infusion of insulin. However, hypoglycaemia should be avoided. Aggressive control of blood glucose—maintaining blood glucose levels at 4.4–6.1 mmol/L (van den Berghe *et al.* 2001)—was found to be unsafe in a multi-centre trial (NICE-SUGAR Study Investigators 2009). Blood glucose levels should initially be checked frequently (e.g. every 1–2 hours), and approximately four-hourly thereafter provided that levels are stable.

Renal management

Diuretics have no effect on improving renal function but can play a useful role in managing fluid balance by increasing urine volumes (see Chapter 7). Renal replacement therapy (RRT) can be used in cases of significant renal dysfunction and to manage severe acidaemia, hyperkalaemia, and fluid overload. There are currently no data to support the use of early RRT. Nephrotoxic and hepatotoxic medicines should be avoided or dosages reduced, with drug levels monitored where possible (e.g. gentamicin).

Gastrointestinal management

Prophylaxis against gastrointestinal bleeding using proton pump inhibitors or H_2 antagonists may be considered, particularly for patients with coagulopathies. However, these agents are associated with increased risks of ventilator-associated pneumonia and *C.difficile* infection, so the risk–benefit ratio for a particular patient needs to be carefully assessed. Restoration and maintenance of adequate organ perfusion is essential.

Provision of appropriate nutrition, based on the individual's requirements, and monitoring and maintenance of electrolyte and trace element levels should be implemented. The enteral route is preferable provided that there is little or no damage or dysfunction of the gastrointestinal tract. Patients not tolerating enteral feed due to large aspirates, abdominal distension, or diarrhoea have a higher mortality; whether this is a reflection of the severity of the underlying illness or direct harm from attempting to feed a dysfunctional gut (with or without the use of prokinetics) remains uncertain. Unless the patient has severe malnutrition, patients not tolerating enteral feed can be starved for up to five days, although hypoglycaemia has to be corrected if present. Parenteral nutrition is an alternative, although in a multi-centre trial early parenteral nutrition started within 48 hours of admission was associated with more complications and a slower recovery rate (Casaer *et al.* 2011).

Haematological support

It has become a standard that haemoglobin levels should be maintained above 70 g/L in critical care (Hébert *et al.* 1999), although it is uncertain whether a 70 g/L threshold should apply to patients with coexisting ischaemic heart disease or ongoing myocardial ischaemia (Hébert *et al.* 2001). A recent multi-centre Scandinavian study in septic shock patients showed no benefit between transfusion thresholds of 70 and 90 g/L.

Severe clotting abnormalities should be corrected to 'acceptably abnormal' levels using fresh frozen plasma, clotting factors, platelet transfusions, etc. In general, a platelet count ≥20 × 10^9/L is acceptable in sepsis if there is no active bleeding, or ≥50 × 10^9/L if bleeding is present. Likewise, an INR up to 1.5–2 times normal is acceptable if there is no active bleeding.

Infection management

Any focus of infection—such as an abscess—should be located and drained. Prevention of secondary infection is essential and strict asepsis, scrupulous care of intravenous cannulae and other invasive devices, and all aspects of infection control should be observed. It should be noted that, contradicting what has become standard practice, a recent meta-analysis found that the use of chlorhexidine mouthwash was implicated in worse outcomes (Price *et al.* 2014).

Musculoskeletal

Pressure areas should be protected from damage by position change where possible and/or special support beds where necessary. Frequent changes in position are also likely to be beneficial for ventilation. Early passive movements and mobilization will assist in preventing contractures and decreased range of movement, and in preserving muscle bulk.

Adjunctive therapies

There have been many encouraging reports of novel treatments that have led to nothing. Numerous agents that modulate inflammatory, immune, coagulant, hormonal, and metabolic pathways have been trialled, but none are currently licensed for use in critical illness. Activated protein C therapy, which offered a combination of anti-inflammatory and anti-coagulant effects, was awarded a licence after an initial positive study (ProWESS) but the drug was subsequently withdrawn after a repeat multi-centre study failed to show any benefit (ProWESS-SHOCK). The complexity of the sepsis process makes it very unlikely that there will be a single therapeutic remedy, and much more work is required to fully understand the mechanisms involved, to clarify the effects of each treatment, and to determine optimal timing and dosing. Until these goals are achieved and genuinely effective interventions are identified, the mainstay of patient care will remain the support of failing organs and the prevention of complications.

Corticosteroids

Annane *et al.* (2002) showed improved survival with 'low dose' hydrocortisone and fludrocortisone in a subset of septic shock patients whose cortisol levels did not respond to ACTH stimulation. However, the subsequent CORTICUS trial, although confirming the finding of earlier cessation of catecholamine therapy with steroid therapy, failed to show any survival benefit (Sprung *et al.* 2008). Post hoc analysis suggested benefit in those requiring high levels of norepinephrine. Current recommendations are that corticosteroid therapy should only be considered in septic shock patients where standard fluid and vasoactive agent regimens have failed to achieve adequate cardiovascular performance (Dellinger *et al.* 2013).

Blood purification techniques

Extracorporeal techniques that remove circulating mediators and toxins have been tested, although mainly in small single-centre studies. Such techniques include plasmapheresis (plasma exchange) that replaces the patient's plasma with fresh frozen plasma (containing potentially beneficial substances). This type of treatment is used with good effect in the removal of harmful antibodies in thrombotic thrombocytopenic purpura

(TTP), Guillain–Barré syndrome, and myasthenia gravis, but at present trials in sepsis are limited. Adsorbers (i.e. filters that bind mediators and/or toxins) have also been tested. Examples include polymyxin B, which showed benefit in a small multi-centre study of 64 patients (Cruz *et al.* 2009), and Cytosorb. However, a recent multi-centre study of coupled plasma filtration adsorption in 192 septic shock patients failed to show any benefit (Livigni *et al.* 2014).

Targeted immunomodulatory therapies

Many therapies targeting specific toxins (e.g. endotoxin) or mediators (e.g. cytokines, such as tumour necrosis factor and interleukin 1, or nitric oxide) have been studied in large multi-centre Phase III studies; all have failed to show outcome benefit and some have even been stopped early because of harm. This is despite promising animal and small scale patient studies. It is being increasingly recognized that a 'one size fits all' approach giving a fixed dosing regimen of drug to a highly variable patient population who differ not only in terms of sepsis source but also in their pro-inflammatory–anti-inflammatory balance is too simplistic. A more targeted approach using biomarkers to identify suitable patients and titrate treatment appropriately is increasingly seen as a more rational approach. However, development of such diagnostics has traditionally lagged behind novel pharmaceutical therapies. Nevertheless, in recent years there has been a marked effort to find new biomarkers that will be available even as point-of-care tests. For example, patients who are immunosuppressed by critical illness could be identified by relatively rapid testing (e.g. testing of decreased monocyte HLA–DR expression) and then given an immune-stimulatory agent such as interferon-gamma, granulocyte macrophage–colony stimulating factor (GM–CSF), or interleukin-7 (IL-7), as well as co-inhibitory molecule blockade (e.g. anti-programmed cell death receptor-1 (anti-PD-1) antibody).

Antioxidants

As damaging reactive oxygen species are produced in excess in sepsis, these appear to be a reasonable therapeutic target. ROS can damage proteins, cell membranes, and DNA, and can alter membrane fluidity, secretory function, and ionic gradients. On the other hand, they play an important role in combating invading pathogens. Endogenous antioxidants that regulate ROS activity can be overwhelmed in sepsis, so the potential for damage by excessive oxidative stress increases. Various antioxidant therapies have been tested, including selenium and glutamine. However, to date none have shown benefit and some have even shown harm, such as the recent Reducing Deaths Due to Oxidative Stress (REDOXS) study in which patients receiving high doses of glutamine had an increased mortality (Heyland *et al.* 2013). Antioxidants targeted to mitochondria may be more effective (Galley 2011).

References and bibliography

Acute Respiratory Distress Syndrome Network (2000). Ventilation with lower tidal volumes as compared with traditional tidal volumes for acute lung injury and the acute respiratory distress syndrome. *New England Journal of Medicine*, **342**, 1301–8.

Annane, D., Sébille, V., Charpentier, C., *et al.* (2002). Effect of treatment with low doses of hydrocortisone and fludrocortisone on mortality in patients with septic shock. *JAMA*, **288**, 862–71.

Annane, D., Sébille, V., Troché, G, *et al.* (2000). A 3-level prognostic classification in septic shock based on cortisol levels and cortisol response to corticotropin. *JAMA*, **283**, 1038–45.

Anon. (1992). American College of Chest Physicians/Society of Critical Care Medicine Consensus Conference. Definitions for sepsis and organ failure and guidelines for the use of innovative therapies in sepsis. *Critical Care Medicine*, **20**, 864–74.

ARDS Definition Task Force (2012). Acute respiratory distress syndrome: the Berlin Definition. *JAMA*, **307**, 2526–33.

ARISE Investigators (2014). Goal-directed resuscitation for patients with early septic shock. *New England Journal of Medicine*, **371**, 1496–1506.

Bednarik, J., Lukas, Z., Vondracek, P. (2003). Critical illness polyneuromyopathy: the electrophysiological components of a complex entity. *Intensive Care Medicine*, **29**, 1505–14.

Bernard, G.R., Artigas, A., Brigham, K.L., *et al.* (1994). The American–European Consensus Conference on ARDS. Definitions, mechanisms, relevant outcomes, and clinical trial coordination. *American Journal of Respiratory & Critical Care Medicine*, **149**, 818–24.

Bernard, G.R., Vincent, J.L., Laterre, P.F., *et al.* (2001). Efficacy and safety of recombinant human activated protein C for severe sepsis. *New England Journal of Medicine*, **344**, 699–709.

Bradley, J.R. (2008). TNF-mediated inflammatory disease. *Journal of Pathology*, **214**, 149–60.

Brealey, D., Brand, M., Hargreaves, I., *et al.* (2002). Association between mitochondrial dysfunction and severity and outcome of septic shock. *Lancet*, **360**, 219–23.

Casaer, M.P., Mesotten, D., Hermans, G., *et al.* (2011). Early versus late parenteral nutrition in critically ill adults. *New England Journal of Medicine*, **365**, 506–17.

Cinel, I., Opal, S.M. (2009). Molecular biology of inflammation and sepsis: a primer. *Critical Care Medicine*, **37**, 291–304.

Combes, A., Bacchetta, M., Brodie, D., *et al.* (2012). Extracorporeal membrane oxygenation for respiratory failure in adults. *Current Opinion in Critical Care*, **18**, 99–104.

Creteur, J., De Backer, D., Sakr, Y., *et al.* (2006). Sublingual capnometry tracks microcirculatory changes in septic patients. *Intensive Care Medicine*, **32**, 516–23.

Cruz, D.N., Antonelli, M., Fumagalli, R., *et al.* (2009). Early use of polymyxin B hemoperfusion in abdominal septic shock: the EUPHAS randomized controlled trial. *JAMA*, **301**, 2445–52.

Dellinger, R.P., Levy, M.M., Rhodes, A., *et al.* (2013). Surviving Sepsis Campaign: International Guidelines for Management of Severe Sepsis and Septic Shock: 2012. *Critical Care Medicine*. **41**, 580–637; *Intensive Care Medicine*, **39**, 165–228.

Dushianthan, A., Grocott, M.P., Postle, A.D., *et al.* (2011). Acute respiratory distress syndrome and acute lung injury. *Postgraduate Medical Journal*, **87**, 612–22.

Ferguson, N.D., Cook, D.J., Guyatt, G.H., *et al.* (2013). High-frequency oscillation in early acute respiratory distress syndrome. *New England Journal of Medicine*, **368**, 795–805.

Flierl, M.A., Rittirsch, D., Huber-Lang, M.S., *et al.* (2010). Pathophysiology of septic encephalopathy--an unsolved puzzle. *Critical Care*, **14**, 165.

Gaieski, D.F., Edwards, J.M., Kallan, M.J., Carr, B. (2013). Benchmarking the incidence and mortality of severe sepsis in the United States. *Critical Care Medicine*, **41**, 1167–74.

Galley, H.F. (2011). Oxidative stress and mitochondrial dysfunction in sepsis. *British Journal of Anaesthesia*, **107**, 57–64.

Gofton, T.E., Young, G.B. (2012). Sepsis-associated encephalopathy. *Nature Reviews Neurology*, **8**, 557–66.

Guérin, C., Reignier, J., Richard, J.C., *et al.* (2013). Prone positioning in severe acute respiratory distress syndrome. *New England Journal of Medicine*, **368**, 2159–68.

Hébert, P.C., Wells, G., Blajchman, M.A., *et al.* (1999). A multicenter, randomized, controlled clinical trial of transfusion requirements in critical care. Transfusion Requirements in Critical Care Investigators, Canadian Critical Care Trials Group. *New England Journal of Medicine*. **340**, 409–17.

Hébert, P.C., Yetisir, E., Martin, C., *et al.* (2001). Is a low transfusion threshold safe in critically ill patients with cardiovascular diseases? *Critical Care Medicine*, **29**, 227–34.

Hermans, G., De Jonghe, B., Bruyninckx, F., *et al.* (2008). Clinical review: Critical illness polyneuropathy and myopathy. *Critical Care*, **12**, 238.

Herridge, M.S., Tansey, C.M., Matté, A., *et al.* (2011). Functional disability 5 years after acute respiratory distress syndrome. *New England Journal of Medicine*, **364**, 1293–304.

Heyland, D., Muscedere, J., Wischmeyer, P.E., *et al.* (2013). A randomized trial of glutamine and antioxidants in critically ill patients. *New England Journal of Medicine*, **368**, 1489–97.

Hotchkiss, R.S., Monneret, G., Payen, D. (2013). Immunosuppression in sepsis: a novel understanding of the disorder and a new therapeutic approach. *Lancet Infectious Diseases*, **13**, 260–8.

Holst, L.B., Haase, N., Wetterslev, J., *et al.* (2014). Lower versus higher hemoglobin threshold for transfusion in septic shock. *New England Journal of Medicine*, **371**, 1381–91.

Lagu, T., Rothberg, M.B., Shieh, M.S., *et al.* (2012). Hospitalizations, costs, and outcomes of severe sepsis in the United States 2003 to 2007. *Critical Care Medicine*, **40**, 754–61.

Langouche, L., van den Berghe, G. (2006). The dynamic neuroendocrine response to critical illness. *Endocrinology and Metabolism Clinics of North America*, **35**, 777–91, ix.

Latronico, N., Shehu, I., Seghelini, E. (2005). Neuromuscular sequelae of critical illness. *C***11**, 381–90.

Levy, M.M., Fink, M.P., Marshall, J.C., *et al.* (2003). 2001 SCCM/ESICM/ACCP/ATS/SIS International Sepsis Definitions Conference. *Critical Care Medicine*, **31**, 1250–6; *Intensive Care Medicine*, **29**, 530–8.

Livigni, S., Bertolini, G., Rossi, C, *et al.* (2014). Efficacy of coupled plasma filtration adsorption (CPFA) in patients with septic shock: a multicenter randomised controlled clinical trial. *BMJ Open*, **4**, e003536.

Matthay, M.A, Zemans, R.L. (2011). The acute respiratory distress syndrome: pathogenesis and treatment. *Annual Reviews of Pathology*, **6**, 147–63.

Mongardon, N., Dyson, A., Singer, M. (2009). Is MOF an outcome parameter or a transient, adaptive state in critical illness? *Current Opinion in Critical Care*, **15**, 431–6.

Mouncey, P.R., Osborn, T.M., Power, G.S., *et al.* (2015). Trial of early, goal-directed resuscitation for septic shock. *New England Journal of Medicine*, **372**, 1301–11.

NICE-SUGAR Study Investigators (2009). Intensive versus conventional glucose control in critically ill patients. *New England Journal of Medicine*, **360**, 1283–97.

Nichol, A., Bailey, M., Egi, M., *et al.* (2011). Dynamic lactate indices as predictors of outcome in critically ill patients. *Critical Care*, **15**(5), R242.

Oddo, M., Carrera, E., Claassen, J., *et al.* (2009). Continuous electroencephalography in the medical intensive care unit. *Critical Care Medicine*, **37**, 2051–6.

Peek, G.J., Mugford, M., Tiruvoipati, R., *et al.* (2009). Efficacy and economic assessment of conventional ventilatory support versus extracorporeal membrane oxygenation for severe adult respiratory failure (CESAR): a multicentre randomised controlled trial. *Lancet*, **374**, 1351–63.

Price, R., MacLennan, G., Glen. J. SuDDICU Collaboration (2014). Selective digestive or oropharyngeal decontamination and topical oropharyngeal chlorhexidine for prevention of death in general intensive care: systematic review and network meta-analysis. *BMJ*, **348**, g2197.

ProCESS Investigators (2014). A randomized trial of protocol-based care for early septic shock. *New England Journal of Medicine*, **370**, 1683–93

Ranieri, V.M., Thompson, B.T., Barie, P.S., *et al.* (2012). Drotrecogin alfa (activated) in adults with septic shock. *New England Journal of Medicine*, **366**, 2055–64.

Rimmelé, T., Kellum, J.A. (2011). Clinical review: blood purification for sepsis. *Critical Care*, **15**, 205.

Sakr, Y., Lobo, S.M., Moreno, R., *et al.* (2012). Patterns and early evolution of organ failure in the intensive care unit and their relation to outcome. *Critical Care*, **16**, R222.

Scully, M., Hunt, B.J., Benjamin, S., *et al.* (2012). Guidelines on the diagnosis and management of thrombotic thrombocytopenic purpura and other thrombotic microangiopathies. *British Journal of Haematology*, **158**, 323–35.

Shahin, J., Harrison, D.A., Rowan, K.M. (2012). Relation between volume and outcome for patients with severe sepsis in United Kingdom: retrospective cohort study. *BMJ*, **344**, e3394.

Sharshar, T., Hopkinson, N.S., Orlikowski, D., *et al.* (2005). Science review: The brain in sepsis—culprit and victim. *Critical Care*, **9**, 37–44.

Shi, Z., Xie, H., Wang, P., *et al.* (2013). Oral hygiene care for critically ill patients to prevent ventilator-associated pneumonia. *Cochrane Database of Systematic Reviews*, **8**, CD008367.

Spieth, P.M., Gama de Abreu, M. (2012). Lung recruitment in ARDS: we are still confused, but on a higher PEEP level. *Critical Care*, **16**, 108.

Sprung, C.L., Annane, D., Keh, D., *et al.* (2008). Hydrocortisone therapy for patients with septic shock. *New England Journal of Medicine*, **358**, 111–24.

van den Berghe, G., Wouters, P., Weekers, F., *et al.* (2001). Intensive insulin therapy in critically ill patients. *New England Journal of Medicine*, **345**, 1359–67.

van der Meer, J.W. (2013). The infectious disease challenges of our time. *Frontiers of Public Health*, **1**, 7.

Vieillard-Baron, A. (2011). Septic cardiomyopathy. *Annals of Intensive Care*, **1**, 6.

Vincent, J.L., Moreno, R., Takala, J., *et al.* (1996). The SOFA (Sepsis-related Organ Failure Assessment) score to describe organ dysfunction/failure. *Intensive Care Medicine*, **22**, 707–10.

Vincent, J.L., Sakr, Y., Sprung, C.L., *et al.* (2006). Sepsis in European intensive care units: results of the SOAP study. *Critical Care Medicine*, **34**, 344–53.

Vincent, J.L., Rello, J., Marshall, J., *et al.* (2009). International study of the prevalence and outcomes of infection in intensive care units. *JAMA*, **302**, 2323–9.

Vincent, J.L., Martinez, E.O., Silva, E. (2011). Evolving concepts in sepsis definitions. *Critical Care Nursing Clinics of North America*, **23**, 29–39.

Vincent, J.L., Opal, S.M., Marshall, J.C., *et al.* (2013). Sepsis definitions: time for change. *Lancet*, **381**, 774–5.

Volakli, E., Spies, C., Michalopoulos, A., *et al.* (2010). Infections of respiratory or abdominal origin in ICU patients: what are the differences? *Critical Care*, **14**, R32.

Ward, P.A. (2008). Sepsis, apoptosis and complement. *Biochemical Pharmacology*, **76**, 1383–8.

Winters, B.D., Eberlein, M., Leung, J., *et al.* (2010). Long-term mortality and quality of life in sepsis: a systematic review. *Critical Care Medicine*, **38**, 1276–83.

Yost, C.C., Weyrich, A.S., Zimmerman, G.A. (2010). The platelet activating factor (PAF) signalling cascade in systemic inflammatory responses. *Biochimie*, **92**, 692–7.

Young, D., Lamb, S.E., Shah, S., *et al.* (2013). High-frequency oscillation for acute respiratory distress syndrome. *New England Journal of Medicine*, **368**, 806–13.

Zanotti-Cavazzoni, S.L., Hollenberg, S.M. (2009). Cardiac dysfunction in severe sepsis and septic shock. *Current Opinion in Critical Care*, **15**, 392–7.

CHAPTER 11
Trauma and major haemorrhage

Introduction

Management of the trauma patient demands considerable skill from the many disciplines involved in patient care. Injuries may range from single-organ damage to severe multiple injuries, with initial management being centred on the immediate identification of life-threatening injuries and maintenance of the airway, breathing, and circulation. Continuous reassessment of the patient's clinical state and adequate monitoring of vital signs are essential from the moment the patient arrives in the emergency department.

The aim of continuous reassessment and intensive monitoring is the early detection of deterioration and the prevention of secondary complications. There are four stages in the initial management of the trauma patient:

(1) primary survey
(2) resuscitation phase
(3) secondary survey
(4) definitive care phase.

These strategies begin at the scene of the trauma and continue until the patient is stabilized prior to transfer to the critical care unit.

Primary survey

This is conducted at the scene by pre-hospital staff and continues on arrival in the emergency department. As the primary survey is concerned with identification and management of life-threatening injuries, the following areas must be *simultaneously* assessed:

- Airway maintenance and cervical spine control
- Breathing and ventilation
- Circulation and haemorrhage control
- Dysfunction of the central nervous system—neurological status
- Exposure—the patient is completely undressed for rapid assessment of injuries.

The patient's vital functions must be assessed quickly and treatment priorities established.

Airway

A patent airway must be established by chin-lift or jaw-thrust manoeuvres. Debris, blood clots, and loose-fitting false teeth should be removed from the mouth. High flow oxygen therapy should be immediately instituted by facemask to restore or maintain an adequate oxygen saturation, if required. Endotracheal intubation, or an emergency cricothyroidotomy or tracheostomy, may be required to maintain a patent airway. The possibility of cervical spine injuries should always be suspected, particularly in patients with multiple trauma or blunt trauma above the clavicle, including whiplash injuries. If a neck injury is a possibility, the patient's head should not be hyperextended to maintain the airway. This is easier to assess in an awake mentally competent patient who can denote neck pain on palpation or self-movement, but particular care needs to be applied to the unconscious or obtunded patient.

Breathing

The chest must be exposed to assess respiratory movement as ventilation may be impaired even though the patient has a patent airway. The following are the most common traumatic conditions that compromise ventilation and must be considered if ventilation is inadequate:

- tension pneumothorax
- open pneumothorax
- large haemothorax
- flail chest with pulmonary contusions
- severe head injuries
- severe blood loss resulting in decreased perfusion of brain, heart, and respiratory muscles.

Circulation

A rapid assessment of the patient's haemodynamic status is essential. Initial observations include heart rate, blood pressure, skin colour and capillary return, and evidence of organ hypoperfusion (e.g. obtunded conscious level). Hypotension following trauma is presumed to be due to hypovolaemia until proved otherwise. External haemorrhage should be controlled by direct pressure on the wound or by the use of pneumatic splints. Pneumatic antishock garments may be useful in controlling haemorrhage from injuries to the abdomen and lower extremities. Haemorrhage into the thoracic and abdominal cavities, and around fracture sites, may account for major blood loss.

Dysfunction of central nervous system

A rapid neurological assessment must be made to evaluate level of consciousness, and pupillary size and reaction. A more detailed examination is performed in the secondary survey.

Exposure and examination

The patient should be undressed and a rapid assessment made of injuries to the trunk and limbs.

Resuscitation phase

The management of shock must be initiated, patient oxygenation reassessed, and haemorrhage control re-evaluated. Hypovolaemic shock is corrected by replacement of lost intravascular volume by blood, colloids, or crystalloids. Bloods should be taken for urgent blood tests (full blood count, biochemistry, clotting studies) and cross-match. If blood loss is considered particularly severe (i.e. >1500–2000 ml), the hospital major bleeding protocol should be enacted with emergency provision of O-negative blood, fresh frozen plasma, and platelets. If not contraindicated (i.e. pelvic trauma with possible damage to urethra and bladder), a urinary catheter should be inserted to monitor urine output. Life-threatening conditions identified in the primary survey should be constantly reassessed as management continues.

Secondary survey

This begins after the life-threatening conditions have been identified and treated, and shock therapy has begun. The secondary survey involves a thorough head-to-toe examination and assessment of the patient where each region of the body is examined in detail. In this phase further laboratory studies, X-rays, ultrasound, CT scans (including FAST—focused abdominal sonography for trauma), and special investigations such as peritoneal lavage are carried out.

Definitive care phase

In this phase, all of the patient's injuries are managed comprehensively: fractures are stabilized, the patient is transferred to the operating theatre if immediate operative measures are necessary, or is stabilized in preparation for transfer to the critical care unit or other specialist area.

Arrival at the critical care unit

The critical care staff should be informed in advance of the impending arrival of the patient. The time prior to receiving the patient must be spent preparing the bed area and assembling the necessary equipment (see Box 11.1). The nurse must anticipate all eventualities.

- If the patient is to remain spontaneously breathing, prepare equipment for administering humidified oxygen.
- If mechanical ventilation is required, ensure that the ventilator is functioning correctly and is set appropriately for delivery of oxygen, minute or tidal volume, and respiratory rate. The patient can then be connected promptly on arrival. If possible, prepare appropriate infusions of sedative and/or analgesic drugs.
- Suction equipment must be tested and ready for use. A manual rebreathing bag should be connected to the oxygen supply.
- Other basic supplies and apparatus should be available as per unit protocol.
- Depending on the patient's injuries, an appropriate bed or pressure-relieving mattress may be required (e.g. Stryker frame for spinal injuries).
- If required, prepare traction in advance and ensure that this can be affixed to the particular bed used.
- Prepare a range of volumetric pumps for the immediate administration of drugs and fluids.
- Pressure bags for rapid volume transfusions may be needed. If continuous pressure monitoring is required, this should also be prepared in advance.
- These patients are often hypothermic on arrival because of exposure and infusion of cold fluid. Blood warmers and body-warming devices may be needed. On the other hand, some hospitals follow the concept of therapeutic hypothermia for certain types of trauma (e.g. head injury) so cooling devices may be needed.
- Continuous ECG monitoring is essential. Ensure that the monitor is working correctly, set the alarm limits, and have skin electrodes ready to attach.

Box 11.1 **Checklist for equipment preparation**

- Humidified oxygen/non-invasive ventilation/mechanical ventilation
- Rebreathing bag
- Suction + catheters
- Skin electrodes for ECG monitoring
- Stethoscope/automated blood pressure recording device/pulse oximeter
- Temperature recording device/skin probes
- Primed transducers for invasive monitoring
- Blood/fluid-warming device
- Volumetric pumps/prepared infusions
- Pressure bags
- Special bed/pressure-relieving matress/traction
- Nasogastric tube
- Trolleys prepared for chest drain/central venous/arterial line insertion

- Ensure that a stethoscope, an automated blood pressure recording device, and pulse oximetry equipment are at the bedside. Pulse oximetry will give an immediate guide to patient oxygenation prior to the insertion of an intra-arterial cannula for blood gas analysis. Temperature recording devices will be required to measure core temperature, and skin probes should be available if there is vascular injury to the limbs.
- Anticipate the need for central vein cannulation or recannulation as emergency insertion may not have been sterile. Prepare a trolley with the necessary catheters (e.g. triple-lumen central venous, pulmonary artery).
- Anticipate the need for nasogastric tube insertion.

When the patient arrives in the critical care unit, their clinical state may vary from conscious, alert, breathing spontaneously, and haemodynamically stable to unconscious, endotracheally intubated, mechanically ventilated, hypoxaemic, and shocked. Therefore the subsequent nursing and medical management will depend entirely on the extent of the patient's injuries and other alterations in their clinical status. Constant reassessment of the patient's condition is essential. Continual monitoring of vital signs is important for the early detection of deterioration and the institution of appropriate treatment quickly and effectively.

The extent of use of invasive and non-invasive monitoring devices will depend on the degree of the patient's injuries and the facilities available on the critical care unit. For a full description of patient monitoring refer to Chapter 5.

When the patient arrives the immediate nursing priorities are airway, breathing, and circulation, all of which should have been stabilized prior to transfer but may have deteriorated en route. If the patient is breathing spontaneously and requires oxygen therapy, they should be connected to the prepared humidified oxygen system at the prescribed concentration and flow. Other non-invasive ventilatory support may be required (eg. BiPAP). If the patient is being mechanically ventilated, confirm that the ventilatory settings are correct and then connect to the ventilator. Ensure that the alarm limits are set appropriately and chest expansion is adequate and symmetrical.

Connect the patient to the ECG monitor and note the heart rate and rhythm. If a central venous catheter is in situ, attach to the prepared transducer or manometer. Ensure that infusions in progress are running correctly and that any wound or chest drains and the bladder catheter are correctly positioned. Check that chest drains are not clamped and ascertain whether suction is required. Check chest drain patency and volume of drainage.

The correct positioning of the patient will depend on the injuries sustained. For instance, a spontaneously breathing patient with a flail chest should sit erect if their cardiovascular status and other injuries allow. Patients with actual or suspected fractures of the neck or spine will need extreme care in positioning and must remain flat with the appropriate area immobilized until cleared by an expert orthopaedic/radiology opinion. Similarly, adequate precautions should be taken when rolling or turning the patient ('log-rolling' with in-line immobilization). Fractured limbs must be carefully positioned and supported. Any traction must be correctly fitted and the end of the bed elevated if appropriate and not contraindicated (e.g. spinal injury).

If the patient is stable at this point and no immediate treatment is necessary, a full nursing assessment should be carried out. If the patient is haemodynamically unstable, ventilatory support is inadequate, or the patient is in pain, these aspects must be corrected first.

General nursing assessment

This involves a thorough head-to-toe examination of the patient by the nurse (including the patient's back) and will provide the starting point from which any change can be determined. The nurse must continually observe and reassess, document and report changes, and be aware of the significance of deviations from the baseline measures.

Respiratory injuries

For a full description of respiratory assessment refer to Chapter 4. The following are essential observations in the trauma patient (see Box 11.2 for a summary).

Respiratory rate and depth

Record the rate if the patient is breathing spontaneously. Note the depth of respirations. Is the patient using accessory muscles to aid breathing? Is there stridor (a sign of upper airway obstruction)? A rate greater than 20 breaths/min should alert to the possibility of respiratory compromise. Pulse oximetry and blood gas analysis should be used as an adjunct to observation and examination.

Chest movements and air entry

Is the chest moving symmetrically with each respiration? Is there air entry in all regions? If chest movement

Box 11.2 Summary of respiratory assessment

- Respiratory rate, depth, pattern
- Chest movements and air entry
- Skin bruising/lacerations/surgical emphysema
- Pain

is unilateral, or air entry is poor in any region, consider intraluminal bronchial obstruction (e.g. blood, clot, tooth), malposition of the endotracheal tube (if intubated), pneumothorax, haemothorax, rupture of a bronchus, or pulmonary contusions. Bear in mind that the patient may have underlying respiratory disease such as asthma or chronic obstructive airways disease.

If the patient has multiple rib fractures and/or a flail segment this may impair movement of the chest wall. If the patient is breathing spontaneously, paradoxical chest wall movement may be evident over the flail segment (see later section on chest injuries).

Respiratory pattern

Note the pattern of respiration. Is it regular? Particular patterns of respiration are characteristic of particular head injuries in spontaneously breathing patients. For example, Cheyne–Stokes respiration (periodic rapid and slow breathing) is seen in bilateral cerebral hemisphere damage, hyperventilation in midbrain injuries, apneustic (prolonged inspiration) in pontine injuries, and ataxic (random) breathing in medullary injuries. For further details see Chapter 8.

Skin

Examine the skin of the chest for bruising, lacerations, and abrasions which may indicate underlying injuries (e.g. seat-belt marks). Feel for subcutaneous emphysema which is due to air leaking into the subcutaneous tissues either from external (e.g. stab wound) or from internal (e.g. fractured ribs lacerating underlying lung) injuries. Observe for cyanosis due to a decreased oxyhaemoglobin level which can occur with rapid deterioration, e.g. due to a tension pneumothorax.

Pain

Does the patient complain of pain or tenderness over any particular area of the chest? Does he/she have pain on inspiration that limits chest movement? If chest drains are *in situ*, note the contents (e.g. blood, haemoserous), and the presence of bubbling and swinging of the fluid level with respiration.

Cardiovascular injuries

A 12-lead ECG should be performed. Continuous ECG monitoring should be in progress to immediately detect any change in rate or rhythm. Feel the pulse from time to time. Is it rapid, thready, irregular, or full and bounding? Are all central pulses present? The patient may have underlying cardiovascular disease that is being treated (e.g. beta-blockers, permanent pacemaker). Limb injuries (e.g. fractures, compartment syndrome) may compromise peripheral perfusion. Peripheral pulses, swelling, and temperature should be monitored frequently.

The frequency of blood pressure recordings will depend on the extent of the patient's injuries. Continuous monitoring using a transduced intra-arterial cannula allows changes in blood pressure to be detected immediately. This is essential in multiply injured or shocked patients if rapid treatment is to be effected. Changes in blood pressure should not be taken in isolation, but always related to changes in other variables such as heart rate, central venous pressure, and stroke volume. Drug therapy (e.g. analgesia or sedation) may be the cause of the change in blood pressure; a fall may be accentuated in a hypovolaemic patient.

Note if there is bleeding over wound sites and drains and measure these losses frequently. See Box 11.3 for a summary of cardiovascular assessment.

Neurological injuries

A full neurological assessment must be undertaken as soon as possible (see Box 11.4 for a summary). This can indicate the severity of the injury and provides a baseline for sequential appraisal and detection of new deterioration. The Glasgow Coma Scale provides a quantitative measure of the level of consciousness and is the sum of the scores of three areas of assessment: eye-opening, best motor response, and best verbal response, each being graded separately. For a full description refer to Chapter 8.

Box 11.3 Summary of cardiovascular assessment

- Heart rate and rhythm
- Blood pressure
- Central venous/pulmonary artery pressure
- 12-lead ECG
- Central and peripheral pulses
- Bleeding (drains, wounds, etc.)
- Limb sweling and temperature differences
- Blood gas analysis

Box 11.4 Summary of neurological assessment

- Conscious level: Glasgow Coma Scale
- Pupillary size and response
- Limb movement and response to stimuli
- Examine head for lacerations/bruising/CSF leakage

Box 11.5 Summary of renal assessment

- Urine output
- Urinalysis
- Urine colour (haematuria/myoglobinuria)
- Examine genitalia

Pupil size and response to light must also be evaluated. A difference in pupil diameter >1 mm is abnormal. A sluggish response, or lack of response, to light may indicate intracranial injury; however, the effect of medications (e.g. atropine, opiates) must be considered.

Observe any spontaneous limb movements for equality, though limb fractures or injuries may inhibit movement. Assess muscle tone for flaccidity and asymmetry. Spasticity (e.g. following spinal cord transection) is a late sign. If spontaneous movements are minimal, determine the response to painful stimuli. A decrease in the amount of movement or the need for more stimulus on one side is significant, and may suggest intracranial, spinal, or nerve injury. Epileptiform movements may be observed in the face and/or limbs and should prompt appropriate investigation and treatment.

The frequency of recording of neurological observations depends on the patient's neurological status and the presence of actual or potential head/cord/nerve injury. The nurse should also examine the scalp for lacerations, bruising, and obvious deformity. Bruising behind the ears may indicate bleeding into the mastoid spaces—a late sign of a basal skull fracture. The presence of otorrhoea or rhinorrhoea is also suggestive of a basal skull fracture. Leakage of cerebrospinal fluid (CSF) is also suggested by measurement of the glucose level which is at least half that of the blood glucose level. Normal nasal secretions do not have such a high glucose level.

Renal injuries

Unless the patient is fully conscious and haemodynamically stable, urine output will usually be monitored hourly by a urinary catheter and collecting system. However, certain conditions contraindicate the use of a urethral catheter, including local trauma (actual or suspected). Urethral bleeding is a clue that there may be local injury. In such cases, a suprapubic catheter is often inserted until or unless damage is excluded.

Routine urinalysis should be carried out on all patients and the urine observed for frank haematuria, clots, debris, and colour change. Haematuria is an important sign of potential genitourinary trauma. Note the urine colour—black urine suggests myoglobinuria, which follows muscle damage and breakdown (rhabdomyolysis). A 'positive' dipstick to haemoglobin may indicate either haemoglobin (related to haemolysis or local trauma) or myoglobinuria. This may prompt a renewed search for rhabdomyolysis and compartment syndrome. Examine the genitalia and note any bruising, lacerations, or oedema, which may indicate underlying injury. Urine output should ideally be maintained at a minimum of 0.5 ml/kg/h in adult patients. See Box 11.5 for a summary of renal assessment.

Gastrointestinal injuries

All mechanically ventilated patients should have a nasogastric tube inserted unless contraindicated (e.g. nasal or basal skull fractures), in which case an orogastric tube should be inserted. Gastric dilatation is common after major trauma. The gastric aspirate should be left to drain freely and should be aspirated regularly. Observe aspirate and test for blood.

Examine the abdomen for bruising, grazes, and lacerations, particularly in the regions of the liver, spleen, and kidneys, which may indicate underlying organ damage. Is the abdomen painful in any particular region? Does the abdomen look distended? Is it rigid on palpation? Is there any evidence of bleeding per rectum (or per vagina)?

Assess the patient's nutritional state and consider the need for early feeding (see Chapter 9). Box 11.6 gives a summary of gastrointestinal assessment.

Skin and limb injuries

Note any bruising, lacerations, or swelling. Feel the skin temperature and note the colour. The hypovolaemic patient may appear ashen-faced with cool pale extremities. Look for cyanosis, both peripherally in the nailbeds and centrally in the lips and tongue. Pressing the tip of a

Box 11.6 Summary of gastrointestinal assessment

- Oro- or nasogastric tube (if not contraindicated)
- Measure nasogastric aspirate and test for blood
- Examine abdomen (bruising/pain/rigidity/distension)
- Note bleeding per rectum

Box 11.7 Summary of skin and limb assessment

- Note bruising, lacerations, swelling
- Skin temperature and colour
- Peripheral perfusion and pulses
- Check plaster casts, splints, traction

digit on the skin to blanch it and observing the return of colour tests the efficiency of capillary refill in each limb. This is immediate in the well-perfused patient. Note if any limb is particularly cool. Check that distal pulses are present, and that pressure dressings, splints, plaster casts, or traction on limbs are not impeding the circulation. Ensure that pressure is not exerted on healthy skin by plaster casts or traction devices (observe for tissue swelling and breaks in the skin). Box 11.7 gives a summary of skin and limb assessment.

The patient and relatives

A concise medical and social history should be taken from the patient, relatives, or friends to aid the planning of your nursing care. Do not ask relatives to repeat information if this is already contained within the medical notes, unless clarification is needed, although it is vital that correct addresses and telephone numbers of next of kin are confirmed.

Establish a short-term plan of action from the medical staff and ensure that this information is relayed to the patient and relatives. Encourage them to ask questions, explain the use of any equipment attached to the patient, and ensure that they are regularly informed of progress and developments. Document any information that the patient or family have been told by medical staff concerning the injuries and outcome. A greater understanding of the patient's injuries and a good rapport with nursing and medical staff will help relatives cope with the frightening environment of the critical care unit.

Trauma is always sudden and unexpected, and, unlike the routine post-operative patient who has a planned admission to the unit, there can be no preparation time to allow the patient or relatives to adjust mentally. The patient's injuries may have a profound effect on normal daily living and family life. Financial and work problems may ensue. Emotional and perhaps professional support will be needed to help the family cope with these. Social workers, ministers of religion, and external organizations (such as those for head- and spine-injured patients) can offer great comfort, support, and advice. Amidst the abundance of wires and tubes is a person who is probably frightened about their injuries and worried about the effects on their future, and who needs your constant care and reassurance.

Head injuries

Head injuries are a common consequence of vehicular or sports accidents, or falls in the home or workplace. Many patients with head injuries are managed in general critical care units that have no facilities for monitoring intracranial or cerebral perfusion pressures, albeit no studies have yet demonstrated that pressure-guided management improves outcomes. Severe head injuries still have a high morbidity and mortality, and the management of such patients must be directed at preventing secondary brain damage and providing the best conditions for recovery from any brain damage already sustained (see Table 11.1 for types of head injury).

Pathophysiology

The detailed anatomy and physiology of the brain is described in Chapter 8. The brain is poorly anchored within the the rigid structure of the skull and its soft

Table 11.1 Types of head injury

Scalp	Abrasions, contusions, lacerations, avulsions	The rich blood supply to the scalp may cause wounds to bleed profusely. Always suspect underlying fractures and potential intracranial damage. Is there any foreign body (e.g. glass) remaining?
Fractures	Simple, linear	Impact causes a simple crack in the bone with no break in the skin.
	Simple, depressed	A portion of bone is pushed inwards.
	Compound, depressed	A violent blow causes pieces of bone fragment to be driven into the intracranial cavity.
	Open	A direct pathway or opening through the scalp laceration into the cerebral substance. The dura is torn, and CSF may leak from the wound or the brain tissue may be visible. This type of fracture is an important potential source of intracranial infection.
	Basal	Characterized by CSF leakage from the ear (otorrhoea) or nose (rhinorrhoea) which may be mixed with blood. Ecchymosis (bruising) in the mastoid area behind the ear (Battle sign) is a late sign appearing several hours after the injury. Peri-orbital ecchymosis (raccoon eyes) is a sign of a cribriform plate fracture
Diffuse	Concussion	Caused by stretching of axonal shafts in white matter with reversible loss of function. Results in temporary confusion or loss of consciousness.
	Diffuse axonal	Microscopic damage throughout the brain caused by tearing or stretching of axonal tracts. Not amenable to surgery. Characterized by prolonged and deep coma, often decerebrate/decorticate posturing, and autonomic dysfunction causing high fever, sweating, and hypertension. Mortality is high.
Focal	Contusion	Macroscopic damage occurring in a relatively local area, often beneath an area of impact (coup contusions) or areas remote from impact (contrecoup contusion). Often prolonged periods of coma, mental confusion, or obtundation. May cause herniation and brainstem compression if large or associated with peri-contusional oedema. Alcoholic patients are prone to delayed bleeding into contusions
	Intracranial haemorrhage: acute epidural	Bleeding from a tear in a dural artery or in the dural sinus. Rare, but may be rapidly fatal. Causes loss of consciousness followed by a lucid period, and then a secondary depression of conscious level. A hemiparesis develops with a fixed dilated pupil on the side opposite the haematoma.
	Intracranial haemorrhage: acute subdural haematoma	Bleeding commonly from rupturing of bridging veins between the cerebral cortex and dura. Also seen with lacerations of the brain or cortical arteries. Often seen as underlying brain injury. Causes decreased level of consciousness and possible epileptic seizures if the clot irritates the cerebral cortex.
Lacerations	Impalements and bullet wounds	Impaled objects must be removed at operation. Outcome depends on location, size of injury, and the patient's condition. Patients in coma following bullet wounds have a high mortality. The larger the calibre and the greater the velocity of the bullet, the more likely death will occur. A bullet that does not penetrate the skull may still result in an intracranial injury

consistency renders it liable to move in response to acceleration or deceleration. Bruising (contusions) can occur when there is contact between the interior skull and the surface of the brain; internal shearing forces can cause axonal tracts within the white matter to stretch and tear. Mild stretch injury, with reversible loss of function, is responsible for the transient disturbance of consciousness known as 'concussion'.

Skull fractures alone do not cause neurological disability, and severe brain injuries can occur without skull fractures. However, a patient with a skull fracture is at risk of having, or developing, intracranial damage. Close observation is necessary to detect early signs of neurological deterioration.

Since the volume within the cranial vault is constant, increasing this volume (by oedema, haemorrhage, or haematoma) will directly increase intracranial pressure (ICP). Increases in ICP are initially compensated by movement of cerebral venous blood into the systemic circulation. As the pressure rises further, brain tissue is compressed and cerebral blood flow falls. If this continues, the ICP rises at the expense of cerebral blood flow, resulting in brain ischaemia. Brain tissue dies when its blood supply is interrupted for only a few minutes. The brain also has minimal metabolic reserves and thus is wholly dependent on an adequate arterial blood flow to meet its metabolic needs. The cerebral perfusion pressure (CPP) is measured by subtracting ICP from mean arterial pressure. CPP is thus decreased by a raised ICP and may fall below the perfusion pressure necessary to maintain cerebral blood flow. Ischaemic injury resulting from a decreased CPP may involve cerebral tissue either globally or focally. When compartmental pressure gradients develop from local areas of injury brain shifts can occur within the skull, the most important being uncal or tentorial herniation (coning) which causes brainstem compression and catastrophic neurological injury.

Changes in vital signs in patients with raised intracranial pressure

As ICP increases, heart rate and respiratory rate decrease, while blood pressure and temperature rise (see Box 11.8). There may be irregular patterns of respiration with Cheyne–Stokes or Kussmaul breathing (see Chapter 4). If brain compression causes the circulation to fail, pulse and respiration become rapid and temperature usually rises, but this does not follow a consistent pattern. The pulse pressure (i.e. difference between systemic systolic and diastolic pressure) widens. Immediately preceding this, there may be a period of rapid and profound fluctuations in heart rate. Death will ensue unless effective interventions are achieved. These changes in vital signs must be assessed in relation to the patient's responsiveness (see Chapter 8 for more details of recognition and management of raised intracranial pressure).

> **Box 11.8 Raised intracranial pressure**
>
> **Cardiovascular signs**
>
> - Decreased heart rate
> - Decreased respiratory rate
> - Raised blood pressure
> - Widened pulse pressure
> - Raised temperature
>
> **Consequences**
>
> - Alteration in level of consciousness
> - Headaches, photophobia, nausea, vomiting
> - Bradycardia and hypertension
> - Coma
> - Brain death

Secondary brain damage

The brain requires continuous perfusion with well-oxygenated blood. A reduction in mean BP below 60–80 mmHg, particularly when ICP is raised, may cause ischaemic neuronal damage if sustained for more than a few minutes. The brain can normally regulate its own blood supply to maintain a constant perfusion pressure despite wide variations in systemic BP. However, when injured, the brain loses this capacity. Thus the brain is particularly vulnerable to ischaemic damage in the presence of hypotension, hypoxaemia, or hypovolaemia (Maas *et al.* 2008).

The primary injury results in shearing and compression of neuronal and vascular tissue, leading to physical disruption of cell membranes and other secondary processes which develop over hours to days and determine the extent of secondary brain damage. These include neurotransmitter release, free-radical generation, calcium-mediated damage, gene activation, mitochondrial dysfunction, and inflammatory responses. The inflammatory response, particularly around the areas of contusions and haemorrhage, is an important component of traumatic brain injury. It leads to disruption of the blood–brain barrier, complement-mediated activation of cell death, and triggering of apoptosis (programmed cell death). Glutamate and other neurotransmitter substances exacerbate leakage of ions from the cell and contribute to brain swelling and raised ICP. Free-radical damage, often mediated by calcium, is a major cause of early necrotic cell death. Secondary brain insults such as seizures, vasospasm, metabolic derangement, and infection will further complicate the primary injury.

Management

Full details of the management of severe traumatic brain injury are given in Chapter 8. The major points are summarized in this section.

Management is aimed at:

- optimizing cerebral oxygenation and perfusion pressure
- preventing intracranial hypertension
- protection from seizures
- preventing secondary brain insults:

- hypoxaemia
- hypo- and hypertension
- hyper- and hypocapnia
- hyper- and hypoglycaemia
- hyper- and hypothermia
- hyponatraemia
- anaemia
- acidaemia and alkalaemia.

The first priority is to stabilize the airway, breathing, and circulation and thus prevent further secondary cerebral damage resulting from hypotension and hypoxia. Management thereafter depends on the patient's condition and the presence of other injuries. Cervical spine injuries should always be suspected. Particular care must be taken to stabilize the cervical spine until neck injury has been excluded by X-rays or CT scans and a specialist opinion sought (Moppett 2007).

Monitoring

The extent of monitoring is determined by the degree of head trauma. A patient with a severe head injury (GCS 3–8) should ideally be admitted to a neurointensive care unit where expertise is greater and facilities exist for specialized neuromonitoring, although the ability to cope with multiple non-neurological traumatic injuries may be limited.

Intracranial pressure monitoring and electrophysiological monoring (EEG) are discussed in Chapters 5 and 8. An explanation of specialized neuromonitoring is outside the scope of this book, but it includes jugular bulb venous oxygen saturation, brain tissue oxygen tension, cerebral microdialysis, transcranial Doppler ultrasonography, infrared spectroscopy, and brain temperature.

Mechanical ventilation, sedation, and analgesia

Many patients with severe traumatic brain injury will develop acute lung injury or acute respiratory distress syndrome (e.g. secondary to massive blood transfusion, pulmonary contusions, aspiration pneumonia, and sepsis) and their ventilatory management can be challenging.

Not all unconscious patients require intubation; a Guedel or nasopharyngeal airway may be adequate to maintain a patent airway as long as a gag reflex is present. As a general rule, most head injuries require intubation and mechanical ventilation if their GCS is <8. Adequate blood gas tensions must be maintained, and so the patient may require mechanical ventilation to prevent or reverse hypoxaemia. Rapidly treatable causes such as a pneumothorax should be excluded. In order to reduce detrimental changes in cerebral and systemic blood pressure, rapid sequence intubation is usually performed with adequate sedation and neuromuscular blockade. The ET tube should not be tied so tightly around the neck that it impedes jugular venous drainage.

Prophylactic hyperventilation was commonly used but is no longer recommended as it results in cerebral vasoconstriction and ischaemia (Coles *et al.* 2002). It is now only used for very brief periods to treat an acute neurological deterioration. However, hypercapnia should be avoided as this causes cerebral vasodilatation and may increase ICP further (Manley *et al.* 2001).

Low tidal volumes and moderate levels of positive end-expiratory pressure (PEEP) have been recommended to prevent ventilator-associated lung injury and increased ICP (Mascia *et al.* 2005). The lowest amount of PEEP necessary to maintain adequate oxygenation and prevent end-expiratory collapse should be used. An increase in ICP secondary to raised intrathoracic pressure is only significant at levels >15 cmH_2O in hypovolaemic patients (Hadad and Arabi 2012).

Suctioning via an endotracheal tube should be as brief as possible and be carried out only as often as is necessary for clearance of secretions. If secretions are minimal, the frequency of suctioning should be reduced. Pre-oxygenate with 100% oxygen prior to suctioning and, if necessary, give additional sedation to avoid desaturation and a sudden increase in ICP.

Adequate analgesia and sedation is essential to limit elevations in ICP due to pain, anxiety, and coughing, and to facilitate mechanical ventilation and nursing procedures. Opiate analgesics are commonly used in the mechanically ventilated patient. Propofol is the hypnotic of choice as it is rapidly reversed when discontinued, allowing periodic neurological assessment, and is easily titratable. Propofol should be used with caution in the hypovolaemic or hypotensive patient because of its vasodilatory effect. Benzodiazepines (e.g midazolam or lorazepam) can be given instead as intermittent boluses or by continuous infusion, but their long half-life may make neurological assessment more difficult. Other alternatives include α_2-adrenergic agonists such as clonidine or dexmedetomidine, or, if deep sedation is required, barbiturates such as thipental can be used. Neuromuscular blocking agents are not routinely used in ventilated patients unless there is refractory intracranial hypertension as they are associated with an increased risk of pneumonia and neuromuscular complications.

Haemodynamic support and fluid management

Hypotension is common in patients with severe head injury. It is usually due to hypovolaemia secondary to haemorrhage from other injuries. Polyuria may result from cranial diabetes insipidus. Other causes of hypotension include myocardial contusions and spinal cord injuries causing spinal shock. Hypotension must be avoided and agressively managed as it is significantly associated with increased mortality. Appropriate fluid administration must be given to correct hypovolaemia. Vasopressors may be required, especially if the patient has underlying cardiovascular disease, or to maintain MAP (or CPP) within a targeted range. Anaemia should be avoided and coagulation abnormalities corrected using appropriate blood products.

Metabolic

Stress-induced diabetes mellitus may be a complication of head injury. Blood and urine should be regularly tested for glucose, and insulin therapy prescribed as necessary. Blood glucose levels must be kept within the normal range. Hyperglycaemia may lead to secondary brain damage both by direct injury and by increasing the osmotic pressure resulting in cerebral ischaemia. Hyperglycaemia is associated with poor neurological outcomes (Meier *et al.* 2008). Diabetes insipidus is caused by damage to the hypothalamus or posterior pituitary gland. It occurs quite commonly in severe head injuries, particularly brain death, but may occasionally follow fairly minor trauma. Failure of appropriate antidiuretic hormone (ADH) secretion results in the passage of large volumes of dilute urine. Intravenous fluid replacement is needed to prevent/reverse hypovolaemia, and therapy with a vasopressin (or an analogue such as desmopressin) is usually required (see Chapter 7). Vital signs and blood electrolytes should be carefully monitored and the urine specific gravity should be regularly ascertained. Fluid balance must be carefully documented. Conversely, inappropriate ADH secretion may occur with head injury, resulting in oliguria and fluid retention.

Seizures

Epileptic seizures may occur with any head injury, either from direct cortical irritation or space-occupying lesions (e.g. haematoma), or from secondary causes such as hypoxia, hypotension, and hypoglycaemia. Prolonged or repetitive seizures may be associated with intracranial haemorrhage. Seizures are usually treated aggressively since they can cause cerebral hypoxia, brain swelling, and raised ICP. Respiratory function, duration of seizure activity, and a description of the seizures must be carefully documented. Appropriate medication should be instituted (e.g. intravenous phenytoin, Keppra). Ensure the safety of the patient at all times; side-rails should be used on the bed and padded with pillows to prevent injury.

Infection

Infection may be a complication of head injury, either directly from an open head wound or skull fracture, especially if CSF leakage is present, or from cannulae and drain sites. This may give rise to meningitis or brain abscesses. Careful monitoring plus microbiological culture of potential sites of infection are needed. Prophylactic antibiotic therapy is now considered only for those with basal skull fractures or compound vault fractures. Tetanus prophylaxis should not be overlooked when lacerations or penetrating injuries occur.

Gastric dilatation

Gastric dilatation is common after trauma and the risk of aspiration is heightened. Vomiting and retching increase ICP and should be avoided by the use of antiemetics such as metoclopramide. All semi-conscious or unconscious patients should have gastric aspiration performed regularly by placement of an oro- or nasogastric tube. A nasogastric tube should not be inserted in patients with frontal basal skull fractures because of the risk of passage of the tube into the cranium. Feeding should be commenced promptly and, ideally, enterally unless contraindicated (see Chapter 9). Early institution of feeding will help prevent the development of stress ulceration. Prophylaxis with H_2 blockers or proton pump inhibitors is often used, especially if there is a coagulopathy and the patient is considered to need prolonged mechanical ventilation; however, these drugs increase the risk of nosocomial pneumonia.

Hyperthermia and agitation

Hyperthermia is harmful to the head-injured patient since elevations in body temperature increase the metabolic rate of the brain. Blood carbon dioxide levels are also raised and the resulting vasodilation may increase ICP further. The higher the temperature, the greater is the risk to the patient. Methods of cooling should be instituted promptly (e.g. antipyretics, fanning, tepid sponging, cooling mattress). Agitation and restlessness may be a sign that the unconscious patient is improving or, more ominously, deteriorating. Hypoxaemia, hypotension, metabolic derangement, a full bladder, and/or pain from other injuries should be sought and excluded. The patient must be assessed for any focal neurological change (e.g. unequal pupils, non-use of one or more limbs) suggesting new or deteriorating intracranial pathology. The patient should be prevented from self-harming (e.g. by using padded side-rails and removing cannulae, tubes, and drains).

Specific nursing procedures

The patient with a raised ICP should not be stimulated unnecessarily and should be nursed in a quiet environment. ICP is raised by agitation, coughing, pain, and nursing and physiotherapy procedures. Efforts should be aimed at minimizing these by using adequate sedation (with bolus doses) if indicated and reducing the ICP response by careful positioning of the patient with 30° head-up tilt and the neck in a neutral position. Cervical collars or tapes securing the endotracheal tube should not be tight as cerebral venous drainage may be impeded, thus increasing ICP. In the unconscious patient, passive limb movements and regular turning must be instituted and a pressure-relieving mattress may be required. Bladder catheterization will also be necessary. Administer a bowel regimen to avoid constipation and an increase in intra-abdominal pressure.

Immobile patients are at high risk of developing thromboembolic events (e.g deep vein thrombosis, pulmonary embolus), so compression stockings are recommended unless contraindicated by lower limb injuries. Low molecular weight (or low dose unfractionated) heparin may be given; however, it is associated with an increased risk of expansion of intracranial haemorrhage and may be contraindicated due to other injuries and any ongoing coagulopathy.

For details of specific treatment strategies for severe traumatic brain injury see Chapter 8.

Maxillofacial and upper airway trauma

Maxillofacial and upper airway injuries are common, and mainly result from vehicular accidents, physical violence, or sporting injuries. There may be other associated injuries, and cervical spine trauma should always be suspected. Consequently, extreme care must be taken to stabilize the neck when the airway is being secured or the patient turned. Sharp trauma, such as knife and gunshot wounds, causes lacerations and penetrating injuries that may damage the air passages, blood vessels, nerves, and oesophagus. Blunt trauma may cause bone fractures and damage to the larynx and trachea leading to severe airway problems.

Injuries to the face and neck can be life-threatening due to airway compromise and/or major haemorrhage. Therefore the management priorities are to secure and maintain a patent airway and to prevent hypovolaemic shock due to massive bleeding from the facial skeleton and soft tissues. Airway management poses particular problems in these patients as access may be obstructed. Once the airway has been secured and haemorrhage controlled, further definitive management should be deferred until other potential life-threatening injuries have been dealt with.

Airway management

Initial management will include assessment of the injury and the patient's conscious level, colour, and ability to maintain a patent airway. Suction can be applied but, depending on the site and extent of the trauma, particular problems may be encountered. Oral intubation or emergency tracheotomy may be required if a patent airway cannot be maintained. This may be particularly necessary in the following circumstances in order to maintain effective gas exchange.

- Bilateral anterior mandibular fracture or symphyseal fracture may cause the tongue to lose its anterior insertion. In the supine patient the tongue may drop back, occluding the oropharynx. To open the airway a suture is placed through the tongue and secured with tape to the side of the face.
- The oral cavity may be blocked by loose teeth, poor fitting dentures, vomitus, bone fragments, blood, or foreign bodies. These can also block the larynx, trachea, or main bronchi. Attempts should be made to scoop out debris with a gloved finger and suction applied with a large-bore Yankauer suction catheter. Bronchoscopy (fibreoptic or rigid) may be needed to remove more distal objects.
- A maxillary fracture may be displaced and block the nasal airway. To open the airway the maxilla needs to be disimpacted by pulling it forwards.
- Haemorrhage resulting from bleeding vessels in open wounds, or from the nose if the maxillary artery or ethmoidal vessels are damaged, may obstruct the airway,. Direct pressure to wounds and suction will be required to open the airway.

- Soft tissue swelling and oedema may obstruct the airway. Although not usually an immediate phenomenon, early intubation may prevent airway obstruction
- Trauma to the larynx or trachea may cause obstruction of the airway by swelling or displacement of structures (e.g. vocal cords or epiglottis). If the airway is threatened and anatomical disruption makes intubation difficult or impossible, an emergency cricothyroidotomy or a tracheostomy must be performed. Nasal intubation is not attempted when mid-facial injuries are present or a basal skull fracture is suspected.

Specific maxillofacial fractures

Mandible

This is easily fractured because of its prominent position. It may cause airway obstruction if fractured bilaterally at the angle or body of the mandible, and often causes haematoma and swelling of the neck and floor of mouth. Definitive treatment consists of internal wiring or plating.

Maxilla

Airway obstruction and fracture of nasal bones, orbit, zygoma, soft tissue injury, and ocular damage often accompany this injury.

- **Le Fort I**—the least severe. A dento-alveolar fracture separates the palate from the remainder of the facial skeleton.
- **Le Fort II** The fracture extends from the lower nasal bridge through the medial wall of the orbit and crosses the zygomatic-maxillary process.
- **Le Fort III**—the most severe. The fracture completely separates the midfacial skeleton from the base of the upper nasal bridge, most of the orbit, and across the zygomatic arch. The fracture involves the ethmoid bone and may affect the cribriform plate at the base of the skull.

Le Fort II and III fractures are often associated with basal skull fractures and may lead to CSF leakage, meningitis, and pneumocranium. Nasal intubation (nasotracheal or nasogastric) should not be attempted because of the risk of passing the tube through the cribriform plate into the cranial cavity. Definitive surgery involves internal fixation with wiring and plating and intermaxillary fixation. External fixation is often required.

Zygoma and orbit

Fracture and displacement of the zygoma can disrupt the lateral wall and floor of the orbit. Subconjunctival bruising and peri-orbital swelling may be present. Unstable fractures require internal or external fixation. Stable fractures can be reduced at operation; no other active management is usually required. Fractures of the orbital walls may tear or compress the optic nerve, and blindness, if it occurs, is usually immediate and permanent.

Nasal

Nasal injuries are very common and haemorrhage may be severe. Packing with gauze, balloon tamponade, and/or closed reduction may be required.

Larynx

Fractures of the larynx are usually caused by blunt trauma. These may severely compromise the airway and necessitate immediate tracheostomy. Surgical exploration and repair is then necessary.

Specific nursing management

Airway and breathing

Careful observation of the airway is essential in any patient with maxillofacial injuries. Soft tissue swelling and oedema rarely present as an immediate problem, but can increase insidiously. Always remember that a patient who does not have an endotracheal tube or tracheostomy in situ is at risk of developing airway problems.

Depending on the type and extent of injuries, the airway may be self-maintained or may require a Guedel or nasopharyngeal airway, an endotracheal tube, or a tracheostomy. Humidified oxygen therapy will usually be required, but the patient may not necessarily require mechanical ventilation unless injuries are severe, there are other injuries necessitating this, or surgery is contemplated.

Ensure that oxygen masks are not tight-fitting if there are facial fractures or wounds. Nasal prongs may be more comfortable but these should not be used if there is rhinorrhoea.

Specific respiratory assessment includes observation for any difficulty in breathing, evidence of stridor, or increasing oedema of the neck, face, and/or mouth. Pulse oximetry is a useful guide to patient oxygenation, but an intra-arterial cannula is often required for blood gas monitoring.

Appropriate imaging and investigations, (e.g. chest X-ray, CT scan, bronchoscopy) will be required if gas exchange is impaired.

In general, patients are best nursed in an upright position if other injuries and their haemodynamic status allow. This encourages drainage of blood, saliva, and CSF away from the airway, reduces venous pressure, and encourages fluid reabsorption.

Circulation

Significant haemorrhage can occur in patients with closed injuries to the bony structures of the middle third of the face (maxilla, nose, and ethmoids). Steady bleeding from the nose and oral cavity into the soft tissues of the face can cause profound swelling of the cheeks and a tense skin. Careful monitoring of blood pressure and heart rate is essential. Even a small puncture wound that is continually trickling blood, which may be overlooked, can cause significant blood loss. It is important to consider the potential for raised intracranial pressure if there are associated head injuries.

Wounds

Obtain clear guidelines from the medical staff regarding specific wound management. Check the scalp for lacerations, bruising, and foreign bodies such as glass fragments. All wounds should be observed for signs of haemorrhage, haematoma formation, and infection. Monitor temperature regularly, and swab and culture any suspected sites of infection. If external fixation has been used to stabilize fractures, ensure that pin sites are kept clean and dry.

Mouth

The mouth must be kept clean, moist, and free of infection. This may be difficult in the patient who has their jaws wired together or is unable to take oral fluids. Patients who have had major oral surgery and have sutures or skin grafts within the oral cavity may require very frequent mouth care (hourly) and this must be carried out with great care in the immediate post-operative period.

If the jaws are wired together wire cutters must be available at the bedside. The nurse must be aware as to which wires should be cut if the airway is compromised. Anti-emetics should be given regularly if the patient is nauseated in order to prevent vomiting. A Yankauer suction catheter should be at hand.

Eyes

Observe for peri-orbital swelling (associated with fractures of the zygoma or maxilla) and subconjunctival bruising which may be due to direct trauma to the globe or a fracture of the zygoma. A 'blow-out' fracture is caused by a direct blow on the eyeball which causes such a rise in intra-orbital pressure that the orbital contents are forced through the orbital floor and herniate into the antrum. As well as bruising and endophthalmus, this causes a tethering of the eyeball where the muscles become trapped, limiting elevation of the eye and causing diplopia. Pooling of tears may indicate damage to the lacrimal apparatus. Proptosis or exopthalmus suggests haemorrhage within the orbital walls. Ask the patient if they can see clearly. Do they have diplopia? Ascertain their normal visual acuity (do they normally wear spectacles?). Is there a contact lens or foreign body in the eye? Small particles that have sufficient force to penetrate the tough wall of the eyeball are generally metallic. Retained iron particles in the eye will gradually dissolve and the brown pigment is then dispersed through the ocular tissues, but the sight is destroyed. Glass may remain inert for years. Pyrogenic infection of the eyeball often follows penetrating injuries.

Nose

Observe for bleeding or rhinorrhoea which suggests a cribriform plate fracture. A nasogastric or nasotracheal tube should not be used as the cranial cavity may be intubated. Ask the patient if they have any difficulty breathing through their nose. Does the nose look deformed in any way?

Ears

Observe for bleeding or otorrhoea (CSF leak from the ear). Look behind the ears for bruising over the mastoid process (Battle sign) which may indicate a basal skull fracture.

Spinal injuries

The most common causes are vehicular accidents (including motorcycles), diving accidents, and falls. Less commonly they occur as a result of gunshot wounds and sporting activities (Figure 11.1).

Spinal injuries are often associated with other injuries, particularly to the head and chest. Any unconscious multiply injured patient must be assumed to have spinal damage until this is excluded by an expert opinion using appropriate imaging. The first aid management is extremely important as considerable damage to the spinal cord can be caused by inexpert care at the scene of the trauma and during hospital transfer.

The spinal cord is most often damaged in the cervical region, but the thoracolumbar region is also at risk.

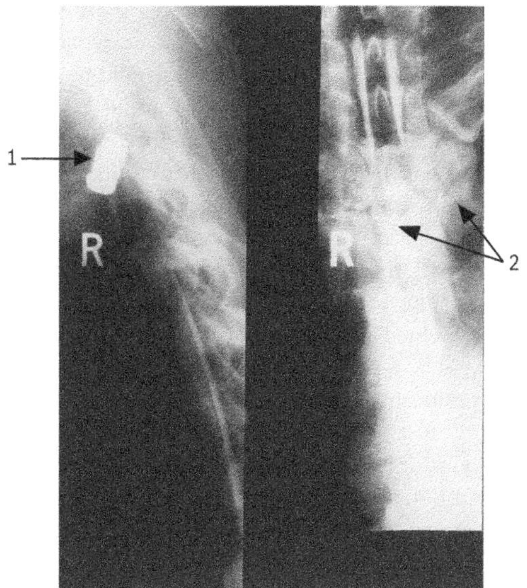

Figure 11.1 Myelogram showing thoracic spinal cord disruption by a bullet injury. The track of the bullet is visible by the debris (arrowed).

Here, the spinal canal is narrower relative to the width of the spinal cord and any vertebral displacement is more likely to cause cord damage. Injury to the cord leads to bruising or mechanical destruction of the nerves, haemorrhage, and oedema. Some of the cord damage may be reversible, but 4 weeks (or more) will be required to fully assess the degree of final damage.

Management of airway, breathing, and circulation must take priority. However, spinal injury must be considered when establishing these priorities, taking precautions to prevent further neurological damage.

Nursing priorities

Airway with cervical spine control

With high cervical spine injuries, endotracheal intubation may be needed to protect the airway and/or provide ventilatory support. Vertebral fractures above C5 may lead to loss of diaphragmatic function and those above C8 to loss of intercostal function. Other injuries to the head or chest may necessitate intubation in order to maintain effective oxygenation and/or secure the airway. The intubation procedure must be carried out by an experienced anaesthetist, with an assistant responsible for controlling the head and neck and minimizing spinal movement. A difficult intubation should be anticipated and necessary accessories such as an intubating laryngoscope or bronchoscope should be at hand. In patients with acute cervical cord injury, pharyngeal stimulation by a Guedel airway, endotracheal tube or suctioning may provoke a vagal reflex causing severe bradycardia or even asystole. This should be anticipated and can be prevented by the administration of atropine or glycopyrrolate prior to the procedure. In patients with actual or suspected cervical spine injuries the neck must be stabilized at all times using a rigid collar of an appropriate size that grips the chin. However, remember that collars alone are inadequate and lateral support must be given by sandbags placed either side of the head (with the head in a neutral position) and manual stabilization during movement of the patient.

Stabilization of the neck and spine must be continued throughout any procedures (e.g. X-rays, insertion of CVP lines) until the risk of cord damage has been ruled out. If imaging confirms spinal damage, more definitive stabilization may be considered (e.g. using skull tongs, halopelvic traction, or spinal fusion).

Breathing

The patient with a cervical spine injury who is breathing spontaneously requires careful observation of their respiratory function. Ascending oedema of the traumatized cervical cord may result in deterioration of respiratory status shortly after admission. Equipment for manual ventilation must be available at the bedside.

Blood gas analysis and/or pulse oximetry should be used to identify hypoxaemia. Vital capacity monitoring may be needed, especially in patients with fractures above C8. A forced vital capacity of less than 10–15 ml/kg body weight may prompt institution of ventilatory support.

Patients with spinal injuries should be nursed on a specific type of bed (e.g. Stoke Mandeville, Parragon, or Stryker frame) capable of lateral tilting and longitudinal elevation while keeping the spine straight. This will ensure that the spine is always in a neutral position and the patient can be tilted head up and feet down to an angle of approximately 45°. This will increase functional residual capacity and is particularly important in patients who have chest trauma but are breathing spontaneously. Atelectasis is common, and the ability to expectorate may be impaired. Regular physiotherapy is essential, and the use of narcotic drugs, which further suppress respiration, should be minimized or avoided.

Circulation

All patients with an acute spinal injury should have continuous ECG monitoring. Patients with injury to the cervical or high thoracic cord may have reduced sympathetic outflow between the T1 and L2 segments. This may cause hypotension and bradycardia, and is known as neurogenic or 'spinal' shock. Atropine or glycopyrrolate may be needed if the heart rate falls below 50 bpm with associated hypotension (systolic BP <80 mmHg). This type of shock must be distinguished from hypovolaemic shock, which may also be present in the multiply injured patient but is usually characterized by hypotension and tachycardia. Aggressive fluid replacement is detrimental in patients with purely neurogenic hypotension as it precipitates pulmonary oedema. Vasopressor support is often required. Patients with bradycardia and hypotension may be given careful fluid challenges with close monitoring of filling pressure (e.g. CVP) or stroke volume.

Abdomino-pelvic trauma may not be easily recognized in the tetraplegic patient since the abdominal wall is anaesthetized and flaccid. The classical signs of a rigid painful abdomen following visceral perforation or haemorrhage may not be apparent. Close monitoring of vital signs and an awareness of potential injury is important. Peritoneal lavage, ultrasound, and X-ray or CT procedures may be performed if abdominal trauma is suspected. Some patients may feel shoulder tip pain from phrenic nerve irritation if abdominal injury is present.

Specific nursing management

Paralytic ileus and gastric dilatation are common after spinal cord trauma. A nasogastric tube should be passed (unless contraindicated) and aspirated regularly. Enteral feeding may take time to become established.

Acute urinary retention will develop in tetraplegic and paraplegic patients unless the sacral segments have been spared. A urethral catheter should be inserted (unless contraindicated) and urine output monitored closely. Urinary tract infection can become a major problem and catheterization should be carried out under strict aseptic conditions. A long-term silastic catheter may be needed and regular urinalysis performed.

Constipation is often problematic and bowel care should be given according to specific unit protocols. This will include regular administration of laxatives and enemas.

Prevention of pressure sores is vital and meticulous attention must be paid to regular changes of position. Proper positioning is important to prevent pressure on heels and bony prominences, with padding (such as a pillow) placed between the inner surfaces of the knees and between the medial malleoli of the ankles. The skin should be kept clean and dry, and hypoalbuminaemia avoided by adequate nutrition. Mattresses and beds appropriate to the risk of pressure sore development should be employed.

The patient will develop wasting of the extremities owing to disuse and as a consequence of their critical illness. If their condition allows, passive exercises should be carried out with a range of movements that preserve joint motion and stimulate circulation. Correct positioning of joints and limbs is important in order to prevent deformities such as footdrop. The patient must be maintained in proper alignment at all times; however, there may be limitations to positioning and limb movements in the multiply injured patient.

Chest injuries

The majority of chest injuries are caused by blunt trauma. Such injuries may result from a high velocity impact (e.g. a rapid deceleration as seen in road traffic accidents), a low velocity impact (e.g. a direct blow to the chest), or crushing trauma to the chest. Less commonly (in the UK), penetrating injuries, such as knife and gunshot wounds, are also seen. Many patients with severe intrathoracic injuries, such as laceration of the heart, aorta, or major airways, do not survive to reach hospital. Patients with chest trauma often have other injuries such as head, spinal, abdominal, and maxillofacial damage. Some will be multiply injured. The priorities of management are, as always, maintenance of airway, breathing, and circulation, with identification and correction of life-threatening injuries.

Nursing priorities

Airway and breathing

A patent airway must be secured and intubation or tracheostomy may be required. Chest injury often leads to hypoxaemia, with causes including failure to ventilate the lungs adequately, ventilation/perfusion mismatch, or changes in intrapleural pressures (e.g. pneumo- or haemothorax) which lead to lung collapse with displacement of mediastinal structures. Hypoxaemia must be corrected with interventions aimed at ensuring that adequate amounts of oxygen are delivered to parts of the lung that are still being ventilated and perfused. CPAP or BiPAP may be useful to avoid atelectasis in spontaneously breathing patients, and to assist breathing in those with a flail chest injury.

Intubation and positive pressure ventilation are necessary in patients who are deeply unconscious and not protecting their airway, and have severe respiratory distress or associated head injuries, where hypoxaemia must be avoided. A chest X-ray will have been taken as a matter of priority in the emergency department in any patient with suspected chest injuries. Serious injuries including fractures, haemo- or pneumothorax, cardiac tamponade, ruptured diaphragm, dissecting aorta, and major airway disruptions need to be diagnosed promptly. Pneumothoraces should ideally be identified and drained before mechanical ventilation is instituted. Close monitoring of arterial blood gases is essential, and appropriate levels of oxygen must be administered to prevent/correct hypoxaemia.

In the self-ventilating patient careful and continuous monitoring of respiratory function should be performed. Signs of respiratory distress may indicate the need for further interventions (see Chapter 4). Central cyanosis may be a late or absent sign of hypoxaemia in patients with decreased haemoglobin as a result of haemorrhage.

Circulation

Patients with major cardiac or vascular lacerations may have had haemorrhage arrested by a tamponade effect. Rapid transfusion and the subsequent increase in arterial and intracardiac pressures may result in uncontrollable and possibly fatal bleeding. Such injuries must be identified before resuscitation elevates the systolic blood pressure above 100 mmHg.

Continuous ECG and monitoring of vital signs are essential. Myocardial contusions are common in chest injuries and may give rise to tachyarrhythmias, conduction abnormalities, and decreased contractility. Large blood losses may result from haemothoraces and tearing of thoracic vessels. Observe for signs of hypovolaemia (see Chapter 5). Is the patient peripherally cool and poorly perfused? Look at the patient's colour. Are they pale? Are there signs of obvious bleeding (e.g. from chest or wound drains)?

Specific chest injuries

Pulmonary contusions

These occur when shearing or crushing forces are applied to the thoracic cage and cause disruption of the microcirculation. Red cells and plasma extravasate and fill the alveoli, resulting in interstitial haemorrhage and alveolar collapse in the contused area. Gas exchange is impaired as perfusion is maintained in the unventilated lung segments, causing intrapulmonary shunting and hypoxaemia. The infiltrates are usually absorbed within 3–5 days but may progress in complicated cases. A chest X-ray or CT scan will reveal localized areas of contusion and haemorrhage.

Management is aimed at ensuring adequate ventilation and treating hypoxaemia. If severe, intubation and mechanical ventilation may be required. Pain control is important and intercostal nerve blocks or epidural analgesia may be very useful. Adequate pain relief allows the patient to breathe more deeply, cooperate with physiotherapy, and clear their secretions more effectively. Supplemental oxygen therapy with or without non-invasive ventilation should be given and blood gases monitored. If the patient is mechanically ventilated, manoeuvres to improve oxygenation are aimed at reducing the shunt (e.g. postural changes), increasing FiO_2, increasing functional residual capacity by the use of PEEP, and improving tracheobronchial toilet by effective suctioning and physiotherapy.

Rib fractures

Blood loss and disruption of the underlying lung tissue are associated with rib fractures. The sharp edges of the fractured rib may lacerate the underlying lung, causing haemorrhage and/or pneumothorax. Any number of ribs may be fractured; if several are fractured in more than one place, or the broken ribs are combined with fracture dislocations of the costochondrial junctions or sternum, this is known as a flail segment and moves independently of the rib cage. The negative intrapleural pressures generated on inspiration will pull this segment inwards. This creates a paradoxical movement which may compromise ventilation by reducing tidal volume. A flail segment itself is not an indication for mechanical ventilation, but the functional consequences must determine the necessity for ventilatory support. Recent studies have shown better outcomes in patients with extensive rib fractures by using a conservative approach and good pain relief, as opposed to routine mechanical ventilation, provided that PaO_2 >6.6 kPa on an FiO_2 of 0.5, vital capacity >10 ml/kg and respiratory rate <40 breaths/min. Non-invasive ventilation may be a useful adjunct.

Adequate analgesia is essential in patients with rib fractures. Pain inhibits adequate breaths, leading to atelectasis in the basal segments, prevents adequate coughing and clearance of secretions, and limits effective physiotherapy. If there are only a few unilateral rib fractures, oral analgesia, intercostal nerve blocks, or thoracic epidural analgesia may be sufficient. With multiple fractures intravenous analgesia may also be needed.

A minitracheotomy may prevent intubation if there is difficulty in clearing secretions. Chest strapping is not recommended, as this only serves to inhibit effective ventilation.

Close monitoring of blood gases and pulse oximetry is required, with careful observation of respiratory function. Assist with physiotherapy and encourage the patient to breathe deeply and cough to clear secretions. Position the patient in an upright and comfortable position if their condition allows. Assess the effect of any analgesia given, and review this if pain persists.

Pneumothorax (simple, open, tension) and haemothorax

Chest injuries are often accompanied by either collection of blood in the chest cavity (haemothorax) from torn intercostal vessels or haemorrhage from lacerated lung tissue, or escape of air from the injured lung into the pleural cavity (pneumothorax). Both blood and air may be found together (haemopneumothorax). The lung on that side of the chest is compressed and ventilation is impaired. A small pneumothorax (<5% of haemothorax volume) can be allowed to resolve spontaneously provided that it is not compromising ventilation and is not enlarging. A chest drain (or needle aspiration) is often performed for larger pneumothoraces, particularly if the patient requires mechanical ventilation (see Figure 11.2).

A tension pneumothorax is a medical emergency and requires immediate decompression. Here, air is drawn into the pleural space from a lacerated lung or through a hole in the chest wall. Air that enters with each inspiration is trapped and cannot be expelled; therefore tension builds up. The lung is compressed and collapses, pushing the mediastinal structures (heart, trachea, and great vessels) towards the unaffected side of the chest (mediastinal shift), impairing ventilation in the other lung and decreasing venous return. Thus tension pneumothorax results in impairment of cardiovascular as well as respiratory function. Collapse and electromechanical dissociation may rapidly result.

Diagnosis of a tension pneumothorax may need to be made clinically as there may not be time to take a chest X-ray before instituting treatment. The patient will become progressively more hypoxaemic and may be tachycardiac and hypotensive. Air entry will be absent over the affected area and chest movement reduced. The trachea will be deviated away from the affected side, the neck veins will be distended, and the patient will become progressively cyanosed.

Immediate decompression is obtained by inserting a needle into the second intercostal space in the mid-clavicular line of the affected hemi-thorax. The ability to aspirate air into a syringe attached to the needle confirms the diagnosis. If the patient is receiving positive pressure ventilation the needle can be left open to air, converting the injury to a simple pneumothorax while a formal chest drain is being inserted. If the patient is spontaneously breathing, be aware that air may be sucked back into the pleura once the initial pneumothorax is decompressed. Again, a formal chest drain is required.

(a)

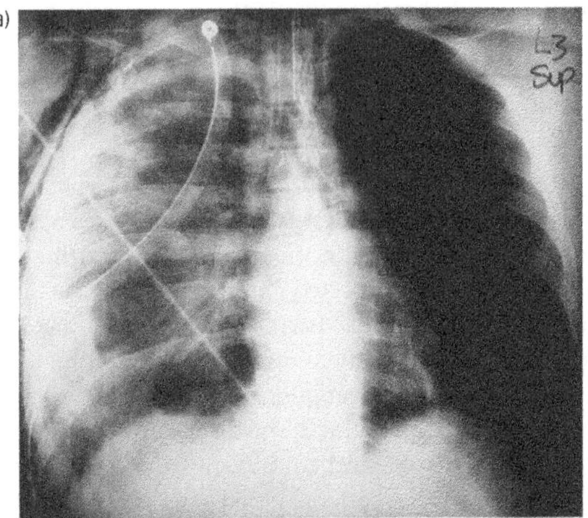

(b)

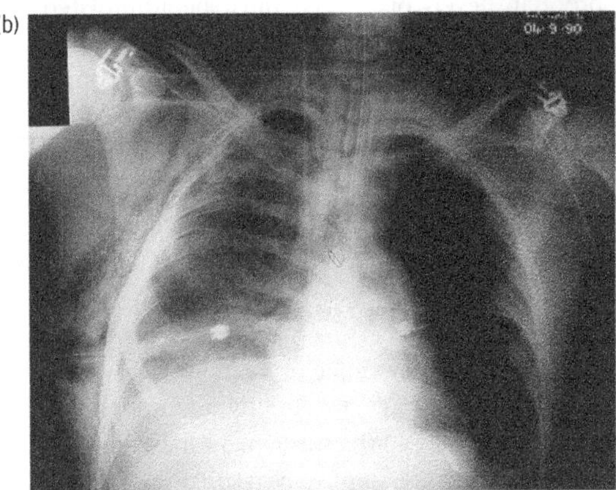

Figure 11.2 X-ray showing fractured ribs, pulmonary contusions, and pneumothorax: (a) before and (b) after insertion of chest drain on left side.

Massive blood loss may result from haemothoraces that are usually caused by penetrating injuries lacerating systemic or pulmonary vessels. Such injuries may be accompanied by hypovolaemic shock, and insertion of a chest drain may reveal a considerable amount of blood in the thoracic cavity. Concurrent drainage of the haemothorax and volume resuscitation is required. Some patients will require surgical intervention; this is usually dependent on the continuing rate and volume of blood loss. Careful measurement of blood loss into the chest drain is required (every 15–30 min) with continuous monitoring of vital signs as fluid replacement is given.

An open pneumothorax is caused by a penetrating injury leaving an open hole between the chest cavity and the atmosphere. Equilibrium between intrathoracic pressure and atmospheric pressure is immediate. If the chest wall opening is more than two-thirds the diameter of the trachea, air will pass preferentially into the chest through the hole (causing a 'sucking' chest wound). Ventilation is impaired and the patient will become hypoxaemic. The hole must be sealed immediately with an occlusive dressing and taped securely on three sides only. Leaving one side of the dressing open will allow air to escape as the patient exhales, but as the patient breathes in the dressing is occlusively sucked over the wound, preventing air from entering. If the hole is sealed completely, air will accumulate in the thoracic cavity resulting in a tension pneumothorax. This is a temporary measure; a chest drain should be inserted remote from the open wound. Surgical closure of the wound is often required.

Low-pressure suction (up to 10 kPa) may be applied to chest drains to aid evacuation of air and blood from the pleural cavity. Pressure levels must be checked regularly and chest drain tubing observed to identify blood clots blocking the tubing and impairing drainage (for comprehensive care of chest drains see Chapter 4). If the patient is making any spontaneous inspiratory effort, two chest drain clamps must be available at the bedside in case of accidental disconnection of the tubing. A tension pneumothorax or a pneumothorax drain that is bubbling (i.e. a bronchopleural fistula) must not be clamped otherwise air will build up in the chest cavity.

Pericardial tamponade

This results from penetrating or blunt trauma which cause the pericardium to fill with blood from the heart or great vessels. The pericardium is a fibrous structure, and even relatively small amounts of fluid in the pericardial sac will restrict cardiac filling.

Cardiac tamponade is characterized by increases in heart rate and central venous pressure, and decreases in blood pressure and cardiac output. Peripheral perfusion will be poor and the neck veins may become distended due to the increase in CVP. Pulsus paradoxus (disappearance or weakening of the radial pulse on spontaneous inspiration, or expiration if mechanically ventilated) may be present. Large cyclical beat-to-beat variations in phase with the respiratory cycle may be seen on the transduced systemic blood pressure trace.

Treatment is by pericardiocentesis where blood is aspirated by a needle sited transcutaenously into the pericardium, usually under echo, electrocardiographic, or X-ray guidance. If the blood in the pericardium is clotted, aspiration may prove impossible. If the patient is moribund, urgent thoracotomy will be required with creation of a pericardial window. Cardiac tamponade caused by penetrating trauma will need surgical exploration and repair.

Myocardial contusion

This is caused by blunt trauma to the chest or by deceleration trauma. ECG abnormalities are usually apparent; these are usually non-specific ST segment and T wave changes. Dysrhythmias (e.g. tachyarrhythmias, multiple premature ventricular ectopics, and conduction disturbances (heart block and bundle branch block)) are common and may be fatal. Cardiac enzymes and troponin levels are also elevated. Continuous ECG monitoring is essential as the onset of dysrhythmias may be sudden. Cardiogenic shock may result from myocardial contusions; if so, inotropic support and mechancial support may be required to maintain an adequate cardiac output and blood pressure.

Diaphragmatic rupture

This usually follows penetrating or blunt trauma to the abdomen and may result in abdominal contents being forced into the chest through a laceration in the diaphragm. The liver usually prevents herniation through the right hemidiaphragm and therefore it is most commonly seen on the left side. Herniation of the stomach into the chest may become evident when a nasogastric tube is seen in the chest cavity on X-ray. Early mechanical ventilation may mask signs of respiratory distress that would be evident in the self-ventilating patient. Penetrating abdominal injuries may lacerate the diaphragm causing a haemothorax. Most patients with a diaphragmatic rupture require surgical exploration and repair.

Major airway injuries

Blunt or penetrating trauma may cause rupture of the trachea or bronchus, or tears and punctures of the lung tissue. The presence of surgical emphysema is a sign of airway injury; with transection of the trachea or bronchus this may be extensive in the mediastinum and subcutaneous tissues. Pneumothorax and haemothorax are commonly associated and usually require drainage. Rupture of a large bronchus may cause haemoptysis and atelectasis of the affected lung. Patients with complete transection of the trachea often die rapidly of asphyxia, but an adequate airway may exist and treatment is by surgical repair. Patients with tracheal rupture may have stridor, aphonia, and/or respiratory distress. Considerable problems may be encountered in endotracheal intubation. Blind intubation may prove fatal and fibreoptic intubation may be required.

Penetrating injuries are often accompanied by injuries to the oesophagus, carotid artery, and jugular vein; missile injuries may cause extensive tissue destruction.

Aortic rupture

This usually occurs as a result of deceleration trauma, but occasionally from penetrating trauma. Tears of the aorta and pulmonary arteries are frequently fatal; 90% of affected patients die at the scene of the injury. Most survivors have the blood loss contained by a haematoma. An intact adventitia (outer wall) may prevent immediate death. Initial severe hypotension will occur with the loss of up to 1000 ml of blood, and the patient will usually respond to rapid fluid resuscitation. However, hypotension may be recurrent or persistent and blood transfusion may be necessary to maintain adequate perfusion and blood pressure. A chest X-ray may show a widened mediastinum, tracheal shift to the right, and blurring of the aortic outline. Early angiography would be indicated if the patient's condition permits, but urgent surgical repair may be required.

Abdominal and pelvic injuries

Penetrating injuries, particularly stab and gunshot wounds, are common causes of abdominal trauma in young men. Blunt trauma most often results from road traffic accidents and falls. There are often associated injuries to the head, spine, chest, and genitourinary system, and these will complicate management. Patients with abdominal injuries have the potential for severe haemorrhage and an increased risk of post-traumatic sepsis. Injuries resulting from blunt trauma to the abdomen are the most difficult to diagnose; in the multiply injured patient, signs of intra-abdominal injury (pain, guarding) may be difficult to assess (sedation, agitation) or be masked by other injuries.

Immediate management is aimed at identifying the presence of abdominal injury rather than making an accurate diagnosis of a specific injury. The liver, spleen, and kidneys are the major organs involved in blunt trauma. Visceral disruption can occur as a result of rapid deceleration, a direct blow, or shearing forces. The compulsory use of seat belts in vehicles has reduced mortality from head and maxillofacial injuries, but has significantly increased the incidence of damage to the thoracic cage, liver, spleen, and mesentery.

Diagnosis can be aided by various procedures such as peritoneal lavage, CT scan, ultrasonography, X-rays, and selective angiography. Peritoneal lavage is performed by installation of a litre of normal saline into the peritoneal cavity through a percutaneous catheter; this fluid is then drained out through the same catheter and examined for blood. The technique accurately detects intra-abdominal haemorrhage (including bleeding from pelvic fractures) in 95% of cases and is helpful in evaluating the need for laparotomy.

Injuries sustained from penetrating trauma will depend on the type of weapon or object, its path or trajectory, and in the case of gunshot wounds the velocity and calibre of bullet. Stab wounds will penetrate adjacent structures, but bullets may have a circuitous or tumbling action causing extensive tissue damage involving multiple organs.

Abdominal injuries

Initial resuscitation priorities are maintenance of airway, breathing, and circulation. Specific treatment of abdominal injuries should not delay correction of hypoxaemia and tissue perfusion. Urgent laparotomy may be indicated if hypovolaemia persists after adequate fluid replacement and the cause cannot be attributed to other injuries.

In the critical care unit the patient must be carefully observed for increasing abdominal pain, rigidity, or tenderness. Continuous monitoring of vital signs is essential. Be alert for haemodynamic changes that indicate haemorrhage (tachycardia, hypotension, low CVP, poor peripheral perfusion, pale colour) or the need for excessive fluid replacement that does not improve the patient's cardiovascular status. The abdominal cavity is a potential reservoir for major occult blood loss; injury must always be suspected if there is bruising or superficial laceration (e.g. from seat belts) that indicates possible damage to underlying organs.

Unless contraindicated, a urethral catheter should be inserted to monitor urine output. The presence of haematuria is an important sign of potential genitourinary damage, although such damage can occur without any subsequent haematuria. Remember that patients whose prime insult is not to the abdomen may still have the potential for abdominal injury. Trauma to the lower chest (e.g. rib fractures or stab wounds) may damage the underlying abdominal viscera. Up to 60% of gunshot wounds and 25% of stab wounds in this region of the chest will cause abdominal injury.

Pelvic fractures

Pelvic fractures may cause massive and sometimes uncontrollable haemorrhage; over 4 L of blood may be lost. However, 75% of patients become haemodynamically stable after initial fluid resuscitation, often because a local tamponade by the blood clot within the pelvis prevents further bleeding. The associated muscles are also very vascular, and major veins and arteries in the pelvis can easily be disrupted by trauma. Bleeding can track down into the thigh. The mortality of patients with open pelvic fractures exceeds 50%, and associated rectal and genitourinary injuries are common. Approximately 30% of patients with pelvic fractures also have a ruptured bladder and torn urethra. Severe haemorrhage may be difficult to control and pneumatic antishock garments may be useful in initial resuscitation. Immobilization and internal external fixation may help control bleeding, but surgical repair of torn vessels, or angiography and embolization may be required.

Genitourinary injuries

Upper genitourinary injuries (kidneys, upper ureters, and renal vessels)

Injuries to the kidneys are most often caused by blunt trauma (sporting injuries, falls, vehicle accidents, and assaults); 40% of patients have associated or multiple injuries that may obscure the signs and symptoms of renal trauma. Penetrating trauma directly to the kidney from stab or gunshot wounds is easy to diagnose but may cause injury to other organs such as spleen, liver, pancreas, bowel, and duodenum, or perforate the diaphragm. Damage from penetrating trauma can be severe and extensive, particularly from gunshot wounds, causing laceration of renal vessels, kidney, and ureters.

Direct blows to the back resulting in bruising and abrasions may indicate underlying renal damage. In any patient sustaining deceleration trauma there is the potential for genitourinary injury. Rapid deceleration (e.g. falls) may cause tearing of the renal vessels, intimal tearing, or rupture of the ureters at the pelvi-ureteric junction. Direct blows to the abdomen can crush the kidney; therefore fractures to the lower ribs or spinal processes should raise suspicion of renal injury. Road traffic accidents may cause renal injury if a seat belt, steering wheel, or other external mechanical force crushes the kidney anteriorly between the abdominal wall and the paravertebral muscles.

Renal trauma can be categorized into minor, major, and critical. Minor injuries are limited to minor parenchymal damage, contusions, and superficial lacerations. These constitute 85% of renal trauma. Major injuries include deep lacerations involving the pelvi-calyceal system and/or tears of the capsule. These result in major parenchymal damage and constitute 10% of renal injuries. Critical injuries include renal fragmentation and pedicle injuries (renal artery thrombosis, pelvi-ureteric rupture, or avulsion of renal vessels) and occur in 5% of renal trauma cases. Major blood loss can occur in these patients with consequent hypovolaemic shock.

A direct blow to the flank may result in signs of bruising or swelling over the lower thoracic, loin or upper abdominal areas. The patient will often complain of loin pain, and the anterior abdominal wall may be rigid on the affected side. Haematuria may be present and painful ureteric colic can occur if blood clots are passed through the ureter.

Initial management depends on the patient's clinical state. Airway, breathing, and circulation must be stabilized before attention is directed to a specific diagnosis of renal injury. Renal trauma alone rarely causes severe hypovolaemic shock or threatens life. If hypovolaemia is present, other injuries must be considered beforehand as the prime cause. Once the patient's breathing and circulation are stabilized, diagnostic X-ray procedures can be undertaken. Intravenous urography or CT scanning with contrast is usually carried out on all patients with haematuria and a systolic blood pressure <90 mmHg. Renal ultrasonography is used on patients who are clinically stable but require evaluation of renal damage. Occasionally, a retrograde ureterogram may be required in patients with suspected disruption of the pelvi-ureteric junction, and selective renal arteriography may be performed in patients with persistent haematuria (longer than a week) or those with vascular pedicle injuries.

Patients with critical renal injuries or penetrating trauma will usually require surgical exploration. Lacerations to the renal vessels may then be repaired, and partial or total nephrectomy will be required for patients with fragmented kidneys. Patients with a renal artery thrombosis identified early may be considered for thrombectomy.

All patients with renal injuries, however minor, must be observed closely. Vital signs should be recorded frequently and urine output monitored and observed for haematuria. Pain must be assessed and adequate analgesia administered. Any loin swelling should be observed for change in size. Strict bedrest is usually enforced until the vital signs are stable, haematuria has ceased, and any peri-renal swelling has clinically resolved.

Lower genitourinary injuries (bladder, urethra, genitalia)

Injuries to the bladder, urethra, and genitalia can be caused by penetrating trauma (particularly gunshots), but are more common from blunt trauma. In patients with suspected lower genitourinary trauma injuries the urethral meatus must be inspected for blood, the abdomen examined for signs of peritonism (a rigid painful abdomen), and the perineum for signs of bruising. A urethral catheter should not be inserted in patients with suspected urotrauma until advised by a urologist. If blood is present in the meatus, intravenous urography (antegrade or retrograde) will be required to detect a perforated or displaced bladder before suprapubic catheterization. Pelvic fractures are a common cause of injury to the bladder and urethra due to perforation from a bony segment. Signs of urethral injury are blood in the urethral meatus, inability to void, and perineal bruising. If these are present, a urethral catheter must not be passed as the urethra is often traumatized and devascularized when torn and may be eroded by the catheter, disintegrate around it, or the catheter may be passed through the tear. The catheter would also prevent haematoma drainage and may introduce infection. Therefore a suprapubic catheter must be inserted.

In patients with pelvic fractures, but no evidence of blood in the meatus, a urethral catheter may be passed and a cystogram used to exclude bladder rupture. Patients who are shocked, have peritonism, and in whom cystography shows bladder rupture will require laparotomy. In women, the shorter urethra is rarely damaged by pelvic fractures and a urethral catheter can usually be passed, following which cystography may be performed to exclude bladder injuries.

Bulbar injuries are usually caused by direct trauma (e.g. a straddle impact) and such patients will have blood in the urethral meatus and perineal bruising. A urethral catheter must never be passed as this will introduce infection and aggravate the injury. The patient should be allowed to pass urine naturally, but if retention occurs a suprapubic catheter should be inserted. Prophylactic antibiotics should be given. Injuries to the scrotum and penis can also occur. Scrotal tears heal very well and do not normally require suturing, but direct blows to the scrotum can cause large scrotal haematomas and damage to the testes which may require surgical repair.

Specific nursing management

The nursing management of the patient with abdominal trauma (including pelvic fractures) depends on the patient's specific injuries. Patients with severe abdominal injuries will probably undergo explorative laparotomy and definitive surgery before being admitted to the critical care unit. Care will then be directed towards anticipating potential problems relating to the specific surgery performed.

All patients will require careful monitoring of vital signs, urine output, wound drainage, and blood gas analysis. It is essential to be aware of potential haemorrhage, even after surgery, as coagulation defects are common after major trauma and large blood transfusions. Anticipate complications arising from the hypoperfusion of major organs if large blood losses have occurred. Management must always be directed to restabilizing vital functions and optimizing oxygenation and tissue perfusion. Blood glucose levels must be monitored, particularly after surgery to the pancreas or liver, and the need for parenteral nutrition should be considered if the enteral route cannot be used for some time.

Patients with pelvic fractures may pose particular problems in the care of pressure areas. Clear instructions must be obtained from the surgeons as to the degree of mobility that the patient is allowed. Nursing is made considerably easier if the fracture is stable or externally/internally fixed. However, some type of pressure-relieving mattress will be required as movement will still be considerably limited.

Patients with abdominal and pelvic injuries are more susceptible to infection, particularly if the injury results from penetrating trauma. Contamination by foreign material (e.g. clothing in missile injuries) may occur, and if the gastrointestinal tract is disrupted the bowel contents may be distributed into the peritoneal cavity. Such patients are at risk from local infection (abscess formation), septicaemia, and multi-organ failure. Patients who have undergone total splenectomy are at risk from overwhelming infection due to diminished humoral immunity; operative measures now attempt to preserve some splenic tissue. Prophylactic antibiotics should be administered to patients with penetrating trauma, and the patient must be monitored for potential infection (e.g. temperature, signs of peritonism, presence of purulent discharge from wounds or drains).

The immobile patient is also at risk of deep vein thrombosis and pulmonary embolus. Unless contraindicated (e.g. ongoing bleeding), prophylactic heparinization should be commenced.

The abdominal cavity is capable of containing a significant amount of blood without distension and large blood losses can occur retroperitoneally. Therefore an increase in girth may be a late sign of haemorrhage, or be due to the presence of excess air and/or fluid either inside or outside the bowel, or to oedematous bowel (see Table 11.2). Girth measurements are generally inaccurate, particularly if wounds are padded. Intra-abdominal pressure measurement is a more useful guide (Webber *et al.* 2002).

Intra-abdominal hypertension and abdominal compartment syndrome

The abdomen and its contents can be considered a closed box; the elasticity of its walls and the character of its contents determine the pressure within. In a healthy individual this intra-abdominal pressure (IAP)is <5–7 mmHg. As the abdomen distends and abdominal wall compliance decreases, the IAP rises. Intra-abdominal hypertension (IAH) is defined as a sustained or repeated pathological increase in IAP >12 mmHg (Carlotti and Carvalho 2009). This can occur as a result of medical and surgical pathologies and may be acute or chronic (see Table 11.2).

Abdominal compartment syndrome (ACS) develops if IAH is not recognized appropriately. It is defined as a pathological state caused by an acute increase in IAH >20–25 mmHg with adverse effects on end-organ function, where abdominal decompression has beneficial effects (Cheatham 2009). ACS is associated with a high incidence of morbidity and mortality because of the effects of the raised intra-abdominal pressure on respiratory, cardiovascular, hepatic, renal, gastrointestinal, and central nervous systems and may result in multi-organ failure (Theodossis *et al.* 2011).

Table 11.2 Causes of intra-abdominal hypertension/abdominal compartment syndrome

Cause	Secondary to:
Trauma	Massive fluid resuscitation Coagulopathy Continued intra-abdominal bleeding Haematoma Intra-abdominal trauma Capillary leak due to release of vasoactive substances Circumferential burns of abdominal area causing abdominal compression from oedema and eschar formation
Abdominal surgery	Presence of intra-abdominal pack Wound closed under tension Continued bleeding Extensive handling of the bowel Development of an ileus Massive fluid resuscitation
Paralytic ileus Bowel obstruction/ infarction/volvulus Gastroparesis/gastric dilatation Pancreatitis GI haemorrhage Post laparoscopy	Gaseous and fluid distention
Liver cirrhosis	Ascites
Peritoneal dialysis	Dialysate fluid
Haemo/ pneumoperitoneum	
Intra-abdominal abscess/sepsis	
Intra-abdominal or retroperitoneal tumour	
Acute respiratory failure	Elevated intrathoracic pressure
Prone positioning	Compression of abdomen
Obesity (BMI >30)	
Pregnancy	

Pathophysiological effects of intra-abdominal hypertension/abdominal compartment syndrome

Respiratory

Respiratory failure may be caused or aggravated by the raised IAP pushing the diaphragm higher than normal into the chest, thus increasing intrathoracic pressure and reducing functional capacity and compliance. This increases peak airway pressures, reduces tidal volume, and causes atelectasis. Compression of the pulmonary parenchyma decreases oxygen and carbon dioxide transport across the pulmonary capillary membrane, resulting in hypoxaemia, hypercapnia, and a respiratory acidosis. High levels of PEEP and inspired oxygen may be required to maintain oxygenation; however, PEEP can exacerbate the cardiac and respiratory complications of IAH.

Cardiovascular

As the diaphragm is pushed upwards, the abdominal pressure is transmitted to, and directly compresses, the heart and major vessels. This decreases preload and increases afterload on the left ventricle, reducing cardiac output and elevating SVR (O'Mara *et al.* 2005).

The central venous and pulmonary artery pressures are elevated, even if the patient is hypovolaemic. This may make it difficult to monitor the patient's response to intravascular fluid boluses unless flow is measured.

The patient should be observed for any impaired distal extremity circulation secondary to compression of the aorta (pedal pulses, limb colour, temperature).

Gastrointestinal

As IAP increases, blood flow to the abdominal organs decreases. Visceral perfusion may start to fall with an IAP as low as 12 mmHg. At pressures >40 mmHg microcirculatory flow decreases and the intestinal mucosa becomes ischaemic. Such patients are at risk of gastrointestinal bleeding.

Hepatic

Blood flow in the hepatic artery and veins and the portal circulation is reduced with altered glucose metabolism and decreased lactate clearance (Cheatham, 2009).

Renal

Direct compression on the kidneys and renal veins cause the glomerular filtration rate to fall. The raised IAP reduces renal perfusion, causing oligo-anuria and, ultimately, renal failure. Glucose reabsorption is decreased, and plasma renin activity, aldosterone, and antidiuretic hormone levels increase (Balogh *et al.* 2007).

Neurological

IAH increases intracranial pressure (ICP) and reduces cerebral perfusion pressure (CPP). The elevated intrathoracic and central venous pressures cause increased resistance to cerebral venous drainage, so CPP decreases as ICP rises. Volume expansion and any fall in mean BP further reduces CPP.

Abdominal wall

Blood flow to the abdominal wall is reduced due to compression and leads to local ischaemia and oedema. This decreases abdominal wall compliance, further exacerbating IAH and contributes to impaired wound healing, wound dehiscence, bowel herniation, and infection, especially if the wound is closed under tension. Table 11.3 summarizes the effects of IAH.

Management of intra-abdominal hypertension and abdominal compartment syndrome

Prevention and early detection of IAH in the high risk patient is essential if the physiological consequences are to be prevented. In patients with intestinal oedema or distension, wound closure may be delayed following

Table 11.3 Summary of the effects of intra-abdominal hypertension

System	Increased	Decreased
Cardiovascular	CVP Heart rate SVR PAWP Afterload	Stroke volume Cardiac output Preload Venous return
Respiratory	Intrathoracic pressure Peak inspiratory pressure P_aCO_2	Functional capacity Tidal volume P_aO_2 Compliance
Gastrointestinal		Intramucosal gastric pH (pH_i) Blood flow to all abdominal organs Mesenteric and mucosal blood flow
Renal		Oliguria or anuria Glomerular filtration rate Renal perfusion Glucose reabsorption
Neurological	Intracranial pressure	Cerebral perfusion pressure

laparotomy, or alternative closures employed such as prosthetic mesh followed by staged abdominal reconstruction.

Supportive therapies include pressure-controlled ventilation with paralysis, and inotropic and renal support.

Non-operative treatments include the use of prokinetic drugs if the condition is secondary to an ileus, and diuretics and/or haemofiltration if it is due to bowel oedema and fluid overload. Rectal and nasogastric tubes, enemas, paracentesis catheters, and CT or ultrasound drainage of abcesses or haematoma are used as appropriate. Neostigmine can be used for severe ileus, but carries a risk of bowel ischaemia.

Definitive treatment of ACS is by abdominal decompression, but there is no clear consensus on optimal timing and clear confirmation of outcome benefit. Patients undergoing surgical decompression are at risk of sudden and severe hypotension and asystolic cardiac arrest when the abdomen is opened. This may be due in part to hypovolaemia and also to reperfusion injury where mediators and free radicals are released following reperfusion of the splanchnic bed. Therefore it is recommended that adequate volume administration be given prior to decompression.

Measurement of intra-abdominal pressure

Intra-abdominal pressure (IAP) can be measured indirectly by placing transfemoral catheters into the inferior vena cava, via intraperitoneal catheters, through gastrostomy or nasogastric tubes, or intrarectally. A quick and simple method is to use an existing Foley catheter to measure bladder pressure. At intravesical volumes <100 ml, the bladder acts as a passive reservoir and reflects IAP reasonably accurately within a range of 5–70 mmHg. It should be recorded two- to four-hourly, according to clinical need. The trend in pressure values can provide useful information regarding clinical progression. Abdominal compartment syndrome cannot be ruled out in the presence of normal pressures if organ dysfunction exists. Bladder pressure may also not capture an elevated abdominal pressure within a localized area.

Measuring abdominal pressure via a urinary catheter

The procedure is relatively straightforward and involves instilling normal saline into the bladder, clamping the tubing, and connecting a transducer to measure the pressure (Figure 11.3). Though the bladder needs to be filled in order to transmit pressure to the transducer, there is no clear agreement regarding how much fluid should be instilled. Many studies correlating intravesical (bladder) pressure with IAP have been carried out in animal models, but human studies are lacking. Generally, 50–100 ml is used; when the bladder volume exceeds 100 ml the intrinsic contraction of the distended bladder wall causes an increase in pressure and so IAP is not

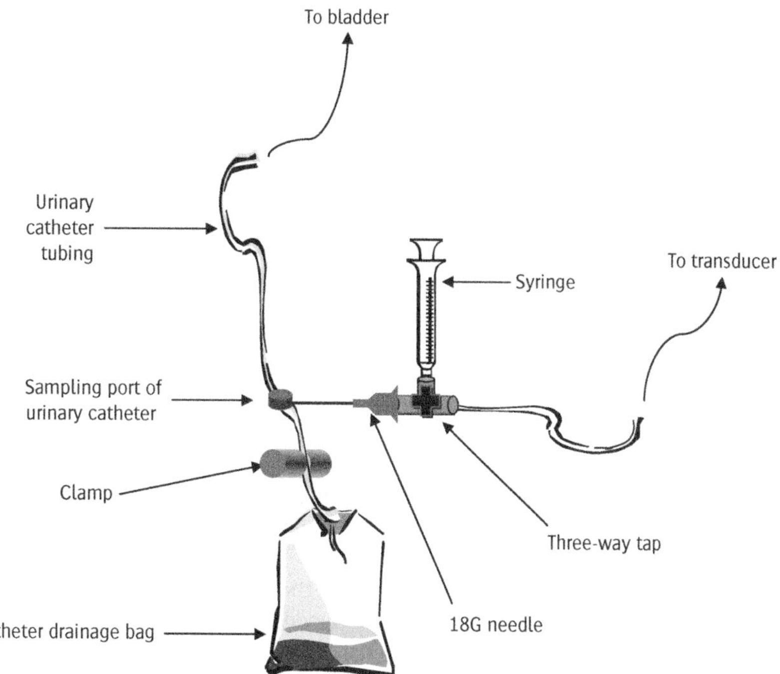

Figure 11.3 Measurement of intra-abdominal pressure.

accurately reflected. Positioning of the patient is important; they should be placed supine so that the weight of the abdominal contents does not press on the bladder. If unable to lie supine, the position at which the first measurement is taken should be recorded, and all subsequent recordings made in the same position. Although the individual reading may not be the 'true' pressure, trends can still be assessed. The transducer should be level with the pubic symphysis bone (this approximates to the mid-axillary line).

There are several methods of measuring IAP using a Foley urinary catheter. Either a two- or three-way Foley bladder catheter can be used. Most patients will have a two-way catheter in situ, as a three-way catheter is mainly reserved for bladder irrigation. The benefit of using a three-way catheter is that the saline can be instilled into the irrigation limb, thus avoiding the need to access a closed system.

- Equipment:
  - transducer primed with normal saline (this does not need to be under pressure)
  - clamp
  - 18-gauge needle
  - 60 ml syringe
  - urinary drainage bag with a sampling port close to the catheter connection
- Method—the procedure must be carried out aseptically, using sterile gloves and placing a sterile towel beneath the catheter connection.
  1. Place the patient supine.
  2. Zero the transducer at the pubic symphysis pubis bone.
  3. Clamp the drainage bag distal to the sampling port.
  4. Draw up 50 ml of sterile saline into the catheter syringe.
  5. Disconnect the drainage bag, inject the saline, and reconnect.
  6. Insert the 18-gauge needle (with the transducer attached) into the sampling port of the Foley catheter.
  7. Release the clamp momentarily until fluid fills the tubing and then reclamp.
  8. Allow the transducer to equilibriate and then record the pressure.

An alternative method is to insert a three-way tap between the needle and transducer. The saline can be injected via this tap instead of disconnecting the catheter drainage bag, thus reducing the risk of infection.

A similar method is used when measuring abdominal pressure via a nasogastric tube.

Musculoskeletal injuries

Musculoskeletal injuries themselves are rarely life-threatening but any associated injuries can be. Up to 70% of multiply injured patients will have injured limbs, fractures, or dislocations. The management of limb trauma is always secondary to resuscitation and control of the airway, breathing, and circulation. Only when the multiply injured patient is stable should attention be directed to the definitive care of the limb injury. At this point a thorough head-to-toe examination is carried out and limb X-rays taken. Certain musculoskeletal conditions are considered life-threatening. These include traumatic amputations (particularly of a whole limb), major haemorrhage from vascular injuries or open fractures, severe crush injuries to the pelvis and abdomen, and multiple long-bone fractures.

Blood loss from open wounds is obvious, though often underestimated, and large amounts of blood can be lost in closed fractures. Major haemorrhage can occur in closed fractures of the humerus and tibia (up to 1.5 L each) and femur (up to 2.5 L). Rapid resuscitation is vital to replace the lost circulatory volume. However, the cause of haemorrhagic shock should never be presumed to originate solely from skeletal injury until other potential injuries have been excluded. Open wounds or fractures may have bled extensively from the time of the injury, and blood loss may be difficult to assess. Generally, the blood loss for open fractures is two- to threefold greater than for closed fractures. Direct pressure should be applied to any open wounds that are bleeding by compression bandage or hand pressure until definitive treatment can be carried out.

A fracture also produces damage to muscles surrounding the injured bone, and to blood vessels and nerves in its vicinity. Penetrating trauma and local contusions may disrupt blood flow, while limb perfusion may be poor in the hypovolaemic patient. Therefore vascular impairment and neurovascular bundle injury may compromise the survival of a limb and must be identified without delay. Bleeding or thrombosis in a blood vessel can impair the distal circulation and cause limb ischaemia. Vascular injury should be identified promptly by close and regular observation before ischaemia develops. Peripheral pulses must be evaluated regularly to assess circulation, and an absent or diminished pulse reported without delay. Skin perfusion should be assessed by capillary return, temperature, and colour of the limb distal to the injury. A low skin temperature indicates inadequate perfusion. Check that plaster casts, traction, and compression bandages are not impairing the circulation.

If nerve damage has occurred, sensation will be impaired. This sensation is lost early if ischaemia is present. Direct severing of nerve fibres by penetrating trauma or by stretching or compression of the nerve fibres, causing variable degrees of paralysis, may cause nerve injury.

Dislocations may produce neurovascular injury by stretching nerves and compressing blood vessels causing muscle injury. Dislocations should be reduced promptly, particularly at the knee, elbow, and ankle. Angiography may be required if vascular injury is suspected. Obvious and complete arterial occlusion will, however, require prompt surgical exploration.

Compartment syndrome and rhabdomyolysis are specific complications following musculoskeletal injuries and are discussed fully elsewhere in this chapter.

Specific management

Open fractures

Here, a wound in the skin communicates directly with the broken bone. The most important factor in management is to prevent infection; thus, ideally, open fractures should be definitively treated within 8 hours of the injury. The fracture should be aligned and splinted and the wound covered with a sterile dry dressing. Antibiotic therapy should be instituted and tetanus prophylaxis administered. Surgery will include thorough cleaning of the wound and debridement of non-viable tissue. Wounds are often left open for 5–7 days to prevent a rise in tissue pressure, which contributes to wound hypoxia and infection. Open fractures are often unstable; rigid stabilization will promote tissue healing.

Closed fractures

Here, there is no open wound (Figure 11.4). In the multiply injured patient early fixation of fractures (within 24 hours) can reduce mortality and morbidity from ARDS, fat embolism, and systemic sepsis. Nursing of the patient is made considerably easier and analgesia requirements can be reduced.

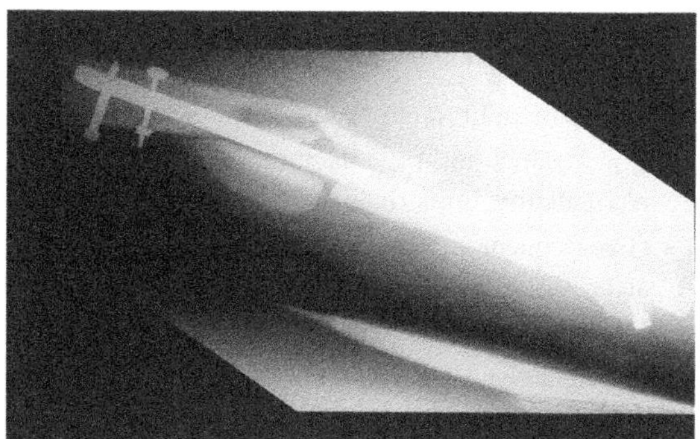

Figure 11.4 Repair of compound femoral fracture with an intramedullary nail

Dislocations

Dislocations must be reduced promptly to prevent potentially irreversible damage to neurovascular bundles and plexus injuries (Table 11.4). All dislocations are extremely painful. Adequate analgesia must be given. The limb should be supported on a pillow or immobilized with traction while awaiting definitive treatment.

Specific nursing management of musculoskeletal injuries

The extent of the injuries and the degree of patient immobility will dictate specific nursing care. Several methods can be used to maintain reduction of fractures, depending on their nature—for example, plaster casts, splints, continuous traction, pin and plaster techniques, and internal fixation devices (nails, plates, wires, screws, rods). Continuous traction can be via skin traction or skeletal traction using wires, pins, or tongs placed through the bone with a system of ropes, pulleys, and weights. Space does not permit a comprehensive description of the nursing management of orthopaedic injuries. However, the patient in the critical care unit frequently has multiple or other serious injuries as well as fractures

Table 11.4 Types of dislocation and associated complications

Dislocation	Associated complication
Knee	Popliteal artery/nerve injuries
Ankle	Skin pressure and necrosis
Elbow	Ulnar and median nerve damage
Shoulder	Brachial plexus injury
Hip	Asceptic necrosis of femoral head

that necessitates their stay on the critical care unit. The following points should be remembered.

- For the patient in traction:
  - Check skin around the traction device for evidence of circulatory impairment.
  - Give frequent and meticulous attention to pressure areas. Use a pressure-relieving mattress.
  - Inspect pin sites daily and keep clean and dry.
  - Passive/active exercises to non-immobilized joints.
  - The knots on the traction rope should be secure and the supporting apparatus free of the pulleys.
  - Check that the ropes are in the wheel groove and the weights hang free.
  - The weights should not be removed when the patient is moved. One nurse must support the weights without relieving the traction if a patient is moved up the bed.
- For the patient with a plaster cast:
  - Constriction due to swelling may cause circulatory impairment, pain, and pressure on healthy tissue. Therefore check skin temperature, colour, pulses, and sensation in the affected limb.
  - Check skin integrity around the edge of the cast. Pressure points may need extra padding.
  - Pain under the cast may be due to pressure on a bony prominence, nerve, or blood vessel.
  - Supracondylar fractures of the elbow are often accompanied by considerable swelling which may impair circulation in the forearm and hand. The radial pulse must be checked frequently. Elevating the limb on a pillow may alleviate swelling, but, if it is severe, the plaster may need to be split.
- Anticipate complications:
  - **Haemorrhage** Monitor vital signs, observe wounds and drains for bleeding, monitor haemoglobin.
  - **Compartment syndrome** Observe the limb frequently for tense swelling, pain, decreased temperature, and diminished sensation.
  - **Infection** Monitor temperature, inspect wounds, cannulae, and pin sites. Swab and culture if necessary.
  - **Deep vein thrombosis** Inspect calves for pain and swelling. Consider anti-embolic stockings and prophylactic anticoagulation. Passive/active limb movements may help prevent thrombosis.
  - **Rhabdomyolysis** Monitor urine output, daily urinalysis, observe urine for myoglobinuria (NB: this gives a false positive test for haemoglobinuria), measure serum creatinine kinase. Keep patient well hydrated and maintain a good diuresis. Monitor urea and electrolytes, including magnesium, calcium, and phosphate.

Musculoskeletal injuries

Check limbs for:

- Colour
- Temperature
- Pulses
- Sensation/pain
- Local compression (splints, bandages etc.).

Flaps

The patient with severe musculoskeletal injuries may require reconstruction using free or pedicled flaps in order to correct an anatomical defect. A free flap is where a section of tissue (which can include a combination of skin, muscle, fascia, or bone) is detached from the body and microsurgically reattached elsewhere. A pedicled flap is where the tissue is transposed elsewhere while still attached to its original blood supply.

The post-operative survival of the flap depends on good perfusion. Close and frequent observation is needed to promptly detect arterial insufficiency or venous congestion, particularly in the first 72 hours.

Factors that may be detrimental to flap survival include:

- hypotension (decreases arterial flow through the flap)
- vasopressors (may decrease flow due to vasoconstriction)
- hypovolaemia
- poor positioning.

Recordings of core, flap, and peripheral temperature should be made. Ideally, the core–flap temperature difference should be <1.5°C. In order to achieve this and to optimize blood flow, the patient and flap both need to be kept warm and the vessels dilated. Vasodilators such as glyceryl trinitrate are often used intravenously, and the haemoglobin level kept below 100g/L (10 g/dl) to reduce blood viscosity. Some protocols also use dextran infusions to reduce viscosity. A body-warming device, such as a Bair Hugger, should be used as necessary, and mean arterial blood pressure and CVP kept within set ranges.

The flap must be inspected regularly and an assessment made of its colour, temperature, capillary refill, turgidity, and the presence of a pulse (using Doppler if necessary). The frequency of these observations should be dictated by the surgeon's instructions and/or unit policy. Many critical care areas will have dedicated flap observation charts.

Any changes in observation must be reported immediately as the salvage rate of a failing flap is dependent on rapid intervention.

Flap observations should include the following.

- **Colour** The flap should have a normal skin colour. A mottled or purple flap indicates venous congestion and a pale flap suggests arterial insufficiency.
- **Capillary refill** Normal capillary refill should take 2–3 sec. Venous congestion is indicated if it is >3 sec and arterial insufficiency if it is >6 sec.
- **Turgidity** The flap should feel soft to the touch. Arterial insufficiency causes the flap to feel flaccid, and if venous congestion is present it will feel turgid or tense.
- **Pulse and temperature** The flap should feel warm and a pulse should be present. An absent pulse indicates arterial insufficiency.

Complications following trauma

Complications secondary to trauma can result from the following.

- Shock causing hypoperfusion of vital organs (e.g. renal and circulatory failure). The origin of the shock may be hypovolaemic (e.g. haemorrhage), septic, neurogenic (e.g. spinal injury), obstructive (e.g. pulmonary embolus), or cardiogenic (e.g. direct myocardial contusion).
- Specific types of trauma causing rhabdomyolysis, compartment syndrome, air embolism, and fat embolism syndrome (e.g. long-bone fractures, chest injuries, crush injuries).
- Transfusion of large amounts of blood causing anaphylactic reactions, ARDS, multi-organ failure, coagulopathies, and hypocalcaemia.
- Infection causing wound breakdown, anastomotic breakdown, or sepsis.
- Immobility causing pressure sores, chest infection, deep vein thrombosis (DVT), or pulmonary embolism.
- Respiratory failure from chest, head, and neck injuries.

Compartment syndrome

Compartment syndrome is due to swelling, bleeding, or ischaemia within the fascial compartments of the arm and/or leg (including buttocks). As these compartments are unable to expand to any significant degree, interstitial tissue pressure rises. When this pressure exceeds that of the capillary bed, local ischaemia occurs and rhabdomyolysis, permanent paralysis through nerve injury, or gangrene may result. This typically occurs after crush injuries, closed or open fractures, or sustained compression of a limb in an immobile patient.

If able, the patient will complain of increasing pain in the affected limb despite immobilization of fractures. Pain on passive stretching of muscles within the affected region may also be evident. There will be tense swelling of the involved fascial compartment(s) and possibly reduced sensation over the dermatomes supplied by the affected nerves. The absence of distal pulses does not identify the early stages of compartment syndrome, as these may be intact until late in the progression of the syndrome after irreversible damage has been done. Development of a compartment syndrome may not be an immediate complication, and careful observation of limbs for swelling, abnormal perfusion, temperature differences, or pain should be performed.

Intracompartmental pressures can be monitored with needle manometry or other invasive devices. Some non-invasive techniques, such as near-infrared spectroscopy, ultrasonic devices and laser Doppler flowmetry, are also available. Pressures >20 mmHg are considered abnormal, but there is no clear consensus on the threshold at which surgical intervention is warranted—this is usually quoted as between 30 and 40 mmHg but the decision must also be based on clinical assessment (Mabvuure *et al.* 2012).

Restricting dressings should be released, and if recovery is not rapid urgent fasciotomy should be carried out to relieve the pressure. The wounds are often left open and closed at a second operation up to 7 days later. Delaying primary closure also allows repeated irrigation and debridement if required. Skin grafts may be needed to close the wounds and considerable blood loss may occur. Complications include permenant muscle or nerve damage; in severe cases amputation may be necessary. Pain is a major feature and adequate analgesia must be given. The patient must be kept well hydrated as muscle necrosis and rhabdomyolysis (see Chapter 7) can cause acute renal failure.

Fat embolism syndrome

Patients with fat embolism syndrome (FES) have emboli of fat macroglobules in the pulmonary and systemic circulations. Organs with high blood flow, such as heart, lungs, brain, and kidney, show evidence of capillary obstruction by fat or microaggregates of platelets, red cells, and fibrin. The syndrome usually presents as respiratory insufficiency, cerebral dysfunction, and petechial skin haemorrhages (see Box 11.9).

FES is associated with bone fractures, particularly of the long bones and pelvis. These fractures result in fat and marrow entering the venous circulation. Massive trauma may also disrupt adipose tissue, causing large fat globules to enter the bloodstream. The onset of signs and symptoms of the syndrome is generally 24–48 hours post-injury.

Mechanical obstruction of the pulmonary capillaries rapidly causes dyspnoea and tachypnoea, hypoxaemia, and occasionally production of blood-stained frothy sputum. A petechial rash develops, classically over the upper thorax, neck, and soft palate, and is seen in up to 50% of patients. Petechiae can sometimes be seen in the retina. Pyrexia often develops, with an associated tachycardia. Occlusion of cerebral vessels causes confusion, drowsiness, decerebrate signs, convulsions, and coma. If these signs become apparent, other causes must be excluded by appropriate investigations (e.g. delayed post-traumatic intracranial injury by CT scanning). Obstruction of renal vessels causes oligo-anuria and there may be a diagnostic presence of fat globules in pulmonary artery blood or urine. Coagulopathy may occur and there may be significant intrapulmonary haemorrhage. ECG changes may reveal right heart strain in fulminant FES. Biopsy of skin or kidneys may reveal microinfarcts associated with fat globules.

Box 11.9 Features of fat embolism syndrome

- Hypoxaemia
- Increased respiratory rate, heart rate, and temperature
- Decreased blood pressure, cardiac output, and urine output
- Poor cerebral perfusion
- Petechiae

Treatment is largely supportive; however, the prognosis in fulminant FES is poor. Supplemental oxygen therapy is used to correct hypoxaemia, but often mechanical ventilation ± PEEP is required. An adequate circulatory volume must be ensured, taking into account blood loss at fracture sites and fluid loss from wounds. Careful haemodynamic monitoring should be instituted. There is often a fall in cardiac output and an increase in pulmonary vascular resistance as the syndrome develops. Inotropic support may be required to maintain arterial pressure (Shaik, 2009).

Renal support will be required if the patient becomes anuric or oliguric with rapidly deteriorating renal function. Close monitoring of serum electrolytes is essential.

The prevention of hypoxaemia reduces the severity of the syndrome. Early institution of oxygen therapy and maintaining good blood gas exchange are important preventative factors in the first 48 hours of patients at risk of FES.

Air embolism

This results from entrainment of air, either from an open operative field or from communication outside the body (e.g. penetrating chest trauma causing alveolar rupture), into the venous or arterial vasculature. Small amounts of air in the circulation can be absorbed, but a large bolus (>100 ml) can lead to a right ventricular air lock and immediate death. Massive air embolism can occur from a bronchopulmonary vein fistula when patients with severe lung injury are mechanically ventilated. Air embolism can also occur during removal or insertion of central venous catheters; there is an increased risk if the patient is in an upright position, hypovolaemic, or takes a deep inspiration. In up to 35% of patients, systemic air embolism is due to a patent foramen ovale, with air passing directly from the right to the left side of the heart (paradoxical air embolism) through a congenital opening. Much smaller amounts of air (0.5–2 ml) can cause symptoms if coronary or cerebral circulations are affected (Shaikh, 2009).

The diagnosis of air embolism can be difficult when there may be other causes of sudden cardiovascular collapse and hypoxaemia. It is uncommon, so other causes such as tension pneumothorax should be excluded first. The main systems affected are the respiratory, cardiovascular, and central nervous systems. Clinical manifestations depend on the amount, nature, and speed of air entrainment. Signs and symptoms include:

- chest pain, arrhythmias, reduced cardiac output, right heart failure, cardiovascular collapse

- dyspnoea, tachypnoea, hypoxaemia, hypercarbia
- cerebral hypoperfusion.

Management is largely supportive. If there is a large air embolism causing cardiovascular collapse the patient can be turned on to their left side in a head-down, feet-up (Trendelenburg) position so that air in the ventricle will not enter the lung or systemic circulation and, hopefully, blood flow obstruction may be (partially) relieved. Air can be aspirated from the ventricle followed by thoracotomy of the injured side.

Hypothermia

Hypothermia is defined as a sustained core temperature below 35°C. It can be further classified as mild (32–35°C), moderate (28–32°C), severe (<28°C) or profound (<20°C).

In the patient with normal thermoregulation, accidental hypothermia may occur when the body is exposed to a cold environment or immersed in cold water. However, in the patient with abnormal thermogenesis a mild exposure to cold can cause hypothermia. This may occur for the following reasons:

- a reduced metabolic rate (e.g. hypothyroidism, hypopituitarism, or malnutrition, where heat production is insufficient to maintain the body's temperature)
- spinal injury where muscle activity cannot be increased
- hypothalamic injuries (e.g. CVA), self-poisoning, alcohol abuse, and sedative drugs which cause cutaneous vasodilatation and increased heat loss
- the elderly, as a consequence of a reduced shivering response, immobility, poor living conditions, reduced subcutaneous fat, and a low metabolic rate.

Core temperature should be measured in hypothermic patients, ideally with a low-reading oesophageal, rectal, or bladder temperature probe. Tympanic membrane thermometers are unreliable in the setting of profound hypothermia. The clinical manifestations of hypothermia vary according to the core temperature, rate of cooling, and duration of hypothermia. Thermoregulatory mechanisms usually remain intact above 33°C, but below this there is progressive physiological deterioration. Loss of consciousness and pupillary dilatation occurs at 30°C. The shivering mechanism is replaced by muscular rigidity at 33°C and a rigor-mortis-like appearance, with cessation of respiration, at 24°C.

The solubility of gases in plasma increases with hypothermia and the oxygen dissociation curve is shifted to the right (due to an increased affinity of haemoglobin for oxygen).

Mortality varies from 6% to 85%, depending on the severity of hypothermia, its duration, the underlying disease conditions, and associated complications (see Table 11.5 for the physioological manifestations of hypothermia).

Rewarming

The rate of rewarming depends on the degree of hypothermia. Rapid rewarming up to 15°C/h can be achieved by extracorporeal circuits, but this is reserved for severe cases who have life-threatening complications. Generally, rewarming is at a rate of 0.5–4°C/h. Rapid rewarming may precipitate 'rewarming shock' where sudden surface peripheral vasodilatation causes hypotension, an increase in metabolic acidosis, and a drop in temperature of up to 4°C due to cool peripheral blood perfusing the central organs. Cool blood perfusing the myocardium may give rise to fatal arrhythmias, such as ventricular fibrillation, during rewarming. The elderly and those with underlying cardiac disease are particularly vulnerable, so rewarming should he controlled and cautious.

Methods of rewarming

Passive rewarming is suitable for mild hypothermia. Rewarming takes place slowly (0.5–1.0°C/):

- warm environment (25–30°C)
- reflective space blanket/warm air blanket
- extra blankets
- cover skin areas through which heat loss may occur (e.g. scalp).

Active rewarming is used in moderate hypothermia, those with impaired thermoregulation, and inability to shiver:

- heated humidified respiratory gases
- warmed intravenous fluids
- electrically heated mattresses or pads/warm air blanket
- hot baths (40–45°C) with limbs out of the water to avoid rewarming shock. These are only suitable for young adults and are usually not practicable. Monitoring is difficult in this situation.

Core warming is used for severe hypothermia:

- peritoneal/haemodialysis
- extracorporeal circuits (as in heart bypass)
- intragastric or bladder irrigation with warm fluids.

Table 11.5 Physiological manifestations of hypothermia

System	Problem	Cause	Treatment
Cardiovascular	Tachycardia/peripheral vasoconstriction/↑ cardiac output	Elevated levels of norepinephrine due to increased sympathetic activity	Monitor vital signs Passive rewarming
	↓cardiac output/ ↓BP (moderate hypothermia)	Bradycardia	Active rewarming. Intravenous fluids. Monitor vital signs
	Dysrhythmias: bradycardia, conduction disturbances, AF + SVT (< 30°C), VF (< 28°C). (VF may also be precipitated by stimulation, e.g. CVP insertion, endotracheal intubation)	Decreased tissue perfusion, acidosis, underlying cardiac ischaemia, direct effect of cold on sinus node	Continuous ECG monitoring. Avoid unnecessary stimulation. Treat bradycardias with atropine/pacing (as necessary). DC cardioversion is needed for VF; however, this may be resistant to electrical or pharmacological interventions until core temperature >28° C. (NB: In cardiac arrest situations, resuscitation must continue until the core temperature approaches normal. Hypothermia does have a cerebroprotective effect even though drugs and defibrillation may be ineffective)
Respiratory	Hypoventilation	Decreased rate and depth of respiration	Monitor blood gases.
	Hypoxaemia	Decreased gaseous diffusion capacity	Ensure patent airway. Use supplemental oxygen and mechanical ventilation as necessary.
	Respiratory acidosis	Increased levels of CO2 due to hypoventilation	Monitor blood gases. Mechanical ventilation may be necessary.
Renal	Polyuria. electrolyte imbalance	Impaired tubular function due to inhibition of enzyme systems and reduced responsiveness to ADH	Measure urine and fluid input. Monitor urine specific gravity, vital signs, blood urea, and electrolytes. Electrolyte replacement as necessary. Some patients develop renal failure (this is usually associated with hypotension). Renal support (e.g. dialysis) may be required.
Neurological	Cerebral depression	Decreased cerebral blood flow (7% decrease per °C)	Neurological observations. Maintain patent airway
Metabolic	Metabolic acidosis	Peripheral vasoconstriction and hypotension causing poor tissue perfusion. Lactate and other metabolites increase. Lactate clearance by liver is decreased. Decreased H^+ ion secretion by kidneys	Monitor blood pH. Intravenous fluid therapy (± vasodilators) as patient warms up
	Hyperglycaemia	Impaired peripheral circulation of glucose, decreased insulin release, glucose metabolized from liver glycogen. (NB: Pancreatitis may occur secondary to hypothermia)	Monitor blood glucose. Insulin infusion if necessary. In prolonged hypothermia, glycogen stores may be depleted and hypoglycaemia may develop

Burn injuries

Burn injuries may have psychological, systemic, and local effects. The wounds range from superficial, where the injury extends only partly into the skin and healing is spontaneous, to full thickness where the burn extends through the dermis, damaging the underlying fat and muscle tissue. Scarring will occur when a certain critical depth of damage to the dermis has occurred; this is permanent, often causing disability and disfiguration. Morbidity and mortality increase with increased body surface area (BSA) percentage of burn, in the very young or old, and when pre-existing morbidity, such as cardiovascular, renal, or pulmonary disorders, is present.

Assessment of severity is traditionally by the percentage of the BSA involved. In adults a minor burn is <10% BSA, a moderate burn 10–20% BSA, and a major burn is >20% BSA. Various methods can be used to determine the percentage of BSA involved, including charts (Lund and Browder charts), and palm size (a person's hand print including palm and fingers is approximately 1% of their BSA). The easiest method is the 'rule of 9' (see Box 11.10), but this can only be used in those aged >16 years (Alharbi *et al.* 2010; Hettiaratchy *et al.* 2004).

The depth of the burn can be classified as follows.

- Superficial (first degree)—involves the epidermis. The skin is red and painful, has no blisters, and heals well (e.g. sunburn).
- Superficial partial thickness (second degree)—extends into the superficial dermis. The skin is red with clear blisters, blanches with pressure, and is very painful. Local infection or cellulitis may develop, but there is usually no scarring.
- Deep partial thickness (second degree)—extends into the deep dermis. The skin may appear yellow or white and there is less blanching. There may be blistering with pain and discomfort on pressure. Scarring and contractures can develop and skin excision and grafting is often required.
- Full thickness (third degree)—extends through the entire dermis. The skin appears white/brown, stiff, and leathery, with no blanching. It is painless as the sensory nerve endings have been destroyed. Scarring and contractures develop and amputation may be necessary.
- Fourth degree—extends through the entire skin and into the underlying fat, muscle, and bone. The skin appears black/charred with eschar. It is painless and requires excision/amputation. There is significant functional impairment.

Areas of particular concern are burns to the face (especially around the nose and mouth which may indicate inhalational injury), circumferential burns of the limbs, and burns to the eyelids (Figure 11.5). The cause of the burn should be taken into account when assessment is made. These may be from a dry source (e.g. flames), from a wet source (e.g. scalds), electrical (e.g. household appliances, pylons), or chemical (acid, alkali, radiation).

Box 11.10 Calculation of total percentage of burned skin: 'the rule of 9'

- Head: 9%
- Arms: 9% each
- Front and back of trunk: 18% each
- Legs: 18% each
- Perineum: 1%

Initial management

If possible, the patient should be nursed in protective isolation and in an environment with humidity

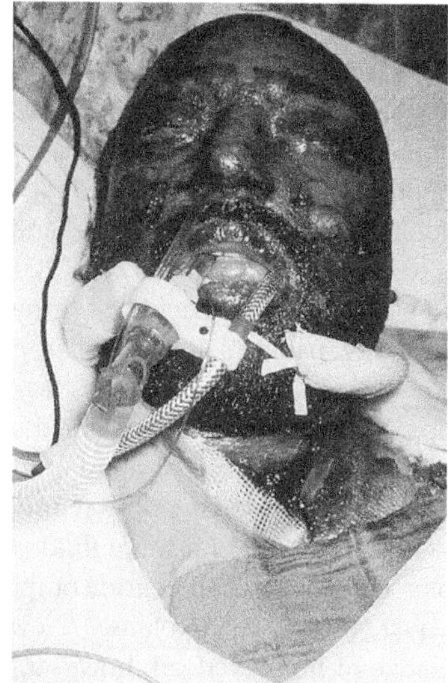

Figure 11.5 Severe burn injury showing generalized swelling of face and upper airway.

and temperature control. An air-fluidized bed may be required for severe burn injuries.

On arrival at the critical care unit, the patient must be assessed and vital signs recorded. A patent airway must be maintained and humidified oxygen therapy instituted. Patients with massive burns or inhalational injury may require urgent endotracheal intubation and mechanical ventilation. Large bore intravenous access, preferably in a non-burned area, must be established. High fluid losses will occur from the burned area; haemodynamic monitoring is required to guide resuscitation. An arterial line should be inserted for systemic pressure monitoring and blood sampling. A nasogastric tube and urinary catheter will also be required in severe cases. Insertion of tubes and cannulae should be carried out at an early stage as the patient will become grossly oedematous within hours due to massive capillary leakage, thus making late instrumentation extremely difficult. For this reason, scrupulous attention should also be paid to the airway, and endotracheal intubation performed on early signs of respiratory distress. Massive swelling may occur around the face and/or neck resulting in respiratory difficulties; an inhalational injury need not necessarily be present.

Various formulae exist for fluid replacement (e.g the Parkland formula and the Muir–Barclay regimen) but these are only general guidelines. The aim is to maintain adequate tissue perfusion guided by cardiovascular monitoring. The greatest fluid loss occurs in the first 8–12 hours after the injury when there is a general shift of fluid from intravascular to interstitial fluid compartments, and external loss. Too little fluid replacement will result in inadequate perfusion, resulting in hypovolaemic shock, renal failure, and the conversion of partial-thickness burns to full-thickness wounds. Similarly, massive volumes of fluid resuscitation have deleterous effects including abdominal compartment syndrome, ARDS, prolonged ventilator dependence, and increased mortality (Klein *et al.* 2007; Sullivan *et al.* 2006).

Haemodynamic variables should be measured continuously and the patient's intravascular fluid status frequently reassessed and adjusted as necessary. A haematocrit of approximately 0.35 is considered satisfactory to ensure adequate oxygen carriage and a non-elevated blood viscosity. A high haematocrit may imply haemoconcentration and the need for more fluid. An increasing metabolic acidosis and a fall in urine output are signs of an inadequate intravascular volume. A low haematocrit is suggestive of fluid overload; however, blood loss should also be considered as a cause of a low haematocrit. This may be due to either haemorrhage from non-burn injuries or haemolysis of blood cells trapped in the burned areas. In general, blood transfusions are not needed in the first 24 hours unless escharotomies are performed (Latenser, 2009).

Coagulation screens should be performed regularly, as massive dilution may occur due to the huge amount of fluid infused; clotting factors may also be consumed and/or production suppressed. Replacement, usually as fresh frozen plasma ± cryoprecipitate, should be considered if significant derangement in coagulation occurs. Likewise, marked shifts may occur in electrolyte status; these should be measured regularly and corrected as necessary.

After 2–5 days the capillary leakage usually slows and the patient often enters a diuretic phase. Excessive tissue fluid is reabsorbed back into the intravascular compartment and thence excreted via the kidney. This diuresis is spontaneous and may be massive; although fluid and sodium input should be reduced at this stage, care must be taken not to allow intravascular depletion and electrolyte imbalance.

Subsequent management

Cardiovascular

The circulation of a burned patient after resuscitation is usually hyperdynamic with an elevated cardiac output. Shock can occur rapidly within the first 48 hours of the injury or later. Hypotension and a fall in cardiac output causes hypoperfusion of vital organs which may lead to organ failure. Vascular permeability in the area of the burn increases and large amounts of fluid, similar in composition to plasma, leak out and are lost through the burned tissue. Oedema is related to vasoactive substances released as a consequence of the injury. This is not just limited to the affected areas; there is widespread generalized swelling, indicative of the whole-body systemic inflammatory response to the burn injury. Thus the circulating intravascular volume is depleted, resulting in hypoperfusion. The released inflammatory mediators may also cause progression to multi-organ failure with cardiovascular collapse. The first step in management is to ensure adequate fluid resuscitation, although vasoactive drugs, such as norepinephrine, may often be required to maintain an adequate blood pressure.

Respiratory

Pulmonary injury may result from inhalation of irritant or noxious gases such as carbon monoxide and cyanide. Heat may cause damage to the upper and lower airways and lung tissue. Smoke inhalation causes thermal injury to the larynx and pharynx only, as hot gases have a low specific heat content. Steam has a much higher heat content and causes injury to the whole respiratory tract. ARDS and pneumonia may be secondary complications of the primary burn injury.

Water-soluble gases found in smoke from burning plastics or rubber react with water in mucous membranes to produce strong acids and alkalis which may cause bronchospasm, ulceration, oedema, and damage to the ciliary mechanism. Lipid-soluble compounds can be transported to the lower airways on carbon particles and produce cell membrane damage and alveolar flooding.

There should be a very low threshold for endotracheal intubation in patients with inhalational injuries, as these patients can quickly progress to complete airway obstruction as oedema develops. Oedema with impaired upper airway patency may develop over the first few hours and can be progressive for the first 18–24 hours.

Indications for intubation are:

- failure to maintain an adequate airway
- respiratory failure
- severe cyanide or carbon monoxide poisoning
- convulsions
- stridor, lip swelling, or hoarseness
- circumferential chest burns
- severe facial burns or full-thickness burns of nose or lips
- deep burns to the neck which may cause external compression of the airway
- evidence of pharyngeal or laryngeal oedema/blistering/erythema, soot.

When intubating, remember not to cut the endotracheal tube too short—leave several inches of endotracheal tube beyond the mouth to allow for facial and lip swelling, which can be extensive. Depolarizing muscle relaxants (such as suxamethonium) are contraindicated after the first few hours because they may cause severe hyperkalaemia; non-depolarizing agents (such as rocuronium or vecuronium) should be used instead.

Several factors can decrease chest wall compliance:

- full-thickness burns to the thorax resulting in loss of elasticity of the skin and scar formation
- full-thickness burns to the abdomen causing abdominal compartment syndrome
- increased capillary leak of fluid, increasing chest wall oedema.

In such cases urgent escharotomy (surgical release of scar tissue) is usually required soon after admission and should extend into the fat and, possibly, through underlying fascia.

Arterial blood gas tensions must be monitored regularly, as pulse oximetry may be inaccurate. Soot in the airways should be promptly removed by aggressive per-endoscopic saline lavage to minimize local inflammation. Samples should be taken for bacteriological analysis and antibiotics (e.g. benzyl penicillin) commenced. Difficulty with the clearance of secretions increases the risk of secretion retention; thus PEEP, bronchodilators, frequent suctioning, patient turning. and physiotherapy are important therapies for minimizing lung injury and deterioration in gas exchange.

Carbon monoxide (CO) poisoning should be considered in any patient burned in an enclosed space such as a building or vehicle. Confusion, drowsiness, or coma may be present, as may the characteristic cherry-red colour. Carbon monoxide levels in the blood may be rapidly measured as carboxyhaemoglobin (COHb) using a co-oximeter. Both arterial blood gas tensions and pulse oximetry will be unreliable as neither will recognize the percentage of haemoglobin molecules bound to carbon monoxide rather than oxygen. Carbon monoxide has 200–250 times the affinity for haemoglobin as oxygen; therefore oxygen transport to the tissues may be severely compromised. High flow, high concentration oxygen should be administered immediately and continued until COHb levels fall below 10%. The half-life of carboxyhaemoglobin is 4 hours when breathing air, but only 45 min on 100% oxygen. Carbon monoxide toxicity may also cause a metabolic acidosis by directly inhibiting mitochondrial respiration and thus production of ATP.

Cyanide poisoning may occur from fires in enclosed spaces. This will also poison the mitochondria. Treatment is to administer 100% oxygen as soon as possible. Antidotes such as sodium thiosulphate or dicobalt edetate have dangers in themselves, and should be reserved for cases where cyanide poisoning is known to have occurred or is strongly suspected and the patient's condition is deteriorating. Clues to making the diagnosis include increasing drowsiness and a progressive metabolic acidosis despite adequate fluid resuscitation. Confirmation by measuring plasma cyanide levels will take several days and there may be insufficient time to wait in life-threatening situations.

Renal

Renal failure can develop in burn injury for several reasons. Most commonly, it results from hypoperfusion of the kidneys, but is also a consequence of systemic inflammation. Rhabdomyolysis can occur as a result of compartment syndrome or from severe burn injury and is diagnosed by an elevated serum creatine kinase and myoglobinuria. To prevent renal failure in the presence of rhabdomyolysis, increased fluid resuscitation, urinary alkalinization, and aggressive diuresis is required. Fasciotomies/escharotomies may be needed. Urine output, urea, and creatinine must be closely monitored. Renal replacement therapy may be required.

Metabolic

Hyperkalaemia can develop early in the burn patient as a result of both the metabolic acidosis and release of potassium from damaged tissue. This will usually resolve with fluid resuscitation and correction of the acidosis. Hypokalaemia is also common during resuscitation and can be exaggerated by nasogastric loss and diarrhoea. Hyponatraemia can occur due to loss of sodium through the burn wound and dilution from fluid administration. Inflammatory mediators may generate a systemic inflammatory response syndrome (SIRS) and increase the potential for circulatory failure.

Burn injuries cause an increase in metabolic rate. This begins at about day 5 and metabolic rate gradually increases until, by day 10, it is about 2.5 times normal. The hypermetabolic state is characterized by increased oxygen consumption, heat production, body temperature, hyperglycaemia, and protein catabolism. Cardiac output and carbon dioxide production can double.

Malnutrition may cause poor wound-healing and an increase in mortality. Therefore adequate and early institution of nutritional support is vital, ideally within 24 hours of the burn injury. If enteral feeding is required, a fine bore polyurethane nasogastric tube should be passed as soon as possible after admission. Vitamin and mineral requirements, particularly zinc, iron, and vitamins B and C, all increase in burn injuries, so these may need to be supplemented. If the gut is inaccessible or non-functioning, total parenteral nutrition must be given.

Pain

Pain can be considerable in all but full-thickness burns. Continuous high dose intravenous opiate infusions are necessary and can be supplemented by benzodiazepines. There is often an increased need during dressing changes and physiotherapy, and Entonox (oxygen–nitrous oxide) or ketamine can be administered if the patient is conscious.

Infection

Sepsis accounts for 50% of deaths from burn injuries. The immune system is globally depressed in severe injuries, but prophylactic administration of antibiotics is not recommended unless there is evidence of an inhalation injury. In this case penicillin should be used as the main threat comes from pneumococcal infection.

In the first few days burn wounds become colonized with Gram-positive bacteria (*Staphylococcus aureus* and *Staphylococcus epidermis*), and within 5 days by predominantly gut flora (*Pseudomonas aeruginosa, Enterobacter cloacae*, and *Escherichia coli*). Colonization does not require systemic antibiotic therapy but should be managed by early debridement and/or excision together with appropriate topical or biological dressings. Wounds should be swabbed and cultured on admission and then serially to monitor for changes in colonization. Strict aseptic techniques during wound redressing, protective isolation, good nutritional support, and avoidance of unnecessary instrumentation will help reduce the incidence of infection.

Thermoregulation

With burn injury the barrier to evaporative heat loss is impaired, promoting heat loss. This can lead to an increased metabolic rate as the burn victim attempts to maintain body temperature. Covering the wounds and maintaining a high room temperature can decrease heat loss.

Gastrointestinal

Gastric dilation and ileus are common in the patient with burn injury >20% of BSA. A nasogastric tube will minimize gastric distension and the risk of aspiration. Increased stress hormone output increases the risk of gastric ulceration, and the patient should be monitored for evidence of gastrointestinal bleeding (melaena, coffee ground aspirate, Hb). Some units routinely use prophylactic agents such as ranitidine or a proton pump inhibitor, though these can increase the risk of pneumonia.

Haematological

Anaemia may follow either haemolysis or blood loss. The plasma concentration of clotting factors may be diluted by the massive fluid replacement needed, and DIC can occur as part of the multi-organ failure syndrome. Treatment is by appropriate replacement of blood products.

Surgical

Urgent escharotomy (or limb amputation) may be required soon after admission. Escharotomy is the surgical release of a constricting area or circumferential burn by incising down to the fatty layer. Anaesthesia may not be required as the skin area affected is usually dead. Debridement and grafting (using cadaveric tissue or the patient's own split skin from an unburnt site) will be indicated for full-thickness burns. If this area is large, debridement may be advisable in the first few days with tangential excision of the necrotic area. Massive bleeding can occur both during and after this procedure.

Wound care

Dressing procedures will vary considerably from unit to unit, and a wide variety of biological, biosynthetic, and synthetic wound dressings are available. The type of dressing used depends on the depth, site, cause, and extent of the burn. Local hospital protocols should be followed and the following notes are intended as guidelines only.

Cleaning and aggressive wound debridement is essential for the removal of potential sources of infection such as bacteria and necrotic tissue, and this is followed by the application of a topical antimicrobial agent to control colonization (e.g. containing silver sulfadiazine such as Flamazine).

Some minor superficial burns can be left uncovered, but if dressings are used they should protect the wound and encourage re-epithelialization (e.g polyurethane semi-permeable films or hydrocolloids). Dead tissue (eschar) must be removed with scissors and forceps or scalpels; small areas can be debrided during routine dressing changes. Scrubbing of wounds during dressing changes can enhance mechanical debridement, and enzymatic debriding agents can be used to loosen eschar and promote removal. Frequent surgical debridement is optimal to remove non-viable tissue.

Most burn experts recommend debridement of all blisters larger than 0.5 cm to reduce the risk of bacterial colonization or infection (Kasten *et al.* 2010).

Grafts

Deep partial-thickness and very small full-thickness burns will heal spontaneously, but large full-thickness burns will require grafting. Autografts (from an uninjured area of the patient's own skin or an identical twin) provide the only permanent graft material. Grafting shortens healing time, improves the cosmetic appearance of deep partial burns, and is mandatory for the healing of full-thickness burns. The decision to graft may be based on the total percentage BSA of the burn and the need to conserve donor sites for full-thickness injuries.

In large area burns, the same graft donor site may need to be used repeatedly as the only source for graft material; therefore protection of this donor site from infection is critical. When autograft sites are sparse, donor skin can be minced and placed in a growth medium to increase the number of epithelial cells, or small pieces of donor skin can be dropped across a large burn in an attempt to increase the benefit from a small donor site.

Cadaver skin (allograft or homograft) can be used as a temporary dressing. Allografts will promote vascular ingrowth to seal the wound against bacterial invasion; however, they will be rejected within about 2 weeks. Xenografts or heterografts (from another species), such as porcine grafts, can also provide temporary wound dressings but should be removed in 3–4 days or if a purulent discharge is noted (porcine grafts may be digested by the wound, becoming a source of infection).

Tubular support dressings are applied 5–7 days after grafting and provide a pressure of 10–20 mmHg in order to minimize contracture formation.

Physiotherapy

This is important in all burn patients in order to maintain joint mobility, muscle strength, and functional joint positions. Chest physiotherapy is useful for inhalational injuries, trunk burns (especially circumferential), bed-bound patients, and before and after surgery. Limbs may need to be splinted to minimize contractures and maintain the functional position of joints. Passive exercises should be carried out frequently to maintain a full range of movement of joints and to maintain muscle power. Prior to physiotherapy, ensure that pain control is adequate. Try to coordinate physiotherapy with dressing changes to avoid excessive use of analgesia. The patient should be mobilized as early as possible, allowing for their general condition.

Psychological aspects

Psychological problems following the injury pose a major challenge. The patient and family need help in coming to terms with disfigurement or disablement. Considerable psychological support will be required over a prolonged period. Burn units have access to specially trained counsellors who should be involved at an early stage.

Drowning

The definition of drowning is the process of experiencing respiratory impairment from submersion or immersion in a liquid. Drowning outcomes are classified as death, morbidity, and no morbidity (van Beeck *et al.* 2005).

Alcohol and epilepsy are sometimes major contributing factors, while deliberate hyperventilation prior to prolonged underwater swimming is also a common cause. Hyperventilation causes hypocarbia and the low levels of P_aCO2 suppresses respiratory effort, even in the presence of severe hypoxaemia; thus consciousness is lost while under water.

Aspiration of fluid is not always necessary to 'drown'. Little or no fluid may be aspirated into the lungs while under water as reflex laryngospasm caused by the presence of water in the larynx prevents fluid entry into the lungs. This glottic spasm persists until death from asphyxiation occurs. The prognosis for drowning victims who have not aspirated fluid is fairly good, provided that they are promptly resuscitated, since they do not develop the secondary complications of fluid inhalation.

The diving reflex and hypothermia are potential protective mechanisms in submersion victims. The diving reflex is initiated by cold water on the face and consists of apnoea, bradycardia, and intense peripheral vasoconstriction. Blood flow is preferentially diverted to essential organs such as heart and brain. Hypothermia decreases cardiac output, cellular metabolism, and oxygen consumption. It is especially protective if it precedes anoxia. Survival without neurological damage has been reported after periods of submersion >20 min. Neither a long submersion time nor the death-like appearance of the victim are reasons for not resuscitating. Resuscitation should be commenced in every victim who has been under water for less than an hour, and should only stop on the basis of objective diagnostic criteria when the patient has reached hospital and has been warmed to normothermia. Cervical spine injuries are frequently associated with diving accidents, and these must be considered during resuscitation.

Submersion is primarily a ventilatory disturbance with hypoxaemia as the cause of cardiac arrest. The nature of the inhaled fluid will cause different physiological effects. In freshwater drowning, fluid in the lungs is quickly absorbed into the circulation, causing dilutional effects that may lead to haemolysis. Pulmonary surfactant is denatured and widespread atelectasis can result. Electrolyte disturbances are usually mild. Salt water contains higher levels of sodium and chloride and this causes mucosal injury and loss of surfactant. As this fluid is hypertonic, water and plasma proteins move rapidly into the alveoli and interstitium, resulting in an osmotic pulmonary oedema.

In most drowning victims, the stomach also fills with water and there is a high risk of inhalation of gastric contents, especially during resuscitation and cardiac compression. Gastric content aspiration will produce further inflammatory reactions in the alveolar–capillary membrane.

Management

There is little difference in management between saltwater and freshwater drowning. Therapy is directed at restoring the circulation and oxygenation, correcting electrolyte imbalance, and maintaining cerebral perfusion.

Hypoxaemia

Full cardiopulmonary resuscitation may be required initially and comatose patients will require endotracheal intubation. Mechanical ventilation, high inspired oxygen concentrations, and PEEP are usually needed. CPAP via a facemask may be used if the patient is conscious and able to maintain a patent airway and an adequate arterial oxygen saturation. Hypoxaemia and intrapulmonary shunting can occur with inhalation of as little as 2.5 ml fluid/kg body weight. Hypoxaemia is usually the major problem with submersion victims and pulmonary oedema may occur soon after endotracheal intubation. Therapy with high levels of PEEP is usually effective. Secondary pulmonary oedema can occur after 24 hours and therefore patients should be closely observed for at least this period of time. Denaturation of surfactant can continue even after resuscitation, and ARDS and pulmonary infection are common. The type of immersion liquid may influence the type of inhaled organism, and in many instances mud, sand, and particulate matter are aspirated. Multiple abscess formation may ensue.

High inflation pressures may be required due to bronchospasm caused by water aspiration and altered surfactant activity, atelectasis, and pulmonary oedema. Extracorporal membrane oxygenation may be useful in patients unresponsive to mechanical or high frequency ventilation who have persistent hypothermia from cold water drowning and a reasonable probability of recovering neurological function.

Circulatory failure

Positive inotropic agents may be required if the patient is hypotensive and not responding to adequate fluid replacement. In theory, salt water should cause hypovolaemia while fresh water should increase the circulatory volume. However, in practice such small amounts of fluid are aspirated that significant changes in blood volume are not seen. Dysrhythmias may result from acidosis, hypoxaemia, hypothermia, and electrolyte imbalance. These usually revert to a normal rhythm once the abnormalities have been corrected.

Hypothermia

Hypothermia is common in submersion victims. Core temperature must be maintained and passive/active rewarming instituted (note that dysrhythmias may occur during rewarming).

Electrolyte imbalance

Plasma levels of sodium, chloride, and magnesium may be elevated in saltwater drowning but serious disturbances are unusual.

Renal failure

In freshwater drowning haemolysis may cause haemoglobinuria and consequent acute renal failure. Urine output must be closely monitored.

Neurological damage

Ischaemic cerebral damage can follow prolonged hypoxaemia and some patients will develop cerebral oedema. Attempts should be made to reduce raised intracranial pressure and maintain cerebral perfusion. Pyrexia must be reduced, oxygenation and circulation maintained, and blood glucose monitored. The patient must be observed for seizures and frequent neurological assessments should be made.

Gastric dilatation

Submersion victims often swallow large amounts of water. A nasogastric tube should be inserted to prevent inhalation and remove swallowed water. The orogastric route should be used if head or facial trauma is suspected.

Metabolic acidosis

Metabolic acidosis may develop following intense peripheral vasoconstriction and hypoxaemia. Lactate levels rise as oxygen delivery to the tissues falls. The acidosis usually improves as the patient is rewarmed and hypoxaemia corrected.

The success rate of resuscitation in submersion victims is relatively high but a multitude of fatal complications may develop, in particular ARDS and multi-organ failure, sepsis, and pneumonia. Prognosis is poor if the patient is comatose following resuscitation.

Trauma scores

Trauma scoring is used to classify the severity of injury. Various scoring systems have been devised and usually combine both anatomical and physiological variables. Some are simple and specific for a particular type of injury such as the Glasgow Coma Scale (GCS) for head injuries. Others are complex and may even combine several individual scoring systems (see later) (Raum *et al.* 2009).

Trauma scoring allows an evaluation of the trauma care provided and a means of comparing outcomes, either over time or between different hospitals. It can aid planning and provision of resources in special units and identify those patients who will benefit most from the specialized care that can be provided in these areas. Scoring is helpful in triage, where patients are categorized into the urgency of treatment need, enabling identification of the most severely injured patients who may require immediate transfer to specialized units or priority treatment. It may also distinguish those with a poor chance of survival, especially when resources are overwhelmed (e.g. following disasters, where treatment could be directed initially at those critically ill patients with a better prognosis) (Yates, 1990).

TRISS

TRISS (Trauma Score—Injury Severity Score) offers consistent and reasonable predictions of outcome. It combines the Revised Trauma Score (RTS) and the Injury Severity Score (ISS), the patient's age, and the type of injury (blunt or penetrating). The score provides a measure of predicted outcome—the probability of survival.

Table 11.6 The Revised Trauma Scale (RTS)

Variable	Score					
	4	3	2	1	0	Weighting factor
Systolic BP (mmHg)	>89	76–89	50–75	1–49	Pulseless	×0.7326
Systolic BP (mmHg)	10–29	>29	6–9	1–5	0	×0.2908
GCS	13–15	9–12	6–8	4–5	3	×0.9368

Note: Add the combined scores for each variable to obtain the RTS.

Table 11.7 Weighted coefficient values

Injury	Constant	RTS	ISS	Age
Blunt	−1.2470	0.9544	−0.0768	−1.9052
Penetrating	−0.6029	1.1430	−0.1516	−2.6676

The RTS (Table 11.6) is composed of the GCS (see Chapter 8) and measurements of cardiopulmonary function. Each variable is given a number and multiplied by a weighting factor (see Table 11.7) derived from regression analysis of a large US trauma database. This reflects the relative value of that variable in determining survival. The numbers are then totalled to provide the patient's RTS, which should be recorded on arrival in hospital.

The ISS provides a numerical measure of injury severity in patients with multiple injuries. Every injury is given an AIS-85 code and classified into one of seven regions: head and neck, face, thorax, abdomen and pelvic contents, extremities, pelvic girdle, and external and burns. The AIS-85 code is an abbreviated injury scale that incorporates codes for assessment of blunt and penetrating injuries. Each injury is assigned a six-digit code based on anatomical site, nature, and severity. The ISS is the sum of the squares of the highest AIS scores from three of the seven body regions. There is a significant correlation between ISS and mortality, morbidity, and length of hospital stay.

The probability of survival (P_s) is calculated as follows:

$$P_s = \frac{1}{1+e^{-b}}$$

where P_s is probability of survival, e = 2.718282 is the base of the natural logarithm, and b is the sum of RTS + ISS + age coefficient (age coefficient = 0 if age ≤54 years, or +1 if age >54 years).

Although this scoring method appears complicated, a TRISS chart has been devised to allow rapid determination of the probability of survival. However, despite being able to predict outcome reasonably well, the quality of life of survivors can vary considerably.

References and bibliography

Alharbi, Z., Piatowski, A., Denbinski, R., *et al.* (2012). Treatment of burns in the first 24 hours: simple and practical guide by answering 10 questions in a step-by-step form. *World Journal of Emergency Surgery*, **7**, 13.

Balogh, Z., Moore, F.A, Moore, E.E., Biffl, W.L. (2007). Secondary abdominal compartment syndrome: a potential threat for all trauma clinicians. *Injury*, **38**, 272–9.

Carlotti, A., Carvalho, W. (2009), Abdominal compartment syndrome: a review. *Pediatric Critical Care Medicine*, **10**, 115–20.

Cheatham, M.L. (2009). Abdominal compartment syndrome: pathophysiology and definitions. *Scandinavian Journal of Trauma, Resuscitation and Emergency Medicine*, **17**, 10.

Coles, J.P., Minhas, P.S., Fryer, T.D., *et al.* (2002). Effects of hyperventilation on cerebral blood flow in traumatic head injury: clinical relevance and monitoring correlates. *Critical Care Medicine*, **30**, 1950–9.

Haddad, S.H., Arabi, Y.M. (2012). Critical care management of severe traumatic brain injury in adults. *Scandinavian Journal of Trauma, Resuscitation and Emergency Medicine*, **20**, 12.

Hettiaratchy, S., Papini, R. (2004). Initial management of a major burn. II: Assessment and resuscitation. *BMJ*, **329**,101–3.

Kasten, K., Makely, A., Kagan, R. (2010). Update on the critical care management of severe burns. *Journal of Intensive Care Medicine*, **26**, 223–6.

Klein, M., Hayden, D., Elson, C. *et al.* (2007). The association between fluid administration and outcomes following major burn. *Annals of Surgery*, **245**, 622–8.

Latenser, B.A (2009). Critical care of the burn patient: the first 48 hours. *Critical Care Medicine*, **37**, 10

Maas, A., Stocchetti, N., Bullock, R. (2008). Moderate and severe traumatic brain injury in adults. *Lancet Neurology*, **7**, 728–41.

Mabvuure, N.T, Malhahias, M., Hindocha, S., *et al.* (2012). Acute compartment syndrome of the limbs: current concepts and management. *Open Orthopaedics Journal*, 6(Supple 3:M7), 535–43.

Manley, G., Knudson, M.M., Morabito, D., *et al.* (2001). Hypotension, hypoxia and head injury: frequency, duration and consequence. *Archives of Surgery*, **136**, 1118–23.

Mascia, L., Grasso, S., Fiore, T., *et al.* (2005). Cerebro-pulmonary interactions during the application of low levels of positive end-expiratory pressure. *Intensive Care Medicine*, **31**, 373–9.

Meier, R., Béchir, M., Ludwig, S., *et al.* (2008). Differential temporal profile of lowered blood glucose levels (3.5 to 6.5 mmol/l versus 5 to 8 mmol/l) in patients with severe traumatic brain injury. *Critical Care*, **12**, R98.

Moppett, I.K. (2007). Traumatic brain injury: assessment, resuscitation and early management. *British Journal of Anaesthesia*, **99**, 18–31.

O'Mara, M.S., Slater, H., Goldfarb, I.W., *et al.* (2005). A prospective, randomized evaluation of intra-abdominal pressures with crystalloid and colloid resuscitation in burn patients. *Journal of Trauma*, **58**, 1011–18.

Raum, M., Nijsten, M., Vogelzang, M., *et al.* (2009). Emergency trauma score: an instrument for early estimation of trauma severity. *Critical Care Medicine*, **37**, 1972–7.

Shaikh, N. (2009). Emergency management of fat embolism syndrome. *Journal of Emergencies, Trauma and Shock*, **2**, 29–33.

Shaikh, N., Ummunisa, F. (2009). Acute managment of vascular air embolism. *Journal of Emergencies, Trauma and Shock*, **2**, 180–5.

Sullivan, S.R., Ahmadi, A.J., Singh, C.N., *et al.* (2006). Elevated orbital pressure: another untoward effect of massive fluid resuscitation after burn injury. Journal of Trauma, **60**, 72–6.

Theodossis, S.P., Athanasios, D.M., Joannis, P., *et al.* (2011). Abdominal compartment syndrome—intra-abdominal hypertension: defining, diagnosing, and managing. *Journal of Emergencies, Trauma and* Shock, **4**, 279–91.

van Beeck, E.F., Branche, C.M., Szpilman, D., *et al.* (2005) A new definition of drowning: towards documentation and prevention of a global public health problem. *Bulletin of theWorld Health Organization*, **83**, 853–6.

Webber, S.J., Mills, G.H. (2002). The abdominal compartment syndrome: an under-recognised and inadequately treated condition. *Care of the Critically Ill*, **18**, 115–17.

Yates, D.W. (1990) Scoring systems for trauma. *British Medical Journal*, **301**, 1090A.

CHAPTER 12
Haematological problems

Physiology of the blood cells

The basic cellular components of blood are:

- erythrocytes (red cells)
- leucocytes (white cells)
- thrombocytes (platelets).

All blood cells are derived from a single cell type in the bone marrow known as a pluripotent stem cell. The pluripotent stem cell gives rise to a myeloid stem cell and a lymphoid stem cell from which erythrocytes, leucocytes, and thrombocytes develop (Figure 12.1).

Erythrocytes (red cells)

These cells have no nucleus and consist mostly of cytoplasm and haemoglobin (see Box 12.1). Haemoglobin constitutes about 34% of the erythrocyte cell mass, but may fall to 20% when its formation in the bone marrow is deficient. Each cell is biconcave in shape with a cell membrane considerably larger than is required; this surplus allows the cell to change its shape as it passes through narrow capillaries.

Red cell formation is stimulated by the hormone erythropoietin, which is produced in the kidneys. Erythropoietin release is influenced by renal hypoxia, but the maximum rate of red cell production is only seen 5 days after its release. Thus it is a long-term rather than an immediate response. Lack of erythropoietin, as seen in patients with renal failure, can cause severe anaemia.

Several vitamins and elements are vital for red cell maturation. Vitamin B_{12} is essential for nuclear

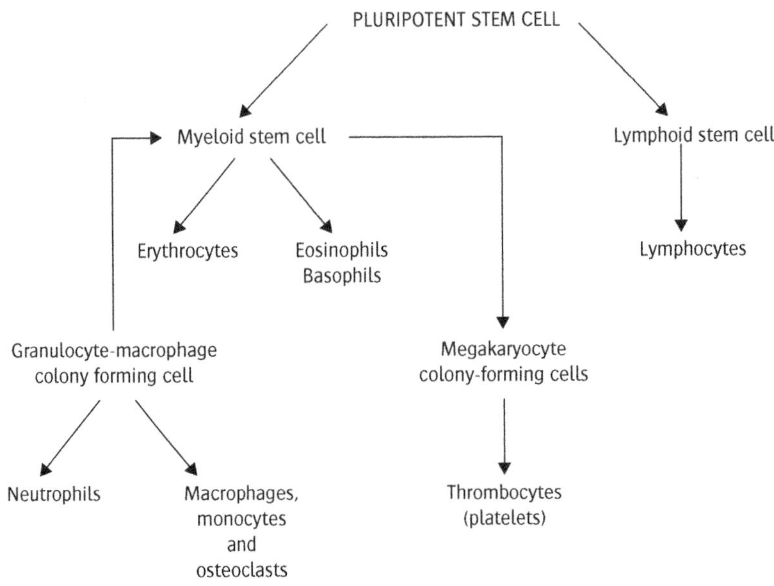

Figure 12.1 Differentation from the pluripotent stem cell

> **Box 12.1 Terms associated with erythrocytes**
>
> **Anaemia** is defined as a haemoglobin level <115 g/L in adult females or <130 g/L in adult males.
>
> **Erythrocyte sedimentation rate (ESR)** is the rate at which red cells settle under gravity in a sample of blood. A blood sample is placed in a standard 100 mm long test tube; after 1 hour the rate of sedimentation should be <10 mm. Diseases involving inflammation, tissue destruction, or blood hyperviscosity increase the ESR, and this can serve as a guide to disease progression.

maturation and cell division, while folic acid is required for DNA formation. Vitamin B_6, thiamine, riboflavin, manganese, and cobalt are also important. Iron is needed for formation of haemoglobin and is obtained either by absorption from the gastrointestinal tract or from the breakdown of old red blood cells by the reticuloendothelial system.

The prime function of erythrocytes is oxygen transport. Haemoglobin has a great affinity for oxygen with 1 g of haemoglobin capable of combining with 1.34 ml of oxygen. Oxygen combines with haemoglobin in the lungs to form oxyhaemoglobin and readily dissociates from it in the tissues (for full details of oxygen transport see Chapter 4).

Red blood cells also contain high levels of 2,3-diphosphoglycerate (2,3-DPG) which plays an important part in oxygen transfer. In the middle range of oxygen tensions this compound combines with deoxyhaemoglobin and decreases the affinity of haemoglobin for oxygen. The more 2,3-DPG present, the more oxygen will be released at a given oxygen tension; thus the oxyhaemoglobin dissociation curve is shifted to the right. Anoxia increases 2,3-DPG levels in the red cells, thus increasing the amount of oxygen released when blood reaches the tissues (see Chapter 4).

Table 12.1 summarizes conditions associated with red blood cell disorders. Only those disorders relevant to the ICU patient are described in detail here.

Table 12.1 Erythrocyte disorders

Disorder	Cause
Increased red blood cell destruction (haemolytic anaemia)	Membrane disorders (e.g. spherocytosis) Enzyme deficiencies (e.g. glucose-6-phosphate-dehydrogenase) Abnormal haemoglobin synthesis (e.g. thalassaemia, sickle cell disease)
Decreased red cell production	Decreased haemoglobin synthesis (e.g. iron-deficiency anaemia) Decreased DNA synthesis (megoblastic anaemia) Stem cell failure (aplastic anaemia) Unknown causes (anaemia of chronic disease)

Polycythaemia

Here, the red cell count increases to >6 × 10^{12}/L or the Hb rises >180 g/L. Primary polycythaemia occurs when the blood cell mass is increased due to excessive production; its aetiology is unknown. Secondary polycythaemia occurs when the red cell count is increased in response to chronic hypoxaemia (e.g. chronic obstructive pulmonary disease, cyanotic congenital heart disease, or adaptation to high altitude) and results from increased erythropoietin production.

Primary polycythaemia (polycythaemia rubra vera)

The bone marrow becomes more proliferative and all cellular factors—red cells, white cells, and platelets—are increased. There is an increase in cell mass and blood volume. The resulting increase in blood viscosity causes vascular occlusion with cardiovascular, neurological, and vascular complications. Immediate treatment is aimed at reducing blood viscosity; this can be achieved by venesection to keep the haematocrit <0.5. Concurrent volume replacement is given using crystalloid or colloid. Aspirin is given to reduce platelet function, while more definitive treatments include cytarabine (to reduce platelet production), radioactive phosphorus, or chemotherapy to depress bone marrow production. Occasionally, primary polycythaemia may transform into acute myeloid leukaemia.

Sickle cell anaemia

Normal adult haemoglobin (HbA) contains two alpha and two beta chains. There are two genes for the synthesis of each chain. Sickle cell haemoglobin (HbS) has two alpha chains and two abnormal beta chains. The beta chain defect involves a single amino acid substitution and is inherited as an autosomal dominant gene. This leads to a chronic haemolytic anaemia. Sickle cell disease is predominantly found in individuals of African, Caribbean, Turkish, Greek, and Indian origin. The prevalence of the gene in these areas is probably because HbS protects against the serious effects of *Falciparum* malaria.

Patients with sickle cell trait have mainly HbA and <50% HbS, while sickle cell anaemia occurs in homozygotes (HbS/HbS). When exposed to a low oxygen tension, the red cells become deformed, rigid, and elongated (sickle-shaped). They then lodge and aggregate in small blood vessels, causing ischaemia or infarction. Abnormal red cells are also prematurely destroyed, resulting in a haemolytic anaemia. Patients with sickle cell anaemia suffer chronic ill health, thrombotic crises, leg ulcers, and infections. Many do not survive beyond 40 years of age. Those with sickle cell trait are usually symptom free unless the oxygen tension is very low, since the HbA prevents the cells from 'sickling'.

Acute haemolytic crises (sickle cell crises) occur from 6 months of age. Haemolysis of the sickled cells produces anaemia and jaundice, causing tachycardia and cardiomegaly; heart failure and arrhythmias may develop in older patients, often as a consequence of iron overload from repeated transfusions. Vaso-occlusion causes infarction of tissues resulting in bone, pulmonary, or splenic infarcts, cerebrovascular accidents, haematuria, swelling (particularly of the toes and fingers), fever, and abdominal pain. Acute splenic sequestration can occur and may be life-threatening in young patients. The spleen enlarges acutely and deformed red cells cannot be filtered and moved back into the circulation. Anaemia rapidly develops and, as splenic function deteriorates, the patient is at risk of overwhelming infection. Pulmonary sequestration can also occur, and can lead to rapid deterioration and death. Oxygen transfer in the alveoli is impaired, leading to hypoxia that promotes further sickling. In combination with pulmonary infarction, consolidation, and infection this is termed 'acute chest syndrome'. Patients may be admitted to the critical care unit for management during these crises. Dehydration and hypoxaemia promote sickling but the crises are unpredictable. Management is aimed at:

- adequate oxygenation
- rehydration
- pain relief
- prevention of infection
- exchange transfusion.

Correction/prevention of hypoxaemia

Blood gases and continuous pulse oximetry must be monitored closely; however, the normal values of haemoglobin and saturation when the patient is clinically well (the steady state) should be used as a guide for treatment. Many patients have steady state haemoglobin levels of only 50–90 g/L. Those with low levels have HbS within the red cells that has a low affinity for oxygen, and maintain normal oxygen delivery because more oxygen can be unloaded per gram of haemoglobin. Therefore a higher level is unnecessary. Oxygen saturations may occasionally be lower than 90% in the steady state, so changes in saturation are more important than absolute values.

It is important to ensure that the patient does not become hypoxaemic, so supplemental oxygen should be given. However, excess oxygen causing hyperoxia should be avoided to prevent further vasoconstriction.

Non-invasive or invasive mechanical ventilation may be required To maintain adequate oxygenation.

Rehydration

Increasing the plasma volume dilutes the blood and decreases the agglutination of sickled cells in small vessels. However, care must be taken not to overload these patients who usually have a cardiomyopathy and can thus be pushed into acute heart failure. CVP or cardiac output monitoring may be required, especially if the patient is known to have poor heart function or becomes symptomatic with heart failure.

Analgesia

Thrombotic episodes may cause severe pain in any part of the body. Oral analgesia or anti-inflammatory drugs such as codeine or diclofenac may be sufficient, but intravenous opiates such as pethidine or morphine may be required. Patient-controlled administration will give more sustained blood levels than intermittent injections. Pain management in sickle cell patients is often difficult and it may be problematic to wean them from analgesics. Strong psychological support is vital.

Infection

Patients often present with fever and a raised white cell count during a crisis. Attempts must be made to rule out an underlying infection which, if found, requires appropriate treatment. Patients with splenic dysfunction are prone to capsulated organisms such as pneumococcus and long-term prophylactic penicillin may be advocated.

Blood transfusion

If a crisis is severe, exchange blood transfusions may be carried out in order to reduce the levels of HbS. This is usually reserved for patients who have a rapid drop in haemoglobin, those who develop chest or cerebral crises, a severe painful crisis not responding to other therapy, or pre-operatively if elective surgery is required.

Leucocytes (white cells)

The function of the leucocyte is to resist infection by phagocytosis or by forming antibodies against foreign material or agents. Phagocytosis is the process by which white cells engulf a foreign agent and then destroy it by the release of digesting enzymes within the cell. Most of the white cells are formed in the bone marrow. There are five types:

- neutrophils
- eosinophils
- basophils
- monocytes
- lymphocytes.

Neutrophils, eosinophils, and basophils are collectively known as granulocytes.

Neutrophils

Neutrophils account for 60–75% of the white cell count. They are an essential part of the defence against infection and tissue damage. An inflamed area of tissue releases inflammatory mediators, such as cytokines and chemokines, to increase the number of neutrophils in the blood by up to fourfold, and to attract them to the required location. They engulf pathogens and, by the process of phagocytosis, release enzymes and reactive oxygen species from granules within the cytoplasm to kill the micro-organism.

The normal number of neutrophils is influenced by age, gender, and ethnic origin. Females have a higher normal range than males, while some non-Caucasian populations have lower ranges. 'Neutrophilia' is used to describe an increase in the number of circulating blood neutrophils. Leucocytosis is also often used in this context, although this strictly means an increase in the number of circulating white cells of all varieties, not just neutrophils. Neutrophilia occurs following infection, trauma, burn injury, or tissue necrosis. Neutropenia—a low neutrophil count—may also occur under these conditions (see later).

Eosinophils

These are weak phagocytes that collect at sites of antigen–antibody reactions in the tissues where they can phagocytose the antigen–antibody complex. Eosinophils also secrete toxic inflammatory mediators that are stored in preformed vesicles and can also be synthesized following cell activation. They increase in number in allergic conditions and collect around areas where histamine is released from mast cells. Eosinophil infiltration into the lung is a hallmark of allergic asthma and may play a role in the development of allergic airway inflammation.

An eosinphil count $>0.45 \times 10^9$/L is termed eosinophila and can be idiopathic or secondary to another disease. Common causes are:

- allergic disorders (asthma, hay fever, drug allergies, allergic skin diseases)
- parasitic infections
- some types of malignancy (Hodgkin's lymphoma, ovarian cancer)
- systemic autoimmune disaese (SLE)

- some forms of vasculitis
- interstitial nephropathy.

Basophils

These resemble mast cells, which are found just outside capillaries and are responsible for liberating heparin into the blood. It is possible that basophils may be transported into the tissues where they become mast cells. Basophils provide a similar function to mast cells, releasing heparin into the blood, which prevents coagulation, and also produce small quantities of bradykinin and serotonin.

Monocytes

These circulate in the bloodstream for 1–3 days and then usually move into tissues and mature into macrophages (e.g. Kupffer cells in the liver). Half are stored as a reserve in the spleen. Monocytes are very active phagocytes and large numbers will infiltrate areas of inflammation The rate of monocyte production in the bone marrow increases with chronic infections (e.g. tuberculosis, endocarditis). They also release inflammatory cytokines such as tumour necrosis factor (TNF) and interleukin 1 (IL-1), and are also involved in antigen presentation to T lymphocytes, which can then mount a specific immune response.

Lymphocytes

There are three types of lymphocyte: B cells, T cells and natural killer (NK) cells. They originate from a common cell type in the bone marrow but then differentiate into their final form in distinct sites. B lymphocytes mature in the bone marrow, while T lymphocytes mature in the thymus. They then enter the circulation and lymphoid organs (e.g. spleen, lymph nodes). B lymphocytes play an important part in the humoral immune response and the formation of antibodies, while T lymphocytes are necessary for cell-mediated immunity. Their role is to identify 'non-self' antigens such as bacteria. The inflammatory reaction is very complex and is discussed in more detail in Chapter 13.

Tissue injury causes a local sympathetic reflex which results in an increased blood flow, a consequent increase in blood cells, and redness and swelling in the area of injury. Macrophage-monocytes release cytokines such as IL-l, TNF, serotonin, and histamine. Histamine causes local swelling. IL-1 and TNF stimulate an increase in basophils, eosinophils, and lymphocytes, and increase production of granulocyte macrophage–colony-stimulating factor (GM–CSF) which, with histamine, results in increased neutrophil and eosinophil chemotaxis. Bacterial products (e.g. endotoxin that comes from Gram-negative bacterial cell walls) stimulates inflammatory mediators (e.g. macrophages to release cytokines) and activates complement (small proteins that help white cells to bind and destroy bacteria).

Leucocyte disorders

Terms associated with leucocytes are summarized in Box 12.2.

Neutropenia

Neutropenia is defined as a neutrophil count below the normal range, i.e. $<1.0 \times 10^9/L$. It occurs when neutrophil survival is decreased due to sepsis or immune destruction and/or there is insufficient production in the bone marrow (see Box 12.3). The most common causes are infection and drug-related.

Patients with neutropenia are at considerable risk of secondary infection. In severe neutropenia, the normal signs of infection may be absent and patients may deteriorate rapidly. Pyrexia may be the only indication that infection is present and early treatment with broad-spectrum antibiotics is considered essential. If serial blood cultures are negative, fungal or other atypical infection should be considered, particularly if the patient has been receiving high dose corticosteroid and/or other immunosuppressive therapy.

Box 12.2 Terms associated with leucocytes

Leucopenia: the white cell count is $<4 \times 10^9/L$. This may be due to a generalized bone marrow disorder (e.g. megaloblastic anaemia, aplasia, acute leukaemia, or metastatic tumour), viral or bacterial infections, or drug toxicity.

Leucocytosis: the total white cell count is $>11 \times 10^9/L$.

Neutropenia: the neutrophil count is $<1.0 \times 10^9/L$ (severe neutropenia is $<0.5 \times 10^9/L$).

Eosinophilia: the eosinophil count is $>0.4 \times 10^9/L$.

Lymphocytosis: the lymphocyte count is $>3.5 \times 10^9/L$.

Lymphopenia: the lymphocyte count is $<1.5 \times 10^9/L$.

Monocytosis: the monocyte count is $>0.8 \times 10^9/L$.

Agranulocytosis: in this condition the bone marrow stops producing white cells, leaving the body open to overwhelming infection. It is often caused by irradiation or drug toxicity (e.g. chemotherapy, carbimazole).

> **Box 12.3 Causes of neutropenia**
>
> **Decreased production**
> - Aplastic anaemia
> - Cancer, leukaemia, myelodysplastic syndrome, myelofibrosis
> - Radiation therapy
> - Hereditary disorders (e.g. congenital neutropenia)
> - Vitamin B_{12}, folate, and copper deficiency
> - Arsenic poisoning
> - Paroxysmal nocturnal haemoglobinuria
> - Medication
> - Infection (including sepis)
>
> **Increased destruction**
> - Sepsis (increased consumption)
> - Anti-neutrophil antibody
> - Systemic lupus erythematosus
> - Medication (e.g. phenothiazines)
> - Autoimmue neutropenia
> - Chemotherapy treatment
>
> **Increased sequestration**
> - Haemodialysis
> - Hypersplenism

The leukaemias

These are neoplastic disorders of the blood-forming tissues (bone marrow, spleen, lymphatic system). Commonly, there is an unregulated accumulation of white cells in the bone marrow, liver, spleen, and lymph nodes with invasion of the gastrointestinal tract, meninges, skin, and kidneys. They are classified according to the cell line involved, and are either acute or chronic. Leukaemias may be caused by irradiation but the cause is often unknown. Some are linked with genetic susceptibilities. Symptoms reflect the infiltration of organs by the white cells and/or bone marrow failure. Infiltration can cause local pain in the liver, spleen, and lymph nodes, as well as bone pain due to expansion of the marrow.

Bone marrow failure results in:

- anaemia causing lethargy and pallor
- leucopenia causing increased risk of infection
- thrombocytopenia causing increased risk of bleeding.

Summary of the types of leukaemia

Acute lymphoblastic leukaemia (ALL) is more common in children where lymph nodes, bone, and nervous tissue can become infiltrated. Therapy aims to induce a remission by cytotoxic agents and irradiation of the central nervous system. The success of therapy has steadily increased; five year survival rates for children are nearly 80% and approximately 40% for adults.

Chronic lymphatic leukaemia (CLL) occurs mainly in adults >55 years, and is often discovered at a routine medical examination or blood test as patients are often symptom free. They may present with enlarged lymph nodes or tiredness. The onset is insidious and is characterized by a progressive accumulation of poorly functional lymphocytes. Occasionally, pleural or peritoneal effusions develop. Chemotherapy is not needed until patients become symptomatic or display evidence of rapid disease progression. Most patients live for 5–10 years, but prognosis depends on the stage at diagnosis and the presence of high risk markers (e.g. chromosomal abnormalities).

Acute myeloid leukaemia (AML) affects people of any age, but is more common in adults. It is characterized by an increase in the number of myeloid cells in the bone marrow and an arrest in their maturation, resulting in leucopenia, thrombocytopenia, and/or anaemia. Even with modern intensive chemotherapy regimens and bone marrow transplantation, only about 40% of patients aged <65 years survive for 5 years. However, survival depends on the subtype.

Chronic myeloid leukaemia (CML) This myeloproliferative disorder is characterized by an increase in proliferation of the granulocytic cell line without the loss of their capacity to differentiate. More than 90% of cases are caused by a single specific genetic mutation (the Philadelphia chromosome). It often occurs in people aged 30–50 years, and the onset is often insidious with fever and weight loss. Splenomegaly, hepatomegaly, and thrombocytopenia may develop later in the disease. The white blood cell count is often very high. Treatment is with chemotherapy. Currently, the 5 year survival rate is >60–80%. CML typically begins in a chronic phase, and progresses to an accelerated phase and, finally, a blast crisis.

The care and management of malignant haematological disease are discussed later.

Thrombocytes (platelets)

Thrombocytes are actually non-nucleated fragments of large cells called megakaryocytes and are formed in the bone marrow. The tips of the cells are thought to extend into the blood sinusoid. Platelets are essential for blood clotting, the mechanism of which is complex and is discussed later.

Thrombocyte disorders

Thrombocytopenia

A platelet count of 150 × 10^9/L is the lower limit of the normal range, but bleeding due to thrombocytopenia is unlikely to occur unless the count is below 50 × 10^9/L. Thrombocytopenia can result from an increased destruction or decreased production of platelets (see Box 12.4). Specific management depends on the underlying cause.

Idiopathic thrombocytopenic purpura (ITP)

This is a rare autoimmune disorder where autoantibodies are directed against platelets so that their lifespan is considerably shortened. There are two types of ITP: an acute form that occcurs in children, and a chronic form (lasting >6 months) that occurs in adults. Symptoms usually begin suddenly with petechiae and mucosal bleeding. The platelet count is low and bleeding time is prolonged, but coagulation times are normal. The acute form is usually post-infectious and recovery can take from weeks to months. The chronic form has a variable course and often does not recover.

Box 12.4 Causes of thrombocytopenia

Decreased production

- Viral or bacterial infection
- Leukaemia or myelodysplastic syndrome
- Vitamin B_{12} or folic acid
- Decreased production of thrombopoietin by the liver (in liver failure)
- Hereditary syndromes

Increased destruction

- Idiopathic thrombocytopenic purpura (ITP)
- Thrombotic thrombocytopenic purpura (TTP)
- Haemolytic-uraemic syndrome (HUS)
- Disseminated intravascular coagulation (DIC)
- Paroxysmal nocturnal haemoglobinuria (PNH)
- Antiphospholipid syndrome
- Systemic lupus erythrematosus (SLE)
- Post-perfusion purpura
- Splenic sequestration of platelets due to hypersplenism
- HIV-associated thrombocytopenia
- Drug-induced—direct myelosuppression (e.g. methotrexate, interferon) or immunological platelet destruction (e.g. heparin-induced thrombocytopenia (HIT), abciximab induced thrombocytopenia)

Treatment is aimed at achieving a platelet count associated with adequate haemostasis. Initial treatment is with corticosteroids, IV imunoglobulin, or anti-D immunoglobulin. Platelet infusions may be given in emergency situations when the platelet count needs to be raised quickly. Subsequent treatment may include splenectomy, rituximab, thrombopoietin receptor agonists (these stimulate platelet production), or more potent immunosuppression.

Thrombotic thrombocytopenic purpura (TTP)

TTP is a rare condition mainly affecting adults. It is life threatening unless adequately treated and can be recurrent, with multiple unpredictable episodes. Spontaneous thrombi consisting mostly of platelets form in the capillaries and arterioles and cause widespread multivisceral ischaemia or infarction, haemolytic anaemia, and severe thrombocytopenia. The gut and cerebral circulation are particularly affected, but also the liver, kidneys, and lung. Clinical manifestations are:

- neurological disturbances—headache, transient paralysis, numbness, altered mental state, seizures, hemiplegia, visual disturbances, stroke, hypertension
- renal abnormalities—haemoglobinuria, haematuria, renal failure
- haemolytic anaemia—pallor, jaundice, fatigue
- thrombocytopenia—petechiae, purpura, bleeding into mucous membranes (though severe bleeding is unusual)
- fever in approximately 50% of cases, abdominal pain.

The pathophysiology is obscure, but in about 90% of cases it is linked to the inhibition of the enzyme ADAMTS13. Patients with TTP have been found to have unusually large multimers of von Willebrand factor (vWF). This is a protein that links platelets, blood clots, and the blood vessel wall in the process of coagulation. Very large vWF multimers are more prone to cause coagulation. The function of ADAMTS13 is to cleave these multimers, and therefore limit their size and haemostatic ability. Most cases of TTP are associated with a severe deficiency of ADAMTS13. Here, the deficiency is acquired via autoantibodies to ADAMTS13; more rarely, it is inherited via ADAMTS13 gene mutations.

The mainstay of treatment is frequent high volume plasma exchange using fresh frozen plasma (see later) to reduce circulating antibodies against ADAMTS13. Platelet infusions should be avoided unless life-threatening bleeding is present. Patients then receive additional immunosupression therapy, for example with glucocorticosteroids, vincristine, cyclophosphamide, rituximab, or splenectomy (or a mixture of these). If untreated, the mortality rate is about 90%, but with plasma exchange this is reduced to about 10%. Cardiac failure or cardiac arrest is a common mode of death for reasons as yet unclear.

Drug-induced thrombocytopenia (DIT)

DIT is a relatively common disorder caused by drugs that either decrease platelet production or accelerate their destruction. Generally, the platelet count falls rapidly within 2–3 days of taking a drug which has been taken previously, or ≥7 days after starting a new drug. The commonest causative agents are heparin and quinine, but others include penicillin, sulphonamides, non-steroidal anti-inflammatory drugs, anticonvulsants, diuretics, ranitidine, and rifampicin. The treatment is to stop the drug. When the drug is stopped, the platelet count usually rises rapidly within 1–2 days of withdrawal. The platelet count is rarely low enough to cause severe bleeding. Platelet transfusions are not routinely given as these can increase thrombosis.

Heparin-induced thrombocytopenia (HIT)

There are two types of HIT. In type 1 the platelet count is reduced rapidly within a few days of starting heparin, but is transient and is not associated with the formation of thrombus. Type 2, however, is an immune process. Heparin binds to a protein called platelet factor 4 (PF4) in the blood and this complex induces the formation of antibodies (called anti-PF4 antibodies). These antibodies are usually of the immunoglobulin G class (IgG) and their development takes about 5 days. If PF4 binds to heparin on the cell surface, the antibodies attack the cells. This causes platelet activation and the formation of platelet microparticles which initiate the formation of venous and arterial thrombi. The platelet count falls as a result, leading to thrombocytopenia. Diagnosis is by a reduced platelet count typically 5–10 days after exposure to heparin. However, critically ill patients may develop thrombocytopenia from other causes. Confirmation of HIT is by the detection of anti-PF4 antibodies or by a serotonin release assay.

HIT-associated thrombotic events are more common in patients treated with unfractionated heparin than in those treated with low molecular weight heparin (LMWH). If HIT is diagnosed, administration of all heparin must be stopped. If the patient still needs anticoagulation a drug with a different mechanism must be used, for example direct thrombin inhibitors or Xa inhibitors (e.g. bivalarudin, fondaparinux). HIT is usually a transient immune response, and after several months have passed it is usually safe to re-challenge with heparin if needed.

Platelet dysfunction in renal failure/uraemia

Patients with renal failure may have a prolonged bleeding time. Although bleeding is typically cutaneous (bruising or mucosal bleeding), epistaxis, gastrointestinal bleeding, or other more severe haemorrhage may develop.

Multiple factors are responsible for impairing platelet function in uraemic patients. Uraemic toxins result in dysfunctional von Willebrand factor (vWF) and vWF–factor VIII complex with impaired platelet aggregation.

Treatment for bleeding in uraemic patients consists of renal replacement therapy to remove uraemic toxins, as well as desmopressin (DDAVP). DDAVP causes release of vWF from tissue stores and reduces bleeding time. Packed red blood cells may be given to improve anaemia and cryoprecipitate to increase the proportion of functional factor VIII, vWF, and fibrinogen. Conjugated oestrogens may also be given (to both men and women) to promote coagulation. Low dose heparin or prostacyclin should be used to maintain the patency of the circuit if renal replacement therapy is required.

The coagulation mechanism and fibrinolysis

The process of coagulation and fibrinolysis is extremely complex, involving a multitude of clotting factors, cofactors, regulators, and feedback mechanisms. Space does not permit a detailed explanation, and therefore the following is a general overview. The diagram of the clotting mechanism and fibrinolytic pathway (Figure 12.2) has also been simplified to show the essential components. The common names of the coagulation factors are given in Table 12.2.

In normal homeostasis, when a blood vessel is damaged the endpoint of the coagulation cascade is the formation of a fibrin clot which seals the vessel. Fibrinolysis prevents too much clot forming and degrades the clot when it is no longer required. There are two pathways that are activated when a vessel is damaged; the intrinsic (also known as contact activation) pathway, and the extrinsic (also known as the tissue factor) pathway. These two pathways merge into the common pathway.

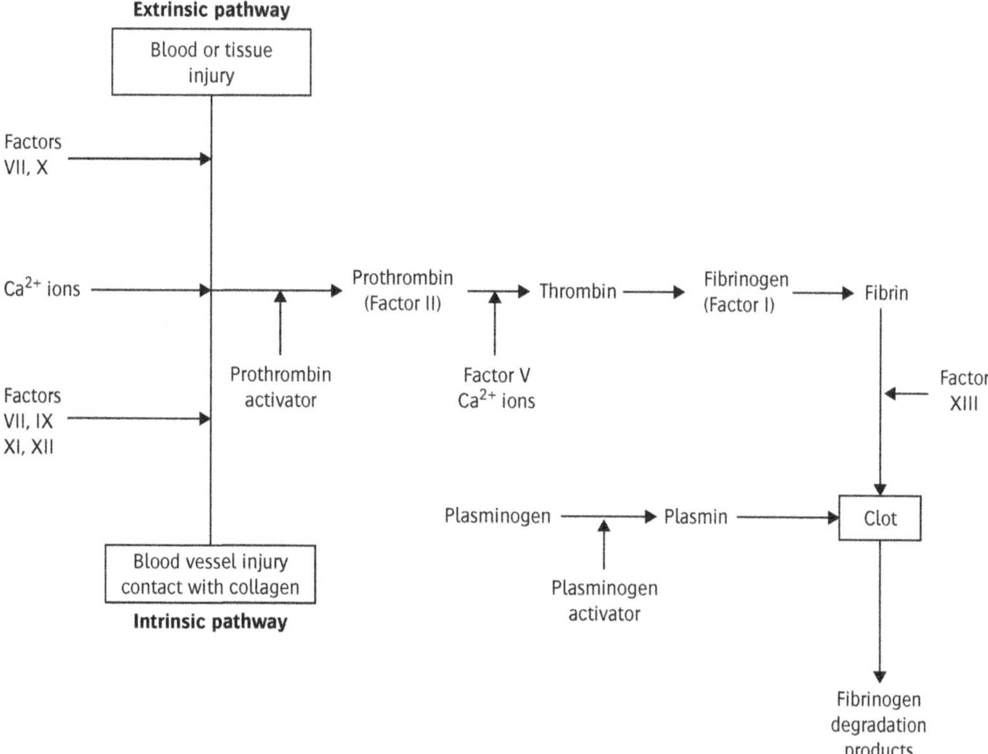

Figure 12.2 The clotting mechanism and fibrinolytic pathway.

The intrinsic pathway

Injury to a blood vessel leads to the exposure of collagen fibres in the vessel wall, and this pathway is activated when factor XII (fibrin stabilizing factor) binds to the negatively charged 'foreign' surface that is exposed to the blood. This sequentially activates factors XI, IX, X, and II (prothrombin to thrombin) which then convert fibrinogen to fibrin. Kallikrein (an enzyme that cleaves peptide bonds in protein) also releases bradykinin from kininogen. This causes vasoconstriction of the vessel which limits blood flow to the area.

The extrinsic pathway

This involves tissue factor (TF) which binds to activated factor VII (factor VIIa). This forms a complex called TF-Factor VIIa which, in turn, activates factor X and IX. Activated factor IX activates more factor X. Activated factor X converts prothrombin to thrombin with activated factor V, anionic phospholipids, and calcium acting as cofactors. Prothrombin factor is then released (see the section on the common pathway). After initial activation the pathway is inhibited by the binding of tissue factor pathway inhibitor (TFPI) to factor Xa, which inhibits formation of the TF–factor VIIa complex. Further coagulation is then dependent on the intrinsic pathway.

The common pathway

This involves factor I (fibrinogen), factor II (prothrombin), and factors V and X. Thrombin converts soluble fibrinogen to insoluble fibrin, forming a fibrin clot. Thrombin may also activate factors XI (part of the intrinsic pathway), V, VIII, and XI, and platelets. Factor XIII crosslinks the fibrin to increase the stability of the clot.

The protein C–protein S anticoagulant pathway

This anticoagulant pathway limits the formation of the blood clot (i.e. fibrinogen to fibrin) at the site of injury. The major anticoagulants are proteins C and S, antithrombin, and tissue factor pathway inhibitor (TFPI). Proteins C and S are anticoagulants produced mainly in the liver and are vitamin K dependent.

Table 12.2 Coagulation factors

Coagulation factor	Common name
Antithrombin	Antithrombin
I	Fibrinogen
II	Prothrombin
III	Tissue factor
IV	Calcium
V	Proaccelerin
VI	Accelerin
VII	Serum prothrombin conversion accelerator
VIII	Anti-haemophilic factor A
IX	Christmas factor
X	Stuart factor or Stewart Power factor
XI	Plasma thromboplastin antecedant
XII	Hageman factor
XIII	Fibrin stabilizing factor
High molecular weight kininogen	Contact activation factor
Prekallikrein	Fletcher factor
Protein C	Anticoagulant protein C
Protein S	Anticoagulant protein S
Thromboplastin	Fetomodulin

The pathway is activated at the site of injury when the endothelial protein C receptor binds a thrombin–thrombodulin complex. This then activates protein C which binds to free protein S on the endothelium or platelet phospholipid surfaces. The protein C–protein S complex degrades factors Va and VIIIa, which reduces the formation of fibrin. Activated protein C also indirectly promotes fibrinolysis.

Antithrombin also functions as an anticoagulant by inhibiting activated factors II (thrombin), IX, X, XI, XII, kallikrein, plasmin, and probably factor VII. Its activity is accelerated a thousand-fold by its interaction with heparin (located on the endothelial cells).

The fibrinolysis pathway

This pathway degrades the clot when it is no longer required and also prevents extension of the clot beyond the site of injury. Its activation occurs immediately whenever the clotting cascade is triggered and runs alongside the coagulation pathway.The pathway is initiated by tissue plasminogen activator (tPA) or urokinase-like plasminogen activator (uPA). These convert plasminogen to plasmin in the presence of fibrin. Plasmin degrades the fibrin clot and intact fibrinogen into soluble fibrin/fibrinogen degradation products (FDPs). Plasmin also inactivates factors Va and VIIa (as do proteins C and S). The endothelial cells of the blood vessel produce tPA, and its activation by plasminogen is a major mechanism for the lysis of fibrin clots. Recombinant tPA is used to treat myocardial infarction, strokes, and some acute thrombosis. uPA is produced by urine and plasma and keeps the renal tract free of blood clots. It is also important for other cell surfaces and initiating the non-fibrinolytic activities of plasmin.

Excessive fibrinolysis is prevented by plasmin inhibitor (antiplasmin) and plasminogen activator inhibitor (PAI)-1. The normal mechanisms of coagulation and fibrinolysis will complement each other until an underlying condition disturbs the body's homeostasis.

Bleeding and hypercoagulopathy disorders

Bleeding disorders are due to defects in clot formation or an over-active fibrinolytic system. Hypercoagulopathy disorders (also known as thrombophilia) cause excessive clotting and are due to defects in the anticoagulant system or an under-active fibrinolytic system. Some disorders (e.g. polycythemia rubra, essential thrombcythaemia) can be associated with both bleeding and thrombosis (see Table 12.3).

Haemophilia

This sex-linked genetic disorder affects men but is carried by women. Haemophilia A is caused by deficiency of factor VIII and haemophilia B (Christmas disease) is caused by factor IX deficiency. Clinically, they are indistinguishable. Haemophilia can cause severe bleeding from minor trauma, and disabling muscle and joint haemorrhages.

Table 12.3 Bleeding disorders and hypercoaguable states

Acquired bleeding disorders	Liver dysfunction (as many coagulation factors are made in the liver) Nephrotic syndrome/renal disease (can cause platelet dysfunction and reduced aggregation) Sepsis/shock (may cause DIC—see later) Vitamin K deficiency (some coagulation factors are vitamin K dependent) Circulating autoantibodies to coagulation factors (e.g. lymphoma, SLE) Amyloidosis (factor X deficiency can occur)
Hereditary bleeding disorders	von Willebrand's disease (reduced vWF) Haemophilia A (factor VIII deficiency) Haemophilia B (Christmas disease—factor IX deficiency)
Acquired hypercoagulable states	Acquired thrombophilia Antiphospholipid antibodies Heparin-induced thrombocytopenia Pregnancy/obesity Prolonged immobility/lengthy air travel Hormone replacement therapy Recent trauma/surgery Cancer/some myeloproliferative disorders Paroxysmal nocturnal haemoglobinuria HIV/AIDS
Hereditary hypercoagulable states	Activated protein C resistance Factor V Leiden Deficiency of natural proteins that prevent clotting (e.g. proteins C and S, antithrombin) Dysfibrinogenaemia Elevated coagulation factor levels in plasma Sickle cell disease

Treatment is by administering purified factor VIII or IX concentrate as soon as possible after the bleeding has started, or prophylactically before dental extractions or surgery. The aim is to raise the factor to >30% of normal. Repeated infusions may be necessary every 8–12 hours.

Fresh frozen plasma (FFP) contains both factors but vast quantities are usually required. It is usually given only if the single factor concentrates are unavailable. Patients with haemophilia should never be given aspirin as this impairs platelet function. Intramuscular injections must be avoided and dental hygiene is important since dental extraction can be hazardous.

von Willebrand's disease

This autosomal dominant disease affects both males and females. It is due to a deficiency of von Willebrand factor (vWF) which is required for platelet adhesion. There is a prolonged bleeding time with variable degrees of bleeding. Commonly, patients have nose bleeds, post-operative bleeding, and bleeding from cuts, but do not suffer from the massive soft tissue/joint haemorrhages seen in haemophilia. Treatment is with transfusion of cryoprecipitate (wich contains factor VIII) or by a purified concentrate of factor VIII. Mild von Willebrand's disease may be treated by DDAVP, and this can also be used for prophylaxis prior to surgery. Patients should avoid aspirin and non-steroidal anti-inflammatory drugs.

Liver disease

The liver produces nearly all the factors involved in the formation and control of coagulation (except factor VIII). Bleeding associated with liver disease can be devastating and difficult to manage. Liver disease may result in reduced synthesis of all of the coagulation factors. Fat-soluble vitamin K, which is necessary for the precursors of factors II, VII, IX, and X, may not be absorbed if there is concomitant cholestasis. Disseminated intravascular coagulation (DIC) can be initiated or exacerbated by the release of tissue thromboplastin from damaged liver cells. The prothrombin time (PT) and partial thromboplastin time (PTT) are both prolonged in liver failure, and the platelet count is low if there is splenomegaly. Fibrin degradation products (FDPs) may be elevated as a result of excessive fibrinolysis or because the liver fails to clear them from the blood.

Bleeding due to vitamin K deficiency may be reversed by administration of vitamin K. Treatment of bleeding episodes associated with abnormal laboratory tests is by transfusions of FFP and platelets to maintain the platelet count >50 × 10⁹/L and to normalize the prothrombin time and increase the low platelet count. Low fibrinogen levels usually indicate severe liver disease or the presence of DIC. Cryoprecipitate can be used to increase fibrinogen levels.

Disseminated intravascular coagulation (DIC)

This is a dysregulated activation of the coagulation cascade leading to the formation of soluble or insoluble fibrin within the circulation. Thrombus formation and haemorrhage occur almost at the same time, and microvascular thrombi can contribute to multi-organ failure. DIC never occurs as a primary disorder, but always arises as a secondary complication of an underlying condition (see Box 12.5). Often, the primary condition that has induced the DIC will dominate the clinical picture, and the development of the syndrome provides a diagnostic and management challenge. Mortality of patients with DIC can be extremely high.

The normal mechanisms of coagulation and fibrinolysis complement each other until an underlying condition or trigger disturbs this fine balance. The pathogenesis of DIC is complex, and the trigger mechanisms can also be complicated by hypoxia, acidosis, and hyper-pyrexia. The three main mechanisms of acute DIC are:

- excessive generation and circulation of thrombin
- impairment of the natural anticoagulation pathway
- suppression of fibrinolysis.

Damage to the vessel wall due to inflammatory cytokines, microbial toxins, or tissue injury exposes collagen fibres, attracts platelets, and triggers the intrinsic coagulation pathway. This causes excessive release of tissue factor and massive generation and activation of thrombin, causing deposition of fibrin within the microvasculature and the release of plasmin and other proteolytic enzymes.

Low levels of protein C and antithrombin result in insufficient coagulation control. The natural defence against this widespread clotting is the fibrinolysis pathway. Activated factor XII, thrombin, and endothelial cells all stimulate the fibrinolytic system to release plasminogen activators. These stimulate plasmin to degrade fibrin into fibrin degradation products (FDPs). FDPs are potent anticoagulants and further potentiate the bleeding cycle. Specific inhibitors of clot formation include activated protein C, antithrombin (formerly called antithrombin III), and tissue factor pathway inhibitor (TFPI) which control the formation of fibrin. Antithrombin also inhibits production of thrombin and promotes release of prostacyclin (PGI_2) from endothelial cells inhibiting platelet aggregation and white cell activation. The result is the formation of small thrombi throughout the body, the consumption of coagulation factors and platelets resulting in bleeding, and further activation of the systemic inflammatory response as thrombin is a potent stimulus. In the patient with DIC the reticuloendothelial system (which normally removes FDPs) is overwhelmed and the patient has a self-perpetuating combination of thrombotic and bleeding activity.

Box 12.5 Disorders that may trigger disseminated intravascular coagulation

- Sepsis/severe infection (any micro-organism)
- Tissue destruction (e.g. burns, crush injuries, head injury, severe pancreatitis, extensive surgery, rhabdomyolysis)
- Malignancy/myeloproliferative disorders
- Severe blood transfusion reactions
- Rheumatological and autoimmune diseases
- Obstetric disorders (e.g. HELLP, amniotic fluid embolism, eclampsia, abruptio placentae, retained dead fetus)
- Vascular abnormalities (e.g. large vascular aneurysms, haemangiomas)
- Severe toxic reactions (e.g. transplant rejection)
- Hyperthermia (e.g. heat stroke)
- Haemorrhagic skin necrosis
- Liver disease (e.g. obstructive jaundice, acute liver failure)
- Snake venom

Box 12.6 Tests used in the detection of DIC

- Prothrombin time—prolonged
- Partial thromboplastin time—prolonged
- Thrombin time—prolonged
- Fibrinogen levels—low
- Platelet count—low
- Fibrogen degradation products—high
- D-dimers—high

There is no single laboratory test that specifically confirms a diagnosis of DIC (see Box 12.6). Interpretation of laboratory tests must be correlated with the clinical presentation of the patient and an awareness of the conditions that predispose to DIC. Serial measurements are required in order to monitor the progression of the disease and to administer the appropriate treatment.

Treatment of DIC

This can present a considerable challenge. There is no single universally accepted treatment regimen and medical management is controversial. However, the agreed aims of therapy are:

- elimination of the underlying cause, although this may not always be possible (e.g. malignancy)
- restoration of haemostasis
- prevention of microemboli
- maintenance of blood volume and prevention of vascular stasis, hypoxia, and acidosis.

Transfusion of blood, FFP, and platelets is reserved for patients who are actively bleeding or who require an invasive procedure. These restore haemoglobin levels and replete the consumed coagulation factors while the underlying condition is brought under control. FFP is particularly useful as it provides all the clotting factors required, however large the volumes needed. A platelet count $<50 \times 10^9$/L in a patient who is actively bleeding would be an indication for platelet transfusion. Fibrinogen concentrates, cryoprecipitate, or antithrombin may be used though supportive data are scanty. The evidence base for factor VIIa, protein C concentrate, and prothrombin complex concentrate is even weaker. In general, antifibrinolytic agents such as tranexamic acid should not be used, though they do have an important role given early in trauma.

Therapeutic (full-dose) heparin doses should be considered where clinical features of thrombosis predominate, but not in those at high risk of bleeding. In >95% of cases of DIC there is no indication for heparin. Prophylactic (low dose) heparin (usually LMWH) is recommended for prevention of venous thromboembolism in critically ill patients who are not bleeding.

Nursing management

The aims of management are:

- identifying the patient at risk of developing DIC (see Box 12.5).
- early detection and management of bleeding.
- preventing further bleeding
- preventing complications associated with decreased tissue perfusion or haemorrhage.
- treating the underlying cause of DIC (if possible).

Problems associated with DIC

Cardiovascular and skin disorders

- **Potential problems** Hypovolaemia due to haemorrhage; skin necrosis due to decreased perfusion and infarction.
- **Action** Haemorrhage can range from an acute large bleed (although this is unusual) to, more commonly, an ongoing ooze from cannulae, drain, and wound sites, or bleeding into the mucous membranes or skin that is visible as purpura—either small (petechiae) or large (ecchymosis). Often there is no clinical manifestation and DIC is diagnosed solely on the basis of abnormal blood tests. Vital signs must be monitored closely to detect hypovolaemia and treated as necessary to prevent organ hypoperfusion. Observe for necrotic areas (particularly on the toes and fingers). Invasive procedures should be kept to the minimum necessary in the patient with DIC. An arterial line in situ will avoid repeated vessel puncture for blood sampling and can be used to monitor blood pressure. If a blood pressure cuff is used, it should be removed between recordings, as traumatic petechiae may develop under the cuff, and alternate arms should be used if possible. Intramuscular injections should be avoided, but if essential, a small gauge needle should be used. Mouth care must be gentle to avoid trauma to the gums. Local pressure or haemostatic dressings may be necessary if there is bleeding from cannulae sites.

Respiratory disorders

- **Potential problems** Respiratory failure due to pulmonary haemorrhage, haemothorax, acute respiratory distress syndrome. It is important to recognize that DIC is not a cause of ARDS (or vice versa); rather these are both concurrent manifestations of multi-organ failure triggered by an insult such as trauma or infection.

- **Action:** Pulmonary bleeding will cause haemoptysis (in the self-ventilating patient) or blood-stained secretions on endotracheal suction. Respiratory function must be monitored closely (see Chapter 4). Oxygen therapy should be administered according to the arterial oxygen saturation, but intubation and ventilation should not be delayed if the patient is hypoxaemic (despite the potential risk of bleeding associated with the procedure).

Renal disorders

- **Potential problem** Renal failure due to hypovolaemia.
- **Action** A common misapprehension of the pathophysiology of acute renal failure is that it is due to microemboli from DIC causing acute tubular necrosis (ATN). While ATN can be seen at post-mortem, it is usually minor and patchy, and rarely widespread. Thus it cannot in itself account for the clinical and biochemical kidney dysfunction seen when the patient was alive. Like ARDS, acute kidney injury is another manifestation of organ system dysfunction concurrent with coagulation abnormalities. Urine output must be monitored and attempts made to maintain output >0.5 ml/kg/hour. Oliguria can result from hypoperfusion of the kidney; therefore hypovolaemia must be treated aggressively and an adequate blood pressure maintained with inotropic or vasopressor support, as needed. If renal failure becomes established, renal support will be required (see Chapter 7). Urine should be tested regularly for protein and blood, and biochemical function should be checked frequently.

Neurological disorders

- **Potential problem** Cerebral ischaemia due to intracranial haemorrhage or thrombosis.
- **Action** The patient must be observed for changes in conscious level, restlessness, agitation, visual disturbances, headaches, and sensory or motor function. Monitor pupillary reaction (see Chapter 8).

Gastrointestinal disorders

- **Potential problem** Bleeding from the gastrointestinal tract.
- **Action** Observe nasogastric aspirate, emesis, and stool for blood. Stools should be tested for occult blood. A mesenteric embolus may cause small bowel infarction and severe abdominal pain. Bleeding into the retroperitoneal space can result in varying degrees of pain, tingling, or numbness due to secondary nerve compression

Anticoagulant therapy

Anticoagulants are used to prevent thrombus formation or the extension of an existing thrombus. Prophylactic anticoagulation is administered to patients at risk of developing thrombi (e.g. prolonged immobilization, chronic atrial fibrillation, previous thromboembolic events, , prosthetic heart valves). Therapeutic anticoagulation is used to treat venous or arterial thrombi (e.g. pulmonary embolus, deep vein thrombosis). The duration of therapy and choice of anticoagulant is determined by the patient's condition. Anticoagulant therapy is commonly used in critical care, but always carries the potential complication of haemorrhage. Patients having anticoagulant therapy must be observed closely for signs of bleeding. This may be overt, with active bleeding from cannulae sites, drains, and wounds, or may be hidden, i.e. occult (e.g. from the gastrointestinal tract—haematemesis, melaena).

Urine should be tested daily for blood, and nasogastric aspirate should also be regularly observed or tested for blood. The skin should be observed for bruising, petechiae, or purpuric haemorrhages. Purpura is the extravasation of blood into the skin causing purple areas, which may be variable in size. Pinhead-sized spots are termed petechiae and larger areas ecchymoses (bruises). Purpura result from the increased fragility of the capillary due to a deficiency in the number or function of platelets, or damage to the capillary wall due to antibodies (allergic purpura), or metabolic/bacterial toxins (bacterial endocarditis and uraemia).

To prevent haemorrhage the effect of the anticoagulant must be monitored carefully and regular laboratory coagulation screens are required. Anticoagulation dosing is titrated to a specific therapeutic range of laboratory values but this strongly depends on the drug used. Thus, the INR (international normalized ratio) or prothrombin time is used for warfarin, while the activated partial thromboplastin time is used for unfractionated heparin or direct thrombin inhibitors such as bivalirudin. Anti-factor Xa activity can be measured in specialized laboratoriess to titrate dosing of LMW heparin or fondaparinux, but this is generally not performed as a routine test. There is no specific test for prostacyclin-type agents (functional monitoring of coagulation is required).

It is possible to measure activated clotting times (ACTs) at the bedside as this is a simple and quick procedure. Some ICUs use the ACT test in patients undergoing renal replacement therapy to titrate the dose of heparin. The desired value varies according to the patient's clinical state and the purpose of the anticoagulation.

Patients with extracorporeal circuits for renal replacement therapy usually require an ACT in the region of 170–200 sec, while those on cardiopulmonary bypass will need levels of 400–600 sec. The ACT cannot be used for determining the anticoagulant action of prostacyclin. Thromboelastography (TEG) is another method of testing the efficiency of coagulation and can also assess platelet function, clot strength, and fibrinolysis. A small sample of blood is rotated gently to initiate sluggish venous flow and active coagulation. When the clot forms a thin wire probe is used to measure the speed and strength of clot formation (by computer). Rotational thromboelastometry (ROTEM) is another version that measures and graphically displays the changes in elasticity at all stages of the developing and resolving clot.

Anticoagulants commonly used in the critical care unit

Heparin

Unfractionated heparin

Heparin works by markedly enhancing the activity of antithrombin, which inhibits activated factors II, IX, X, XI, XII, kallikrein, and probably factor VII. It is commonly used, for example, in patients with pulmonary embolus, deep vein thrombosis, and those undergoing heart surgery or renal replacement therapy. Unfractionated heparin is administered intravenously and acts rapidly, but has a short half-life of about 90 min so generally needs to be given by continuous infusion. Heparin may prolong the clotting time if heparin-induced antibodies block platelet aggregation. Heparin overdose can be corrected by stopping the heparin and, if necessary, by the intravenous administration of protamine sulphate. When used alone, protamine sulphate has an anticoagulant effect but when given in the presence of heparin, a stable salt is formed and the anticoagulant activity of both is lost; 1 mg of protamine sulphate will neutralize 100 IU of heparin. This is usually given in small doses with laboratory monitoring to assess the effect. A complication of unfractionated heparin is heparin-induced thrombocytopenia or HIT (see earlier) which may occur in 3% of patients.

Low molecular weight heparin (LMWH)

These subcutaneous agents (e.g. dalteparin, enoxaparin) can be used instead of fractionated heparin with similar efficacy. They have a more predictable anticoagulant effect and there is much less need for laboratory monitoring. They can also be reversed by protamine, though not as effectively as with unfractionated heparin. Unlike standard heparins, LMWHs do not inhibit thrombin or factor IXa, but acts predominantly on factor Xa. They have a longer half-life (4 hours) than standard heparins, but this is prolonged in renal failure so the risk of bleeding will increase. Thus they are not generally recommended for patients in renal failure or receiving renal replacement therapy. LMWHs have a lower incidence of heparin-induced thrombocytopenia than unfractionated heparin. They are given once or twice daily with dosing depending on whether a prophylactic or therapeutic action is sought.

Warfarin

Warfarin is given orally and must be administered for 3–5 days before full anticoagulation is achieved. Heparin therapy (LMWH or unfractionated) should be co-administered until the INR is within the therapeutic range for 2–3 days. Warfarin is commonly used in, for example, patients with poorly controlled atrial fibrillation or prosthetic heart valves to prevent thrombus formation. It antagonizes the effects of vitamin K, which is a cofactor for an enzyme essential for the synthesis of prothrombin and factors VII, IX, and X.

Warfarin readily combines with plasma proteins in the blood, but its metabolism can be affected by many drugs including aspirin, non-steroidal anti-inflamamtory agents, and drugs commonly used for treating atrial fibrillation such as amiodarone. Thus patients receiving such drugs in combination with warfarin are subject to increased sensitivity and bleeding risk, and must be monitored carefully. The ICU pharmacist can advise on interactions.

Dosage of warfarin is controlled by regular measurements of the INR, which is the ratio of the prothrombin time measured in the patient's blood to that of a World Health Organization standard reagent. The INR should generally be kept between 2 and 3. Warfarin overdose should be treated by stopping warfarin treatment; the INR will generally correct within a few days. For more urgent reversal, vitamin K can be used to antagonize the effect of warfarin on the liver's production of clotting factors. However, a vitamin K dose ≥10 mg should only be used for severe bleeding as it will prevent warfarin from acting for several weeks. If the patient is actively bleeding, FFP can be transfused to provide an immediate supply of the deficient clotting factors. Small amounts of vitamin K (e.g. 1 mg) can be given to offset the warfarin effect without affecting its long-term use. Specialist haematology advice should be sought.

Thrombolytics

Thrombolytics are fibrinolytic drugs that are used to break down a thrombus that has already formed (e.g. in acute myocardial infarction, pulmonary embolism, thrombotic/embolic stroke). The classic agents included streptokinase and urokinase, but nowadays recombinant tissue plasminogen activator (tPA) agents such as alteplase and tenecteplase are predominantly used because of their ease of use (shorter infusion, more rapid onset of effect) and fewer allergic reactions. The risk of an allergic reaction is much higher if the patient has previously had streptokinase or urokinase. tPA specifically activates fibrin-bound plasminogen, while streptokinase can also activate circulating plasminogen. Plasminogen is usually inactive until triggered. It is the circulating precursor of plasmin, a proteolytic enzyme that dissolves fibrin. Bleeding can be a major problem with fibrinolytic therapy. The infusion should be stopped and fibrinolysis corrected, if necessary, by the intravenous administration of tranexamic acid (plus FFP, cryoprecipitate, and blood transfusion, as necessary).

Epoprostenol sodium (prostacyclin, PGI_2)

Epoprostenol is a naturally occurring prostaglandin. It is a potent inhibitor of platelet aggregation and the degree of inhibition is dose related. The effect on the platelets usually disappears within 30 min of discontinuing the infusion. It can be used as an alternative to heparin in renal support therapy where a high risk of bleeding from heparin exists. It must be given as a continuous infusion either intravenously or into the extracorporeal circuit.

Epoprostenol is also a vasodilator affecting both systemic and pulmonary circulations. It is used therapeutically for pulmonary hypertension; however, hypotension may occur. If so, the dose should be reduced or discontinued and supportive measures instituted.

Aspirin

Aspirin supresses the production of prostaglandins and thromboxanes by its irreversible inhibition of the cyclo-oxygenase enzyme required for prostaglandin and thromboxane synthesis. Therefore it inhibits platelet aggregation and the ensuing coagulation.

Direct thrombin inhibitors (DTIs)

DTIs act by directly inhibiting thrombin to delay clotting and are classified as either univalent (e.g. argatroban, dabigatron) or bivalent (e.g. hirudin, bivalirudin, lepirudin, and desirudin). Bivalent DTIs have a limited use where heparin would be indicated but cannot be used (such as heparin-induced thrombocytopenia or acute coronary syndromes) but are less suitable for long-term treatment. There is currently a lack of standardized laboratory tests for monitoring these anticoagulants and there are no reversal agents; therefore elevated levels of these drugs carry the risk of life-threatening bleeding complications.

Factor Xa inhibitors

These directly inhibit factor Xa in the coagulation cascade. Factor Xa is generated by both the intrinsic and extrinsic coagulation pathways and activates prothrombin to thrombin (which activates the final components of the coagulation pathway to form clots). Factor Xa inhibitors (e.g. fondaparinux) do not require frequent monitoring and offer an alternative to vitamin K antagonists such as warfarin or LMWH/unfractionated heparin. They are generally used as prophylaxis to prevent deep vein thrombosis and pulmonary embolism. An advantage of using fondaparinux is that the risk of heparin-induced thrombocytopenia is substantially lower than with LMWH or unfractionated heparin. However, it cannot be used in patients with renal dysfunction. Currently, there is no antidote against factor Xa inhibitors.

Coagulation tests

See Appendix for normal ranges of coagulation tests.

Prothrombin time (PT) and international normalized ratio (INR)

The PT is the time taken for plasma to clot after the addition of tissue factor. It measures the effect of a reduction in the vitamin-K-dependent coagulation factors II, V, VII, and X which are involved in the extrinsic pathway. The PT is prolonged in patients with vitamin K deficiency (e.g. due to warfarin or malabsorption from the intestine), poor synthesis of vitamin K (in liver failure), or increased consumption (in DIC).

PT measurements vary according to the type of analytical system used owing to variations in the different batches of manufacturers' tissue factor that is used as a reagent. The INR is a derived measure of the PT that is used to standardize the results. Each manufacturer assigns an internal sensitivity index for their tissue factor product, and this indicates how a particular batch compares with an international reference tissue factor. PT and INR are most commonly used to monitor oral anticogulant therapy.

Thrombin time (TT)

The TT is the time required for fibrin clot to form following addition of a standard amount of thrombin to plasma. It measures the conversion of fibrinogen to fibrin after thrombin is added, and therefore is greatly affected by the level and/or the presence of inhibitors (e.g. heparin, FDPs). It may be prolonged in liver disease, DIC, and dysfibrinogenaemia.

Partial thromboplastin time (PTT)—also known as activated partial thromboplastin time (aPTT)

The PTT evaluates the coagulation factors XI, XII, IX, VIII, X, V, II, and I, and prekallikrein and kininogen.

It is used to monitor unfractionated heparin or fondaparinux therapy. The PTT is also prolonged in the presence of abnormal factor inhibitors (autoantibodies) such as lupus anticoagulant.

Fibronogen degradation products (FDPs) and D-dimers

These measure the activity of the fibrinolytic system. FDPs are fragments produced when either fibrin or fibrinogen is broken down by plasmin. When a fibrin clot breaks down, four principal fibrin degradation products (called X, Y, D, and E) are liberated in various amounts. The last fragment to be degraded is called the D-dimer and is produced from fibrin but not fibrinogen degradation. FDPs and D-dimers will be present in fibrinolysis or thrombosis and therefore are elevated in DIC, thrombolytic drug therapy, and thrombotic disorders.

Blood transfusion and blood component products

Transfusion of blood and blood products is commonplace in the critical care environment for the management of anaemia, haemorrhage, and a range of haematological disorders where specific components of the blood are needed. Donated blood is collected and stored in closed plastic packs which can then be kept for up to 35 days at 4°C. Whole blood can be separated into its component parts after donation and stored separately. This is an economical way of using a valuable resource as several different patients can benefit from a single unit of blood. Specific blood components, once separated, have different uses and storage needs and these are detailed later.

Blood screening

All donated blood is screened for infectious risk (e.g. hepatitis B, HIV) and cross-matched with the recipient's blood for immunological compatibility. The purpose of cross-matching blood before transfusion is to ensure that there is no antibody present in the recipient's plasma that will react with any antigen on the donor's cells. The most frequent causes of giving incompatible blood are incorrect labelling of samples, confusion between patients with the same name, and failing to check from the label on the blood pack that the blood being transfused is the blood cross-matched for the patient. Scrupulous and rigid checking procedures must be carried out at the bedside before any unit of blood or blood product is transfused. The patient identification details on the blood pack must be checked against those on the patient's wristband before the infusion is connected, no matter how urgent their need for the blood, as the consequences of giving mismatched blood can be dire (see section on 'Hazards of blood transfusion'). The pack should also be checked carefully for expiry time and date.

Blood and blood products

Stored whole blood

Donated blood is stored at 4°C in a special blood refrigerator from where it should not be removed for more than 30 min prior to the transfusion. Depending on the anticoagulant used in the blood pack, it can be kept for up to 35 days. The main use of stored whole blood is for the restoration of red cells and circulating blood volume in acute haemorrhage. After 3 days the platelets will not function, and after 3 weeks the levels of 2,3-DPG will diminish. There are normal concentrations of albumin and clotting factors, except factors V and VIII which are reduced to 20% of normal. Whole blood is usually separated within a few hours of donation so that plasma, platelets, and concentrated red cells can be stored under optimal conditions. The consequences of giving large volumes of whole stored blood are discussed later.

Packed red cells (red cell concentrate)

Much of the plasma is removed from whole blood, leaving a concentrated solution of red cells to which 80 ml of anticoagulant nutrient solution is added. It can be kept for 35–42 days depending on the preservative used. There are no platelets and 2,3-DPG levels remain normal for up to 14 days. Generally, in the anaemic patient, the transfusion of 4 ml/kg of packed cells (one bag) should raise the haemoglobin level by approximately 10 g/L. Packed red cells should be stored at 4°C until use.

It is not given where volume replacement is needed but is used for blood loss or bone marrow failure (e.g. anaemia, leukaemia). It was previously thought necessary to maintain haemoglobin levels above 100 g/L for optimal oxygen delivery, but there are no data to support this concept. Studies have shown that a transfusion trigger of 70 g/L is adequate for most critical care patients, though subsets with cardiac disease, COPD, or cerebrovascular disease may need a higher threshold for transfusion. These studies were performed using blood that was not leucodepleted, i.e. where most of the white cells and leucocyte antigens have been removed. The risk of immune and allergic reactions, both overt and covert, and potential transmission of infection is considered to be lower with leucodepleted blood. This is now the norm for blood transfusion in many countries, including the UK. Studies are currently ongoing to determine whether the optimal transfusion trigger differs with leucodepleted blood.

Frozen red cells

These are red cells, uncontaminated by other cells or plasma, in a suspending medium (usually saline). They are used in patients who have a rare blood group as a supply of blood. The patient donates the blood and then the red cells are frozen for future use. Once frozen, they can be stored for up to 10 years but, when thawed, should be used within 12 hours.

CMV-negative red cells

Red cell concentrates can also be specifically CMV-negative or irradiated. CMV-negative products are from donors who have been screened for cytomegalovirus (CMV) and found to be seronegative. They are used in patients who are (potential) recipients of bone marrow transplants. Irradiation is used to destroy lymphocytes which can cause third-party graft versus host disease in the immunosuppressed patient. The CMV load can be reduced in leucocyte-depleted blood by using a filter.

Platelets

These are obtained either from whole blood or by passing blood through a cell separator (apheresis). They may come from either single or multiple random donors. A pack of random donor platelets contains platelet concentrate in 30–50 ml of donor plasma and is usually issued in pools of six to eight packs. A single donor pack may contain up to 300 ml of platelets in plasma. Platelet transfusions are used:

- in patients with symptomatic thrombocytopenia due to chemotherapy, radiotherapy, bone marrow failure, or congenital platelet defects
- if the patient is bleeding (surgical or non-surgical conditions) and they have taken aspirin, clopidogrel, or a similar long-acting anticoagulant in the previous 10 days
- in patients with disseminated intravascular coagulation (DIC)
- following massive blood transfusion
- in patients with platelet dysfunction or thrombocytopenia disorders prior to surgery or invasive procedures
- prior to invasive procedures such as lumbar puncture, liver biopsy, CVP line insertion, or epidural if the platelet count is <50 × 10^9/L.

Ideally, IBO ± RhD group-compatible platelets should be given, but in practice any ABO group can be given if there is a shortage of ABO-compatible platelets. Rhesus-compatible platelets should be given to female patients of child-bearing age. If this is not possible, anti-immunoglobulin should be given (50 IU per adult bag of platelets).

Once prepared, platelet function is best preserved at room temperature. Platelets should be used within 5 days to avoid bacterial contamination and must be continually agitated to prevent clumping (check the expiry time carefully on the pack). Each pack of platelets should be transfused via a 170 mm in-line filter, and specific platelet giving sets are available which have small filter surfaces and drip chambers to reduce the loss of platelets from volume left in the infusion line. Platelets can be infused as rapidly as the patient tolerates but infusion should be completed within 30 min.

Fresh frozen plasma (FFP)

FFP is prepared in blood banks as a by-product of red cell concentrate preparation. The plasma is separated in a low temperature centrifuge at 4°C and then deep frozen to –50°C within 30 min. It is stored at –20°C and, when needed, can be prepared in about 15 min by immersion in a water bath at 37°C. After thawing, the potency of the replacement factors deteriorates and therefore it should be given as soon as possible and at least within 4 hours. A pack of FFP is usually has a volume of about 150–250 ml. It should be given through an infusion set with a 170 mm filter. There is no added benefit in using microaggregate filters. It can be transfused as fast as the patient can tolerate.

FFP contains normal amounts of all clotting factors and plasma proteins. The ABO group should be compatible with that of the recipient. RhD-compatible FFP should be given to women of child-bearing age. If this is not possible anti-D immunoglobulin should be given.

FFP is used as a source of clotting factors for the treatment of coagulopathy, the reversal of the effects of warfarin, and in conjunction with rapid large volume blood transfusions, although replacement should be subsequently guided by clotting studies. FFP is also given to treat clotting factor deficiencies, either when the deficient factor is not known or the specific factor is unavailable. FFP is useful in the treatment of liver disease where there is defective synthesis of coagulation factors.

Cryoprecipitate

Cryoprecipitate is prepared from FFP by collecting the precipitate that forms during controlled thawing and resuspending it in 10–20 ml plasma. It can be stored for 12 months at –30°C and thawed at room temperature immediately before use. It contains high levels of factor VIII, fibrinogen and von Willebrand factor. Cryoprecipitate is used to provide these replacement factors in haemophilia and von Willebrand's disease, or in patients with bleeding associated with hypofibrinogenaemia (<0.8g/dl) or uraemia. In particular in the ICU situation, it is used in the bleeding patient with a severe coagulopathy where FFP alone is considered inadequate. It is usually prepared in pools of six units, with each unit containing approximately 20 ml of donor plasma. ABO + RhD groups should be compatible between donor and recipient. Cryoprecipitate must be filtered because it contains cellular material from leucocytes, red cells, platelets, and fibrin. Transfuse through a 170 mm filter as rapidly as the patient's condition allows.

Specific notes on administering blood transfusions

1. If *any* discrepancies are found when checking the identification details between the blood pack and the patient, do *not* connect the transfusion. Inform the haematology department immediately.
2. Gloves should be worn when handling blood or blood products in order to avoid skin contact.
3. Blood and component products should be administered through a 170 mm filter (standard blood giving set) in order to remove particulate material. A fine 40 mm filter should be used in patients who are neutropenic as these will also remove leucocytes and leucocyte debris.
4. Do not use the pack if it is perforated, clots are visible, or it is past its expiry date.
5. Do not mix any drugs with whole blood or red cell concentrate transfusions.
6. If a unit of blood is left out of the storage refrigerator or cooled transport box for more than 30 min, it should be returned to the laboratory.
7. Do not store blood in the ward or kitchen refrigerator, even temporarily. It must be stored at 4°C (± 2°C) in a specified blood refrigerator.
8. When the transfusion is in progress be alert for transfusion reactions.
9. It is usually necessary to warm blood during infusion if the flow rate exceeds 50 ml/kg/hour (in adults). Only specifically designed warming devices may be used. Never use hot water, radiators, microwaves, etc.
10. Blood and blood products are not compatible with dextrose, which lyses red blood cells.

Adverse reactions to blood transfusions

Blood transfusions are common so it is easy to overlook the associated hazards. Unfavourable reactions usually occur within 20 min of starting the transfusion, and it is during this time that particular attention must be paid. However, careful continuous monitoring is vital throughout the transfusion, particularly in critical care where circulatory overload can easily occur in patients with renal or cardiac impairment. Immediate transfusion reactions are usually due to pyrogens, allergens, bacteria, or incompatible blood, but delayed reactions can occur over days, weeks, or even months. The acute reactions are:

- febrile non-haemolytic (due to cytokines released from transfused white cells).
- acute haemolytic (due to incompatible blood).
- allergic/urticarial.
- anaphylactic.

Febrile non-haemolytic reactions

Monitoring of temperature is vital while a transfusion is in progress. Pyrexia may be due to reactions to pyrogens, leucocytes, or platelet antibodies. Pyrogens are polysaccharides produced by bacteria and can be present in distilled water, citrate, dextrose, and saline. Strict infection control procedures mean that contamination has now been reduced, but febrile reactions may be caused by the presence of anti-HLA (human lymphocyte antibody), granulocyte-specific antibodies, and platelet-specific antibodies in the recipient as a result of sensitization during pregnancy or from previous transfusions. Since pyrexia due to pyrogens is now rare, if it occurs it should be presumed to be due to incompatibility of the red cells, white cells, or platelets that have been transfused, or to plasma proteins. Plasma proteins are the main cause of transfusion reactions. Urticaria and pruritis often develop in these reactions.

The fever should respond to antipyretics, such as aspirin or paracetamol. Antihistamines such as chlorphenamine

(10 mg IV) in addition to hydrocortisone (100 mg IV) should also be administered. If mild, the transfusion may continue slowly. However, if accompanied by rigors and a temperature exceeding 38°C, the transfusion should be stopped.

Acute haemolytic reactions

These occur when red cells are destroyed (haemolysed) in the circulation following transfusion. Haemoglobin is released, while complement activation causes platelet aggregation and the release of vasoactive substances. The reaction may be delayed or immediate and the consequences can be fatal. Most delayed haemolytic reactions are immune related and severity will depend on the red cell antibody involved. Most immediate reactions have an avoidable and identifiable cause and these can be the most dangerous. Immediate haemolysis can be caused by incompatible ABO blood groups, usually as a result of identification error (there is a 10% mortality associated with this). Other immediate causes are incorrectly stored or out-of-date blood, over-heated, frozen, or infected blood, mechanical destruction of the red cells by administering the infusion under pressure, and mixing of the blood with hypotonic infusion fluids.

The signs and symptoms of haemolysis can be immediate and severe. The patient may complain of pain at the infusion site, facial flushing, dyspnoea, headache, and chest, abdominal, or loin pain. Nausea, vomiting, pyrexia, and rigors usually develop. Tachycardia and hypotension are common and may lead to complete circulatory collapse. Oliguria and consequent renal failure may follow. Other features of the reaction include the development of DIC.

When a haemolytic reaction is suspected the blood transfusion must be stopped immediately. The blood bag must be retained and returned to the laboratory, together with samples of blood from the patient for checking the blood group and cross-match, full blood count, coagulation screen, fibrinogen, urea and electrolytes, and direct antiglobulin test. Blood cultures should be taken if sepsis is suspected. A full blood count, urea and electrolytes, and coagulation screen should be repeated two- to four-hourly. Full resuscitative measures may be required in order to restore cardiovascular stability. An ECG should be performed and urine output maintained at 0.5 ml/kg/h. A urine sample should be taken to test for haemoglobinuria. If DIC develops, replacement of clotting factors will be required. Delayed haemolytic reactions are less severe and may occur over a period of days following the transfusion; symptoms include anaemia and jaundice.

Close monitoring of vital signs is essential for early detection of an immediate haemolytic reaction in any patient receiving a blood transfusion. The sooner it can be identified, the transfusion stopped, and supportive treatment begun, the better the prognosis. Careful rigorous attention to the correct procedures of storing and checking may prevent many such reactions.

Circulatory overload

This is not usually a problem in patients with normal cardiac and renal function. However, those with impaired function, the elderly, or the pregnant patient may not tolerate the fluid load associated with blood transfusions, and this may lead to development of pulmonary oedema and heart failure. Careful monitoring of vital signs is essential if this is to be recognized early. Dyspnoea and tachypnoea, and elevated blood pressure, CVP, and heart rate may indicate fluid overload. In patients at risk, this complication may be avoided by administrating a diuretic at the time the transfusion begins, and by the use of red cell concentrate instead of whole blood when volume replacement is not required.

Transfusion-associated graft versus host disease

This is a rare, but usually fatal, complication of transfusion. It is due to engraftment of viable T lymphocytes, which cause widespread tissue damage. Patients who are immunosuppressed, such as those with malinancy, bone marrow transplant recipients, and those with congenital immunodeficiency, are particularly at risk. Typical symptoms include fever, profuse diarrhoea, abdominal pain, maculopapular rash, and toxic epidermal necrolysis in extreme cases. Transfusion-associated graft versus host disease can be prevented by gamma irradiation of blood products (red cell, platelet, and white cell transfusions) prior to transfusion.

Hazards of blood transfusion

Bacterial contamination

Contamination of the blood by bacteria is rare but may be lethal. Contaminants from the donor's skin may enter the blood while it is being donated. Usually, the bacteria responsible are staphylococci, which do not grow at 4°C and are killed during storage. However, any Gram-negative bacteria entering the blood will grow slowly at 4°C (their number doubling in 8 hours), and over several weeks of storage may be sufficient to cause a lethal septicaemia. It is essential that blood is stored at 4°C to minimize this risk, as bacterial growth accelerates considerably at room temperature. The onset of pyrexia and circulatory collapse can be rapid if transfused blood is infected.

Transmission of disease

Donor selection criteria and the testing of donor blood for infectious agents have decreased the transmission of disease but can never completely eradicate it. Many of the organisms responsible for transmitting infection have a long incubation period and are stable in blood and blood products.

In 1983, the first deaths associated with transfusion-related HIV were reported. From 1986, those in high risk groups were excluded from giving blood and all donor blood was tested for the presence of anti-HIV antibodies. However, the average delay in the appearance of the antibody after the time of infection is 2–3 months, with 95% of infected people having seroconverted by 6 months. Thus donors giving blood within about 6 months of infection may not be detected. Factor VIII and IX concentrates used today in the UK carry a negligible risk of HIV transmission because of the use of anti-HIV screened plasma for their preparation. Furthermore, HIV appears to be inactivated by the heat treatment now applied to such concentrates. Certain populations have a high incidence of viral carriers of hepatitis, and post-transfusion hepatitis remains one of the most common hazards of blood transfusion. Screening tests have been devised for hepatitis B surface antigen and the incidence of such carriers in the UK is fairly low. Transmission of hepatitis C is the cause of the majority of cases of post-transfusion hepatitis and there is now a serological test to diagnose this.

Cytomegalovirus (CMV) is a herpesvirus present in white cells and found free in the plasma. It can persist latently after infection. Up to 3.5% of blood transfusion units have the potential for virus transmission. The main danger of CMV is to infants and immunocompromised patients; the only way to avoid transfusion transmission is by using anti-CMV-negative blood.

Malaria can be transmitted via transfused blood or products that contain the parasites which can remain viable for a week at 4°C. Careful vetting of potential donors and screening for malarial antibodies is necessary now that travel to tropical countries is widespread. All donor blood in the UK is tested for syphilis, so transmission by transfusion is now very rare.

Hazards associated with massive blood transfusion

Massive transfusion is defined as the transfusion of the patient's own volume of blood within 24 hours or the acute administration of more than half the patient's estimated blood volume per hour. Stored blood is deficient in platelets and coagulation factors. It is cold (4°C), acidic (pH 6.6–6.8), and contains citrate anticoagulant. Therefore transfusions of large volumes of blood can lead to metabolic and cardiac disturbances.

Hypothermia

A thermostatically controlled blood warmer should always be used when giving more than a few units of blood to a normothermic patient, as blood transfused at 4°C can rapidly cool the patient. If the patient is pyrexial and the blood is not transfused rapidly, it may not be necessary to warm the blood until the patient is normothermic. Hypothermia increases the risk of cardiac arrhythmias, reduces metabolism, and shifts the oxygen dissociation curve to the left, causing a reduction in oxygen delivery to the tissues. Citrate toxicity (see below) is also more likely to occur when the patient is hypothermic.

Acid–base disturbances

Stored blood is acidic mainly due to the citric acid used as an anticoagulant and the lactic acid generated during storage (red cells contain 1–2 mmol of lactate per unit, and whole blood contains 3–10 mmol per unit). In the well-perfused patient, lactic and citric acid are rapidly metabolized by the liver. However, with hypoperfusion, metabolism will be depressed and lactic acid production may continue, increasing the metabolic acidosis. Frequent acid–base measurements are necessary to monitor this. Citrate (see below) can also contribute to metabolic alkalosis when large volumes of blood components are transfused.

Electrolyte disturbances

Sodium

The sodium content of whole blood and FFP is higher than that of normal blood due to the sodium citrate anticoagulant (FFP contains approximately 35 mmol per unit, and whole blood contains 49–53 mmol per unit, depending on the number of days it has been stored). This should be remembered when giving such products to patients with renal failure or hypernatraemia.

Calcium

FFP and platelets contain citrate anticoagulants (red cells in additive solution contain only traces of citrate). Citrate binds to ionized calcium in the blood and may cause hypocalcaemia. The healthy liver can metabolize citrate rapidly, so this is rarely a problem unless transfusion rates exceed one unit every 5 min or the patient has impaired liver function. Manifestations of hypocalcaemia include tetany, muscle tremors, paraesthesia, and cardiac dysfunction. Prolongation of the Q–T interval is seen on the ECG. The routine use of intravenous calcium supplements during large volume blood transfusion is controversial. Some authorities recommend that 2.2 mmol of calcium gluconate should be given for every 4 units of blood transfused. Others recommend that plasma ionized calcium levels should be monitored and supplements given as needed.

Potassium

The plasma or additive solution in a unit of blood stored for 4–5 weeks may contain 5–10 mmol of potassium and this may cause hyperkalaemia with massive transfusions.

Haemostatic failure

Transfusion of large volumes of red cells can lead to dilutional thrombocytopenia and haemostatic failure. Since stored blood contains no viable platelets and few of the clotting factors, the platelet count will be reduced, and the PT and PTT prolonged. Laboratory monitoring is necessary to guide therapy; however, if this is unavailable, it is recommended that 2 units of FFP should be given per 10 units of blood transfused, while platelet administration should be given according to the platelet count. A more aggressive platelet and FFP transfusion regimen is used in massive bleeding following trauma.

Transfusion-related acute lung injury (TRALI)

TRALI is due to a reaction with antibodies against one of the blood components in a transfusion that triggers a cascade of inflammatory events resulting in non-cardiogenic pulmonary oedema and ARDS. It occurs within 6 hours following transfusion and is typically associated with FFP and platelet administration, although it can occur in recipients of packed cells due to the residual plasma present in the unit. It can only be diagnosed if the chest X-ray was normal before the transfusion so many cases probably pass unrecognized. Treatment is supportive, and many patients will require respiratory support. Since it is associated with microvascular damage and not fluid overload, diuretics are not generally indicated.

Plasma exchange (plasmapheresis)

In plasma exchange, an extracorporeal circuit is used to remove blood from the patient (in a similar way to haemodialysis). This is then passed through a cell separator where plasma and large molecular weight and protein-bound toxic substances are extracted (e.g. cryoglobulins, anti-glomerular basement membrane antibodies, myeloma light chains, immune complexes). Red cells and platelets are then returned to the patient in plasma or plasma substitute fluid. The same volume of plasma that is removed is replaced with 5% albumin or FFP, or a mixture of both. Additional crystalloid may also be given. Albumin causes fewer sensitivity reactions and does not transmit infections, but FFP is used in patients with thrombocytopenic purpura in order to replace von Willebrand factor cleaving enzymes. The frequency of plasma exchange varies according to the condition being treated, and may range from daily (or more often), in treating thrombotic thrombocytopenic purpura, to weekly. Plasma exchange should not generally be the sole treatment of a disease; concomitant immunosuppressive therapy is usually given to reduce the rate of re-synthesis of pathological antibodies.

Anticoagulation using heparin or acid citrate dextrose is necessary during the procedure. If citrate is used, hypocalcaemia can occur because citrate binds to calcium in the blood. Prophylactic supplementation in the form of boluses or continuous infusion of 10% calcium gluconate is often given during the procedure; the patient should be observed for signs of hypocalcaemia (shivering, parasthesiae, tremors, carpopedal spasm, tetany). Cardiac monitoring should be in progress as arrhythmias may occur secondary to hypokalaemia. If the replacement fluid is albumin, there may be a 25% drop in serum potassium levels in the immediate post-pheresis period.

Indications

Some conditions for which plasma exchange may be used are:

- acute demyelinating (Guillain–Barré) polyneuropathy
- chronic inflammatory demyelinating polyneuropathy
- myasthenic crisis
- thrombotic thrombocytopenic purpura
- hyperviscosity syndromes
- Goodpasture's syndrome
- post-transfusion purpura
- antineutrophil cytoplasmic antigen (ANCA) positive nephritis
- cryoglobinaemias
- bullous pemphigoid and pemphigus vulgaris
- myeloma cast nephropathy
- ABO-incompatible marrow transplantation
- sepsis.

Complications

- Haemorrhage or haematoma at venepuncture site due to reduction in plasma levels of coagulation factors

- Hypocalcaemia (if citrate anticoagulation is used)
- Hypokalaemia
- Hypotension—usually due to hypovolaemia secondary to inadequate replacement of fluid
- Infection
- Hypothermia—replacement fluid can be warmed if necessary
- Allergic/anaphylaxis/urticarial/sensitivity reaction to replacement fluids
- Membrane incompatibility (ethylene oxide hypersensitivity reactions)
- Thrombocytopenia
- Fluid overload
- Metabolic alkalosis (with citrate anticoagulation)

The critical care patient with haematological malignancy

Advances in therapy have meant that the long-term prognosis has improved for many patients with malignant disease. Although the mortality rate for some cancers remains high, despite aggressive treatment, selected patients with life-threatening but potentially reversible complications can benefit from intensive care. Many of the reasons for their transfer to the critical care unit result from complications of the malignancy itself or from its treatment. These include:

- infection/sepsis
- haemorrhage
- respiratory failure
- cardiac disturbances
- graft versus host reactions
- tumour lysis syndrome
- hypercalcaemia
- fluid overload/renal failure
- following extensive surgical procedures.

Infection

Patients with haematological malignancy have an increased susceptibility to infection. This may be related directly to the cancer affecting the immune system, or to the effects of the therapy. Although neutropenia. (neutrophil count $<0.5 \times 10^9$/L) increases the risk further, and many critical care areas advocate reverse barrier nursing for neutropenic patients, the non-neutropenic patient is still at high risk of developing infection. Thus scrupulous attention to handwashing and other infection control measures is vital to minimize secondary infection.

Such patients with neutropenia are susceptible to infection by bacteria (including atypical bacteria such as mycobacteria), viruses, protozoa, and fungi. Frequently, the infection originates endogenously from the patient's own gut, airways, or skin. Broad-spectrum antibiotics suppress the normal bacterial flora; in the gut this can promote the overgrowth of pathogenic Gram-negative organisms and fungi. Chemotherapy can also cause areas of ulceration in the gastrointestinal tract and tracheobronchial mucosa. These areas can act as a focus for local colonization by hospital organisms and may lead to invasion into deep tissues and sepsis. There is a high incidence of fungal infection (commonly Candida and Aspergillus) in these immunosupressed patients, causing sepsis and pneumonia. Herpes simplex and cytomegalovirus are common viral infections, and *Pneumocystis jiroveci* is the most common protozoan infection.

Invasive procedures should be kept to a minimum and performed when the patient requires them rather than by virtue of simply being an ICU patient. Large bore, soft Teflon catheters, such as Hickman and PICC (peripherally inserted central catheter) lines, are often used for intravenous drug administration to minimize infection from skin flora. Scrupulous attention must be paid to cannula insertion sites to keep them free of infection, and lines must be dated and changed according to hospital policy. Consider non-invasive methods of monitoring where possible (e.g. pulse oximetry, see Chapter 5).

Fungal infections (e.g. Candida) are common in warm moist areas such as the groin, vagina, axilla, and mouth. The skin should be kept clean and dry, and local antifungal cream applied as appropriate. Mouth care is very important, and a variety of antifungal preparations are available (such as lozenges, suspensions, and mouthwashes) and should be used at least five times a day. Prophylactic antifungal drugs (such as fluconazole) and antiviral drugs (such as aciclovir) have also been used with success in recipients of bone marrow transplants.

Selective decontamination of the gastrointestinal tract by the use of oral non-absorbable antibiotics to reduce the endogenous flora has been advocated. This reduces only the aerobic organisms, and leave anaerobes to confer colonization resistance. However, this strategy has not been specifically examined in this patient population. There is also a theoretical risk of promoting the emergence of resistant organisms.

Treatment of (suspected) infection should be prompt. Any likely source such as an infected intravenous catheter should be removed, though clotting products may be required first if the patient is coagulopathic. Antibiotics are usually commenced quickly, though the choice depends on local guidelines. This will be dictated by the presumed causative organism, local resistance patterns, previous cultures, and the types of antibiotic that have been used before. Broad-spectrum antibiotics, which may or may not include antifungal agents, are usually commenced initially, with de-escalation once cultures or other tests identify the infecting pathogen.

Haemorrhage

Thrombocytopenia is the most common cause of haemorrhage and can result from bone marrow suppression by cytotoxic drugs, bone marrow infiltration by tumour, or sequestration of platelets in the spleen (especially in patients with chronic lymphatic leukaemia). DIC is common and may be a complication of sepsis, drugs, or the malignancy itself. Patients with leukaemia often have reduced levels of factors V, VII, and X, and production of clotting factors by the liver may be impaired in patients with liver metastases. With graft versus host disease or infective colitis there may be bleeding from the gastrointestinal tract. Most patients with bone marrow failure will require multiple transfusions, particularly of red cells, platelets, and clotting factors. If DIC is present, FFP and cryoprecipitate may also be required.

Cardiac disturbances

Cytotoxic drugs can cause serious cardiac disturbances. Adriamycin in large cumulative doses is particularly cardiotoxic, causing congestive cardiac failure and a cardiomyopathy. This may occur idiosyncratically after much lower doses. Some drugs cause a variety of acute dysrhythmias, particularly if the patient has existing cardiac disease. Cardiac tamponade can result from metastatic tumour, particularly those originating in the bronchus or breast. If the tumour extends around the heart a constrictive pericarditis can develop (this can also be caused by radiotherapy).

Graft versus host disease

This is an autoimmune reaction that can occur in allogenic bone marrow transplants. Immunocompetent donor T lymphocytes recognize the host histocompatability antigens as 'foreign' and produce a cell-mediated reaction against sensitive tissue, particularly the skin, gastrointestinal tract, liver, and bone marrow. It causes fever, diarrhoea, severe skin rashes, and jaundice. Mortality is high at approximately 25%. Management is with steroids, other immunosuppressive agents (e.g. cyclosporin, rituximab), and appropriate supportive care. Clofazimine or thalidomide may help with sore throat if particularly troublesome. See Chapter 13 for further details.

Tumour lysis syndrome

The rapid lysis of malignant cells by cytotoxic drugs can cause hyperkalaemia, hyperuricaemia, hyperphosphataemia, and acute renal failure. This usually occurs in patients who present with a very high white cell count ($>100 \times 10^9$/L). The patient must be kept well hydrated with a good diuresis. They are usually given rasburicase or allopurinol prophylactically prior to commencing cytotoxic therapy to reduce uric acid levels resulting from the purine release following cell lysis. For patients with high white counts, leukapheresis may be performed prior to the first dose of chemotherapy to reduce the circulating white cell count. See chapter 13 for more information.

Hypercalcaemia

Hypercalcaemia is common in patients with malignant disease, particularly those with multiple myeloma. This can be due to invasion of the bone by tumour cells or stimulation of osteoclastic activity by mediators, such as osteoclastic-activating factor which causes bone reabsorption. Immediate treatment is aimed at reducing the calcium level by rehydration (3–6 L/24 h), furosemide (which prevents calcium reabsorption in the loop of Henle), calcitonin (which inhibits osteoclastic bone reabsorption), and sodium etidronate. Steroids are useful in reducing calcium reabsorption but may take up to a week to show effect. Oral sodium phosphate is also effective, but should be administered after hydration. For the long-term treatment of hypercalcaemia the cause must be removed by specific therapy (surgery, radiotherapy, or chemotherapy). Hypercalcaemia is discussed in more detail in Chapter 14.

Fluid overload/renal failure

This is discussed in detail in Chapter 7.

Following extensive surgical procedures

Intensive care can benefit many patients undergoing lengthy radical surgery to remove tumours. Such surgery (e.g. pelvic exenteration) can involve considerable blood loss, and patients are often hypovolaemic on transfer from theatre. Continuous haemodynamic monitoring can permit optimal fluid replacement and preserve renal function. Analgesia can also be administered by intravenous infusion and titrated to achieve adequate pain control. Patients at high risk of respiratory failure are often electively ventilated post-operatively, especially if surgery is prolonged or the patient has pre-existing pulmonary disease.

Respiratory failure

A variety of factors may precipitate respiratory failure in the patient with malignant disease (see Table 12.4). Patients with malignant disease may develop respiratory failure secondary to infection, pleural effusions, fluid overload, cardiac failure, or pneumothorax, or may require endotracheal intubation following diagnostic surgical procedures such as mediastiotomy.

Mortality rates are high in critically ill patients with haematological malignancy. Those requiring prolonged ventilation and/or renal support have a particularly poor prognosis. Before such patients are admitted to the critical care unit the nature and progress of the underlying malignancy must be taken into account and the impact of the admission on the patient's quantity and quality of life must be considered. Ideally, critical care admission should be discussed with the patient while they are mentally competent, and with their next-of-kin, explaining the risks and possible benefits in the context of their disease, the acute problem requiring possible admission, and the likely prognosis. The patient/family can then express their own wishes regarding admission (or not) and the extent of treatment to be offered. Such conversations should take place with both the haematologist and the intensivist. If ICU admission is considered futile, the patient/family should be informed of this as the requirements of life-sustaining therapy may simply prolong the patient's suffering, especially if the underlying malignancy has not been cured or is in remission, or other comorbidities such as severe chronic respiratory disease make survival unlikely.

Table 12.4 Causes of respiratory failure in the patient with malignant disease.

Infection	Bacterial	*Klebsiella, E.coli,* Proteus, Staphylococcus, Pseudomonas, Pneumococcus
	Fungal	Aspergillus, Candida
	Protozoan	*Pneumocystis carinii*
	Viral	Cytomegalovirus
Drug-induced lung disease		A variety of cytotoxic drugs (e.g. bleomycin) can cause interstitial inflammation
Radiation pneumonitis		Occurs approximately 8 weeks following radiotherapy
Pulmonary haemorrhage		Usually occurs only in patients with thrombocytopenia
Malignant lung disease		Metastatic spread of lymphoma or carcinoma
Tracheobronchial compression		Due to airway compression by tumour or haematoma formation
Acute respiratory distress syndrome (ARDS)		Secondary to sepsis, DIC, pulmonary aspiration, radiation pneumonitis, or haemorrhage
Pleural effusions		
Fluid overload, cardiac failure		Some chemotherapies are cardiotoxic and nephrotoxic
Pneumothorax		

Bibliography

Cartese, I., Chaudrey, V., So, V.T., *et al.* (2011). Evidence-based guideline update: plasmapheresis in neurologic disorders. Report of the Therapeutics and Technology Assessment Subcomittee of the American Academy of Neurology. *Neurology*, **76**, 294–300.

Gando, S., Sawamura, A., Hayakawa, M. (2011) Trauma, shock and disseminated intravascular coagulation: lessons from the classical literature. *Annals of Surgery*, **254**, 10–19.

Kusama, B., Schultz, T. (2009) Acute disseminated intravascular coagulation. *Hospital Physician*, March–April, 35–40.

Malluche, H.H., Sawayan, B.P., Hakim, R.M., Sayegh, M.H. (2009). *Clinical Nephrology. Dialysis and Transplantation*. Ober-Haching: Dustri-Verlag.

Neunert, C., Lim, W., Crowther, M., *et al.* The American Society of Hematology 2011 evidence-based practice guideline for immune thrombocytopenia. *Blood*, **117**, 4190–207.

Sadler, J.E. (2008). Von Willbrand factor, ADAMTS13 and thrombotic thrombocytopenia purpura. *Blood*, **112**, 11–18.

Simon, D., Simon, H.-U. (2007). Eosinophilic disorders. *Journal of Allergy and Clinical Immunology*, **119**, 1291–1300.

Thompson, C.A., Kyle, R., Gertz, M., *et al.* (2010). Systemic AL amyloidosis with acquired factor X deficiency: a study of perioperative bleeding risk and treatment outcomes in 60 patients. *American Journal of Haematology*, **85**, 171–3.

Tsai, H.-M. (2006). Current concepts in thrombotic thrombocytopenic purpura. *Annual Review of Medicine*, **57**, 419–36.

Visentin, G.P., Lui, C.Y. (2007). Drug induced thrombocytopenia. *Hematology and Oncology Clinics of North America*, **21**, 685–96.

Wada, H., Thacil, J., Di Nisio, M., *et al.* (2013). Guidance for diagnosis and treatment of disseminated intravascular coagulation from harmonization of the recommendations from three guidelines. *Journal of Thrombosis and Haemostasis*, **11**, 761–7.

Warkentin, T., Greinacher, A., Koster, A. *et al.* (2008). Treatment and prevention of heparin-induced thrombocytopenia. American College of Chest Physicians evidence-based clinical practice guidelines (8th edition). *Chest*, **133**(6 Suppl), 340S.

Warkentin, T., Levine, M., Hirsh, J., *et al.* (1995). Heparin induced thrombocytopenia in patients treated with low-molecular weight or unfractionated heparin. *New England Journal of Medicine*, **332**, 1330–6.

CHAPTER 13
The immune system and the immunocompromised patient

Introduction

In health, the immune system utilizes non-specific (innate) and specific (adaptive) defence systems to protect the body against insults on a daily basis. An understanding of the immune system is essential in order to understand many of the disease processes in the critically ill patient. Since immunosuppressive therapy is commonly used in treatment strategies, it is also important to be aware of any side effects and its effects on patient care.

The immune system is extremely complex and limited space does not permit more than an overview. Chapter 10 contains additional information, which expands on the concept of the immunocompromised critical care patient, and should be read in conjunction with this chapter.

The immune system

The immune system consists of many different tissues and cell types that collectively protect the body against infectious micro-organisms, development of tumour cells, and transplanted organs or grafts. At certain sites, the cells of the immune system are organized into specific structures. These can be classified as central lymphoid tissue (bone marrow and thymus) and peripheral lymphoid tissue (lymph nodes, spleen, Peyer's patches, appendix, tonsils, and adenoids).

The organs of the immune system

Lymph nodes

These are small bean-shaped structures lying along the course of the lymphatic network and are aggregated in particular locations. They are embedded within connective tissue, so they are not always easily seen, and range in size from 1 mm to more than 20 mm in diameter. Clinically, the most significant groups are the pre-auricular, submental and submandibular, superficial cervical, superficial cubital, auxiliary, and iliac and inguinal lymph nodes.

Lymph is interstitial fluid that is collected by the lymphatic vessels after bathing the tissues of the body. Lymph contains white cells, chiefly lymphocytes, and is immunologically filtered by the lymph nodes before returning into the circulation. Lymph nodes are composed of mostly T cells, B cells, dendritic cells, and macrophages. B cells enter the node and, if activated by antigenic stimulation, proliferate and remain there. If not stimulated, they pass out of the node to return to the general circulation. Various types of T cell enter lymph nodes which, when activated, form lymphoblasts. These divide to produce a clone of T cells that will respond to a specific antigen. Activated T cells then pass into the circulation to reach peripheral sites.

Bone marrow

The bone marrow produces red blood cells, platelets, and all cells of the immune system by the process of haematopoiesis. Stem cells residing in the bone marrow differentiate into either mature cells of the immune system or precursors of cells that mature elsewhere. Some develop into myeloid cells, a group typified by large particle-devouring white cells known as phagocytes. These include monocytes, macrophages, and neutrophils. Other myeloid descendants become granule-containing inflammatory cells such as eosinophils and basophils. Lymphoid precursors develop into lymphocytes. The two major classes of lymphocytes are B and T cells. B cells mature in the bone marrow, while T cells, which originate in the bone marrow as immature thymocytes, mature in the thymus.

Thymus

The thymus serves as the final site of lymphocyte development before birth and produces mature T cells from immature thymocytes that have migrated from the bone marrow. Mature T cells are then released into the circulation.

Spleen

The spleen is the largest lymphoid organ and is the site of both lymphocyte proliferation and immune surveillance. The spleen contains B cells, T cells, macrophages, dendritic cells, natural killer cells, and red cells. It acts as an immunological filter and also destroys old red blood cells. In addition to capturing antigens as blood passes through, migratory macrophages and dendritic cells also bring antigens to it. When these cells present the antigen to the appropriate B or T cell, an immune response is initiated. The B cells become activated in the spleen and produce large amounts of antibodies.

Non-specific immunity (innate or natural immunity)

The non-specific immune response provides the first level of defence against micro-organisms and is capable of being activated at any time. It does not require previous exposure nor does it involve memory or recognition. Non-specific immunity is in place at birth and, in many cases, can defend against invading pathogens on its own.

Examples of non-specific protection are:

- skin and mucous membranes
- pH of body secretions

- antimicrobial enzymes
- complement proteins
- respiratory cilia.

The result of an activated non-specific immune response is inflammation. This involves the actions of neutrophils, monocytes, mast cells, basophils, and macrophages.

Surface barriers: skin and mucosa

These are the body's first line of defence and are highly effective provided that they remain intact. The skin is a heavily keratinized layer of epithelial cells with a surface area of approximately 2 m^2. Keratin is resistant to most bacterial enzymes, toxins, weak acids, and bases. The mucosa lines all cavities that are open to the external environment, such as the digestive, respiratory, and reproductive tracts. Its surface area is approximately 400 m^2. Although essentially non-specific, the epithelial membranes also have specific defence mechanisms such as the production of locally protective chemicals.

Skin secretions have an acidic pH of 3–5, hence inhibiting bacterial growth. Gastric mucosa produces hydrochloric acid and protein-digesting enzymes that destroy micro-organisms. Within the oral cavity saliva not only cleanses the area but also contains enzymes and other anti-bacterial compounds. Lysozomes found in the lacrimal fluid in the eye also destroys bacteria. Mucus-coated hairs within the nose trap particles, inhibiting their entry into the respiratory tract. Cilia within the respiratory tract sweep particles and bacteria towards the mouth and away from the lower respiratory tract, thereby preventing infection.

Internal defences: cells and chemicals

These are important components of the internal defence mechanisms. Various specialized cells (Figure 13.1) are crucial in the immune response.

Phagocytes and granulocytes

Phagocytes are large white cells that can engulf and digest foreign invaders by a mechanism known as phagocytosis. In many organs of the body, 10–15% of cells are phagocytes. They include monocytes (which circulate in the blood), macrophages (found in tissues throughout the body), and neutrophils (cells that circulate in the bloodstream but move into tissues when needed). Macrophages are the predominant phagocytes and are very versatile. They act as scavengers and can secrete a wide variety of powerful chemicals and mediators. They also play an essential role in activating T cells.

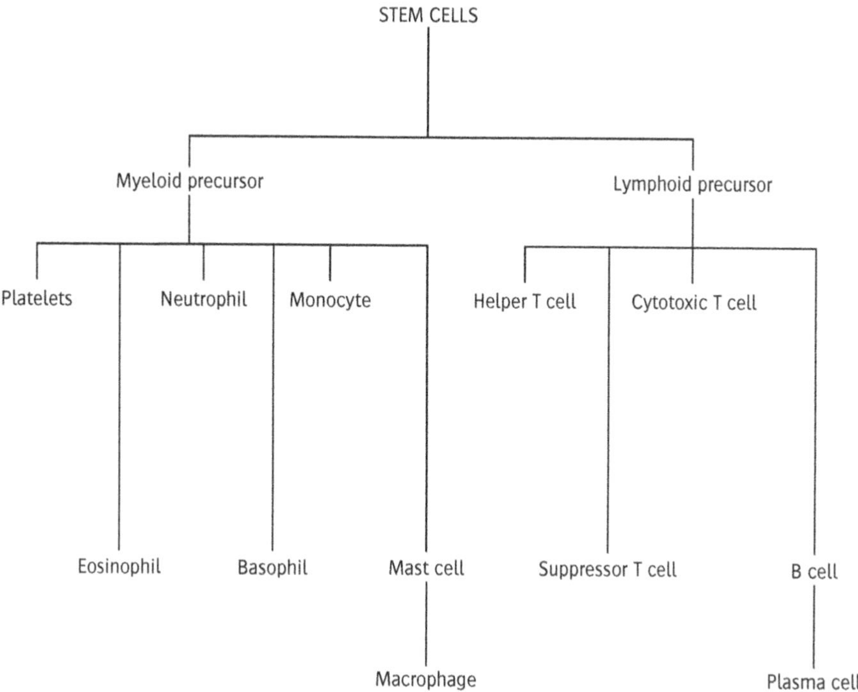

Figure 13.1 Cells of the immune system.

Neutrophils are the most abundant white blood cell. They are both phagocytes and granulocytes as they contain granules filled with potent chemicals and enzymes which, in addition to destroying micro-organisms, play a key role in acute inflammatory reactions. Release of these chemicals outside the cell is known as degranulation. Other types of granulocyte are eosinophils and basophils. Mast cells are granule-containing cells situated within tissue.

Dendritic cells

Dendritic cells are another type of phagocyte. They originate in the bone marrow but are found particularly in the peripheral lymph nodes, thymus, and spleen. They are also found elsewhere in the body, including the bloodstream and tissues in contact with the external environment such as the skin and mucous membranes. They have long cytoplasmic processes that localize and present antigens to responsive T and B cells. They are more efficient antigen-presenting cells (APCs) than macrophages.

Natural killer cells

Natural killer (NK) cells are distinct from B cells and T cells yet are also produced in the bone marrow. They constitute approximately 15% of the lymphocyte count. NK cells circulate in blood and lymph and directly kill certain tumours such as melanomas, lymphomas, and cell-infecting viruses such as cytomegalovirus and herpes. NK cells are less specific than the lymphocytes of the adaptive immune system and can destroy a variety of cells. They are not phagocytic but use several different ways of killing, mainly involving a chemical trigger. When in direct contact with a cell they can induce programmed cell death or apoptosis. If previously activated by T helper cells ($CD4^+$ T cells), they can kill their targets more effectively.

The inflammatory response

Chemical mediators

In response to injury, mast cells (histocytes if fixed in tissue, or basophils if free flowing in blood) release histamine. Histamine causes dilatation of local blood vessels, increased permeability, and contraction of smooth muscle. This causes fluid to move from the blood vessels into the tissues. Histamine also causes bronchoconstriction and mucous production, which becomes evident in allergic reactions.

When the injury releases clotting factors, bradykinin is formed. This also causes increased permeability, vasodilatation, and smooth muscle contraction, and can cause pain. When tissue cells are injured, arachidonic acid is released from the cell membranes and is metabolized into a variety of prostaglandins, thromboxanes, and leukotrienes. These have often opposing actions such as vessel dilatation and constriction, or platelet aggregation and reduced adhesiveness. Some increase vessel permeability, whereas others act as a chemotactic factor to attract neutrophils to the site of injury. Increased blood vessel permeability and vasodilatation allows plasma proteins, neutrophils, oxygen, and glucose to reach the site of injury more easily. This is a protective response with local injury but can become damaging if the response is systemic.

The classical signs of inflammation are redness and heat (due to vasodilatation and increased local metabolic reactions), oedema (due to increased permeability), and pain (due to pressure and chemical irritation on the nerve endings).

Cellular actions

Chemotactic factors stimulate release of neutrophils from the bone marrow and attract them to the site of inflammation. Neutrophils are highly phagocytic, and engulf organisms and debris. Monocytes also arrive, again attracted by chemotaxins, to assist the neutrophils. Inside these cells are lysosomes which contain lytic enzymes and reactive oxygen species, such as hydrogen peroxide and superoxide, that digest whatever the cell has engulfed and cause an increased use of oxygen by the cell (the 'respiratory burst').

Healing

When debris has been removed the neutrophils self-destruct and fibrin is laid down where capillaries have broken. This provides a framework for new tissue growth using collagen produced by fibroblasts. The monocytes release a substance that promotes the growth of endothelial cells and these become new capillaries. Gradually, fibrin is changed to granulation tissue. The fluid provides nutrition for the new tissue but, as the granulation tissue matures, it can dry and contract to produce scar tissue. Scar tissue is white or pale in colour, and is dense with many collagen fibres. It has less flexibility and function than normal tissue and can become pathological depending on where it is formed (e.g. in the lungs, heart, or brain).

Fever

When inflammatory mediators trigger a systemic response, the patient may develop a fever. However, especially in the young or old, this may not occur and the patient may present with a hypothermic response. A raised temperature may inhibit reproduction of some microbes and aid some immune reactions, including phagocytosis. The benefits and risks of modifying the patient's temperature (e.g. with antipyretics) are poorly understood.

Complement

The complement system is a group of over 25 enzymes mainly produced by the liver that circulate in the plasma. They are activated by chemical reactions generated by antigens, but also by antigen–antibody complexes as part of the adaptive immune system. Once activated, they greatly assist ('complement') antibodies and phagocytic cells to clear pathogens, forming membrane attack complexes on the surface of bacteria. This process is called opsonization. They also have a chemotactic role, attracting neutrophils and macrophages to the site of inflammation, and can directly lyse the membrane of foreign cells.

The specific immune response (adaptive immunity)

This response aims to attack specific antigens that have been recognized as foreign. The specific immune response is delivered by two different classes of lymphocyte that are involved in the cellular (T cell) and humoral (B cell) immune response.

In order to initiate an immune response, an antigen-presenting cell (APC), usually a macrophage or dendritic cell, needs to be present in combination with a B or T cell. When an APC presents an antigen on its cell surface to a B cell, the B cell is signalled to proliferate and produce antibodies that specifically bind to that antigen. If the antibodies bind to antigens on bacteria or parasites, this acts as a signal for polymorphonuclear leucocytes (PMNLs) or macrophages to phagocytose them. Antibodies also initiate the complement activation cascade and signal NK cells and macrophages to kill cells infected by viruses or bacteria.

When the APC presents the antigen to T cells, they become activated and proliferate into different subsets. They become secretory 'helper cells' if they express the CD4^{+} receptor on their surface. If they are CD8^{+} they kill target cells that specifically express the antigen presented by the APC. The production of antibodies and the activity of CD8^{+} 'killer T cells' are regulated by the CD4^{+} helper cells. These produce and secrete growth factors and cytokines that signal other cells to proliferate and function more efficiently. CD4^{+} T cells are essential to ensure the activation of NK cells, macrophages, CD8^{+} T cells, and PMNLs.

B cells

About a billion B cells are produced daily in the bone marrow. These produce antibodies in response to the foreign proteins of bacteria, viruses, and tumour cells. The antibodies circulate in blood and lymph, specifically recognizing and binding to one particular protein and thus marking it for destruction by other cells. They are part of what is known as antibody-mediated or humoral immunity.

The antibodies produced by B cells are basic templates with a highly specific region that can target a given antigen. Each mature B cell produces one kind of antibody with receptors that are also different, thus enabling the cell to recognize any organic molecule.

When some antibodies combine with antigens they can activate the complement system to form a partnership that helps to destroy foreign invaders. Other types of antibodies can block viruses from entering cells.

T cells

T cells are produced in the bone marrow and mature in the thymus. They circulate in blood and lymph and account for approximately 70% of circulating lymphocytes. In addition to marking antigens for destruction, they can attack and destroy any diseased cells recognized as foreign. This recognition of antigen depends on unique cell surface molecules called the major histocompatibility complex (MHC).

There are three main T-cell subsets: killer cells, helper cells, and regulatory cells. They may be further categorized as either effector or regulatory cells. The killer T cell (also known as T cytotoxic (Tc) or CD8^{+} T cell) is an effector cell as it has a direct cytotoxic effect on other cells, such as certain tumour cells, virally infected cells, and sometimes parasites. They are also important in the downregulation of the immune response to terminate inflammation. The T helper (Th) subset, also called the CD4^{+} T cell, is a coordinator of immune regulation. Its main function is to augment or potentiate immune responses by secreting cytokines such as interleukin 2

(IL-2) that activate other white cells to fight infection. They alert B cells to make antibodies, activate macrophages, and can influence the type of antibody produced. The roles of the regulatory T cell (also known as T_{reg} or suppressor T cells) are to suppress immune activation and offer self-tolerance to prevent the immune system turning on its own host.

Cytokines

Cytokines are diverse and potent chemical messengers secreted by immune cells that trigger or regulate both innate and adaptive immune responses. Tumour necrosis factor (TNF), interleukins (ILs), leukotrienes, and interferons (IFNs) are examples of cytokines. B and T lymphocytes secrete lymphokines, while monocytes and macrophages secrete monokines such as TNF and interleukin 1 (IL-1). Cytokines recruit many other cells and substances by binding to specific receptors on target cells. They encourage cell growth, promote cell activation, direct cellular traffic, and destroy target cells including cancer cells.

Antibodies

These are a family of large protein molecules known as immunoglobulins and are composed of long chains of amino acids (polypeptides). Each antibody is made up of two identical heavy and light chains, shaped to form a Y. The sections that make up the tips of the Y's arms vary greatly from one antibody to another. This is the variable region where the unique contours in the antigen-binding site allow the antibody to recognize a matching antigen. The stem of the Y links the antibody to other participants in the immune defence system. This area—the constant region—is identical in all antibodies of the same class.

Function of antibodies

Antibodies provide antibody-mediated (humoral) immunity and are an important defence mechanism against bacteria and viruses. They function by recognizing and tagging the invader in preparation for destruction. The antibodies can bind to viruses outside cells, thus preventing them from entering the cell or inhibiting their replication within the cell.

Classes of antibodies

There are nine distinct classes of human immunoglobulins: four types of IgG, two types of IgA, IgM, IgE, and IgD. Immunoglobulins G, D and E are similar in appearance.

IgG

The most abundant and diverse immunoglobulin in blood, IgG can also enter tissue spaces. It accounts for 75–85% of antibodies in the circulation and has a half-life of 3 weeks. It coats micro-organisms and enhances their uptake by other immune cells. It is antiviral, antibacterial, and can neutralize toxins. IgG can cross the placenta in the last 3 months of pregnancy and is responsible for immunity in the newborn until it begins to produce its own IgG several months after birth.

IgM

IgM is the first antibody type to develop in response to an infection. It is found only in serum and has a half-life of approximately a day. It agglutinates and precipitates proteins, but its main function is to protect against bacteria in the bloodstream. IgM is located on the B cell wall and acts as a B-cell receptor for antigens. It also binds to viruses and neutralizes them, hence preventing them from infecting cells.

IgE

IgE is found on the cell membranes of basophils and mast cells where it acts as an antigen receptor. Although it is the least abundant immunoglobulin, it can cause the most potent reactions. When it binds with an antigen it causes degranulation of basophils and mast cells with release of histamine, serotonin, leukotrienes, and other chemicals that can give rise to allergic or even life-threatening anaphylactoid reactions. It is particularly associated with Type I hypersensitivity reactions. IgE is also involved in the immune response to parasitic worms and protozoan infections (e.g. malaria).

IgD

IgD is predominantly found within the membrane of mature B cells, usually in co-location with IgM. A secreted form is present in the blood in small amounts. It signals B-cell activation but can also stimulate basophils and mast cells. The highest levels are found during childhood.

IgA

IgA guards the 400 m^2 of mucosal surfaces in the body. It is contained in secretions (tears, saliva, and mucus) and serum, and prevents entry of bacteria into the body. IgA can cross membranes to enter the respiratory, gastrointestinal, and genitourinary tracts and is particularly important in defending against respiratory infections. It is also found in breast milk, where it is passed into the newborn's intestinal tract, coating the mucosa and protecting against pathogens.

Antigen receptors

B and T cells carry customized receptor molecules that allow them to recognize and respond to their specific targets. The B cell's antigen-specific receptor recognizes the antigen in its natural state.

The immunocompromised patient

An individual's resistance to infection may be reduced by many general factors, such as extremes of age, nutritional state, and previous exposure to vaccination or infection. Profound impairments in the immune response can be caused by autoimmune diseases, genetic disorders, immunosuppressive drug therapy, and certain infections such as the human immunodeficiency virus (HIV).

A person whose resistance to infection is reduced due to an abnormality in the immune response is said to be immunocompromised. Such patients are extremely vulnerable to bacteria, viruses, and opportunistic infections from, for example, *Pneumocystis jirovecii* or fungi such as *Candida albicans*. In healthy individuals these organisms are not generally able to cause a serious infection. Table 13.1 lists factors that increase the risk for the development of immunocompromised states.

Table 13.1 Risk factors for immunocompromise

Risk factor	Considerations
Age	• Declining immune function • Decreased nutritional intake
Chronic disease	• Diabetes • Aplastic anaemia • Cancer • Chronic hepatic failure • Chronic renal failure
Immunosuppressed states	• Haematological conditions (e.g. leukaemia, lymphoma, multiple myeloma) • Immunodeficiency syndromes (HIV) • Autoimmune diseases
Medication and treatment	• Antibiotics • Corticosteroids (decreased lymphocyte and antibody concentration) • Sedatives and opiates • Proton pump inhibitors • Non-steroidal anti-inflammatory agents • Chemotherapy • Cyclosporin and other post-transplantation immunosuppressives • Radiotherapy to spine, long bones, sternum, etc. (reduced bone marrow production)
Nutritional status	• Inadequate protein and calorie intake (alters immune responses and resistance to infection due to decreased lymphocyte and antibody production)
Skin integrity	• Breaches in skin (wounds, burns, pressure-related injury) • Vascular access devices, urethral catheters, endotracheal tubes, chest and abdominal drains, etc.

The immunocompromised critical care patient

There are many causes of immunosuppression in the critical care patient. It may occur simply as a result of being critically ill, and/or having a condition that predisposes to impaired immunity (e.g. leukaemia, liver dysfunction), and/or as a consequence of the drugs and treatments being given, either directly (e.g. chemotherapy, radiotherapy) or indirectly (e.g. sedation).

Critical illness itself causes depression of the protective immune mechanisms of the body. After initial activation of the immune system in response to an inflammatory insult (e.g. infection, haemorrhage, trauma, burns), the immune system is deactivated and the patient may become severely immunosuppressed. This is usually an appropriate response to quench the fires of inflammation, but after significant and prolonged inflammatory activation this downregulation may be profound. The patient enters a state of immunoparesis (or immune paralysis) and is far more susceptible to new infections. This is particularly relevant in the critical care environment where more virulent and resistant micro-organisms reside, where the patient's normal defence barriers have been breached with multiple tubes, catheters, and drains, and where standard drug therapies may additionally compromise immune function.

Endogenous anti-inflammatory mediators (such as IL-10), certain prostaglandins (such as E2), and nitric oxide are produced at the same time as pro-inflammatory mediators following an insult, but take longer to peak. The relative balance between pro- and anti-inflammatory mediators dictates whether the patient is in an overall state of activation or suppression. The situation is more complex in that some immune cell types may be activated at the same time as others are suppressed.

In addition, many commonly used drugs are implicated in direct immune suppression. These include gastric protectants such as the proton pump inhibitors (e.g. omeprazole) and H_2 blockers (e.g. ranitidine), antibiotics, catecholamines, steroids, non-steroidal anti-inflammatory drugs (NSAIDs), heparin, opiates, benzodiazepines, and propofol. This list can be extended further to include blood transfusion and both crystalloid and colloid fluids.

Malnutrition also predisposes to infection and poor wound healing by reducing the number of T cells and depressing antibody responses. Thus early nutritional replacement (including vitamins and trace elements) is very important in patients with severe malnutrition. However, this requirement is less clear cut in other critically ill patients, even though they lose considerable amounts of protein and fat. Recent studies have shown worse outcomes when early institution of parenteral nutrition is commenced to achieve protein-calorie targets. This may be related in part to immune modulation. Hyperglycaemia also decreases neutrophil function and stimulates bacterial growth.

Patients with renal and liver failure will also have impaired immune function. Acute or chronic renal failure reduces neutrophil bactericidal activity, affects macrophage activation, impairs macrophage antigen presentation, and causes defective T-cell function. Uraemia also has a direct immunosuppressive effect. Cirrhosis results in depression of antigen presentation and a decrease in the number of circulating T cells. Acute and chronic alcohol consumption is associated with decreased phagocytic activity and depressed cellular immunity.

Patients who have undergone chemotherapy and/or bone marrow transplantation (BMT) for tumour therapy or who receive immunosuppressive drugs, such as corticosteroids and cyclosporin, to prevent rejection after solid organ transplantation are all at considerable risk of developing infection and sepsis related to their immunocompromised state. BMT may be needed to replace the patient's haematopoietic stem cells after ablative chemotherapy, for example for treating haemato-oncological diseases such as the lymphomas and leukaemias. Neutrophil function may still be impaired even when the bone marrow and the neutrophil count recover after chemotherapy ± BMT. Indeed, critical care survival data are similar for neutropenic and non-neutropenic haematology patients.

Specific immunosuppressive drug therapy

Immunosuppressive drug therapy can be extremely beneficial for a wide range of conditions within the critical care area. However, since the drugs are not specific to targeted cells, they can also have many deleterious effects.

Intentional (therapeutic) immune suppression is used to treat a variety of conditions:

- malignant disease
- prevention of organ rejection following transplantation
- asthma and inflammatory bowel disease

- autoimmune diseases (e.g. rheumatoid arthritis, SLE, glomerulonephritis)
- skin diseases (e.g. pemphigus)
- neurological diseases (e.g. multiple sclerosis)
- anaphylactoid reactions
- septic shock and specific infections.

The actions of different types of immunosuppressive drugs are complex and affect the immune system in different ways. For example, corticosteroids decrease the number of lymphocytes and block production and release of proinflammatory cytokines, but increase the number of neutrophils. Cyclosporin is used to prevent the rejection of transplanted organs and acts primarily on T cells. It blocks production of lymphokines and thus the response to new antigens, but not the response of old memory cells to previously encountered antigens. Cytotoxic drugs have profound effects on the bone marrow by non-specifically interfering in cell division. Monoclonal antibodies can bind specifically to B- and T-cell subtypes, modulating their function. One such example is rituximab that targets the CD20 receptor primarily found on the surface of B lymphocytes. This agent is increasingly being used in the treatment of many lymphomas and leukaemias, in transplant rejection, and in a variety of autoimmune conditions

Nursing considerations

When nursing any immunosuppressed patient, regardless of whether they are neutropenic, great care must be paid to infection control practices. Protective isolation is an important tool in minimizing the risk of exposure to the immunocompromised patient. This should be considered if the white blood count is less than 1.0×10^9/L. Single-room accommodation is preferable for those at most risk where the room can be pressurized to prevent infections being transferred into it via the ventilation system. A high efficiency particulate air (HEPA) filtered air supply is also important. Personal protective equipment (PPE) and infection control procedures such as adequate handwashing will help to prevent nosocomial infections.

Microbiological screening should be instituted if there is any deterioration in the patient's condition. Invasive procedures and manipulations should be kept to a minimum, and non-invasive monitoring should be used where possible. Line insertion sites, wounds, and secretions must be observed carefully for signs of infection. Cannulae and catheters should be changed regularly according to unit policy. Long-term Vascular access devices (VAD's), such as Hickman, Portacath, or PICC lines, are a common source of infection. These should be considered for removal if the patient develops ongoing pyrexia or severe sepsis, even if vascular access is difficult and platelet pool/clotting product cover is required if they are concurrently thrombocytopenic and/or coagulopathic.

Infective complications can be difficult to diagnose as a temperature rise may not be evident. Protocols for prophylactic antibiotics and antifungals should be followed. However, overuse of antibiotics should be avoided as this predisposes the patient to new infections with fungal or resistant bacterial organisms. This is particularly problematic in immunosuppressed patients as they often develop pyrexia and other signs that are suggestive of infection but are actually caused as a side effect of their drug therapy, by transfusion of blood or blood products, or by graft versus host reactions.

Altered immune response

Table 13.2 outlines a number of complications related to altered immune responses.

Immunodeficiency disorders

Human immunodeficiency virus (HIV)

The human immunodeficiency virus is a retrovirus that causes acquired immune deficiency syndrome (AIDS), resulting in destruction of the immune system. Patients infected with HIV are at risk of illness and death from opportunistic infectious and neoplastic complications. The variant of HIV that causes most infections is HIV-1.

Table 13.2 Complications related to altered immune responses

Type of reaction	Response
Type 1: Hypersensitivity reactions	Allergic responses
Type 2: Cytotoxic hypersensitivity	Incompatible blood transfusions Autoimmune haemolytic anaemia Drug-induced reactions
Type 3: Immune complex hypersensitivity	Rheumatic heart disease Glomerulonephritis Goodpasture's syndrome Serum sickness Rheumatoid arthritis
Type 4: Cell-mediated delayed hypersensitivity	Contact dermatitis Allograft rejection Graft versus host disease (GvHD)
Autoimmune disorders	Antibody-mediated: • autoimmune haemolytic anaemia • myasthenia gravis • Graves' disease Immune complex autoimmune disease: • systemic lupus erythematosus (SLE) • rheumatoid arthritis Antibody and T-cell-mediated autoimmune disease: • primary immunodeficiency syndromes • secondary immune deficiency syndromes (HIV)
Unregulated immune excess disorders	Multiple myeloma

The virus primarily infects cells with CD4 surface receptor molecules. In some cells that lack CD4 receptors, such as macrophages and fibroblasts, an Fc receptor site or complement receptor site can be used instead. The primary targets for the HIV are blood monocytes, tissue macrophages, T, B and NK lymphocytes, dendritic cells, haematopoietic stem cells, microglial cells in the brain, endothelial cells, and gastrointestinal epithelial cells.

After entry of the virus into the cells, replication may first occur within inflammatory cells at the site of infection or within peripheral blood mononuclear cells. However, the major site of replication then becomes the lymphoid tissues. Viral replication is stimulated by a variety of cytokines such as interleukins and tumour necrosis factor, which activate CD4 lymphocytes and make them more susceptible to HIV infection.

Viral replication actively continues following the initial infection, and there is progressive destruction of the CD4 lymphocytes. The immune system is gradually destroyed but the HIV infection may appear clinically latent as this process may take some years. During this time, enough of the immune system remains intact to prevent most infections but, eventually, the production of new CD4 cells cannot match their rate of destruction and the clinical picture of AIDS appears. This stage is marked by the appearance of one or more of the typical opportunistic infections or neoplasms that are diagnostic of AIDS.

Complications of HIV infection and admission to critical care

Advances in antiretroviral medication have significantly increased life expectancy and reduced the incidence of illnesses associated with AIDS. However, there is an increased frequency of diseases not directly related to the underlying HIV disease. These include cardiovascular, renal, neurological, and neurocognitive conditions which may be related to the virus and/or the therapy.

HIV patients may require critical care for a number of reasons. Acute respiratory failure following opportunistic infection is the most common reason for admission, although the number of such cases has been in decline. Patients with neurological manifestations, such as central nervous system (CNS) toxoplasmosis, primary CNS lymphoma, and cryptococcal meningitis, may require critical care for managing an altered level of consciousness or for intractable seizures. HIV-infected patients may also present to the critical care unit with medical or surgical issues unrelated to their HIV infection.

Infected individuals are susceptible to a diverse collection of bacteria, viruses, fungi, and protozoa that represent a major cause of death. However, as a result of effective antiretroviral therapies and the use of opportunistic infection prophylaxis, co-infections have emerged as important complications in HIV infection. Hepatitis B and C virus co-infections are becoming increasingly prevalent, and chronic liver disease now represents a major cause of morbidity and mortality.

Respiratory complications

Respiratory failure remains the commonest reason for patients with HIV requiring critical care admission. Both

Table 13.3 Other causes of respiratory failure in HIV positive patients.

Disease	Subgroup
Bacterial pneumonia	*Streptococcus pneumoniae* *Staphylococcus aureus* *Haemophilis influenzae* *Pseudomonas* species (e.g. *Serratia marcescens*)
Atypical pneumonia	*Mycobacterium tuberculosis* (and atypical mycobacterial species) *Mycoplasma pneumoniae*
Fungal pneumonia	*Cryptococcus neoformans* *Histoplasma capsulatum* *Coccidioides immitus* *Aspergillus fumigatus*
Cytomegalovirus pneumonia	
Lymphocytic interstitial pneumonia	
Toxoplasmosis gondii pneumonitis	
Non-Hodgkin's lymphoma and pulmonary Karposi's sarcoma	
Pulmonary embolus	

Pneumocystis jirovecii pneumonia and tuberculosis (TB) continue to be important infections associated with the onset of respiratory failure. While infection with opportunistic organisms is more likely, standard bacterial infections should not be overlooked. Respiratory failure may also be related to the development of the immune reconstitution inflammatory syndrome (IRIS). This occurs due to an over-reaction of the immune system (in particular, reconstitution of antigen-specific T-cell-mediated immunity) to a new or latent opportunistic infection following its recovery after antiretroviral therapy. The consequence is a far greater inflammatory response with high levels of fever and sometimes, respiratory failure with an ARDS-like picture. Other causes of respiratory failure are listed in Table 13.3.

Pneumocystis jirovecii pneumonia

Pneumocystis jirovecii pneumonia (previously known as *Pneumocystis carinii* pneumonia (PCP)) commonly occurs in patients infected by HIV, but also affects immunocompromised patients who:

- are receiving myelosuppressive chemotherapy
- have undergone organ transplantation
- have general immunosuppressive diseases such as Hodgkin's disease.

It is the leading cause of death in HIV positive patients, and their commonest cause of admission to the critical care unit. Affected patients tend to have prolonged prodromal illnesses for weeks or months before respiratory failure occurs. Patients who are immunocompromised but HIV seronegative tend to present more acutely. The causative agent, *Pneumocystis jirovecii*, is a fungus-like organism that is widespread in the environment and is transmitted through the air. When inhaled, it commonly infects both the upper and lower respiratory tract.

Clinical presentation Typically, the patient presents with fever (usually >38.5°C), tachycardia, and a cough which is usually dry and non-productive in HIV seropositive patients. There is exertional dyspnoea, followed by dyspnoea at rest as the disease progresses. As respiratory failure develops, the patient becomes severely tachypnoeic and hypoxaemic.

Diagnosis Chest X-ray and CT scan may be normal in the early stages, but later on bilateral interstitial 'ground-glass' shadowing, most prominently in the mid-zones, is commonly seen. This may resemble the radiological appearance of ARDS but tends to spare the subpleural areas. Pneumatocoeles (thin-walled cysts filled with air) may be present or can develop over the course of the disease. These can be multiple and large, and predispose the patient to single or multiple pneumothoraces. Arterial blood gases usually show an abnormally low P_aO_2 out of keeping with the patient's symptoms.

Sputum samples for microscopic examination are often difficult to obtain because of the non-productive nature of the cough. Hypertonic saline solutions are sometimes used to generate a deep cough and a productive sample. In the ventilated patient, or in the non-intubated patient able to tolerate bronchoscopy safely, a bronchoalveolar lavage (BAL) can be performed with samples sent to microbiology and, importantly, histology for immunofluorescent or histochemical staining. Polymerase chain reaction (PCR) will identify the organism by DNA screening, but a positive PCR result does not necessarily imply PCP infection as the organism can colonize healthy individuals.

Treatment Antibiotic therapy is given, preferably intravenous cotrimoxazole. Alternatives include pentamidine, clindamycin plus primaquine, or trimetrexate plus folinic acid. High dose corticosteroids are usually given concurrently. Large volumes of dilution (especially with cotrimoxazole) should be avoided as these patients are susceptible to pulmonary oedema. The degree of respiratory support required will be dictated by the patient's symptoms. Many will manage on supplemental oxygen by mask or CPAP. Some will need BiPAP, whereas severe cases require intubation and mechanical ventilation.

Cardiovascular complications

Cardiac complications include acute coronary syndromes. It is unclear why there is an increased incidence, but antiretroviral drugs are associated with insulin resistance and diabetes, and these may contribute to the increased risk of cardiovascular complications. Of note, HIV patients who undergo percutaneous coronary interventions are more likely to develop further coronary artery disease or restenosis than those without HIV.

Neurological complications

HIV is a neurotrophic virus that can cause a variety of neurological insults including acute myelopathy, peripheral neuropathy, HIV encephalopathy, meningitis, dementia, and cerebral mass lesions.

Gastrointestinal complications

HIV patients can develop CMV-related peritonitis from small bowel or colonic enteritis, with or without perforation. AIDS cholangiopathy, caused by a variety of infectious and neoplastic processes, can lead to biliary sepsis.

Renal complications

HIV-associated nephropathy can lead to end-stage renal failure. Where appropriate, it is managed with renal replacement therapy and renal transplantation. Treatment with antiretroviral therapies may slow the progression of the HIV-associated nephropathy.

AIDS-related malignancies

Combination antiretroviral therapy (cART) has reduced the mortality and morbidity of AIDS-related malignancy. Previously, Kaposi's sarcoma (KS), non-Hodgkin's lymphoma (NHL), and invasive cervical carcinomas had a higher incidence in HIV positive patients. NHL remains the most common AIDS-defining malignancy, although the incidence is declining from 8.6 per 1000 person-years in 1993–1994 to 2.8 per 1000 person-years in 2006. In their place, other non-AIDS defining malignancies have emerged. These include Hodgkin's lymphoma (HL), lung cancer, invasive anal cancer, melanomas, and hepatoma. Patients with AIDS and cancer have a higher risk of death then those without AIDS. The malignancy appears to be more severe and less likely to be cured.

Autoimmune diseases

In autoimmune disease the normal protective mechanisms of the immune system are reversed. Antibodies are produced against the cells, organs, and tissues of the body. The aetiology of autoimmune disease is not fully known though is probably related to a combination of genetic, environmental, and/or infectious factors.

Systemic lupus erythematosus (SLE)

This chronic, potentially fatal, disease is nine times more common in women aged between 10 and 50 than in men. It occurs in approximately 40–400 per 100,000 individuals and a higher prevalence and severity is seen in those with Hispanic and African ancestry. The disease may vary from a mild episodic illness to severe disease affecting multiple organs including joints, kidney, skin, brain, heart, lung, and gastrointestinal tract. It is a complex disorder but its aetiology remains unknown. Regardless of the trigger, it results in the production of antinuclear antibodies, the generation of circulating immune complexes, and activation of the complement system. B- and T-cell tolerance breaks down, resulting in production of IgG antibodies. These autoantibodies form self antigen–antibody complexes that subsequently occlude some of the organ vascular beds. The disease manifestations result from recurrent vascular injury due to immune complex deposition, white cell deposition, or thrombosis. In addition, the cytotoxic antibodies can mediate an autoimmune haemolytic anaemia and thrombocytopenia, while antibodies to specific cellular antigens can disrupt cell function. The health of the patient is affected not only by disease activity but also by the consequences of recurrent episodes (e.g. deforming arthropathy, chronic renal failure) and the side effects of treatment such as infection and avascular necrosis of bone. Failed or compromised pulmonary, renal, or central nervous systems may be the presenting complications to intensive care. The most frequent causes of mortality are progressive renal failure and sepsis.

Manifestations of SLE

General Patients complain of tiredness and malaise. In 50%, there is fever in exacerbations.

Central nervous system 60% develop neurological involvement including psychosis, personality disorder, dementia, coma, and isolated nerve palsies.

Cerebrovascular accidents can occur due to inflammatory, non-inflammatory, or thrombotic vasculopathy.

Respiratory At least 50% have lung involvement, including recurrent pleurisy with pleural effusions, pneumonitis, pulmonary fibrosis, pulmonary hypertension, alveolar haemorrhage, diaphragmatic dysfunction, or phrenic nerve palsy.

Cardiovascular 25% develop endocarditis, myocarditis, and/or pericarditis with chest pain and arrhythmias. Cardiac tamponade can result from pericardial effusions. The incidence of atherosclerosis increases due to the effects of endothelial cell activation and treatment with corticosteroids.

Gastrointestinal Mouth ulceration is most commonly seen. Peritonitis (± ascites and pancreatitis) and mesenteric ischaemia can result from vasculitis. Inflammatory liver disease may occur.

Renal Most suffer renal impairment. Long-term dialysis or transplantation may be needed. Lupus nephritis occurs in 50%.

Musculoskeletal Most develop joint pain and arthritis, frequently affecting fingers, hands, wrists, and knees. Bone necrosis can occur in hips and shoulders. Half present with myalgia but myositis is rare.

Serositis Half develop inflammatory serositis within pleura, pericardium, and peritoneum producing pleurisy, pericarditis, or peritonitis, respectively. Large effusions sometimes occur.

Skin and mucosa 75% develop photosensitive flushing on the cheeks and bridge of the nose ('butterfly rash'). Other parts of the body may develop rashes or skin lesions. Alopecia occurs in 50%, particularly during exacerbations. Mucosal ulcers can occur on the soft and hard palate and nasal septum.

Haematological Anaemia is common and autoimmune thrombocytopenic purpura may occur. There is an increased incidence of antiphospholipid antibody syndrome where circulating antibody (lupus anticoagulant) places patients are at risk of recurrent arterial and venous thrombosis, causing strokes and pulmonary embolism. Long-term anticoagulation may be required. However, platelets are often decreased, or antibodies are formed against clotting factors, which may result in significant bleeding.

Treatment

Systemic corticosteroid therapy is particularly useful in the treatment of pneumonitis, pleural effusion, and alveolar haemorrhage. NSAIDs are useful for arthralgia, arthritis, fever, and serositis. Cytotoxic drugs have been used in patients refractory to corticosteroid therapy. SLE may be induced by a number of drugs (e.g. procainamide and hydralazine) that commonly induce pulmonary and pleural problems. Cessation of these drugs usually leads to resolution.

Wegener's granulomatosis

This disease can affect many organs (classically nose, eyes, lung, and kidney) and is characterized by necrotizing vasculitis affecting predominantly small but also medium-sized vessels. Necrotizing glomerulonephritis occurs in up to 80%. Circulating antineutrophil cytoplasmic autoantibodies (ANCAs) are directed against white blood cells and endothelial cells, forming clumps of immune complexes which then accumulate in the tissues, leading to granulomatous inflammation of the vessels. This reduces blood flow to the different organs and tissues, causing damage.

Symptoms vary in severity. Patients may complain of weight loss, fever, malaise, pleuritic pain, and myalgia. Most develop upper airway disease such as sinusitis, a purulent or bloody nasal discharge, and epistaxis. The cartilage of the nasal septum may be destroyed (saddle-nose deformity). Haemoptysis (from tracheal and laryngeal ulcers), pleurisy, pneumonia, and subglottal stenosis can develop and pulmonary haemorrhage can be life threatening. Lung granulomas may coalesce into large cavitating masses. Retro-orbital inflammation can cause proptosis, conjunctival haemorrhage, keratitis, or ocular muscle paralysis. Other areas of the skin and nervous system may also be involved.

Treatment

Immunosuppressants such as corticosteroids and cyclophosphamide are used to manage the disease. The prognosis is now much improved with 70–90% achieving complete remission. Success has been reported utilizing monoclonal antibodies such as rituximab for refractory disease.

Polyarteritis nodosa (PAN)

The aetiology of this disease is unknown, but some drugs (e.g. penicillin), bacterial infections, vaccines, and viral infections (hepatitis B and C, HIV) are associated with its onset. It is a vasculitic disease with an incidence of less than one in a million. In areas where the hepatitis virus is endemic the incidence can be up to 77 per million. The disease is characterized by segmental inflammation and necrosis of small- and medium-sized arteries. Secondary thrombosis and vessel occlusion can lead to ischaemia and infarction of multiple organs. Small aneurysms can develop in the weakened tissue wall and healing can result in fibrosis. The kidneys, liver, heart, and gastrointestinal tract are most commonly affected, but it rarely affects the respiratory system. Cutaneous symptoms occur in 25–60%.

Clinical manifestations

There is no specific laboratory test. Diagnosis is made by clinical findings and the presence of necrotizing arteritis in a lesion biopsy. The course of the disease may be acute, resulting in death within a few months, or chronic, leading to debilitating illness. Severity is determined by the organs affected, but multi-organ failure often develops. Initial manifestations are fever, abdominal pain, weakness, weight loss, hypertension, oedema, and oliguria.

Neurological Both central and peripheral nervous system may be affected causing sensory changes (such as numbness and tingling), headaches, strokes, and seizures.

Gastrointestinal Abdominal involvement may cause nausea, vomiting, pain, bloody diarrhoea, and retroperitoneal bleeding. Mesenteric artery thrombosis and bowel infarction may necessitate surgery.

Cardiac Involvement can result in myocardial infarction, pericarditis, and heart failure.

Renal The patient may develop haematuria and proteinuria and can progress to renal failure.

Muscle and joints Myalgia, with areas of focal ischaemia and arthralgia are common.

Skin Lesions can occur with palpable nodules along the course of the affected blood vessel.

Treatment

High doses of corticosteroids are given, but as these have to be taken for long periods the side effects often cause further damage. Other immunosuppressive drugs may be needed, for example cyclophosphamide in patients who are unable to tolerate, or are refractory to, corticosteroids.

Rheumatoid arthritis

This chronic inflammatory disease can present from early childhood up to old age, but most commonly between 30 and 50 years. There is a genetic predisposition to the disease and it is immune mediated, though it remains unknown whether it is primarily an autoimmune disease or whether the initiating agent is infectious, a self-antigen, or both. Synovial inflammation is caused by T-cell activation and both IgM and IgG antibodies and activated macrophages can be found in arthritic joints. The main inflammatory reaction is caused by tumour necrosis factor (TNF) produced by the macrophages.

The disease usually presents with pain and signs of inflammation in small and/or large joints and can spread to additional joints with subsequent irreversible tissue damage causing deformity and instability. Tendons, ligaments, muscle, and fascia may also be affected. Damage and displacement of tendons give rise to typical deformities such as ulnar deviation of the fingers and 'z deformity' of the thumbs. The spine can be affected with compression of the spinal cord. Instability of the cervical spine may preclude extension of the neck and is an important consideration when patients require tracheal intubation. Rheumatoid arthritis may affect other body systems (Table 13.4); most patients are admitted to the critical care unit because of pulmonary involvement or complications of their treatment (e.g. renal failure, bleeding disorders, immunosuppression). Rheumatoid pleurisy, often with large pleural effusions, occurs commonly. Another serious complication is diffuse interstitial pneumonitis and fibrosis, also known as rheumatoid lung. This causes restrictive lung dysfunction with reduced lung volumes. Laryngeal nodules, which may be asymptomatic, may pose problems if tracheal intubation is required.

Treatment

The disease is primarily controlled using NSAIDs which act on the cyclo-oxygenase pathway. Disease modifying anti-rheumatic drugs (DMARDs) reduce inflammation by inhibiting proinflammatory cytokines. Corticosteroids and other immunosuppressant drugs such as methotrexate, gold, and cyclophosphamide are employed, but their use may be limited by side effects. New treatments such as anti-TNF antibody have produced major improvements in some patients though, again, its side-effect profile and cost may limit its use.

Goodpasture's syndrome (anti-glomerular basement membrane disease)

This is a rare disease affecting adults which commonly begins after an upper respiratory tract infection. It is caused by antibodies formed against the glomerular basement membrane, resulting in rapidly progressive global and diffuse glomerulonephritis. The antibodies also cross-react with the lung's basement membrane, leading to pulmonary haemorrhage and haemoptysis, particularly in smokers. Other symptoms include tiredness, anaemia, and potentially massive bleeding.

Table 13.4 Non-articular manifestations of rheumatoid arthritis

	Complication
Neurological	Carpal or tarsal tunnel syndrome
	Peripheral neuropathy
	Compression of nerve roots or cervical spine
	Scleritis and episcleritis
Respiratory	Pleurisy and pleural effusion
	Fibrosing alveolitis
	Laryngeal nodules
	Pulmonary hypertension
	Obstructive bronchiolitis
	Pulmonary vasculitis
Cardiovascular	Pericarditis
	Endocarditis
	Conduction defects
	Mitral valve disease
	Raynaud's syndrome
	Felty's syndrome (splenomegaly and neutropenia)
Gastrointestinal	Bowel infarction (due to necrotizing arteritis of mesenteric vessels)
Renal	Nephrotic syndrome and renal failure (caused by amyloidosis)
	Proteinuria
Skin	Cutaneous vasculitis
	Palmar erythema
Musculoskeletal	Subcutaneous nodules
	Tenosynovitis
	Muscle wasting

Treatment

Daily plasma exchange via plasmapheresis is used to remove the antiglomerular basement antibodies. Corticosteroids combined with cyclophosphamide are given to treat the glomerular inflammation and prevent resynthesis of the antibodies. If left untreated, the disease is fatal.

Hypersensitivity reactions (including drug allergy)

These are immunologically mediated responses to drugs, chemicals, foodstuffs, or natural substances. Generally, the structural characteristics of the allergen determine the type of hypersensitivity reaction that results. Reactions to proteins and peptides, for example, are most often mediated by IgE antibodies or immune complex responses, while topical exposure to fats and oils (e.g. lanolin, beeswax, camphor oil) can cause contact dermatitis. These reactions must be distinguished from anaphylactoid reactions that are caused by direct release of mediators from mast cells and basophils.

The Coombs and Gell classification system of human hypersensitivity (Marieb and Hoehn 2010) can be used to categorize the clinical manifestations and mechanisms of drug allergy reactions.

Anaphylactic and anaphylactoid reactions

An anaphylactic reaction is a potentially life-threatening, systemic response that occurs after re-exposure to an antigen (Table 13.5). It is IgE mediated with immediate release of potent mediators (e.g. histamine, kinins, leukotrienes, serotonin, tryptase) from tissue mast cells and peripheral blood basophils. These mediators cause clinical manifestations of anaphylaxis by inducing mucus production, pruritus, increased vascular permeability, and smooth muscle constriction in various organs.

Anaphylactoid reactions are clinically indistinguishable from anaphylactic reactions but are not IgE mediated and the mechanism of mediator release differs. In this type of reaction the mast cell can be induced to react:

- directly by exercise, stress, opiates, and radiocontrast agents
- by some drugs (e.g. aspirin and other NSAIDs) which inhibit cyclo-oxygenase activity, thus disturbing arachidonic acid metabolism

Table 13.5 Causes of anaphylactic reactions

Type of reaction	Cause
IgE mediated	Foods (e.g. nuts, shellfish, eggs)
	Venoms (insect stings and bites)
	Vaccines
	Latex
	Drugs (e.g. thiopental)
Complement activation	Blood products
	Immunoglobulins
Direct activation	Radiocontrast media
	Opiates
	Dextran
	Exercise
Cyclo-oxygenase inhibitors	Non-steroidal anti-inflammatory drugs (NSAIDs)

- following complement activation by immune complexes, which may be caused by reactions to blood, blood products, and immunoglobulins).

Any drug can potentially cause anaphylactic and anaphylactoid reactions. Antibiotics are the most frequent cause of severe reactions. Other causes include enzymes (e.g. streptokinase), insulin, protamine, vaccines, blood products, plasma expanders (e.g. dextrans, starches, and gelatins) and anaesthetic agents (e.g. thiopental, suxamethonium, and non-depolarizing muscle relaxants).

Clinical manifestations

Symptoms usually occur within 20 min of exposure to the stimulus but can occur within seconds (Table 13.6). Progression can be variable, from a weak response (e.g. nasal congestion, conjunctivitis, pruritus, and abdominal symptoms such as diarrhoea, nausea, and vomiting) to the most severe form with cardiovascular collapse, myocardial depression, angioedema, laryngeal obstruction and severe bronchospasm. These can lead to death within minutes of allergen exposure.

The response is initiated by the release of vasoactive mediators from basophils and mast cells. Histamine binds to histamine H_1 receptors in the lung causing bronchospasm, and to H_2 receptors in the upper respiratory tract causing vasodilation and inflammation. Leukotrienes induce the production of copious amounts of mucus in the lungs which then plugs the constricted bronchioles and causes asphyxiation. Respiratory symptoms are further exacerbated by severe angioedema, pulmonary oedema and oedema of the tongue, larynx, and glottis< causing upper airway obstruction.

The systemic release of histamine and other vasodilating mediators can cause shock due to generalized vasodilation of the arterioles and increased vascular permeability. Rapid fluid shifts to extravascular spaces may result in loss of blood volume and severe hypotension, though the circulation often tries to compensate by vasoconstriction due to release of angiotensin and catecholamines. Hypotension can also cause myocardial ischaemia, arrhythmias, and cardiac arrest. Activation of H_1 receptors in the gastrointestinal tract causes contraction of the smooth muscle, resulting in abdominal cramps, nausea, vomiting, and diarrhoea.

Table 13.6 Clinical manifestations of anaphylaxis

Airway	Oedema of the glottis, tongue, larynx
	Dysphagia
	Hoarse voice
	Stridor
	Bronchospasm
Breathing	Dyspnoea
	Pulmonary oedema
	Tachypnoea
	Wheeze
	Cyanosis
	Respiratory arrest
Circulation	Signs of shock
	Tachycardia
	Hypotension
	Myocardial ischaemia
	Vasodilation
	Arrhythmias
	Cardiac arrest
Disability	Impending sense of doom
	Decreased level of consciousness related to altered airway, breathing, and circulation
	Anxiety
Exposure	Flushing of the skin
	Urticaria
	Angio-oedema
	Erythema

Management of a severe reaction

Treatment is the same for both anaphylactic and anaphylactoid reactions and consists of immediate emergency management followed by less urgent secondary treatments. In a severe reaction, early intervention is critical for a favourable outcome. ABC principles of resuscitation should be followed.

A: Airway and epinephrine

- Stop administration of the causal agent.
- Maintain an adequate airway and administer 100% oxygen.
- If possible, monitor oxygen saturation using pulse oximetry.
- Give epinephrine (adrenaline). This blocks the physiological effect of the mediators and should be given at the earliest opportunity. If no IV access is available it can be given intramuscularly (IM) in the thigh. Intravenously, 0.5–1.0 ml increments of 1:10,000 solution can be repeated as required. Intramuscularly, injections of 500 μg (0.5 ml of 1:1000 solution) can be repeated every 5 min as

required. Intravenous epinephrine is preferable in life-threatening situations, but can cause myocardial ischaemia and arrhythmias and therefore must be given slowly in low doses. Patients with a history of anaphylaxis should carry a pre-filled syringe of epinephrine (e.g. Epipen, Ana-Guard) for immediate injection outside the hospital setting.

B: Breathing

- If breathing is inadequate, endotracheal intubation, cricothyroidotomy, or emergency tracheostomy may be required, depending on the extent of upper airway oedema.
- Nebulized bronchodilators (e.g. salbutamol 5 mg) or IV aminophylline may be required for bronchospasm (loading dose 6 mg/kg followed by 0.5 mg/kg/h). Nebulized epinephrine may also be useful for laryngospasm, bronchospasm, and laryngeal oedema. Intra-tracheal epinephrine can be instilled in intubated patients with severe bronchospasm.

C: Circulation

- Assess circulatory status and commence cardiopulmonary resuscitation if necessary.
- Establish IV access and rapidly infuse normal saline or colloid 500–1000 ml (unless it is the cause of the anaphylaxis).
- Continue to administer epinephrine if hypotension persists. An epinephrine or norepinephrine (noradrenaline) infusion may be necessary, avoiding the dangerous surges in blood pressure seen with IV boluses.
- Monitor ECG and cardiac output if prolonged.

Secondary management

When airway, breathing, and circulation have been stabilised, further management is as follows.

- Antihistamine agents to antagonize the effects of histamine. Chlorphenamine (chlorpheniramine) 10mg IM or slow IV bolus is a histamine H_1 antagonist and is useful for urticaria and oedema, while ranitidine, an H_2 antagonist, is gastro-protective.
- Corticosteroids (e.g. hydrocortisone 200 mg IM or slow IV) helps to dampen the inflammatory response and block a potential late phase response where the physiological manifestations of anaphylaxis can re-occur several hours later without additional exposure to the allergen.
- In patients already taking beta-blockers, anaphylaxis may be severe and refractory to treatment, and additional therapy may be required. Beta-blockers act as competitive inhibitors of catecholamines and therefore high doses of β_1 and/or β_2 agonists may be needed.
- The patient should be transferred to a critical care area, if not already there, for full cardiovascular monitoring and respiratory support.

Cancer and the immune system

When multiple control systems of cells fail, cancer may arise. The two main systems that tend to become problematic relate to proliferation (the cell growth system) or normal cell death (which inhibits or protects against abnormal cell growth). Cell proliferation is essential to life; however, most proliferation slows down or ceases with age. When cells proliferate inappropriately this can be a step towards the cell becoming cancerous. When a gene is mutated it can cause inappropriate proliferation and is called a proto-oncogene. A mutated gene is called an oncogene.

Immune surveillance of cancer

Normally, the immune system responds to and destroys any cancerous cells. However, when it is overwhelmed due to high mutation and proliferation levels it may miss some of these cells. Patients with a weak immune system are more susceptible to haematological or virus-associated cancer. Most cancers are solid tumours and spontaneous in onset. Killer T cells may provide surveillance, as may macrophages and NK cells. Macrophages secrete tumour necrosis factor (TNF) and as they are located within tissue can hence kill some cancer cells at an early stage.

Stem cell transplantation

Stem cell transplantation (SCT) is the transfer of pluripotent haemopoietic stem cells and may be either allogeneic (from a donor) or autologous (from the host). The aim of SCT is to either repopulate stem cells after myelo-ablative chemotherapy or chemo-radiotherapy during treatment of haemato-oncological diseases, or to replace any congenital or acquired life-threatening abnormalities with the bone marrow. Stem cells can be obtained from the bone marrow; however, this often requires sedation. They can also be obtained peripherally after cells have been mobilized by granulocyte colony stimulating factor (G-CSF) treatment. They are then collected utilizing apheresis. Peripheral blood stem cell transplant (PBSCT) has a faster grafting time, but it carries a higher incidence of chronic graft versus host disease (cGvHD).

Allogeneic stem cell transplantation

Stem cells are obtained from a donor who may be either a volunteer (matched unrelated donor (MUD)) or a matched sibling. If a twin donates stem cells, this is known as a syngeneic SCT. An allogeneic SCT is indicated for those with acute or chronic myeloid leukaemia (AML/CML), severe aplastic anaemia, stage II or III multiple myeloma (MM), sickle cell disease, and relapsed non-Hodgkin's lymphoma (NHL).

The mortality for matched sibling allografts is between 15% and 30%, but can be up to 45% for an unrelated donor SCT. Early complications are generally dominated by infection from bacterial, viral, fungal, or atypical organisms due to the general immune dysfunction and myelosuppression. GvHD is also a relatively early complication.

Autologous stem cell transplantation

Similarly to autologous blood donation the patient may donate their own stem cells. Stem cells may also be obtained from placental cord blood. An autologous SCT is indicated in relapsed and aggressive NHL, HL, AML, and MM. it can also be considered in the treatment of neuroblastoma and autoimmune diseases such as multiple sclerosis and rheumatoid arthritis.

The mortality rate is approximately 5–10%; however, other complications such as mucositis and other forms of mucosal damage occur due to the conditioning treatments. Longer-term complications tend to be associated with relapse of the disease.

Cancer in critical care

Patients with cancer are admitted into critical care for either cancer-related complications or treatment-associated side effects. Increasing numbers of patients with cancer are admitted into critical care because of the early diagnosis of complications, early admission, and aggressive management, both medically and surgically. This includes chemotherapy-related organ toxicities and immunosuppression-related infection.

Oncological emergencies such as disseminated intravascular coagulation (DIC), tumour lysis syndrome (TLS), and gastrointestinal obstruction or perforation may also require admission. Overall, there has been an improvement in ICU survival for cancer patients. This includes patients who have required life-sustaining therapies for acute respiratory failure, acute renal failure, and shock. However, selection of suitable patients who would potentially benefit from advanced levels of care is an important consideration.

Organ supportive measures are required, as in the general critical care population. Sepsis and septic shock remain a common cause for admission into critical care, with the most common sites of infection being the lungs and intravascular access. Approximately 20% of cancer patients die of respiratory failure; however, this excludes pulmonary emboli and pneumonia. Patients with cancer are generally more susceptible due to the higher incidence of neutropenia. Neutropenia is often related to the treatment of haematological cancers where the immune system is suppressed due to chemotherapy and or radiotherapy. Neutropenic sepsis and severe sepsis are discussed further in Chapter 10.

Occasionally, chemotherapy may be administered during a patient's stay in critical care. However, there are only a few studies showing the benefits of chemotherapy to those receiving mechanical ventilation, inotropes, and renal replacement therapy. Chemotherapy prevents wound healing and is generally not advised until several weeks after surgery.

Associated states of immunosuppression and coagulopathy further complicate their management. Such patients generally require strict isolation and infection control procedures. Further details with regard to infection in immunocompromised patients and DIC can be found in Chapters 10 and 12, respectively.

Complications of cancer treatment

Tumour lysis syndrome

Tumour lysis syndrome (TLS) is a group of metabolic complications that occur when a large number of tumour cells are destroyed rapidly. It can occur with any form of cancer where the cancer cells are bulky or there is a large volume of cells. This can also occur with tumours that are very chemosensitive and respond very well to chemotherapy. Patients particularly affected are those with haematological cancers such as acute lymphocytic leukaemia (ALL), Burkitt's lymphoma, and acute myelogenous leukaemia (AML). It is less common in solid tumours, but has been seen in patients with cancers such as small cell lung cancer, testicular cancer, and metastatic breast cancer. Patients are at greater risk if they are dehydrated, have a poor urine output, or have any pre-existing renal impairment.

Clinically, the three major symptoms are hyperuricaemia, hyperkalaemia, and hyperphosphataemia. They may occur individually or in combination. Potassium and phosphate are released from the destroyed cells while the uric acid is a product of nucleic acid (DNA) breakdown. ECG changes such as T wave inversion and other dysrhythmias may occur due to the electrolyte abnormalities. Secondary complications include hypocalcaemia, elevated serum lactate dehydrogenase (LDH), and acute kidney injury (AKI). Identifying patients at risk and preventing TLS is the ideal situation. TLS usually occurs within 1–5 days post chemotherapy with non-specific symptoms such as nausea, vomiting, weakness, and fatigue.

Patients at risk should be hydrated prior to commencement of the chemotherapy. Adequate hydration before and during chemotherapy will promote the excretion of metabolic products, reduce the production of uric acid, and prevent renal failure. Treatment with allopurinol or rasburicase as part of the chemotherapy protocol will prevent TLS in most cases. If TLS occurs, haemodynamic monitoring, fluid therapy, and haemodialysis may be required.

Graft versus host disease

Acute graft versus host disease (GvHD) occurs in patients who have had an allogeneic haematopoietic stem cell transplant (HSCT) and usually occurs within 100 days of the transplant. It is more commonly seen in patients who have received HLA identical matched but unrelated transplants. It generally affects the skin, liver, gastrointestinal tract, and haematopoietic systems.

There are four stages of acute GvHD. The most common and initial sign is a rash on the neck, ears, shoulders, soles of the feet, and palms of the hands. The second most commonly affected organs are the liver and gastrointestinal tract. The small bile ducts in the liver are damaged, leading to cholestasis and obstruction of bile flow from the liver. Abnormal liver function tests, such as an elevated serum conjugated bilirubin and alkaline phosphatase, are non-specific so other causes of liver injury must be investigated. Within the gastrointestinal tract severity is determined by the volume of diarrhoea. Watery diarrhoea occurs initially; however, this can become bloody, resulting in a need for blood transfusion and complex fluid management.

General treatment includes organ supportive therapies, nutritional support, fluid balance and weight maintenance, antibiotics, antifungals and corticosteroids. Optimal skin and pressure area management are essential. The skin becomes compromised to a greater degree in the later stages of GvHD. The persistent large volumes of diarrhoea further compromises skin integrity. Bowel management systems should be used with due caution and discussed with a haemato-oncologist and intensivist.

Non-incrementing platelet count (platelet refractoriness)

Platelet refractoriness may occur as a result of immune or non-immune platelet destruction (Table 13.7). Many patients with cancer, but particularly haemoncology patients, become resistant to platelet transfusions. The platelet count does not increase or increment despite

Table 13.7 Causes of platelet refractoriness

Immune	Non-immune
Platelet antibodies HLA Human platelet antigen (HPA)	Infection
Other antibodies Platelet autoantibodies Drug-dependent platelet antibodies ABO	Splenomegaly
Immune complexes	DIC and other bleeding

transfusion with platelets. In the absence of fever, severe bleeding, infection, DIC, and splenomegaly, it can be defined by a failure of two consecutive transfusions to give a corrected platelet count of >7.5 × 10^9/L up to an hour after transfusion. This problem cannot be prevented or corrected in a small group of patients.

Identifying patients with platelet refractoriness due to HLA alloantibodies is important as HLA-matched platelets may produce a greater increment. If the platelet count fails to remain >10 × 10^9/L despite transfusion, further investigation should occur. If bleeding occurs, other drugs such as tranexamic acid may be considered.

References and bibliography

Azoulay, E., Afessa, B. (2006). The intensive care support of patients with malignancy: do everything that can be done. *Intensive Care Medicine*, **32**, 3–5.

Daya, M., Thomas, C.R. (eds) (2009). *Emergency Medical Clinics of North America: Cancer Emergencies, Part I*. Philadelphia, PA: WB Saunders.

Graham, R.R., Cotsapas, C., Davies, L., *et al.* (2008). Genetic variants near TNFAIP3on SQ23 are associated with systemic lupus erythematosus (SLE). *Nature Genetics*, **40**, 1059–61.

Gonce Morton, P., Fontaine, D.K. (2009). *Critical Care Nursing: A Holistic Approach* (9th edn). Philadelphia, PA: Wolters Kluwer Health/Lippincott Williams & Wilkins.

Keogh, K.A., Ytterberg, S.R., Fervenza, F.C., *et al.* (2006). Rituximab for refractory Wegener's granulomatosis. *American Journal of Respiratory and Critical Care Medicine*, **173**, 180–7.

Kumar, P., Clark, M. (2009). *Clinical Medicine* (6th edn). London: Saunders Elsevier.

Laurence, H., Quartin, A., Jones, D., Havlir, D.V. (2006). Intensive care of patients with HIV infection. *New England Journal of Medicine*, **355**, 173–81.

Marieb, E.N., Hoehn, K. (2010). *Human Anatomy and Physiology* (8th edn), pp.767–803. San Francisco, CA: Pearson.

Nakamura, T., Kanazawa, N., Ikeda, T., *et al.* (2009). Cutaneous polyarteritis nodosa: revisiting its definition and diagnostic criteria. *Archives of Dermatological Research*, **301**, 117–21.

Patton, K.T., Thibodeau, G.A. (2010). *Anatomy and Physiology* (7th edn), pp.730–55. St Louis, MO: Mosby Elsevier.

Pratt, R.J. (2003). *HIV & AIDS* (5th edn). London: Hodder Arnold.

Provan, D., Singer, C.R.J., Baglin, T., Lilleyman, J. (eds) (2007). *Oxford Handbook of Clinical Haematology* 2nd edn. Oxford: Oxford University Press.

Resuscitation Council UK (2008). *Emergency Treatment of Anaphylactic Reactions*. http://www.resus.org.uk/anaphylaxis/emergency-treatment-of-anaphylactic-reactions/ (accessed 19 September 2016).

Rusznak, C., Peebles, R.S., Jr (2002). Anaphylaxis and anaphylactoid reactions. A guide to prevention, recognition and emergent treatment. *Postgraduate Medicine* **111**, 101–14.

Savage, C.O., Harper, L., Cockwell, P., *et al.* (2000). Vasculitis. *British Medical Journal*, **320**, 1325–8.

Shah, M.K., Hugghins, S.Y. (2002). Characteristics and outcomes of patients with Goodpasture's syndrome. *Southern Medical Journal*, **95**, 1411–18.

Singer, M., Webb, A. (2007). *Oxford Handbook of Critical Care*. Oxford: Oxford University Press.

Sompayrac, L. (2008). *How the Immune System Works* (3rd edn). Oxford: Blackwell.

Spano, J.P., Costagliola, D., Katlama, C., *et al.* (2008). AIDS-related malignancies: state of the art and therapeutic challenges. *Journal of Clinical Oncology*, **26**, 4834–42.

Spence, R.AJ., Hay, R., Johnson, P. (eds) (2006). *Infection in the Cancer Patient: A Practical Guide*. Oxford: Oxford University Press.

Spiro, D.M., Daya, M. (eds) (2009). *Emergency Medical Clinics of North America: Cancer Emergencies, Part II*. Philadelphia, PA: WB Saunders.

Taccone, F.S., Artigas, A.A., Sprung, C.L., *et al.* (2009). Characteristics and outcomes of cancer patients in European ICUs. *Critical Care*, **13**, 15–20.

Taylor, S.R.J., Salama, A.D., Joshi, L., *et al.* (2009). Rituximab is effective in the treatment of refractory ophthalmic Wegener's granulomatosis. *Arthritis and Rheumatism*, **60**, 1540–7.

Thiery, G., Azoulay, E., Darmon, M., *et al* (2005). Outcome of cancer patients considered for intensive care unit admission: a hospital-wide study. *Journal of Clinical Oncology*, **23**, 4406–13.

Watts, R.A., Scott, D.G.I. (2010). *Vasculitis in Clinical Practice*. London: Springer.

Wilson, J. (2006). *Infection Control in Clinical Practice*. London: Baillière Tindall Elsevier.

CHAPTER 14

Endocrine, obstetric, and drug overdose emergencies

Endocrine disorders

Endocrine syndromes usually produce classical signs and symptoms but these may be difficult to identify in the critically ill patient. Appropriate investigations are needed to diagnose and treat these disorders promptly. Knowledge of normal endocrine physiology is vital for understanding the systemic effects caused by their failure, the interactions between the endocrine glands and other body systems, and the impact of severe illness.

Endocrine emergencies and related conditions that require admission to the critical care unit are described in this chapter.

The adrenal glands

The adrenal glands consist of an inner medulla and an outer cortex. These areas function independently of each other, producing different hormones with different functions.

The adrenal medulla (the inner core of the gland)

The medullary cells are derived from the sympathetic nervous system and secrete epinephrine (adrenaline) and norepinephrine (noradrenaline) in response to sympathetic stimuli. Norepinephrine is the transmitter substance of the sympathetic nervous system and preganglionic sympathetic fibres innervate the medulla. Stressors that activate the sympathetic nervous system (e.g. fear, hypoxia, hypotension, anger, cold, pain, etc.) lead to the release of norepinephrine and epinephrine (collectively known as catecholamines). The medulla normally secretes epinephrine and norepinephrine in a 4:1 ratio. These hormones prepare the body for action ('fight or flight') in response to a stressor.

Epinephrine

This hormone constricts blood vessels in the skin and mucosa and dilates those in skeletal muscle and the eye. It relaxes the bronchioles, thereby increasing lung capacity, and increases heart rate and cardiac output. Epinephrine also dilates the blood vessels of the brain, muscles, and myocardium, ensuring that blood flow is maintained to these crucial areas. Liver glycogen is mobilized and converted to glucose, providing an immediate source of energy.

Norepinephrine

This raises the blood pressure by constricting arterioles and veins, except those in crucial areas where epinephrine counteracts this effect.

The adrenal cortex

The cortex secretes three categories of hormones: mineralocorticoids, glucocorticoids, and sex hormones. All are steroids and are derived from cholesterol. Box 14.1 lists the effects of a lack in these hormones.

Mineralocorticoids

These regulate sodium and potassium concentrations in the extracellular fluid. The most important is aldosterone which accounts for 95% of mineralocorticoid secretion.

Box 14.1 The effects of a lack of aldosterone, cortisol or androgens

Effects of lack of aldosterone

- Polyuria, dehydration, thirst
- Hyponatraemia, hyperkalaemia
- Hypotension (often postural)
- Cardiac arrhythmias

Effect of lack of cortisol

- Muscle weakness, fatigue, weight loss
- Hypoglycaemia
- Gastrointestinal disturbances (nausea, vomiting, diarrhoea, abdominal pain)
- Emotional disturbances (irritability, depression)
- Low resistance to infection, inability to cope with any type of stress)

Effect of lack of androgens

- Loss of body hair
- Loss of libido

The effect of aldosterone is to increase extracellular fluid sodium and chloride ion concentration, and to decrease potassium levels. Aldosterone causes reabsorption of sodium in the distal loops and collecting ducts of the kidney (see Chapter 7). Since sodium and potassium transport mechanisms in the epithelial cells are linked in a partial exchange process, potassium is also excreted at the same time. This sodium–potassium pump is stimulated by aldosterone. However, as the sodium–potassium ion exchange is unequal, this usually leads to more sodium being reabsorbed than potassium being excreted.

A secondary effect of aldosterone is to decrease chloride loss in the urine. The increase in sodium and chloride reabsorption by the tubules also results in more water being reabsorbed.

Aldosterone secretion can be stimulated by:

- elevated levels of potassium ions in the plasma
- a persistently low plasma sodium level
- a prolonged decrease in extracellular fluid volume
- angiotensin: plasma angiotensin rises when renal production of renin is increased as a result of a low plasma sodium level or reduced renal blood flow.

Therefore excess aldosterone secretion causes sodium retention, hypokalaemia, and alkalosis, while aldosterone deficiency causes sodium loss, hyperkalaemia, and acidosis.

Glucocorticoids

These regulate metabolism of fat, protein, and carbohydrate, and enhance resistance to physical stress. The most important glucocorticoid is cortisol. Cortisol production is stimulated by adrenocorticotrophic hormone (ACTH) secreted from the anterior pituitary via a negative feedback mechanism. Cortisol shows a diurnal variation in secretion, being highest in the morning and lowest at about midnight. The primary stimulus for secretion is physical stress (injury) which activates the hypothalamus via nerve impulses from the site of injury. The rise in cortisol increases availability of fat, glucose, and amino acids to repair the damage.

Effects of cortisol

- Increases fat metabolism. Cortisol mobilizes fat from adipose tissue cells, thus providing an important source of energy during starvation states. Excessive fat breakdown can cause ketosis.
- Increases use of protein. Cortisol suppresses the rate of protein production in non-liver cells; thus plasma amino acid levels rise, increasing their availability in times of stress. Chronically, this causes weakening of capillaries, skin atrophy, and muscle wasting. However, the rate of protein formation within the liver is increased by cortisol.
- Increases blood glucose level by:
  - decreasing cellular utilization of glucose (i.e. antagonistic to insulin).
  - stimulating liver cells to convert fat and protein into glucose (by gluconeogenesis). Gluconeogenesis is increased because cortisol causes amino acids to be mobilized from tissue protein and fat (in the form of glycerol) from adipose tissue. This provides the liver with substrate that can be converted into glucose. Therefore excess cortisol can cause insulin resistance and hyperglycaemia.
- Decreases absorption of vitamin D from the intestine. Osteoporosis and delayed development of cartilage occurs with chronically high cortisol levels (e.g. in Cushing's disease or steroid treatment).
- Anti-inflammatory—cortisol inhibits formation of pro-inflammatory mediators such as cytokines and nitric oxide, decreases the number of lymphocytes and eosinophils in the blood, and suppresses allergic responses and the body's reactions to injury, inflammation, and infection. However, neutrophil levels are elevated by corticosteroids.
- Can cause sodium (and water) retention and potassium depletion.

Sex hormones

Androgens, oestrogens, and progesterone are secreted by the adrenal cortex but less than in the gonads. Occasionally, oestrogen-secreting tumours of the adrenal cortex develop.

Disorders of the adrenal medulla

Phaeochromocytoma

This tumour of chromaffin cells usually involves the adrenal medulla (90%) resulting in excess levels of epinephrine, norepinephrine, and dopamine. In 10% of cases extra-adrenal phaeochromocytomas may occur anywhere along the sympathetic chain (aorta, bladder, pelvis, abdomen, thorax). About 10% of phaeochromocytomas are malignant, and up to 25% may have a hereditary predisposition.

Catecholamine secretion is usually intermittent. During acute attacks the patient develops pulsating headaches, sweating, tachycardia, hyperglycaemia, tremor, blurred vision, bowel disturbances, and very severe hypertension. Between attacks the blood pressure may be only slightly raised (see Box 14.2).

Up to 30% of patients present with hypotension due to a greater release of dilating catecholamines. Thus it may mimic septic shock (see Box 14.3).

Precipitants of a hypertensive crisis include anaesthesia induction, opiates, dopamine antagonists, radiographic contrast media, drugs that inhibit catecholamine re-uptake (e.g. tricyclic antidepressants), and childbirth.

Box 14.2 Complications of phaeochromocytoma

- Dilated cardiomyopathy
- Myocarditis
- Pulmonary oedema
- Myocardial infarction
- Hypertensive encephalopathy
- Cerebral infarction
- Embolic events secondary to a mural thrombus from dilated cardiomyopathy
- Intracerebral haemorrhage
- Hypertensive retinopathy

Box 14.3 Diagnosis of phaeochromocytoma

- Raised blood catecholamine levels and 24-hour urinary measurements of vanillylmandelic acid (VMA), a metabolic product of catecholamines. NB: this test is not useful in critical illness where levels are increased because of severe underlying stress.
- MIBG (meta-iodobenzylguanidine) radionuclide scan.
- Computed tomography.

Treatment is by surgical removal (laparoscopically, if possible) but the blood pressure must be controlled well in advance of surgery using α- and β-adrenergic blocking agents. α-Blockade should begin before β-blockade or a severe hypertensive crisis can be precipitated. Phentolamine or phenoxybenzamine are commonly used for short-term pre-operative α-blockade and propanolol for β-blockade. Alternatively, labetolol can be used as it has both α- and β-adrenergic blockade effects. During a severe hypertensive crisis an intravenous infusion of sodium nitroprusside can be used to control blood pressure. Magnesium is also an effective therapy for maintaining blood pressure control.

Post-operative care is as for any major abdominal surgery with continuous monitoring of fluid balance, blood pressure, and heart rate. Removal of the catecholamine source during surgery can cause hypovolaemic collapse unless the patient has been well prepared with α- and β-blockade. If this occurs, large volumes of fluid may need to be infused rapidly to restore blood pressure. Post-operative hypotension can also occur from the persisting action of antihypertensive agents used in the pre- and peri-operative period and the adrenoceptor downregulation resulting from chronically high levels of circulating catecholamines. Norepinephrine may be required in the early post-operative period. Hypoglycaemia can occur and blood glucose levels should be monitored regularly.

Disorders of the adrenal cortex

Disorders causing adrenal insufficiency can be classified as follows.

- Primary causes—autoimmune disease, congenital adrenal hyperplasia, adrenal adenoma, tuberculosis, AIDS, metastatic disease, sarcoidosis.
- Secondary causes—impairment of the pituitary gland (e.g. cancer, head injury, hypopituitarism) resulting in deficiency of ACTH.
- Tertiary causes—disease of the hypothalamus resulting in a deficiency of corticotrophin releasing factor.

Addison's disease (primary adrenal insufficiency)

This results from a chronic deficiency of cortical hormones. Symptoms tend to develop insidiously and reflect the lack of cortisol, aldosterone, and androgens (see Box 14.4).

Treatment of Addison's disease is by lifelong cortical hormone replacement therapy. Maintenance therapy consists of hydrocortisone, usually 20 mg in the morning and 10 mg in the evening. The difference in the 12-hourly dose reflects the normal diurnal variation in secretion of cortisol. Fludrocortisone may be added if a mineralocorticoid effect is required. This is a synthetic form of aldosterone given as a single dose in the morning (usually 0.05–0.3 mg). Dosages are prescribed according to plasma urea and electrolytes, and lying and standing blood pressure.

In a healthy subject, cortisol levels are increased in times of stress (e.g. surgery, trauma, infection). However, a patient with Addison's disease is unable to increase secretion of cortisol, and maintenance therapy is adequate only for normal states. Thus their usual dose of hydrocortisone must be increased.

Addisonian crisis

If an acute demand for cortisol cannot be met, an Addisonian crisis may develop. It may occur as a result of previously undiagnosed Addison's disease, a disease process suddenly affecting adrenal function (e.g. adrenal haemorrhage), an intercurrent problem (e.g. infection or trauma) in a patient known to have Addison's disease, or the sudden withdrawal of long-term steroids. It is one of the most life threatening of the endocrine emergencies, and the patient will progress to complete circulatory collapse unless prompt treatment is instituted. The signs and symptoms of an Addisonian crisis result mainly from the deficiency of aldosterone:

- hypovolaemia
- hypotension

Box 14.4 Signs and symptoms of Addison's disease

- Fatigue, muscle weakness, joint pain, weight loss, fever, headache, sweating
- Nausea, vomiting, diarrhoea, hyperpigmentation of the skin
- Mood and personality changes, orthostatic hypotension

- tachycardia, arrhythmias
- hypoglycaemia
- hyponatraemia
- hyperkalaemia
- hypercalcaemia
- confusion, psychosis, slurred speech
- syncope
- severe lethargy
- fever
- convulsions.

Immediate management of an Addisonian crisis.

- Correct hypovolaemia—urgent rehydration with colloid followed by 0.9% sodium chloride (3–4 L will often be required over the first few hours). Central venous or cardiac output monitoring is often necessary to monitor the response and to titrate fluid requirements accurately.
- Correct hypoglycaemia.
- Cortisol administration—intravenous hydrocortisone must be administered without delay. A blood sample should be taken (before treatment is instituted) for baseline plasma cortisol levels. Hydrocortisone 100–200 mg four times daily. (or dexamethasone 4 mg four times daily) should be given intravenously for the immediate crisis, followed after stabilization by an oral maintenance regimen of twice daily hydrocortisone ± fludrocortisone.
- Correct electrolyte imbalance.
- Identify and treat the precipitating cause of the crisis.

Nursing management

- **Problem** Cardiovascular instability (hypotension, tachycardia, arrhythmias) due to hypovolaemia and/or electrolyte imbalance.
  - **Management** Continuous ECG monitoring—12-lead ECG. Monitor serum electrolytes (particularly potassium, sodium, and calcium) regularly. Administer IV fluids according to monitored variables. If hypotension or low cardiac output persists after adequate rehydration, inotropic or pressor agents may be required (remember that the precipitating cause of the crisis may be sepsis).
- **Problem** Oliguria due to hypotension and dehydration.
  - **Management** The patient should be catheterized and urine output measured hourly. Long periods of hypotension and hypovolaemia may precipitate renal failure. Oliguria should improve as the patient is rehydrated and becomes normotensive. Monitor blood urea and electrolytes.
- **Problem** Respiratory failure (due to convulsions/underlying condition).
  - **Management** Respiratory failure is not directly caused by an Addisonian crisis but may result from the underlying cause (e.g. chest infection, pulmonary embolus). Oxygen requirements and ventilatory support will be dictated by the patient's condition and blood gas analysis. There may be an increased sensitivity to opiates and sedatives in patients with Addison's disease; these should be used with caution in the spontaneously breathing patient.
- **Problem** Hypoglycaemia.
  - **Management** Regular monitoring of blood glucose. Continuous infusions of 10% or 20% glucose may be required. Administer IV boluses of hypertonic glucose (20% or 50%) as required. Aim for blood glucose levels of 5–9 mmol/L.
- **Problem** Pyrexia (if infection is the cause of the crisis).
- **Management** Monitor core temperature. Identify the source of infection by appropriate cultures. Give antibiotics as indicated. Cool the patient (e.g. fanning, tepid sponging, antipyretics) and aim for temperature <37.5°C.

While Addisonian crisis is rare, it should be considered in a shocked patient who is resistant to conventional treatment and where the cause cannot be identified.

The thyroid gland

The thyroid gland has two lobes situated either side of the larynx and trachea, and joined at the midline by an isthmus. It produces three active hormones: thyroxine, triiodothyronine, and calcitonin.

Thyroid hormones

Thyroxine (T_4) and triiodothyronine (T_3) are synthesized from iodide and the amino acid tyrosine, and stored as thyroglobulin. Thyroglobulin is released into the blood under the influence of thyroid-stimulating hormone (TSH) released from the anterior pituitary gland. T_4 dissociates from the thyroglobulin, while T_3 is formed by cleavage of one iodine atom from T_4 by a deiodinase enzyme. Most T_3 and T_4 is bound to circulating plasma proteins, mainly thyroxine-binding globulin (TBG); the remainder circulates free in the plasma. Free T_3 and T_4 can diffuse out of the vascular spaces and be metabolically effective. T_3 and T_4 are virtually identical, but T_3 is much more potent, has a shorter duration, and is present in smaller amounts than T_4. The normal level of plasma T_4 is 60–150 nmol/L and that of T_3 is 1–3 nmol/L.

Reverse T_3 (rT_3) is also produced by deiodination of T_4 but here a different iodine atom is cleaved off. Reverse T_3 is not physiologically active and its production prevents excess catabolism. Levels of rT_3 are elevated during critical illness (e.g. burns, sepsis) and are related to a poor outcome.

Both T_3 and T_4 regulate the metabolic rate of all body tissues. They direct growth, tissue differentiation, and mental and physical development. A third hormone, calcitonin, is also secreted by the thyroid gland and is responsible for lowering the serum calcium level. This is achieved by reducing the rate of calcium release from bone, removing calcium from the extracellular fluid by increasing calcium deposition in bone, and reducing the rate of formation of new osteoclasts. Calcitonin can correct high serum calcium levels fairly quickly, and its secretion is enhanced when blood calcium levels are elevated. Calcitonin is used for short-term control of hypercalcaemia, while parathormone is used for longer-term regulation (see section on 'Hormonal control').

Regulation of T_3 and T_4

The hypothalamus and anterior pituitary control the release of T_3 and T_4 by a negative feedback mechanism (see Figure 14.1).

The anterior pituitary is stimulated to synthesize and secrete thyroid-stimulating hormone (TSH) by thyrotrophin-releasing hormone (TRH) produced by the hypothalamus. TSH stimulates the thyroid gland to synthesize and secrete the thyroid hormones T_3 and T_4. In turn, the secretion of T_3 and T_4 inhibits the release of further TSH. In hypothyroidism (where there is insufficient T_3 and T_4) the cause can be at the level of the hypothalamus, the anterior pituitary, or the thyroid gland itself (see Box 14.5).

Investigations of thyroid function (TSH, T_3, T_4) determine at which level the cause of hypothyroidism is to be found. Serum TSH is increased in primary hypothyroidism (the pituitary gland is trying to stimulate the underactive thyroid), but decreased in secondary and tertiary hypothyroidism. In hyperthyroidism the serum TSH is decreased if there is primary thyroid overproduction, and increased if a pituitary tumour is responsible.

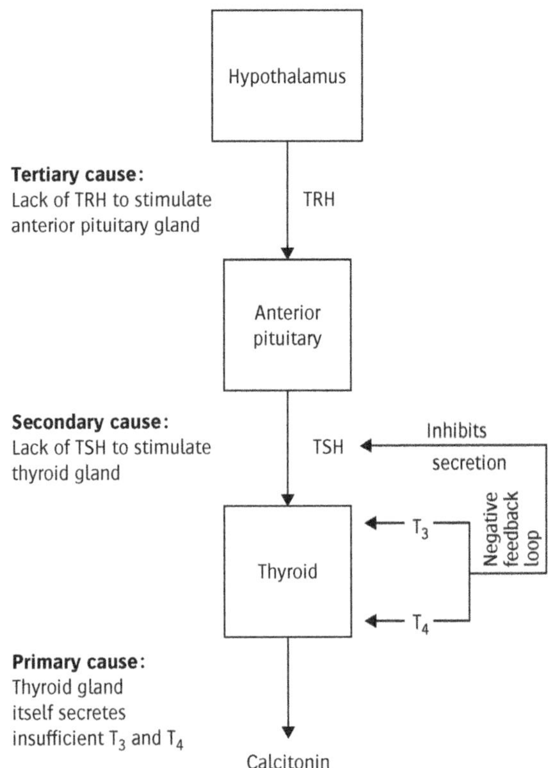

Figure 14.1 Diagram showing negative feedback control of thyroid hormones.

TRH can be given intravenously and the TSH response measured. In pituitary hyperthyroidism there is a high basal level of TSH and a very marked increase in response to TRH. If hypothyroidism is caused by pituitary or hypothalamic disease there may be a reduction in response.

> **Box 14.5 Classification of hypothyroidism**
>
> - Primary—due to disease of the thyroid gland
> - Secondary—where the anterior pituitary secretes insufficient TSH
> - Tertiary—where the hypothalamus secretes insufficient TRH

Disorders of the thyroid gland

Hypothyroidism (myxoedema)

This results from decreased thyroid hormone secretion. Causes include previous thyroid surgery, ^{131}I therapy for hyperthyroidism, viral and autoimmune causes, and certain drugs (e.g. carbimazole, amiodarone). The signs and symptoms reflect the lack of thyroid hormone and a hypometabolic state (see Table 14.1). Once identified, hypothyroidism is treated by oral thyroxine (T4) supplements (or, occasionally, intravenous T_3). However, the cause of the disease must be ascertained by appropriate investigations. If the hypothyroid state continues, myxoedema coma can result. Although rare, this necessitates critical care admission.

Myxoedema coma (or crisis)

This severe life-threatening form of decompensated hypothyroidism arises when a patient with long-standing hypothyroidism (which may be undiagnosed or undertreated) encounters an additional significant stress. Infections and discontinuation of thyroid supplements are the major precipitating factors (see Box 14.6).

The low intracellular T_3 leads to cardiogenic shock, respiratory depression, hypothermia and coma. Arrhythmias, hyponatraemia, coagulation disorders, and effusions secondary to increased vascular permeability may also occur.

Table 14.1 Signs and symptoms of hypothyroidism (myxoedema)

Cardiovascular	Bradycardia Decreased cardiac output Decreased cardiac contractility
Central nervous system	Slow mental function Dementia Slowed speech Hoarse voice Fatigue Excessive sleep
Gastro-intestinal tract	Constipation Weight increase
Other	Dry scaly skin Oedema of hands and feet Face puffiness and peri-orbital oedema Coarse, easily broken hair Poor wound-healing Night blindness

Box 14.6 Factors precipitating myxoedema coma

- Hypothermia
- Infection/systemic illness
- Trauma/burns
- Cerebrovascular accident
- Myocardial infarction
- Congestive cardiac failure
- Drugs with an anti-thyroid action (e.g. lithium and amiodarone)
- Hypoglycaemia
- Gastrointestinal haemorrhage
- CO_2 retention/respiratory acidosis

Treatment of myxoedema coma

The aims of treatment are to:

- support vital functions
- identify precipitating factors
- return to the euthyroid state.

Support of vital functions

- **Problem:** Hypotension, low cardiac output, bradycardia, and other arrhythmias. A low T_3 causes depressed cardiac function with vasoconstriction, decreased contractility, and a slow heart rate. This may result in cardiogenic shock which may be unresponsive to vasopressors without replacement of thyroid hormone and glucocorticosteroids if there is concomitant adrenal insufficiency.
  - **Management:** Continuous ECG monitoring. Observe and treat arrhythmias—bundle branch blocks, complete heart block, and non-specific ST segment changes can occur. No specific treatment is usually required for bradycardia, as the heart rate should increase once treatment is instituted. Perform a 12-lead ECG and measure serum troponin to exclude myocardial infarction. Monitor arterial blood pressure and treat hypotension initially with IV fluid; sodium chloride 0.9% is used if the patient is hyponatraemic. These patients are usually elderly and may have compromised cardiac function; therefore fluids should be infused cautiously and under appropriate monitoring. Central venous ± cardiac output monitoring may be useful, particularly if the patient has existing cardiac disease. Pericardial effusion is a recognized problem and may progress to cardiac tamponade.

- **Problem**: Respiratory failure. This occurs due to decreased central nervous system sensitivity to hypoxia and hypercapnoea. Other contributary factors include respiratory muscle dysfunction, obesity, pleural effusion, and pneumonia.
  - **Management**: Ensure airway is protected. Administer humidified oxygen to maintain adequate oxygenation. Non-invasive ventilation or endotracheal intubation and mechanical ventilation may be required. Antibiotics may be needed to treat infection.
- **Problem**: Hypoglycaemia due to decreased gluconeogenesis.
  - **Management**: Monitor blood sugar regularly. Correct hypoglycaemia with glucose infusions or boluses of 50% glucose as required.
- **Problem**: Hypothermia.
  - **Management**: Monitor core temperature. Rewarm patient (0.5–1°C/h unless very hypothermic) using a rewarming blanket and, if necessary, warming IV infusion fluids. Be aware that the accompanying vasodilatation may cause hypotension. Nurse in a warm environment and warm humidified oxygen if administered. Observe ECG for potential arrhythmias while rewarming. Hyperlactataemia is often present due to hypoperfusion of tissues. This should resolve as the patient is rehydrated, rewarmed, and adequately oxygenated.
- **Problem**: Seizures and decreased level of consciousness Generalized depression of cerebral function, hypoglycaemia, hypoxaemia, hyponatraemia, and reduced cerebral blood flow can precipitate seizures and worsen the level of consciousness.
  - **Management**: Observe and report seizures. Maintain patient safety at all times (cot sides on bed, ensure patent airway during seizures). Monitor serum sodium levels and aim to correct hyponatraemia slowly by IV infusion of 0.9% sodium chloride. If having seizures and serum sodium is <120 mmol/L, more aggressive sodium replacement should be given using frequent small volumes of hypertonic saline. The level of consciousness is always depressed and some patients may be deeply comatose. Regular neurological assessments should be performed. A CT scan should be performed if a cerebrovascular accident is suspected.
- **Problem**: Paralytic ileus due to decreased gut motility.
  - Management: A nasogastric tube should be inserted, regularly aspirated, and left to drain freely.
- **Problem**: Oliguria. Renal function may be severely compromised due to low cardiac output and vasoconstriction causing a low glomerular filtration rate.
  - Management: Maintain adequate blood pressure and cardiac output. Urinary retention can occur, so the bladder should be catheterized and urine output monitored hourly. Oliguria should correct as the patient is rehydrated and normotensive. Monitor and correct serum electrolytes. Renal replacement therapy may be required.

Identify predisposing factors

All potential sites of infection should be cultured (sputum, urine, blood, wounds, etc.). Other precipitating factors, such as hypothermia and trauma, will be obvious. The patient's own drug therapy should be considered as a potential precipitating factor.

Return to the euthyroid state

Thyroxine supplements will be required, but sudden introduction is potentially dangerous as an abrupt increase in metabolism can cause angina, myocardial infarction, and arrhythmias. Many patients with long-term hypothyroidism have ischaemic heart disease to some degree. While oxygen demand to the heart is low in the hypothyroid state, a reduction in blood supply has little effect. However, when thyroid hormone is administered, oxygen demand is increased and requirements may not be met by increased delivery.

Most authorities recommend that small quantities of thyroxine are given initially and then gradually escalated.

If T_4 is administered, it has to be converted to T_3 by the body. This conversion is not efficient in the seriously ill and its half-life in the circulation can be >7 days. T_3 can be administered directly. Its onset of action is also not immediate and may take days to weeks to take effect. It can be given intravenously in slowly increasing doses.

Patients in myxoedema coma usually have an impaired glucocorticoid response to stress since the adrenals share the general hypometabolism of the body. Myxoedema coma may also be secondary to hypopituitarism, in which case there may also be an associated adrenal insufficiency. Corticosteroids (usually IV hydrocortisone 50–100 mg four times daily) are usually given concurrently until adrenal sufficiency can be demonstrated.

Sick euthyroid syndrome

A combination of low TSH, T_3, and T_4 occurs in patients during serious illness that is not caused by primary thyroid or pituitary dysfunction. The progression of thyroid hormone abnormalities generally follows the severity of the underlying illness and can be seen within the first few hours of critical illness. The pathogenesis is multifactorial and includes decreased peripheral conversion of T_4 to T_3, decreased clearance of reverse T_3, and decreased binding of thyroid hormones to thyroxine-binding globulin (TBG).

Interpretation of abnormal thyroid function tests in the critically ill patient is also complicated by the effects of various drugs. Amiodarone impairs peripheral conversion of T_4 to T_3, while dopamine, dobutamine, ocreotide, and high dose corticosteroids depress pituitary secretion of TSH resulting in low serum TSH levels and, subsequently, reduced T_4 secretion. Furosemide and some non-steroidal anti-inflammatory drugs displace T_4 from binding proteins and consequently decrease T_4 levels.

Critically ill patients may manifest many abnormalities mimicking hypothyroidism (e.g. hypothermia, hyponatraemia) that do not reflect actual thyroid pathology. The magnitude of depression of thyroid hormones correlates with the severity of the illness and is associated with a poor prognosis.

Treatment is of the underlying condition; thyroid hormone levels gradually normalize as the patient recovers. It is essential that sick euthyroid syndrome is distinguished from true thyroid disease as thyroid replacement therapy may actually worsen this condition.

Hyperthyroidism (thyrotoxicosis)

Hyperthyroidism results from an excess of T_3 and/or T_4. It may be caused by primary disease of the thyroid gland (e.g. Graves' disease or thyroiditis, or a thyroid adenoma) or can be secondary to a pituitary tumour (where excess TSH is produced) or excess administration of thyroxine.

Effects of hyperthyroidism

These reflect the increase in metabolism caused by the thyroid hormones.

- Cardiovascular:
  - Thyroid hormones increase myocardial contractility and sinoatrial firing, and reduce the electrical threshold of atrial excitation. Sinus tachycardia, atrial fibrillation, or other tachyarrhythmias can develop and may impair cardiac performance.
  - Blood pressure is often elevated, but also may be low if systemic vascular resistance (SVR) is excessively decreased.
  - Cardiac output is increased due to an increase in heart rate and myocardial contractility. This hyperdynamic circulation imposes an increase in cardiac work, which can lead to myocardial hypertrophy as the heart functions near to its limit. Heart failure can result from a combination of reduced myocardial contractile reserve and tachyarrhythmias. 'High output' heart failure can also result from the failure of the heart to meet the excessive metabolic demands of the body.
  - Management of thyrotoxic heart failure is by vasodilation, control of heart rate and any tachyarrhythmia (e.g. with β-blockers—NB: higher than normal doses are often required), and treating the underlying cause of the hyperthyroidism. Remember that amiodarone itself interferes with thyroid hormone metabolism and may cause either hyper- or hypothyroidism.
  - SVR may be decreased. Blood flow is not uniformly distributed in the body; it is greatly increased in the skin, skeletal muscle, and coronary arteries, although not to the cerebral, hepatic, or splanchnic vessels. This may result in a fall in blood pressure.
  - Hyponatraemia and hypovolaemia may result from excess sodium and water loss related to pyrexia, sweating, diarrhoea, etc.
  - Angina may be aggravated due to the increase in myocardial oxygen demand. The risk of thrombosis is also increased in patients with atrial fibrillation and prophylactic anticoagulation should be given.
- Gastrointestinal tract:
  - Nausea, vomiting, diarrhoea (due to increase in gut motility).
  - Weight loss.
- Central nervous system:
  - Nervousness, agitation, confusion.
  - Hyperactivity and tremors.
- Other effects of hyperthyroidism:
  - Frequent micturition.
  - Exophthalmus (see below) and corneal ulceration.
  - Increased body temperature, warm moist skin.
  - Heat intolerance.
  - Goitre (see below) may result in swallowing or breathing difficulties.

Exophthalmus results from an excess growth of tissue and the formation of oedema behind the eye sockets, causing the eyeballs to protrude. The eyelid retracts and the patient cannot lubricate their cornea by blinking. The cornea is then prone to drying and ulceration. Specialist advice should be sought at an early stage if the eyes appear inflamed, as this is a serious complication and can cause blindness.

Goitre is an enlargement of the thyroid gland, which generally becomes visible and palpable though it can enlarge retrosternally. This can be associated with hypothyroidism, hyperthyroidism, or a euthyroid state.A non-toxic goitre occurs when the gland hypertrophies in response to an increase in secretion of TSH secondary to a diminished output of thyroid hormones. In hypothyroidism the thyroid gland enlarges in an attempt to produce adequate quantities of thyroid hormone, while in the euthyroid state a simple non-toxic goitre can result from a dietary lack of iodine.

Some goitres became nodular and can cause hyperthyroidism (toxic goitre) or become malignant. The enlarged gland can also compress the larynx and trachea causing hoarseness of the voice and airway compression with an inspiratory stridor. This may constitute a medical emergency.

Treatment of hyperthyroidism

- Propanolol, metoprolol, esmolol, or other β-blocker agents to reduce sympathetic activity.
- Anti-thyroid drugs. Agents that interfere with the synthesis of thyroid hormones (e.g. carbimazole, propylthiouracil) can be given However, if these are discontinued the underlying hyperthyroidism often returns and permanent treatment (radioactive iodine or surgery) is usually required. Carbimazole can result in agranulocytosis and an increased risk of infection, so the white blood count should be monitored.
- Radioactive iodine (131I). Thyroid cells take up the radioactive iodine and are then destroyed by it. This reduces the vascularity of the gland and hence its size. It is a long-term treatment and results may not be apparent for several months.
- Surgery to remove part of the gland. This is not done as an emergency procedure, but is delayed until metabolic and cardiovascular status have stabilized.

Patients with hyperthyroidism will not usually require critical care admission unless symptoms are severe. Rapid atrial fibrillation may require synchronized cardioversion if unresponsive to anti-arrhythmics. Severe heart failure will also require intensive monitoring.

Thyroid crisis (or thyroid storm)

This exaggerated form of hyperthyroidism occurs acutely, in any age group, and is an extreme life-threatening condition. Advances in diagnostic methods have made this condition very uncommon, and it is usually only seen in patients who have undiagnosed or inadequately treated hyperthyroidism. In these patients a precipitating factor such as infection or trauma is usually required to trigger the acute crisis.

Whatever the predisposing factor, the features and management of the crisis are the same and treatment must be rapid and aggressive. Patients presenting in a thyroid crisis are extremely ill and mortality for this condition remains at 15–20%.

Features of thyroid crisis

- Hyperpyrexia: may be extreme (>40°C) and could be wrongly attributed to sepsis.
- Cardiac failure: often refractory to conventional treatment and may be fatal. Cardiomegaly and ECG changes of left ventricular hypertrophy may be apparent.
- Tachycardia: can be sinus but atrial fibrillation is frequently seen. The heart rate often exceeds 160 bpm and there may also be ventricular arrhythmias.
- Neurological features: extreme agitation, tremors, and confusion which may lead to convulsions and coma.
- Abdominal features: epigastric pain, vomiting and diarrhoea, and, later, liver dysfunction and jaundice.
- Skin: usually hot and moist with increased sweating.

Management of thyroid crisis

- Drug therapy to stop the synthesis of new thyroid hormone, the release of stored hormone from within the thyroid gland, and to prevent the conversion of T_4 to T_3.
  - Iodine (in the form of Lugol's solution or IV potassium iodide) inhibits synthesis and release of thyroxine, reducing the vascularity and size of the thyroid.
  - Drugs such as carbimazole (or propylthiouracil) are used to inhibit the synthesis of T_3 and T_4, and work by blocking the reaction of tyrosine and and iodine.
  - Corticocosteroids (e.g. IV hydrocortisone or dexamethasone) have an inhibitory effect on the conversion of T_4 to T_3 and may also be used to treat a possible coexisting adrenal insufficiency.
  - Cholestyramine (an ion exchange resin) can decreases reabsorption of thyroid hormone from the extra-hepatic circulation. Other therapies such as plasmapheresis and charcoal perfusion can also rapidly reduce plasma thyroid hormone levels.
- β-Adrenergic blockade (e.g. IV propanolol or esmolol) can be used to control the peripheral effects of thyroid hormone. The large quantities of T_3 produced in a thyroid crisis have a similar effect to catecholamines, and are the most commonly used β-adrenergic receptor antagonists. Chlorpromazine or haloperidol are often used in combination for their sedative effect.

- Supportive treatment and the control of cardiovascular manifestations (see below).
- Identification and appropriate treatment of the precipitating cause.

Before treatment begins blood samples should be taken for measurement of TSH, free and total T_3, and T_4. Treatment should not be delayed while results are awaited.

Support of vital functions

- **Problem:** Tachycardia
  - **Management:** Continuous ECG and blood pressure monitoring, 12-lead ECG. Observe for arrhythmias. Atrial fibrillation can be resistant even to large doses of anti-arrhythmics. Serum potassium must be monitored and hypokalaemia corrected, particularly before anti-arrhythmic drugs are given. Administer β-adrenergic blockade, either orally or intravenously according to the severity of illness.
- **Problem:** Heart failure and/or hypovolaemia
  - **Management:** Monitor filling pressures ± cardiac output—there may be considerable fluid loss from sweating, diarrhoea, vomiting, and hyperpyrexia, so hypovolaemia should be corrected. Treatment for heart failure depends on whether it is associated with a 'high' or 'low' cardiac output state. Low output states are managed conventionally with intravenous nitrate infusions, CPAP, etc. For high output states, carefully monitor while giving β-blocker therapy. Hypotension is not usually a problem if cardiac filling pressures are maintained, but continuous BP monitoring should be carried out.
- **Problem:** Pyrexia
  - **Management:** Monitor core temperature. Actively reduce pyrexia by fanning, tepid sponging, cooling blankets, and antipyretics. Salicylates should be avoided as they displace thyroid hormones from their binding proteins, causing an increase in free thyroid hormone.
- **Problem:** Hypoglycaemia
  - **Management:** Monitor blood sugar levels. Give glucose infusions or boluses of 50% glucose as required. Early enteral nutrition should be encouraged, but intestinal absorption is often impaired during a crisis.
- **Problem:** Agitation
  - **Management:** These patients can be very irritable and agitated. Chlorpromazine, haloperidol, or a benzodiazepine should be given as required for sedation. If untreated, convulsions may occur and progress to coma. Observe for seizures; maintain patient safety (cot sides, airway control). Protect patient from additional stresses and nurse in a quiet environment.
- **Problem:** Dyspnoea (secondary to heart failure)
  - **Management:** Monitor respiratory rate and blood gases. Treat heart failure. Administer humidified oxygen therapy as required. CPAP or mechanical ventilation may be required to maintain adequate oxygenation.
- **Problem:** Corneal ulceration due to exophthalmia or lid retraction
  - **Management:** Protect the exposed cornea by frequent application of hypromellose eye drops. Local or systemic steroids may be required for exophthalmos with tarsorraphy (surgical closure of the eyelids) in severe cases. Lid retraction usually responds to treatment of the thyrotoxicosis.

Calcium abnormalities

Calcium is important for a range of functions including vascular tone and permeability, nerve conduction, ventricular contractility and relaxation and blood clotting. There is no direct correlation between the severity of symptoms and the plasma calcium level in hypercalcaemia. Generally, symptoms appear at a level above 3.0 mmol/L (ionized fraction >1.5 mmol/L) and can be fatal above 4–5 mmol/L (ionized fraction 2-2.6 mmol/L). Hypocalcaemia usually becomes symptomatic when levels drop below 1.8 mmol/L (ionized <0.9mmol/L).

Hormonal control

Four parathyroid glands are situated adjacent to the posterior and lateral aspects of the thyroid gland. They produce parathyroid hormone (PTH) which is an important regulator of the plasma calcium level. PTH raises serum calcium and is itself regulated by a negative feedback mechanism so that calcium levels remain constant. PTH and calcitonin (released from the thyroid gland) have opposing effects; together, they maintain a plasma calcium level of 2.15–2.55 mmol/L and an ionized calcium level (non-protein-bound) of 1.18–1.3 mmol/L. Approximately 40% of the calcium is bound to protein (primarily albumin), while 50% is ionized and is in the physiological form. The remaining 10% is complexed to anions. Changes in serum protein concentration alter the total serum calcium level but not the unbound fraction. Laboratories usually report total calcium and give an albumin-corrected value of total calcium, whereas blood gas machines report the ionized fraction, which is more useful in clinical management. PTH increases plasma calcium by increasing renal reabsorption of calcium, release from bone, and absorption from the gut.

Hypercalcaemia

The signs and symptoms of hypercalcaemia are shown in Box 14.7

Management of hypercalcaemia

Symptomatic hypercalcaemia requires immediate treatment and, if severe, admission to the ICU will be necessary for monitoring purposes. The aims of treatment are to:

- lower plasma calcium levels (see Table 14.2)
- monitor and support vital functions
- identify the cause and treat where possible (e.g. malignancy, primary hyperparathyroidism, sarcoidosis).

Box 14.7 Signs and symptoms of hypercalcaemia

- ECG changes: short Q–T interval, prolonged P–R interval, AV block, VF
- Hypertension
- Ureteric stones may form and can lead to obstructive uropathy
- Polyuria, renal failure
- Muscle weakness and general malaise due to neuropathy
- Drowsiness, coma
- Headaches, confusion, myalgia
- Bone pain, joint effusions
- Nausea and vomiting
- Abdominal pain, pancreatitis
- Anorexia, thirst, constipation, peptic ulceration
- Psychiatric disorders

Table 14.2 Methods of reducing plasma calcium levels

Treatment	Reason
Volume replacement followed by low dose loop diuretic (e.g. IV furosemide)	Often volume-depleted due to polyuria. Following rehydration the administration of a low dose diuretic increases renal excretion of calcium. Avoid. thiazide diuretics as they increase reabsorption of calcium.
Glucocorticoid therapy (hydrocortisone or dexamethasone)	Reduces intestinal absorption of calcium.
Bisphosphonates (e.g. pamidronate)	Potent inhibitors of bone resorption and formation, i.e. inhibit osteoclast activity.
Mithromycin (IV)	Inhibits mobilization of calcium from the skeleton. However, cannot be given continuously for more than a few days due to toxicity to bone marrow, liver, and kidney.
Calcitonin (IV or SC)	Inhibits bone reabsorption and increases excretion of calcium. Action seen within a few hours but is short-lived.
Peritoneal dialysis or haemodialysis	Effectively reduces the calcium level and avoids the dangerous side effects of drug therapy. A calcium-free dialysate should be used.

Monitoring and support of vital functions

- **Problem:** Volume loss due to polyuria.
  - **Management:** Monitor filling pressures. Rehydrate using colloid, 0.9% sodium chloride, or Hartmann's solution. Monitor urine output.
- **Problem:** Potential arrhythmias due to hypercalcaemia.
  - **Management:** Continuous ECG monitoring. Observe for and treat arrhythmias. Note that hypercalcaemia enhances the action of digoxin and can cause digoxin toxicity (particularly if there is concurrent renal impairment).
- **Problem:** Potential renal failure due to renal tubular damage or (long-term) stone formation/nephrocalcinosis.
  - **Management:** Monitor urine output, plasma urea and electrolytes, arterial pH, and bicarbonate. Renal replacement therapy if required.

Box 14.8 Signs and symptoms of hypocalcaemia

- Tetany, muscle twitching, tremors, facial spasms
- Brocho- or laryngospasm
- Paraesthesiae (tingling) of extremities and mouth
- ECG changes: prolonged Q–T interval
- Muscle weakness
- Hypotension
- Convulsions
- Confusion, psychosis, fatigue, anxiety

- **Problem:** Hypertension due to hypercalcaemia.
  - **Management:** Correct hypercalcaemia. Monitor blood pressure. Antihypertensive therapy (e.g. calcium antagonists) if necessary.

Hypocalcaemia

Box 14.8 lists the signs and symptoms of hypocalcaemia.

Management of hypocalcaemia

Tetany is the major symptom, with the patient usually complaining of numbness, stiffness, tremor, or tingling in the hands and feet. This can progress to generalized muscle hypertonia causing spasmodic and uncoordinated muscle contractions, particularly of the elbows, wrist, and carpophalangeal joints (carpopedal spasm). If untreated, this can progress to photophobia, bronchospasm, laryngeal spasm, cardiac arrhythmias, dysphagia, and, ultimately, convulsions. There may also be psychiatric disturbances such as anxiety, irritability, and neuroses.

Hypocalcaemia is generally better tolerated than hypercalcaemia; however, the onset of tetany or myocardial dysfunction requires rapid treatment. This is relatively easy to correct by administration of calcium salts. If hypocalcaemia is symptomatic, this is done by intravenous injection of 10–20 ml of 10% calcium chloride or calcium gluconate. If asymptomatic, calcium supplements can be given orally (e.g. calcium gluconate tablets (Sandocal)).

Note that hypermagnesaemia (e.g. from excess diuretics, diarrhoea) may also cause a resistant hypocalcaemia which does, however, respond to magnesium replacement.

Nursing management

- **Problem:** Neuromuscular instability/anxiety.
  - **Management:** Reassure patient and use calm manner. Nurse in an environment with minimum noise and avoid bright lights. Protect patient from injury (padded cot sides, remove articles that may cause harm). Anticonvulsive therapy may be required.
- **Problem:** Potential cardiac arrhythmias.
  - **Management:** Continuous ECG monitoring. Note that calcium potentiates the effect of digoxin and both increase systolic contractions. Observe for arrhythmias and monitor blood pressure.

Hypocalcaemia associated with critical illness

There are many reasons why critically ill patients develop hypocalcaemia including acute or chronic renal failure, hypomagnesaemia, hypoalbuminaemia, medications, pancreatitis or transfusions with citrated blood. Hypocalcaemia can also occur with sepsis.

Disorders of the parathyroid glands

Hyperparathyroidism

Excess parathyroid hormone (PTH) causes hypercalcaemia and hypophosphataemia as PTH also causes increased excretion of phosphate ions by the kidney). Causes include primary (e.g. due to a parathyroid adenoma), secondary (in response to hypocalcaemia resulting from another disease (usually chronic renal failure), and tertiary where longstanding secondary hyperparathyroidism can lead to autonomous function in one or more parathyroid adenomas. Treatment is by the management of hypercalcaemia (see Table 14.2) and, for primary hyperparathyroidism, parathyroidectomy. Calcium levels should be monitored carefully postoperatively as short term hypocalcaemia can result.

Hypoparathyroidism

This is caused by insufficient secretion of parathyroid hormone and may be due to primary idiopathic and autoimmune disease, or secondary to parathyroid surgery or total thyroidectomy. Hypocalcaemia and hyperphosphataemia are usually present.

The pancreas

The pancreas secretes insulin and glucagon from the islets of Langerhans. Insulin is secreted by β cells, and glucagon by α cells. Both hormones have profound effects upon metabolism.

Insulin

The functions of insulin are shown in Box 14.9.

Insulin secretion

Insulin is secreted from the pancreas as a direct effect of raised levels of glucose on the β cells. As insulin facilitates transport of glucose into cells, the glucose level falls and secretion is inhibited (negative feedback mechanism).

Glucagon

Many of the actions of glucagon are opposite to those of insulin and its effect is to raise the blood glucose level. This is achieved by causing the breakdown of stored glycogen (glycogenolysis) and converting proteins into glucose (gluconeogenesis). Glucagon secretion is stimulated when the α cells detect subnormal blood glucose levels. Once released, glucagon causes blood glucose levels to rise within minutes as glucose is released from stored glycogen. As the blood glucose rises to normal, glucagon secretion is inhibited. By the opposing actions of insulin and glucagon, blood glucose levels are kept within a fairly constant range.

Diabetes

Diabetes mellitus

Hyperglycaemia occurs due to deficiency, destruction (due to antibodies), or impaired effectiveness of insulin. There are two types.

- Type 1: insulin-dependent diabetes mellitus. This accounts for approximately 10% of diabetes and usually has its onset in childhood or adolescence. It results from an autoimmune destruction of the β cells in the pancreas and usually leads to absolute insulin deficiency. There may be a genetic predisposition and an identifiable viral trigger (e.g. Coxsackie B, mumps). The condition may present acutely as hyperglycaemic ketoacidosis. Lifelong insulin therapy will be required.
- Type 2: non-insulin-dependent diabetes mellitus. This usually affects those over 40 and tends to occur in the overweight. It encompasses individuals who have insulin resistance and usually have relative (rather than absolute) insulin deficiency. Patients are often asymptomatic and may first present with related complications. This type of diabetes is usually controlled by a combination of diet, weight loss (if appropriate), and oral hypoglycaemic drugs.

Secondary diabetes (insulin resistance)

This occurs secondary to drug therapy, metabolic/endocrine disease, or critical illness, and includes gestational diabetes. The term 'insulin resistance' is usually applied to these states and may be due to problems of decreased secretion, decreased responsiveness of cellular insulin receptors, or modification of pathways further downstream. Increased release of stress hormones (e.g. cortisol, catecholamines, glucagon, growth hormone) also antagonize insulin's metabolic actions (see Box 14.10).

Diabetic emergencies

There are three main diabetic emergencies:

- diabetic ketoacidosis (DKA) characterized by hyperglycaemia, ketosis, and acidosis, often with coma

Box 14.9 Functions of insulin

- Promotes transport of glucose into cells, and hence lowers blood glucose level
- Converts glucose into fat
- Promotes glycogen storage in liver and muscle cells
- Inhibits fat metabolism
- Promotes tissue growth by protein deposition

Box 14.10 Causes of insulin resistance

- Drugs: glucocorticoids, epinephrine, thiazide diuretics, thyroid hormones, oral contraceptives
- Metabolic/endocrine: Cushing's syndrome, Conn's syndrome (primary hyperaldosteronism), phaeochromocytoma
- Other: acute or chronic pancreatitis, pancreatic cancer, pregnancy, 'stress' (e.g. sepsis), major trauma, burns, head injury

- hyperosmolar hyperglycaemic states (HHS) usually characterized by hyperglycaemia but with minimal or no ketosis, often accompanied by profound coma (hyperosmolar non-ketotic coma)
- hypoglycaemic coma.

Diabetic ketoacidosis

Approximately a third of patients presenting with DKA are newly diagnosed. Causes include infection, myocardial infarction, or, commonly, non-compliance with treatment. Coma is not always a feature and the conscious level varies according to the,degree of increased plasma osmolality. Hyperglycaemia (see Box 14.11) and ketosis are always features of DKA, though the blood sugar level does not have to be particularly elevated. The diagnostic criteria include ketonaemia 3 mmol/L or >2+ ketones on standard urine testing, venous bicarbonate <15 mmol/L and/or venous pH < 7.3, and blood glucose levels >11 mmol/L or known diabetes mellitis (Savage *et al.* 2011).

This condition can be life-threatening even if the patient is not comatose. The UK mortality rate is reported as approximately 2%. Cerebral oedema is the most common cause of death (particularly in children), while hypokalaemia, ARDS, and comorbidities (such as pneumonia, myocardial infarction, and sepsis) are associated with increased mortality.

Principal features of DKA

- **Hyperglycaemia** Insulin facilitates transfer of glucose into cells. Therefore lack of insulin results in an inability to utilize glucose derived from carbohydrate metabolism. Other 'stress' hormones, such as epinephrine, norepinephrine, glucagon, cortisol, and growth hormone, are also released in stress states and their antagonistic action against insulin further exacerbates the hyperglycaemia.
- **Volume loss** When the blood glucose concentration exceeds the renal threshold (approximately 8.5–10.5 mmol/L), the kidney does not reabsorb excess glucose which is then excreted in the urine. An osmotic diuresis results and large volumes of water and electrolytes are lost. The patient experiences extreme thirst and becomes polydipsic but nevertheless still rapidly dehydrates. Dehydration initially depletes the intracellular compartment as this is the largest of the body's fluid spaces. Initially there is little effect on the intravascular volume, but as the fluid loss becomes more severe, the intravascular volume falls and the patient can progresses to hypovolaemic shock. Fluid may be lost not only through an osmotic diuresis but also via hyperventilation, nausea, vomiting, sweating, and fever. There may be decreased fluid intake due to coma.
- **Electrolyte loss** This is associated with polyuria and, in particular, sodium, potassium, phosphate, and magnesium ions are lost. Hypokalaemia can be a fatal complication resulting from haemodilution following fluid resuscitation, the correction of hyperglycaemia by insulin infusion (shifting the potassium into the cells), and through inadequate potassium replacement. However, the serum potassium may be elevated on patient admission because of the extracellular shift of potassium caused by insulin deficiency, hypertonicity, and acidaemia. Patients with a low or normal serum potassium on admission have a severe total body potassium debt and require vigorous potassium replacement. Low serum concentrations of potassium and magnesium can cause cardiac arrhythmias or asystole, particularly if there is pre-existing cardiac disease.
- **Ketoacidosis** As the patient cannot utilize glucose derived from dietary carbohydrate because of insufficient insulin, energy is increasingly provided by fat breakdown (lipolysis). Some of the free fatty acids released by lipolysis are converted into ketone bodies by the liver (acetone, acetoacetate, and 3-β-hydroxybutyrate), and these can cause a profound metabolic acidosis. The patient compensates for this acidosis by hyperventilation (Kussmaul respiration).

Management of DKA

While hospital guidelines usually recommend rigid regimens of fluid and insulin, it is important to recognize that patients may vary markedly in their degree of hypovolaemia, blood glucose levels, and level of

Box 14.11 Signs and symptoms of hyperglycaemia

- Restlessness
- Thirst
- Vomiting
- Abdominal pain
- Hot, dry, flushed skin
- Drowsiness
- Tachycardia
- Deep sighing respiration (Kussmaul)
- Hypotension
- Coma

consciousness. They may also have an underlying condition, such as sepsis, which has triggered the illness or an important comorbidity such as renal failure or cardiac impairment. Therefore a fixed volume and rate of fluid infusion may lead to considerable iatrogenic harm. Thus resuscitation must be guided by measured cardiovascular variables and the response to treatment. The patient requires intensive monitoring (usually a central venous line and, if indicated by the precipitating condition or past medical history, cardiac output monitoring with frequent reassessment).

Nursing management

- **Problem:** Inadequate airway protection due to decreased level of consciousness.
  - **Management:** Ensure patent and protected airway—endotracheal intubation may be necessary. Mechanical ventilation may be needed for deeply comatose patients or for concurrent lung pathology. A nasogastric tube should be inserted as gastric atony, which is associated with DKA, increases the risk of pulmonary aspiration. Observe the respiratory rate and pattern. Monitor blood gases and give oxygen therapy as indicated. Note that elderly patients may have underlying respiratory disease or may have been immobile at home prior to admission, thus increasing the risk of atelectasis or infection (this may also be a precipitating factor), or thromboembolism.
- **Problem:** Hypovolaemia due to fluid depletion.
  - **Management:** This must be promptly corrected, particularly in patients with pre-existing renal dysfunction where adequate organ perfusion must be maintained. Care should be taken not to overload the patient, especially if there is a pre-existing history of cardiac disease. Monitor blood pressure and filling pressures ± cardiac output. Average fluid requirements will be 5–10 L in the first 24 hours, but replacement should be governed by filling pressure or stroke volume measurement. Fluid is not lost equally from the three body spaces—intracellular space (ICS), interstitial space (ISS), and intravascular space (IVS). Fluid is initially lost from the largest space (ICS) and least of all from the IVS. Therefore it is logical to rehydrate using a fluid similar in sodium concentration to the fluid lost (e.g. 0.9% sodium chloride or Hartmann's solution). If fluid loss is more severe and has caused hypovolaemia and shock (hypotension, tachycardia, low filling pressures), considerable fluid has also been lost from the IVS. The circulating fluid must be rapidly replaced with either a colloid (e.g. gelatin, albumin) or a salt-containing crystalloid solution to restore the circulating blood volume. Cardiovascular variables must be continuously monitored. The rate of fluid infusion can be gauged by measuring the variables before and after 200 ml aliquots and assessing the response (see Box 14.12).

The choice of fluid used for replacement is controversial. While 0.9% sodium chloride has been the mainstay of therapy for decades, the excessive chloride it contains (154 mmol/L compared with a normal plasma chloride range of 95–105 mmol/L) can result in a rapid-onset hyperchloraemic metabolic acidosis. The unwary practitioner may then treat the unresolving or even worsening acidosis with even more normal saline, thus exacerbating the problem. Hartmann's solution, which contains lactate and a more physiological level of chloride, is a more appropriate fluid, though potassium supplementation will need to be given separately. Guidelines still suggest empirical regimens such as a litre of fluid in the first 30 min, then a litre in the next hour, then a litre in the next two hours, etc. However, a more logical approach, especially in a monitored critical care environment, is to

Box 14.12 A summary of suggested fluid replacement for DKA in a critical care environment

- If the patient is hypovolaemic and shocked, rapidly restore intravascular volume using colloid or salt-containing crystalloid (e.g. normal saline, Hartmann's solution) to acceptable levels of heart rate, blood pressure, filling pressures, and (if monitored) stroke volume.
- Thereafter replace total body fluid deficit with Hartmann's solution or normal saline (e.g. 150–200 ml/h). Infusion rates of fluid should be adjusted according to monitored parameters. Beware of hyperchloraemic metabolic acidosis if using normal saline. Hypotonic (0.45%) saline may be needed if the plasma sodium level rises excessively.
- Switch to 10% glucose (e.g. 100 ml/h) when the blood sugar level is <10 mmol/L.

NB: If following a fixed-rate fluid regimen recommended in diabetic emergencies guidelines, beware of fluid overload, heart failure, and pulmonary oedema, particularly in patients with imparied cardiorespiratory reserve.

manage the fluid balance as for any other ICU patient, with initial rapid infusion as needed to correct hypovolaemia and then a steady background infusion (e.g. 150–200 ml/h) to gradually replete total body fluid volume.

Once glucose levels are corrected to normogylcaemia (<10 mmol/L), by which time the sodium debt has been largely replaced, the type of fluid is usually switched over to 10% glucose until the patient is take food and drink enterally.

Total body water losses are difficult to assess and will differ with each patient. If intravascular replacement needs are high, then water loss will generally be high.

A urinary catheter will usually need to be inserted and urine output should be measured hourly. Persisting hypotension and/or oliguria is not automatically due to hypovolaemia. Care should be taken to give adequate but not excessive fluid replacement.

- **Problem:** Hyperglycaemia.
  - **Management:** The adminstration of intravenous insulin should be as per local unit protocol. The Joint British Diabetes Societies guidelines (Savage *et al.* 2011) recommend a fixed rate IV infusion at a rate of 0.1 units/kg/h. However, the rate of insulin should be regularly reviewed as blood glucose levels should not fall abruptly. This increases the risk of cerebral oedema, particularly in children and young adults, due to rapid changes in osmolality. The ideal rate of fall in glucose level is 3 mmol/L/h. If blood ketones are measured, this should also ideally fall by at least 0.5 mmol/L/h. Thus, rapid correction of hyperglycaemia must be avoided and the aim should be to achieve a gradual smooth reduction of serum glucose. An initial intravenous bolus of insulin is unnecessary if the insulin infusion is started promptly. If the patient is on a long-acting insulin, this can be continued subcutaneously once the patient is resucitated (it will be poorly absorbed in a hypoperfused patient) and the short-acting insulin restarted once glycaemic control has been achieved and the patient is eating/drinking normally. Urine should be tested regularly for ketones and glucose.
- **Problem:** Electrolyte depletion due to polyuria.
  - **Management:** Continuous ECG monitoring; observe for arrhythmias. With the accompanying acidosis the patient is usually hyperkalaemic, though total body potassium is depleted. The potassium level may fall rapidly with insulin and fluid. Thus blood levels should be monitored one- to two-hourly and maintained between 4.0 and 5.3 mmol/L. Give IV supplements accordingly (usually 5–20 mmol/h is required). Higher infusion rates are occasionally needed but there is an increased risk of cardiac arrhythmias or asystole with rapid changes in plasma potassium level. Plasma magnesium levels should be measured on admission and then daily until normal. The osmotic diuresis of DKA results in large losses of magnesium. Supplements can be given IV if the patient is hypomagnesaemic normalized. Plasma phosphate levels may also be low and supplementation may be considered.
- **Problem:** Metabolic acidosis due to ketosis.
  - **Management:** Measure arterial pH, bicarbonate, and base excess/deficit hourly initially. IV sodium bicarbonate is not recommended because of the dangers of paradoxical intracellular acidosis, sodium overload, and rebound alkalosis. The acidosis usually corrects naturally with insulin therapy and fluid replacement. As mentioned earlier, excess normal saline can cause a hyperchloraemic metabolic acidosis. Monitoring of blood or urine ketones can be undertaken at the bedside
- **Problem:** Increased risk of thromboembolism due to dehydration, immobility, and possible pre-existing vascular disease.
  - **Management:** Observe for thrombotic episodes (DVT, pulmonary embolus). Give prophylactic subcutaneous heparin.
- **Problem:** Precipitating factor.
  - **Management:** The cause of the DKA should be identified and treated appropriately. Potential sites of infection (urine, sputum, wounds, etc.) should be cultured. A 12-lead ECG should be taken to exclude a myocardial infarction.

Hyperosmolar hyperglycaemic states (HHS)

HHS typically occurs in older patients with diabetes mellitus (usually Type 2, but often undiagnosed) and develops over a period of days to weeks. Often a predisposing factor such as infection triggers the condition, in particular those that cause considerable fluid loss (e.g. diarrhoea). Such illnesses can cause severe dehydration, resulting in oliguria which prevents glucose excretion by the kidneys, thus exacerbating hyperglycaemia. Patients with pre-existing renal dysfunction and/or congestive cardiac failure are at increased risk.

HHS is characterized by hyperglycaemia, hyperosmolarity, and dehydration but, unlike DKA, patients do not develop a significant ketoacidosis as there is continued secretion of small amounts of insulin. This reduces the availability of the free fatty acids which are needed to produce ketones.

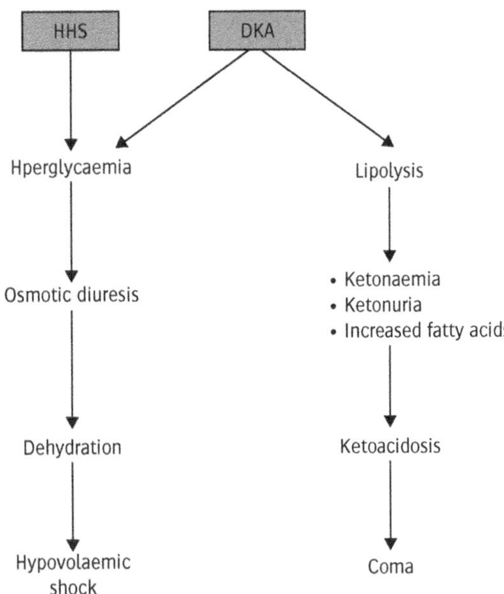

Figure 14.2 Diagram showing the effects of HHS and DKA.

Mortality (10–20%) is higher than for DKA and death is usually as a consequence of the underlying precipitating cause or pulmonary embolism secondary to immobility and blood hyperviscosity (see Figure 14.2).

Management of HHS

The management is similar to that for DKA, although there are some principal differences as detailed in the following.

1. **Neurological/respiratory care** The incidence of coma is higher than in DKA (approximately 10%) but may last longer (up to a week). Therefore active management is usually longer. Airway maintenance and prevention of pneumonia are paramount. Early endotracheal intubation may be needed for airway protection, tracheal toilet, and intensive physiotherapy. There may be a higher incidence of chest infection in these patients since they are usually elderly, and have been immobile or semi-comatose prior to admission for an extended period. Whereas patients with DKA often do not require supplemental oxygen, patients with HHS are often hypoxaemic and may benefit from mask CPAP or BiPAP if intubation is not required. Be aware that respiratory complications may worsen, or develop, as the patient is rehydrated (e.g. ARDS, pulmonary oedema). Hyperventilation is not a major feature of HHS since the acidosis, if present, is usually mild.
2. **Neurological monitoring** should be carried out if the patient's mental staus is impaired. Phenytoin is not usually used if seizures occur as it inhibits endogenous insulin secretion and is generally ineffective in patients with HHS.
3. **Insulin therapy** is the same as for management of DKA, but patients with HHS are often more sensitive to insulin. Lower infusion rates (e.g. 1–2 units/h) are started initially and altered as needed to ensure a slow steady decline (approximately 2–3 mmol/L/hour) and avoid any rapid fall. Monitor serum glucose carefully.
4. **Fluid replacement** Dehydration is often more severe than in DKA and the patient is more likely to be hypovolaemic and shocked. However, the same principles of fluid replacement apply. Treat severe hypovolaemia to restore an adequate circulating blood volume and then, more gradually, replace the total body fluid deficit. The rate of overall rehydration should be slower than for DKA because of the danger of rapid intracerebral fluid shifts precipitating cerebral oedema. The plasma sodium level is often elevated and, despite appropriate treatment, may even continue to rise for a few days, sometimes exceeding 170 mmol/L. However, the total body sodium is grossly depleted so the patient usually requires either 0.9% or 0.45% saline, or Hartmann's solution, for electrolyte replacement. Potassium supplementation is also necessary to correct the large potassium deficit. Particular care must be paid to titrating fluid replacement against cardiovascular variables since these patients are often elderly and may have existing cardiac or renal dysfunction.
5. **Anticoagulation** Pulmonary embolus and other thromoembilic events (e.g. coronary, cerebral, mesenteric) are considered to be the major causes of morbidity and mortality in these patients. They arise due to prolonged immobility and the hyperviscosity of the circulating blood. Most authorities recommend anticoagulation with heparin, although whether this should be prophylactic or full-dose therapy is still contentious.

Hypoglycaemic coma

Patients who develop hypoglycaemia are usually known diabetics controlled by insulin or oral sulphonylurea hypoglycaemics (e.g. glibenclamide). Occasionally, fulminant liver failure or, less commonly, Addison's disease or an insulinoma may precipitate hypoglycaemia.

Hypoglycaemic symptoms (see Box 14.13) result from a low blood glucose level. This may be caused by insulin overdose (deliberate or accidental) or when the diabetic

Box 14.13 Sign and symptoms of hypoglycaemia

- Headache
- Hunger
- Faintness
- Cool, moist skin
- Sweating
- Slurred speech
- Tachycardia/bradycardia
- Irrational behaviour, agitation
- Coma

patient takes excessive exercise, has an inadequate food intake, or ingests excess alcohol.

The onset of coma is usually rapid, but most patients are aware of the onset of symptoms and can prevent an impending hypoglycaemic attack by taking sugar.

Hypoglycaemic patients admitted to the emergency department in coma can easily be diagnosed by bedside blood glucose analysis. Treatment must be rapid as hypoglycaemia can cause irreversible brain damage. Symptoms can be reversed in minutes by the IV administration of aliquots of 20–50 ml of 50% glucose. If venous access proves impossible glucagon 1 mg IM can be given, but this is ineffective in hepatic dysfunction and alcohol ingestion.

Hypoglycaemic patients rarely require ICU care once the coma is reversed, except those patients who have taken an insulin overdose (particularly if a long-acting insulin) or who are in liver failure, where close monitoring of blood glucose levels will be required.

The pituitary gland

The hypothalamus and pituitary gland are anatomically and functionally closely linked. The hypothalamus lies below the third ventricle of the brain and extends down as the pituitary stalk to join the posterior pituitary gland. The anterior pituitary lies adjacent to the posterior pituitary but its secretions and functions are independent. The pituitary stalk contains nerves and capillaries through which hormones produced in the hypothalamus pass for storage in the posterior pituitary gland.

The anterior pituitary gland

Hormones produced by the anterior pituitary include:

- growth hormone (GH)—affects fat, protein, and carbohydrate metabolism
- thyroid-stimulating hormone (TSH)—stimulates the thyroid gland to secrete thyroid hormones
- adrenocorticotrophic hormone (ACTH)—controls the secretion of adrenocortical hormones.
- prolactin—produced during pregnancy and stimulates breast growth and secretory functions.
- gonadotrophic hormones—involved in sexual functions: *in women* follicle-stimulating hormone (stimulates development of follicles in the ovaries) and luteinizing hormone (causes oestrogen and progesterone secretion by the ovaries and allows rupture of follicles); *in men* interstitial cell-stimulating hormone stimulates the testes to produce androgens

The posterior pituitary gland

Two hormones are released from the posterior lobe. These are produced in the hypothalamus and stored in the posterior pituitary gland:

- oxytocin—stimulates contraction of the uterus and the muscles of the milk ducts in the breast.
- antidiuretic hormone (ADH, vasopressin)—stimulates reabsorption of water from the distal tubules of the kidney.

Water balance in the body is regulated by a complex negative feedback system involving thirst, ADH secretion, and the kidney, which maintains plasma osmolality at 275-295 mOsmol/kg. The major stimuli for ADH secretion are as follows.

- Hyperosmolality—sensed by osmoreceptors in the hypothalamus. Normally, ADH secretion ceases when plasma osmolality falls below 275 mOsm/kg. This increases water excretion and produces a dilute urine. When the plasma osmolality rises, ADH is secreted causing increased water reabsorption by the kidney and a more concentrated urine.
- Hypovolaemia—sensed by baroreceptors in the carotid sinus, aortic arch, and left atrium. An 8–10% reduction in blood volume significantly increases ADH secretion.
- ADH secretion is also increased in response to stressful stimuli (pain, anxiety), some drugs (e.g. angiotensin II),

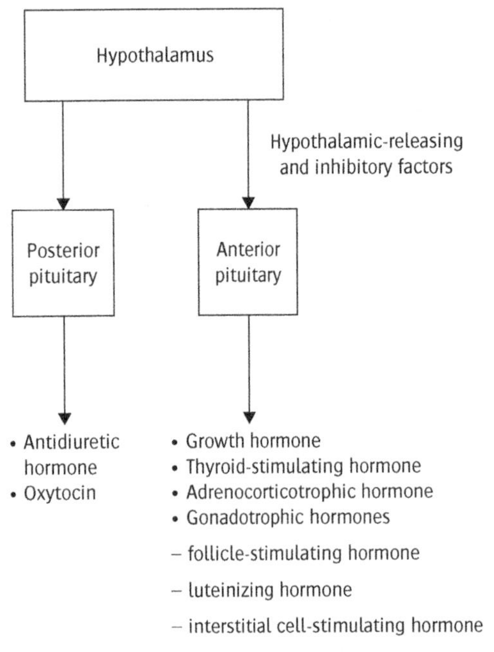

Figure 14.3 Diagram showing the anterior and posterior pituitary hormones.

hyperthermia, exercise, and positive pressure ventilation.

Figure 14.3 shows the hormones secreted by the pituitary gland.

Disorders of the posterior pituitary

Central diabetes insipidus

There are two main forms of diabetes insipidus; central and nephrogenic.

- Central diabetes insipidus results from a lack of ADH causing polyuria and polydipsia. The main causes are after neurosurgery, head trauma, and hypoxic brain injury.
- Nephrogenic diabetes insipidus, on the other hand, is a primary renal tubular defect of water reabsorption in which there is a poor response to ADH. Main causes are drug-induced (e.g. lithium toxicity), and also hypokalaemia and renal disease.

Effects of diabetes insipidus

Failure of adequate secretion of ADH in response to plasma hyperosmolality results in passage of huge volumes of dilute urine (6–30 L/day). If the thirst mechanism or water intake are impaired, the plasma becomes hyperosmotic and hypernatraemic. However, total body sodium is decreased due to renal losses and inadequate intake. Gross dehydration will cause hypovolaemic shock and death. Hypernatraemia can result in delirium, lethargy, convulsions, and coma.

Other causes of polyuria should be excluded by appropriate investigations, particularly hyperglycaemia, recovery from fluid overload, polyuric renal disease, and psychogenic polydipsia.

Box 14.14 Investigations for diagnosis of diabetes insipidus

- Urine specific gravity
- 24-hour urine volume measurement
- Serum urea and electrolytes
- Plasma ADH level
- Simultaneous plasma and urine osmolality

Investigations

Diagnostic investigations are listed in Box 14.14.

Management of diabetes insipidus

Mild polyuria (<250 ml/h) may simply require oral fluid replacement of urine losses. However, if oral intake is inadequate or hypernatraemia is present, losses should be replaced with a crystalloid infusion such as 5% glucose. This replacement fluid should be hypo-osmolar relative to the patient's serum. Hypernatraemia must not be corrected too rapidly; aim to reduce serum sodium by 0.5 mmol/h.

If the urine output persists or is more excessive, specific drug therapy will be required. In central diabetes insipidus, where the primary problem is hormone deficiency, the drug of choice is desmopressin (DDAVP), a synthetic analogue of antidiuretic hormone. It can be given intravenously, subcutaneously, orally, or by nasal inhalation. For nephrogenic diabetes insipidus, any offending drugs should be removed. Non-hormonal drugs can be used for treating this condition, for example non-steroidal anti-inflammatory drugs such as indomethacin or ibuprofen. These inhibit prostaglandin synthesis and reduce the delivery of solute to the distal tubules, thus reducing urine volume and increasing urine osmolality. The dose and frequency depends on the clinical response and can vary. When urine volume has been lowered to about 2 ml/min an infusion of 0.9% sodium chloride should be used to maintain plasma osmolality at 280–300 mOsmol/kg. Measurements of plasma and urine osmolality should be made every 8 hours.

Monitor cardiovascular variables (CVP, BP, heart rate), urine output, serum urea and electrolytes, and glucose (to avoid hyperglycaemia from replacement fluid). Urine specific gravity should be measured regularly. See Chapter 8 for diabetes insipidus in head injury.

Obstetric emergencies

The near-term pregnant patient is unique as the feto-placental unit has major effects on her physiological function. When treating the critically ill pre-term patient, the welfare of the fetus must always be considered, though the mother's life should generally take priority. Pregnancy-associated emergencies that require admission to the ICU are uncommon, but an understanding of the underlying pathological mechanisms is essential.

Major physiological changes occuring during pregnancy

Respiratory

- Minute ventilation increases by 40%. This results in a decline in P_aCO_2 and a respiratory alkalosis. Therefore an arterial blood gas in a normal pregnant women will reflect a slightly increased pH, decreased P_aCO_2 and decreased bicarbonate (respiratory alkalosis with compensatory metabolic alkalosis). As the pregnancy advances, the increasing abdominal girth causes the diaphragm to displace upwards. This causes a decrease in functional residual capacity (FRC), alveolar collapse, and decreased gas exchange.
- Oxygen consumption increases by up to 15% due to demands from the developing fetus, uterus, placenta, and breasts. This is met by an increase in minute ventilation, an increase in cardiac output, and a shift of the maternal oxyhaemoglobin dissociation curve to the right.

Cardiovascular

- Maternal blood volume increases by 1–1.5 L during pregnancy and reaches its maximum by 24–34 weeks. There is increased sodium retention and an increase in total body water. About a third of the extra blood fills the sinuses of the placenta and the remainder stays in the circulation. The increase in plasma volume exceeds that of the red cell volume, creating a dilutional anaemia.
- Cardiac output rises gradually from the first trimester due to the increase in blood volume and an increase in heart rate (up by 20%) and stroke volume. By 30 weeks it can be 30–50% above non-pregnant values.
- Systemic vascular resistance decreases due to smooth muscle relaxation induced by oestrogen and progesterone,.
- Immediately after delivery, cardiac output rises due to autotransfusion by uterine contractions and the relief of venocaval obstruction.
- Within 3 weeks of delivery the expanded blood volume has been reabsorbed and cardiac output is restored to normal values.

Utero-placental perfusion

- The uteroplacental circulation is a pressure-dependent system lacking its own regulatory mechanism. Any factor decreasing maternal venous return or cardiac output will impair uterine flow (e.g. mechanical ventilation or venocaval compression).
- Hypotension can develop due to compression of the iliac vessels, inferior vena cava, and aorta by the enlarging uterus. This is most evident during the second half of pregnancy and maximal when the patient is supine (up to 30% reduction in blood volume). Hypotension can critically impair uteroplacental blood flow, so patients beyond 20 weeks' gestation should not be nursed in a supine position. Such patients must be nursed in the left lateral position in order relieve compression, or a pillow or wedge can be placed under the right hip to tilt the uterus. This is the position in which cardiopulmonary resuscitation is performed since, owing to inferior vena cava occlusion, an adequate cardiac output cannot be achieved if the patient is left supine.
- Hypoxaemia, acidosis, and vasopressors all cause uteroplacental constriction and impair perfusion.
- Utero-placental perfusion can be increased by correct positioning, volume infusion, and leg raising.

Obstetric disorders

Hypertensive disorders of pregnancy

These occur in women with pre-existing primary or secondary chronic hypertension (e.g. due to chronic renal failure), and in those who develop new-onset hypertension in the second half of pregnancy.

Pre-eclampsia is one of the most serious complications of pregnancy, and a leading cause of maternal and perinatal mortality. It is more common in the first pregnancy (2–8% are affected) with an incidence of severe pre-eclampsia of about 1%. Women at high risk of developing pre-eclampsia include those with a history of hyptertensive disease in a previous pregnancy, chronic kidney disease, autoimmune disease, diabetes mellitus, or chronic hypertension.

Pre-eclampsia is defined by gestational onset of hypertension presenting after 20 weeks with significant proteinuria. Severe pre-eclampsia is pre-eclampsia with severe hypertension (systolic ≥160 mmHg, diastolic ≥110 mmHg) with/without symptoms and/or biochemical and haematological impairment. Pre-eclampsia evolves into eclampsia when maternal seizures develop. A severe form of pre-eclampsia is characterized by microangiopathic haemolytic anaemia (HELLP syndrome.

Women who have had gestational hypertension or pre-eclampsia are at an increased risk of developing hypertension and its complications later in life.

Pre-eclampsia

Pre-eclampsia is a progressive multi-organ disorder with delivery of the fetus and placenta being the only cure. However, Preterm delivery may adversely affect the neonate with complications resulting from prematurity and low birth weight.

The precise aetiology is still unclear. It is postulated that the spiral arteries which supply the placenta fail to undergo physiological dilatation in the first trimester, leaving the uteroplacental circulation in a state of high resistance. This can lead to placental ischaemia as the pregnancy progresses, stimulating release of pre-eclamptic factors that lead to endothelial cell damage. This contributes to the platelet activation and vasoconstriction seen in pre-eclampsia. There is an increased response to vasoconstrictor agents, greater cell permeability, reduced plasma volume, coagulation activation, and fibrin deposition in the systemic vascular beds. Thrombosis and vasospasm develop, exacerbating the ischaemia and worsening endothelial cell dysfunction, and this can lead to multi-organ involvement.

Clinical features of pre-eclampsia

Many women develop signs of pre-eclampsia (hypertension and proteinuria) but can remain asymptomatic and deliver at term (See Table 14.3). However, a small proportion progress rapidly through the phases of pre-eclampsia and develop clinical features of severe pre-eclampsia, increasing their risk of developing the numerous complications. Attempts will be made to prolong the pregnancy by close maternal and fetal surveillance, but this is rarely possible for more than a few weeks and, for some women, only a matter of hours before delivery is necessary.

Complications of pre-eclampsia

Complications of pre-eclampsia include:

- eclampsia
- renal failure
- HELLP syndrome (Haemolysis, Elevated Liver enzymes, Low Platelets)
- hepatic rupture

Table 14.3 Clinical features of pre-eclampsia

Cardiovascular/ haemotological	Hypertension Thrombocytopenia Prolonged clotting ime Increased packed cell volume and elevated haemoglobin
Renal/biochemical	Hyperuricaemia Proteinuria Oedema (paticularly hands, face, feet) Rise in creatinine and urea Oliguria
Neurological	Headache Visual disturbances Hyper-reflexia
Hepatic/gastric	Elevated liver function tests Epigastric pain/pain below ribs Nausea/vomiting
Utero-placental	Reduced fetal growth Possible intra-uterine death

- cerebral haemorrhage
- cerebral oedema
- disseminated intravascular coagulation (DIC)
- pulmonary oedema
- ARDS
- placental abruption.

Nursing management

Women with severe pre-eclampsia will require admission to a critical care unit if they require more intensive monitoring or their clinical deterioration is rapid. The majority will have delivered pre-admission to critical care but will still require close monitoring as there is likely to be further clinical deterioration for at least 48 hours after delivery.

Hypertension

The single largest cause of death is cerebral haemorrhage. This generally reflects a failure of effective antihypertensive treatment. The blood pressure must be monitored closely; automated blood pressure recording systems can underestimate blood pressure in pre-eclampsia and therefore arterial pressure monitoring should be considered.

Administer antihypertensive drug therapy. Treatment choices include an infusion of magnesium sulphate (especially if there is severe hypertension or pre-eclampsia), intravenous hydralazine (a peripheral vasodilator), or intravenous or oral labetalol (an α- and β-adrenergic blocker). Monitor the response and review dosage as necessary. Systolic blood pressure should be maintained <150 mmHg and diastolic pressure between 80 and 100 mmHg. In severe pre-eclampsia intravenous volume expansion should be given if the patient is hypovolaemic or if there are ongoing fluid losses (e.g. from haemorrhage). Otherwise, maintenance fluid should be limited to 80 ml/h and fluid balance closely monitored.

The level of proteinuria should be regularly monitored. In the recovery phase patients have a large diuresis, clearance of oedema and proteinuria, and resolution of their hypertension.

Intravenous nitrates are useful if there is evidence of pulmonary oedema. Sodium nitroprusside is useful for acute hypertensive crises complicated by pulmonary oedema and left ventricular failure. However, this should be avoided in the antenatal period because of the risk of fetal toxicity from cyanide poisoning.

Sudden falls in mean blood pressure or hypotension must be avoided, as this will be detrimental to both uteroplacental and cerebral perfusion.

Anticonvulsant therapy

Intravenous magnesium should be given prophylactically to patients with severe hypertension, with severe pre-eclampsia, who have previously had an eclamptic fit, or if birth is planned within 24 hours.

Corticosteroids

Administration of betamethasone (IM) for fetal lung maturation should be considered if birth is likely within 7 days in women with pre-eclampsia.

Potential haemorrhage due to DIC

Observe for evidence of bleeding. Correct the coagulopathy using fresh frozen plasma and cryoprecipitate. Significant thrombocytopenia may require platelet transfusion.

Cerebral haemorrhage can occur if coagulopathy and blood pressure are not controlled. However, thromboembolism remains a risk in pre-eclampsia.

Eclampsia

Eclampsia is a grand mal convulsion occurring in association with features of pre-eclampsia. It occurs in 1–2% of women with pre-eclampsia. Forty-four per cent of convulsions occur post-natally; the remainder areantepartum (38%) and intrapartum (18%).

Eclampsia is thought to be attributed to cerebral vasospasm, ischaemia, cerebral oedema, disruption of the blood–brain barrier, or microemboli in the cerebral circulation. Cerebral haemorrhage can occur irrespective of an elevated blood pressure.

Intravenous magnesium sulphate is the drug of choice for primary prophylaxis in severe pre-eclampsia, especially in those with continued signs of cerebral irritation. Magnesium acts as a cerebral vasodilator and relieves vasospasm.

If a convulsion occurs, the priorities of care are maintenance of the airway, oxygenation, and control of the seizures. Endotracheal intubation and ventilation may be required. Neurological management of these patients includes maintenance of cerebral perfusion and control of intracranial pressure. If the patient remains in coma, cerebral oedema or haemorrhage must be suspected.

Magnesium also acts as a central nervous system depressor. Therapeutic maternal blood levels are 2–3.5 mmol/L but respiratory paralysis can occur when levels exceed 5 mmol/L. Careful observation of respiratory rate and depth will be required to avoid respiratory arrest. Magnesium also increases the patient's sensitivity to neuromuscular blocking agents.

HELLP syndrome (Haemolysis, Elevated Liver enzymes and Low Platelets)

HELLP syndrome usually develops as a complication of pre-eclampsia, but can occur independently. Seventy per cent develop the condition pre-delivery (usually before 37 weeks). Its aetiology is unknown, but it results in endothelial injury with fibrin deposition, resulting in a microangiopathic haemolytic anaemia, and platelet activation and consumption that leads to thrombocytopenia. The fibrin deposits cause obstruction in the hepatic sinusoids which leads to areas of haemorrhage and eventual necrosis in the liver. The haemorrhage can develop into large haematomas and cause liver capsule rupture.

Hypertension and proteinuria are common (since most patients have pre-eclampsia) but are not always present. Epigastric or right upper quadrant pain, malaise, and nausea often occur. Any woman presenting with these symptoms should have platelet and liver function tests performed irrespective of the blood pressure. Prognosis is unpredictable, and immediate delivery is usually indicated if >34 weeks gestation. There may be particular problems with haemorrhage, so transfusion of red cells, fresh frozen plasma, cryoprecipitate, and platelets may be required (See Box 14.15).

Acute fatty liver of pregnancy (AFLP)

This rare, but potentially fatal, condition usually occurs in the third trimester or early post-partum period. It is characterized by progressive lipid accumulation within the hepatocytes. The exact pathophysiology is unclear, but in some cases it is associated with an inherited deficiency of a mitochondial enzyme that allows build-up of long-chain fatty acids resulting in mitochondral dysfunction and subsequent liver failure. Kidney, brain, pancreas, and bone marrow may also demonstrate microvesicular fat infiltration.

The patient presents with several weeks of non-specific symptoms (see Box 14.16) and becomes jaundiced as the condition progresses. Some patients also have pre-eclampsia, with hypertension and oedema. Transient diabetes insipidus can occur, but this is uncommon. The diagnosis of AFLP is made primarily on history, physical examination, laboratory data (increased transaminase levels, decreased platelet count, increased prothrombin time), and in some cases liver biopsy, though this may not be possible due to coagulation abnormalities.

In severe cases, multi-system involvement ensues and may cause:

- acute renal failure
- liver failure
- encephalopathy
- coagulopathy
- gastrointestinal bleeding (from gastric or duodenal lesions or secondary to the coagulopathy)
- pancreatitis—may develop afer the onset of hepatic and renal dysfunction.

Management

Management of AFLP is by intensive supportive care and early delivery of the fetus. Stabilization of the mother must be achieved before delivery. Maternal and fetal death may occur if treatment is delayed (fetal death remains approximately 25%).

Support of vital functions includes the following.

- Airway management—positive pressure ventilation may be required. Endotracheal intubation must be performed quickly because pregnant patients have lower oxygen reserves due to decreased functional residual capacity. Avoid respiratory alkalosis as it may decrease uterine blood flow and therefore oxygenation. Avoid high ventilatory pressures at the expense of a rise in P_aCO_2 (maternal hypercapnoea has not been reported to be harmful to the fetus). Intubation and suctioning may lead to mucosal injury and bleeding because the nasopharyngeal, oropharyngeal, and respiratory mucosa swell during pregnancy.

Box 14.15 Complications of HELLP syndrome

- Disseminated intravascular coagulation (DIC)
- Pulmonary oedema
- Acute renal failure
- Liver failure and haemorrhage
- Placental abruption
- Acute respiratory distress syndrome
- Stroke

Box 14.16 Non-specific symptoms of AFLP

- Right upper quadrant abdominal pain
- Anorexia
- Nausea and vomiting
- Malaise/fatigue
- Headache

- Correction of hypoglycaemia—this must be monitored carefully and infusions of 50% dextrose will often be required. Hypoglycaemia can still occur in the recovery period.
- Correction of coagulation abnormalities—careful administration of IV fluid and blood products.
- Treatment of hypertension.
- Correction of electrolyte abnormalities.
- Renal support.

During the post-partum period haemodynamic monitoring is essential as these patients are at high risk of gastrointestinal bleeding or severe postpartum haemorrhage secondary to coagulation abnormalities. Other complications include sepsis, renal failure, circulatory collapse, pancreatitis, or gastrointestinal bleeding. In extreme cases patients with fulminant hepatic failure or those who have irreversible liver failure despite aggressive supportive care may require liver transplantation.

Thromboembolism

Thromboembolism is a leading cause of maternal mortality in the UK; pulmonary embolism in pregnancy and the puerperium kills 8–10 women each year. Pregnancy increases the risk of thromboembolism sixfold and Caesarean section further increases the risk approximately 10- to 20-fold. The risk of a deep vein thrombosis (DVT) following Caesarean section is around 1–2% and persists for at least 6 weeks post-partum. In 85% of cases pregnancy-associated DVT ocurs on the left side, probably due to compression of the left iliac vein. Less commonly, a pelvic vein thrombosis can occur.

Additional risk factors are:

- age (risk 10-fold greater if >40 years)
- obesity
- smoking
- increased parity (four or more)
- operative delivery
- previous thromboembolism
- prolonged bedrest
- pre-eclampsia
- gross varicose veins.

Pregnancy is a hypercoagulable state with an increased potential for coagulation and thrombosis. This is due primarily to changes in clotting factors (an increase in factors V, VII, VIII, IX, X, and XII) and an increase of 50% in fibrinogen levels. Plasma fibrinolytic activity also decreases as a result of placental inhibitors, but can return to normal within an hour after delivery. When the placenta separates, tissue thromboplastin is released into the circulation, increasing the chance of thrombosis. These physiological changes serve to control blood loss at delivery.

Pulmonary embolism

The size, number and location of the emboli determine the clinical features of pulmonary embolism (PE). The signs and symptoms of pulmonary embolism are:

- dyspnoea and tachypnoea
- hypoxaemia/cyanosis
- pleuritic chest pain (sudden onset)
- haemoptysis
- cardiovascular collapse.

Management

A correct diagnosis is vital because of the major implications of long-term anticoagulation in pregnancy, the potential need for prophylaxis in any future pregnancy, and concerns regarding future use of contraceptives and hormone replacement therapy. Imaging methods that utilize radiation are used with caution owing to concerns with teratogenicity. Investigations such as CT pulmonary angiography or a V/Q (ventilation/perfusion) scan may be required to confirm the diagnosis. D-dimer levels may not be diagnostic as these rise gradually during pregnancy, reduce in the post-partum period, and do not return to normal until 4-6 weeks post-partum.

Routine haemodynamic and respiratory monitoring should be instituted according to the severity of the condition. The aims of treatment are to maintain adequate oxygenation according to blood gas analysis and promote the resolution of the thrombus by intravenous anticoagulation. Low molecular weight heparin is the treatment of choice. Unfractionated intravenous heparin is preferred in patients with renal failure or if urgent anticoagulant reversal is anticipated (e.g. high risk of bleeding or surgery is anticipated).

Anticoagulation should continue for at least 6 weeks' post-partum or until 3 months of anticoagulant therapy has been given. Warfarin is contraindicated during pregnancy because it crosses the placental barrier, is teratogenic, and may cause bleeding in the fetus and placental abruption. It can be commenced post-partum and heparin discontinued once an adequate INR (international normalized ratio) has been achieved. Thrombolytic drugs (e.g. tPA) can be considered in patients who are haemodynamically unstable or who have severe hypoxaemia.

Massive obstetric haemorrhage

Life-threatening haemorrhage occurs in approximately 0.1% of deliveries. Usually, the myometrial fibres contract, causing an occlusive action that stops bleeding. Most serious haemorrhage occurs in the post-partum period when the uterus is unable to contract (see Box 14.17). This may be further exacerbated by thrombocytopenia and coagulopathy secondary to sepsis, amniotic fluid embolism, pre-eclampsia, placental abruption, or intra-uterine death.

Risk factors for massive obstetric haemorrhage are:

- antepartum haemorrhage (additional likelihood of DIC)
- grand gmultiparosity
- pre-eclampsia
- previous post-partum haemorrhage
- multiple pregnancy
- previous Caesarean section
- large baby
- fibroids
- placental site disorders, i.e. praevia, accreta, increta, percreta.

With placenta praevia haemorrhage is due to the inability of the lower uterine segment to contract effectively. With the other abnormalities the placenta cannot be fully removed, thus preventing contraction of the uterus and allowing bleeding to persist.

The normal expected blood loss at delivery is 500 ml for a vaginal delivery and 1000 ml for a Caesarean section. This is usually well tolerated, but excess may result in hypovolaemic shock. In the antepartum patient this may diminish uteroplacental perfusion and induce fetal distress. Systolic blood pressure below 80 mmHg usually indicates a blood loss >1500 ml. Catecholamine-induced vasoconstriction will maintain maternal blood pressure at the expense of the fetus; therefore fetal distress is an important sign.

Box 14.17 Causes of massive obstetric haemorrhage

- Tears of uterus, cervix, or vaginal wall
- Uterine atony (inability to contract)
- Retained placenta or placental fragments
- Coagulation defects

Management

The essentials of management are to identify the cause of the bleeding, stop it, and replace the circulating blood volume. The contents of the uterus must be emptied. This is achieved in the third stage by early clamping and cutting of the cord, prophylactic administration of an oxytocic drug, and controlled cord traction. If bleeding persists, further techniques include vaginal packing, a Foley catheter to induce tamponade, surgical exploration to repair lacerations, radiographic embolization, or hysterectomy.

Intensive haemodynamic monitoring will be required while the patient is resuscitated and blood volume rapidly replaced. Uterine rupture and placenta praevia may cause massive blood loss (4–5 L). Coagulopathy must be corrected using fresh frozen plasma, platelets, and cryoprecipitate. If the airway is not patent or oxygenation is inadequate, endotracheal intubation and ventilation will be required. Monitor for the effects of massive blood loss such as renal failure, ARDS, and DIC.

In the antepartum patient continuous fetal heart monitoring should be instituted to detect fetal distress or hypoxia; if present this should lead to prompt fetal delivery by the safest method.

Amniotic fluid embolism (AFE)

This uncommon disorder has an estimated incidence of 1 in 20,000–30,000 pregnancies. However, it has become one of the top three causes of maternal deaths in industrialized countries, with a mortality rate of up to 80% and accounts for 10% of maternal deaths.

There are no clear risk factors associated with the condition and it is not preventable. Its pathophysiology remains unclear, but it is not thought to be caused by an embolic episode and is more likely to be immunological in nature. Some authorities suggest that the term 'amniotic fluid embolism' should be changed to 'anaphylactoid syndrome of pregnancy'. However, the only diagnostic test available is the finding of fetal material in the maternal circulation at autopsy; therefore it is diagnosed on clinical grounds only. AFE can be described as the entrance of amniotic fluid, containing fetal cells and debris, into the maternal circulation. It is suggested that it is not the amniotic fluid per se, but the woman's individual response to amniotic fluid that is the crucial factor in the development of AFE.

The release of soluble mediators into the maternal circulation results in a syndrome with haemotological and cardiovascular manifestations including pulmonary vasoconstriction, coronary vasoconstriction, a reduction in cardiac output, and increased vascular permeability. Clark *et al.* (1996) proposed that the syndrome had two phases. In the first phase, there is pulmonary artery spasm with pulmonary hypertension leading to right heart failure causing hypoxaemia. This causes heart and lung damage, with the left ventricle failing due to possible coronary artery spasm; myocardial ischaemia and ARDS develop. This initial period of hypoxaemia might account for 50% of patients who succumb in the first hour. The second phase consists of non-cardiogenic pulmonary oedema due to increased alveolar capillary permeability, and a haemorrhagic phase characterized by massive haemorrhage with uterine atony (lack of contracting ability) and DIC.

Signs and symptoms of AFE

- Sudden dyspnoea in late stages of labour or shortly after birth
- Hypotension (shock)
- Hypoxaemia/cyanosis
- Cardiorespiratory arrest
- Seizures
- Pulmonary oedema/ARDS
- DIC causing massive haemorrhage

Management of AFE

Management is entirely supportive.

- Initiate cardiopulmonary resuscitation—over 80% of patients experience cardiorespiratory arrest at the onset.
- Maintain oxygenation. Direct therapy according to arterial blood gas analysis. Endotracheal intubation and ventilation are usually necessary.
- Restore the circulation as directed by haemodynamic monitoring. Rapid volume infusion and inotropic support may be necessary. Use appropriate intravenous fluid. This may include blood transfusion in the presence of haemorrhage.
- Correct coagulopathy using blood component therapy (fresh frozen plasma, cryoprecipitate, platelets).
- Expedite delivery, if undelivered, and perform corrective surgery to control haemorrhage.
- Renal support may be required.
- More aggressive support may be necessary in some patients (e.g. inhaled nitric oxide, cardiopulmonary bypass, extracorporeal membrane oxygenation, and a ventricular assist device).

Peri-partum cardiomyopathy

This life-threatening disorder presents in the last month of pregnancy or in the first 5 months after delivery. It is a form of dilated cardiomyopathy which presents with signs of heart failure. The aetiology is uncertain, but several mechanisms have been proposed including hormonal changes of pregnancy, nutritional deficiencies, and autoimmune or viral processes. Risk factors include:

- multiparity
- maternal age—there is a greater incidence in women aged >30
- multifetal pregnancy
- pre-eclampsia
- gestational hypertension
- African American race.

The patient usually presents with classic signs of left or bi-ventricular failure. There is severe impairment in left ventricular performance and gross dilation of the left ventricle. A major complication is pulmonary or cerebral emboli. Mortality is 25–50%, with death being caused by ventricular arrhythmias, diminished cardiac output, or the consequences of emboli.

This condition can recur with subsequent pregnancies, particularly in patients whose heart size does not return to normal within 6 months of delivery.

Management is as follows.

- Systemic anticoagulation in patients with severe left ventricular dysfunction, evidence of systemic embolism, or cardiac thrombosis.
- Conventional treatment for congestive cardiac failure. Angiotensin-converting enzyme (ACE) inhibitors are contraindicated in pregnancy as they are teratogenic, but are the main treatment in post-partum women with heart failure. Digoxin, loop diuretics, and drugs that reduce afterload (e.g. nitrates and hydralazine) have been proved to be safe in pregnancy. The aim of treatment is to reduce preload by diuretic therapy, reduce afterload with vasodilators, and improve contractibility with inotropic agents.
- Cardiac transplantation in patients with severe heart failure despite maximal drug therapy. Ventricular assist devices or intra-aortic balloon counter-pulsation can be used as a bridge to transplanation.

Other high-risk disorders of pregnancy

Grown-up congenital heart (GUCH) disease

Approximately 85% of patients born with congenital heart disease now survive to adulthood, and increasing numbers of women are reaching child-bearing age. Although most of these patients tolerate pregnancy well, it can become a major issue; GUCH disease is one of the commonest causes of maternal mortality. Management must be based on their functional status before pregnancy and knowledge of the underlying pathophysiological changes that occur in pregnancy and their haemodynamic consequences (increase in cardiac output, blood volume, and heart rate; decreased peripheral vascular resistance; anaemia).

High risk conditions include severe pulmonary hypertension, severe left heart inflow–outflow obstruction, poor systemic ventricular function, and aortic root dilation (e.g. Marfan and Ehler–Danlos syndromes) The risk of complications during pregnancy is determined by:

- the severity of the cardiac lesion
- cyanosis—there is a 50% incidence of fetal death if the arterial oxygen saturation is <85%
- left ventricular ejection fraction <40%
- New York Heart Classification >11
- left heart obstruction
- prior cardiac event (heart failure, arrhythmias)
- anticoagulation during pregnancy.

Mitral stenosis in the pregnant patient

Mitral stenosis is sometimes diagnosed during pregnancy when the additional burden on the previously unchallanged heart causes atrial fibrillation and/or pulmonary oedema. Once the valve area is <1.5cm^2 filling of the left ventricle during diastole is severely limited, resulting in a fixed cardiac output. It is essential that tachycardia is prevented and left ventricular preload maintained. As the heart rate increases, less time is allowed for the left atrium to empty adequately and fill the left ventricle during diastole. The left atrium may become over-distended and can result in pulmonary oedema or arrhythmias (primarily atrial fibrillation, which increases the risk of thromboembolic events). However, adequate preload is essential to maintain left ventricular filling pressure. Patients with severe limitation of valve opening may not tolerate the normal increase in cardiac output, blood volume, and increased heart rate of pregnancy. Management is aimed at treating arrhythmias, β-blockers to control heart rate, and careful use of diuretics. In severe cases percutaneous mitral valvoplasty may be required during pregnancy. Patients with severe mitral stenosis often require elective Caesarean section.

Aortic stenosis in the pregnant patient

This usually develops secondary to childhood rheumatic fever. The major concern during pregnancy is the maintenance of an adequate cardiac output because, as gestation advances, an increased demand is made on the heart. It does not become significant until valve opening is decreased by at least a third. The increased blood volume during pregnancy is usually well tolerated in patients with mild disease, but as the orifice becomes more stenotic, the cardiac output becomes more fixed and patients are unable to maintain adequate coronary or cerebral perfusion. Angina, myocardial infarction, syncope, and sudden death may occur, particularly during delivery when it is crucial that adequate cardiac output and venous return to the heart is maintained. Venous return may be decreased by excess blood loss, regional anaesthetic block, hypotension, or vena caval occlusion in the supine position.

Breastfeeding in the ICU

Many mothers are keen to commence breastfeeding in the critical care unit, but this must be balanced against their level of illness and any drugs that are being administered to them. Breastfeeding works on a supply and demand basis, i.e. the more the baby feeds or the mother expresses, the more milk is produced. Mothers should be encouraged to rest; if they wish to express milk this should be done two to four times during the day in order to promote sleep at night. However, in order to feel comfortable, they may need to express during the night, especially on the third day post-delivery when full milk production occurs. If the mother has been sedated for several days, she can be reassured that she will be able to breastfeed but it will take several attempts to obtain milk. There may be a decrease in milk supply following a massive haemorrhage. Breast pump kits can be used, but they must be sterile if the milk is to be used by the baby. The milk can be kept in sterile plastic bottles for 24 hours if refrigerated. Drugs that are being administered to the mother must be taken into account, as many can be transferred into the milk. Always check the drug prescribing information or consult the unit pharmacist for advice. Medical staff should be encouraged to use drugs that are safe for breastfeeding, particularly if these will be required long-term such as antihypertensive therapy. Many obstetric departments will have a breastfeeding advisor who can offer advice and practical support.

Drug overdose and toxic substance ingestion

Poisoning may follow deliberate or accidental exposure or ingestion and may be acute or chronic. Substances include therapeutic drugs, plant or animal toxins, industrial or agricultural chemicals, and substances found in the home such as cleaning materials.

Self-administered drug poisoning accounts for over 10% of acute medical admissions to hospital. Death from acute poisoning is relatively uncommon, except in children under 4 years of age where accidental poisoning remains an important cause of death.

In deliberate drug overdose, often more than one drug will be ingested and alcohol is a common co-agent. Complications can be unexpected and require prompt action and specific treatments. Supportive therapy in the critical care unit can be life-saving (see Box 14.18).

General principles

The consequences of a drug overdose depend on a variety of factors including:

- the patient's age, weight, health
- the drug
- the route of ingestion
- how long ago the drug was taken and over what period of time
- the quantity taken,
- other drugs that may have been taken at the same time (e.g. alcohol).

For some drugs that require specific treatment (e.g. antidotes) recovery is dependent on the time interval between ingestion and the commencement of therapy.

Box 14.18 Conditions that require admission to the critical care unit

- Cardiovascularly unstable (hypotensive, hypertensive cardiac arrhythmias)
- Unconscious
- Requires (or likely to require) endotracheal intubation or mechanical ventilation
- Requires specialist therapy (e.g. Haemodialysis/ filtration, temporary pacing)
- Suffers seizures

Therefore definitive treatment must begin as soon as resuscitation is completed.

Resuscitation and immediate care

- Vital functions must be assessed and the principles of resuscitation applied in order to stabilize the patient before a general assessment is made.
- The airway must be kept patent. If the patient is comatose with no cough or gag reflex, endotracheal intubation will be required.
- Establish intravenous access.
- Give oxygen by mask; if spontaneous respiration is inadequate, endotracheal intubation and mechanical ventilatory support will be required.
- Take baseline measurements of heart rate and rhythm, respiratory rate, and blood pressure. Assess peripheral perfusion and skin colour.
- Correct hypovolaemia
- Treat hypotension—once hypovolaemia has been corrected use appropriate inotropic or pressor agents (e.g. norepinephrine in poisoning that produces peripheral vasodilation, epinephrine where there is direct toxin-related myocardial depression).
- Carry out a bedside blood glucose test and correct hypoglycaemia.
- Assess conscious level and manage seizures.
- Measure core temperature—if >39°C actively cool the patient.
- Take blood samples for glucose, urea, creatinine, and electrolytes, liver function tests, full blood count, coagulation screen, arterial blood gases, and drug assays. Paracetamol concentration should be measured in all patients who present after overdose. Repeat samples may need to be performed regularly depending on the results and their trends.
- Take urine and blood samples for drug screen.
- Chest X-ray and ECG.
- Continually reassess the patient for impaired vital functions.

Physical examination

Self-poisoning is the cause of undiagnosed coma in approximately 15% of patients aged between 15 and 55 years. Although other causes of coma must be excluded, overdose should always be suspected.

A careful history must be obtained from the patient (if conscious), ambulance personnel, and relatives or friends. Empty bottles, drugs, or a suicide note may have been found with the patient. The patient's general practitioner can provide details of recently prescribed medication or any history of depressive illness.

A good physical examination can provide important clues. Assessment should be made of:

- the central and autonomic nervous system
- the appearance of the skin and mucous membranes, e.g. colour (jaundice, cyanosed, cherry red), blisters, lesions, venepuncture marks
- odours—particular toxic substances cause specific odours—e.g. cyanide causes a bitter almond odour, isopropyl alcohol, phenol, and salicylates an acetone odour, and heavy metals and organophosphates a garlic odour.

Urine, blood, and gastric contents should be sent for analysis, but urgent laboratory drug screening is usually limited to paracetamol and salicylate screening. Bedside kits will detect the presence of recreational drugs, including opiates and cannabis, though reliability is variable. A more comprehensive drug screen can be carried out by a specialized poisons unit. When the cause of coma is unknown, a blood sugar should always be performed urgently. Appropriate measures should be taken if meningitis is suspected.

Some examples of the clinical manifestations of toxic substances are given in Table 14.4, but the list is by no means exhaustive. The clinical manifestations of some substances have characteristic features and are termed toxidromes. This may help to determine which substance has been taken. Some examples of common toxidromes are:

- amphetamine/ecstasy/cocaine: fever, tachycardia, hypertension, hyperactive/delirious, tremor, convulsions, sweating
- Opiates/clonidine: bradycardia, slow depressed respirations, hypotension, hypothermia, pinpoint pupils, hyporeflexia, reduced level of consciousness, coma

Table 14.4 Clinical manifestations of toxic substances

Clinical manifestation	Toxic substance
Bradycardia	Digoxin, opiates, cyanide, carbon monoxide, clonidine, organophosphates, calcium-channel blockers, β-blockers
Tachycardia	Alcohol, amphetamines, tricyclic antidepressants, theophylline, salicylates, cocaine
Hypotension	Nitrates, cyanide, carbon monoxide, tricyclic antidepressants, barbiturates, iron, theophylline, opiates, clonidine, β-blockers, calcium-channel blockers, phenothiazines
Arrhythmias, heartblock	Chloroquine, tricyclic antidepressants, class 1 anti-arrhythmics
Atrioventricular block	β-blockers, digoxin
Hypertension	Amphetamines, monoamine (MAO) inhibitors, antihistamines, clonidine, cocaine
Respiratory depression	Opiates, alcohol, benzodiazipines, barbiturates
Hypothermia	Ethanol, amphetamines, barbiturates, opiates, clonidine, carbamazipine, sedatives
Hyperpyrexia	Quinine, salicylates, amphetamines, tricyclic antidepressants, monoamine oxidase inhibitors (MOAIs), theophylline, cocaine
Hypoglycaemia	Insulin, oral hypoglycaemic drugs
Hyperkalaemia	Digoxin, potassium supplements, excess liquorice
Hypokalaemia	Theophylline, chloroquine, diuretics
Coma	Opiates, anticholinergics, alcohol, anticonvulsants, carbon monoxide, salicylates, organophosphates
Convulsions, agitation	Alcohol, lead, organophosphates, salicylates, antihistamines, tricyclic antidepressants, cocaine, ecstasy, amphetamines
Paralysis	Botulism, alcohol, carbon monoxide, barbiturates, heavy metals, hydrocarbons, organic solvents

- Barbiturates/benzodiazipines: hypotension, bradypnoea, confusion, coma, ataxia, hypothermia, skin vesicles and bullae
- Salicylates: tachypnoea, pyrexia, lethargy/coma, vomiting.

Management

After basic resuscitation, treatment is aimed at:

- decreasing further drug absorption
- increasing drug excretion
- administration of specific antidotes
- supportive therapy.

Decreasing further drug absorption

The traditional technique of gastric lavage is now rarely used because doubts exist over its efficacy and it carries recognized complications, particularly in obtunded patients (e.g. oesophageal perforation, gastric rupture, hyponatraemia, water intoxication, aspiration pneumonia). It is only considered in patients presenting within an hour of ingestion of a potentially life-threatening overdose.

- **Activated charcoal** is the treatment of choice to prevent absorption of the drug/substance from the stomach into the bloodstream. It should ideally be given as early as possible following ingestion of a substantial amount of toxin, but it may still be effective for up to 24 hours, especially with drugs such as aspirin that are absorbed slowly. Repeated doses are given for some drugs, which may help reduce their toxicity. It is an effective adsorbent of many kinds of substances such as phenobarbital, theophylline, and phenytoin, but is ineffective for others such as alcohol, heavy metals, lithium, and petroleum solvents. The airway must be protected as there is a risk of pulmonary aspiration. but other side effects are relatively rare. It can be given to unconscious patients via a large bore nasogastric tube after endotracheal intubation. It should not be given to patients with an ileus or bowel obstruction.
- **Whole bowel irrigation** A solution of polyethylene glycol is given orally or via a nasogastric tube at a rate of 2 L/hour (adults) until the rectal effluent becomes clear. It is used when patients have ingested a potentially serious substance (such as enteric-coated preparations) or those for which activated charcoal is ineffective (such as iron). It is also sometimes used for the intact elimination of 'body packer' packets of cocaine and heroin. Polyethylene glycol is not absorbed and does not produce fluid or electrolyte imbalance. It cannot be used in patients who have unprotected airways, bowel obstruction, ileus, perforation, or gastrointestinal haemorrhage.

Increasing excretion of the drug

- **Forced diuresis** Large volumes of intravenous fluid are infused, often in combination with diuretics, to promote urinary excretion of the drug.
- **Urine alkalinization** An infusion of sodium bicarbonate is given to alkalinize the urine and prevent reabsorption of the drug in the kidney. It is useful in salicylate and barbiturate overdose. It can be potentially hazardous in patients with cardiac or renal dysfunction, and can cause electrolyte imbalance and cerebral oedema, so vigilant monitoring of vital signs, electrolytes, and arterial blood pH is essential. Urinary pH should be monitored and maintained >7.5. Potassium supplementation is necessary to correct renal potassium loss.
- **Extracorporeal elimination** This includes haemodialysis, haemofiltration, haemodiafiltration, and haemoperfusion using a charcoal filter.

In order for these methods to be effective the toxin must have limited protein binding, small volumes of distribution, and a plasma concentration that relates to toxicity.

Antidotes/alteration of drug metabolism

Specific antidotes can be given for certain overdoses/poisons. These compete for the same receptors (e.g. naloxone for opiates, flumazenil for benzodiazepines), block metabolism by using the same enzyme (e.g. ethanol for methanol), or protect body tissues (e.g. *N*-acetylcysteine provides sulphydryl groups to prevent liver damage by paracetamol).

Supportive therapy

The action and side effects of the drug taken (if known) should be documented in order to anticipate and observe any problems that may occur. Specific supportive treatments will vary according to the drug taken (see Table 14.5). The basic principles are as follows.

- **Respiratory** Maintain airway (depends on level of consciousness): oropharyngeal (Guedel) airway, endotracheal intubation, patient positioning. Monitor blood gases, acid–base status, and oxygen saturation. Give oxygen therapy or ventilatory support as indicated. Hypoxaemia may indicate additional pulmonary pathology such as aspiration, infection, oedema, atelectasis.
- **Cardiovascular** Monitor cardiovascular status: continuous ECG recording, observe for arrhythmias, perform 12-lead ECG, monitor vital signs. Circulatory failure can result from a variety of causes (hypovolaemia, myocardial insufficiency, vasodilatation, or reduced cardiac output due to negative inotropy or

Table 14.5 Specific manangement strategies for drug overdose and poisons

Drug/poison	Toxic effect	Management
Antidepressants:		
Tricyclic	Hypertension, tachycardia, tremors, seizures, hyperthermia, respiratory, and CNS depression.	Supportive. Benzodiazepines for seizures. Activated charcoal if within 2 hours of ingestion. Maintain serum pH >7.5 with bicarbonate if cardiotoxic effects.
Monoamine oxidase inhibitors (MOAIs)	Dilated pupils, dry mouth, urinary retention, ileus, agitation, convulsions, hyperpyrexia. Cardiotoxic effects may appear for up to 3 days—hypotension, AV conduction disturbances, sinus tachycardia, ventricular fibrillation or tachycardia.	Supportive. Acivated charcoal. Seizure control. Active cooling if hyperthermic.
Amphetamines	Tachycardia, arrhythmias, hypertension, coronary vasospasm, seizures, confusion, psychosis, hyperthermia, cardiogenic pulmonary oedema.	Supportive. Activated charcoal. Whole-bowel irrigation if suspected 'body packer'. Aggressive cooling if hyperthermic. Seizure control. Glyceryl trinitrate/diuretics if pulmonary oedema.
Antihistamines and anticholinergics	Sinus tachycardia, arrhythmias, hypotension, urine retention, ileus, hyperthermia, delerium, seizures.	Supportive. Activated charcoal. Seizure control. Aggressive cooling if hyperthermic.
Barbiturates	CNS and respiratory depression, coma, hypotension.	Supportive. Activated charcoal. Alkalinization of urine hastens elimination of phenobarbital.
Benzodiazepines (BZD)	CNS and respiratory depression, hypotension.	Supportive, including mechanical ventilation. Activated charcoal. Administer flumazenil to antagonize BZD effects—use with caution as BZD withdrawal can precipitate seizures. NB: flumazenil is short-acting so apart from its bolus use as a diagnostic tool or for rapid reversal of severe respiratory depression, it needs to be given by continuous infusion.
β-blockers	Bradycardia, hypotension, arrhythmias, hypothermia, hypoglycaemia, seizures.	Supportive. Activated charcoal. Glucagon, High dose glucose–insulin–potassium (GIK) infusion. Catecholamine inotropes and chronotropes—though may be ineffective for large overdose. Temorary ventricular pacing may be required. Haemodialysis if pharmacotherapy fails.
Carbon monoxide	Displaces oxygen from haemoglobin, producing carboxyhaemoglobin and hypoxaemia. Also blocks mitochondral respiration. Cerebral and pulmonary oedema, hypertonicity, agitation, coma. Oral and skin mucosae may be cherry red in colour.	Supportive. 100% oxygen. Mechanical ventilation often necessary. Consider hyperbaric oxygen therapy (if available) if HbCO levels >40% (>15% if pregnant). Cerebral oedema may require ICP monitoring.

Caustic ingestion	Causes tissue injury by chemical reaction. Acid ingestion causes coagulation necrosis with gastric and intestinal perforation and haemorrhage. Alkali ingestion causes liquefactive necrosis with airway obstruction, oesophageal perforation, tissue oedema.	Supportive. Airway management—may need tracheostomy or cricothyroidotomy if upper airway swelling severe. Regular irrigation may be needed to affected skin areas. Injury to airway and GI tract should be assessed by imaging and endoscopy. Emergency or semi-emergency surgery may be needed to deal with GI complications
Chlorine gas	Pulmonary irritant causing acute inflammation and local oedema of respiratory tract, hypoxia, ARDS/non-cardiogenic pulmonary oedema, broncospasm, laryngospasm. Corneal abrasions.	Supportive (ventilatory support often required). Fibreoptic endotracheal intubation if laryngospasm. Eye and skin irrrigation.
Cocaine	Cardiotoxic effects—tachyarrhythmias, myocardial infarction, acute coronary syndrome, intraventricular conduction disturbances, hypo/hypertension, asystole. Stroke, seizures, delirium, hyperthermia, rhabdomyolysis, acidaemia, pulmonary oedema.	Supportive. Treat heart failure and arrhythmias. Aggressive cooling if hyperthermic. BZDs for seizure control. Activated charcoal, laxatives, whole-bowel irrigation if 'body packer'.
Cyanide	Prevents mitochondrial respiration. Circulatory failure due to cellular hypoxia. Seizures, respiratory failure. Death often rapid.	Supportive. 100% oxygen. Administer hydroxycobalamin if diagnosis strongly suspected (combines with cyanide to form cyanocobalamin which is renally cleared), or sodium thiosulphate and sodium nitrite if uncertain.
Chloroquine	Cardiotoxic effects—AV conduction disturbances, ventricular fibrillation, neagtive inotropic effects, vasodilation, hypotension, sudden cardiac arrest.	Supportive. Epinephrine for hypotension.
Digoxin	May take 24–36 hours for toxic effects. Sinus bradycardia, ventricular tachycardia and fibrillation, AV conduction disturbances, vomiting, hypokalaemia, hypomagnesaemia.	Supportive. Acivated charcoal, haemodialysis if severe effects. Administer digoxin-fab fragments (Digibind—a receptor antagonist), magnesium and potassium supplementation. Temporary ventricular pacing if necessary.
Ethylene glycol (antifreeze)	Severe metabolic acidosis due to oxalic acid, acute renal failure, hypocalcaemia, inebriation.	Supportive. Administer ethanol or fomepizole which both reduce breakdown of ethylene glycol by alcohol dehydrogenase. IV crystalloids to enhance renal clearance. Correct hypocalcaemia. IV bicarbonate if acidosis severe. Haemodialysis.
Iron	Extremely corrosive to GI tract—nausea, vomiting, diarrhoea, abdominal pain, haematemesis, hypovolaemia, gastric perforation. Cellular toxicity—metabolic acidosis, liver, lung, kidney, and heart impairment.	Supportive. Whole-bowel irrigation (activated charcoal does not bind iron). Correct hypovolaemia. Administer desferrioxamine mesylate.
Lead	Liver and renal failure, diarrhoea, vomiting, abdominal pain, seizures, coma.	Supportive. Chelation therapy—dimercaprol or calcium disodium edetate (EDTA).

(continued)

Table 14.5 Continued

Drug/poison	Toxic effect	Management
Methanol	Methanol is metabolized to formaldehyde and then to formic acid which causes blindness and metabolic acidosis.	Supportive. Haemodialysis. Antidote—ethanol or fomepizole.
Opiates	CNS depression. Pinpoint pupils. Respiratory depression—hypoxia and hypercarbia.	Supportive–endotracheal intubation and mechanical ventilation may be required. Antidote–naloxone
Organophosphates	Respiratory depression, bronchospasm. Muscular weakness/paralysis, fasiculations. Bradycardia/tachycardia, asystole, hyper/hypotension. Agitation. Coma	Supportive—mechanical ventilation. Atropine to control parasympathetic activity and an oxime (e.g. pralidoxime—an anticholesterase reactivator).
Paracetamol	Nausea, vomiting, abdominal pain, sweating. Progressive liver damage develops 24–72 hours after ingestion; 3–5 βdays after ingestion hepatocellular necrosis may lead to liver failure, hypoglycaemia, hepatic encephalopathy, cerebral oedema, multi-organ failure, and death. Acute renal failure may also occur.	Supportive. Activated charcoal if <8 hours after ingestion. Antidote—*N*-acetylcysteine. Its protective effect is time dependent, but can still be given up to 48 hours after overdose with some benefit.
Phenothiazines	As for tricyclic antidepressants.	Supportive
Phenytoin	Hypotension, bradycardia, decreased conscious level, encephalopathy, myocardial depression, VF, asystole, coma, seizures	Supportive. Activated charcoal. Haemodialysis may be of some benefit.
Salicylates	Metabolic acidosis, hypokalaemia, hyponatraemia, hypoglycaemia, fever, cardiac arrrhythmias, pulmonary oedema, tinnitus, deafness, renal failure.	Supportive. Activated charcoal. Alkalization of urine. Haemodialysis.
Thallium	Abdominal pain, vomiting, peripheral neuropathy (after 2–5 days), ataxia, cranial nerve palsies, seizures, coma.	Supportive. Activated charcoal and Prussian blue (potassium ferric hexacyanoferrate)—both absorb thallium. Whole-bowel irrigation. Haemodialysis or haemoperfusion may be of benefit in early poisoning.

cardiac arrhythmias). The mechanism of shock must be ascertained by appropriate monitoring of cardiovascular variables and acid–base status to institute optimal therapy.

- **Neurological** Assess neurological status. Perform full neurological assessment, and document regular neurological observations until fully conscious. Observe for and report convulsions. Convulsions may occur as an effect of the poison taken or following a hypoxic episode. Exclude hypoglycaemia or other metabolic causes. Ensure that the airway is protected and consider hypercapnoea as a cause of obtunded level of consciousness.
- **Renal** If the patient is unable to take oral fluids, an IV infusion will be required. Monitor urine output, blood urea, electrolytes, and creatinine. Perform urinalysis. Rhabdomyolysis can be a complication of some poisonings, particularly when the patient is comatose, but also with drugs that cause 'hyper-exercise' (strychnine, cocaine, amphetamines including ecstasy). Diagnosis is usually confirmed by grossly elevated plasma levels of creatine kinase and creatinine, as well as myoglobinuria ('positive' dipstick to blood or formal laboratory confirmation). Circulatory and renal failure can develop (for further details see Chapter 8) as can compartment syndrome (see Chapter 11).
- **Other** Monitor blood glucose regularly and correct hyper/hypoglycaemia. Monitor body temperature. Hypothermia is a common manifestation of many poisonings (often accompanied by hypotension and oliguria). Such patients must be rewarmed with close monitoring of volaemic status. If plasma expanders are vigorously overinfused, they may cause circulatory overload and pulmonary oedema. Caution is required, especially when the core temperature is <32°C (see Chapter 11 for further details on hypothermia). Aggressive cooling should be used if the patient is hyperthermic.

Specific management of common drug overdoses

Table 14.5 details the management of specific drug overdoses. During the recovery period patients who have made a deliberate suicide attempt may become withdrawn and uncommunicative, or aggressive and uncooperative. Skill and understanding is needed by the nurse during this difficult period. A psychiatric referral should be arranged as soon as possible so that the acute problem can be alleviated and further suicide attempts prevented. Assistance from other support agencies may be required (e.g. social workers, ministers of religion).

References and bibliography

Abadi S, Ginarson A, Karen G. (2002) Use of Warfarin during Pregnancy. *Can Fam Physician* 48:695–97.

Adler JT, Meyer-Rochow GY, Chen H, Benn D *et al* (2008) Phaeochromocytoma: Current Approaches and Future Directions. *The Oncologist* 13(7):779–793.

Bahn R, Burch H, Cooper D, Garber J. *et al* (2011) Hypothyroidism and other causes of thyrotoxicosis; management guidelines of the American Association of Clinical Endocrinologists. *Thyroid* 21(6):593–646.

Bates SM, Greer IA, Middeldorp S *et al* (2010) VTE, Thrombophilia, Antithrombotic therapy, and Pregnancy: Antithrombotic Therapy and Prevention of Thrombosis, 9th ed: American College of Chest Physicians Evidence-Based Clinical Practice Guidelines. *Chest* 141 (no 2 suppl):e691S–3736S.

Bilezikian JP, Khan A, Potts J. *et al* (2011) Hypoparathyroidism in the adult: epidemiology, diagnosis, pathophysiology, target organ involvement, treatment and challanges for future research. *J Bone Miner. Res.* 26(10):2317–37.

Boelan A, Kwakkel J, Fliers E. (2011) Beyond low plasma T3: local thyroid hormone metabolism during inflammation and infection. *Endocr Rev* 32(5):670–93.

Board JB, Graber AL, Christma JW, Powers AC. (2001) Practical Management of Diabetes in Critically ill Patients. *Am J Resp. Crit. Care Med* 164(10):1763–1767.

Bourjeily G, Paidas M, Khali H, Rosene-Motella K, Rodger M. (2010) Pulmonary Embolism in Pregnancy. *Lancet* 375:500–512.

Baumgartner H, Bonhoeffer P, De Groot N. *et al* (2010) ESC Guidelines for the management of grown up congenital heart disease. The Task Force on the management of grown up congenital heart disease of the European Society of Cardiology (ESC) *European Heart Journal* 31: 2915–57.

Clark SL, Hankins GD, Dudley, DA *et al* (1996) Amniotic fluid embolism: analysis of the National Registry. *Am J Obst & Gynecol* 172(4, Part 1), 1158–67.

Clark SL. (2010) Amniotic fluid embolism *Clin Obst Gynecol* 53(2);322–8.

Dutta P, Bhansali S, Masood S. *et al* (2008) Predictors of outcome in myxoedema coma: a study from a tertiary care centre. *Critical care*, 12:R1.

Ecomidou F, Douka E, Tzanela M. *et al* (2011) Thyroid function during critical illness. *Hormones (Athens)* 10(2):117–24.

Eddleston M, Buckley NA, Eyer P, Dawson AH. (2008) Management of acute organophosphorus pesticide poisoning. *Lancet* 371(9612):597–607.

Fahy KM. (2001). Amniotic fluid embolism: a review of the research literature. *Australian Journal of Midwifery* **14**(1), 9–13.

Gist RS, Stafford IP, Leibowitz AB, Beilin Y. (2009) Amniotic fluid embolism. *Anaesth Analg* 108(5);1599–1602.

Greene SL, Dargen PI, Jones AL. (2005) Acute poisoning: understanding 90% of cases in a nutshell. *Postgrad Med J* 81: 204–16

Hypertension in pregnancy. National Institute of Clinical Excellence Guideline 107, 2010.

Karamermer Y, Roos-Hesselink JW. (2007) Pregnancy and adult congenital heart disease. *Expert Rev Cardiovasc Ther* 5(5): 859–69.

Kitabchi AE, Umpierrez GE, Miles JM, Fisher JN. (2009) Hyperglycaemic crisis in adult patients with diabetes; a concensus statement from the American diabetes Association. *Diabetes Care* 32: 1335–43.

Klauer KM, Schraga E. (2008) Adrenal crisis in Emergency Medicine. *Am J Emerg Med.* 26(2):251 e3–4

Ko H, Yoshida E. (2006) Acute fatty liver of pregnancy (AFLP) *Can J Gastroenterol* 20(1):25–30.

Leung AN, Todd M, Jaeschke R, Lockwood CJ. (2011) An official American Thoracic Society/Society of Thoracic Radiology clinical practice guidelines:evaluation of suspected pulmonary embolism in pregnancy. *Am J Resp Crit Care Med* 184:1200–1208.

Lovell AT. (2004) Anaesthetic implications of grown up congenital heart disease. *Br J Anaesth* 93(1):129–39.

McKeown NJ, Tews MC, Gossain V. *et al* (2005) Hyperthyroidism. *Emerg Med Clin N Amer* 23 669–85

Magpie Trial Collaborative Group (2002). Do women with pre-eclampsia, and their babies, benefit from magnesium sulphate? The Magpie Trial: a randomised placebo controlled trial. *Lancet* **359**, 1877.

Martin SR, Foley M. (2006) Intensive Care in Obstetrics: An evidence-based review. *Am J Obst Gyn* 195, 673–80.

Mathew V, Misgar A, Ghosh S. *et al* (2011) Myxedema Coma: A New Look into an Old Crisis. *Journal of Thyroid Research*, vol 2011, Article ID 493462.

Meyer S, Schuetz P, Wieland M. (2011) Low triiodothyronine syndrome: a marker for outcome in sepsis? *Endocrine* Apr;39(2):16–74.

Mokhlesi B, Leiken JB, Murray P. *et al.* (2003). Adult toxicology in critical care. Part I: General approach to the intoxicated patient. *Chest* **123**, 577–92.

Mokhlesi B, Leiken JB, Murray P. *et al.* (2003). Adult toxicology in critical care. Part II: Specific poisonings. *Chest* **123**, 897–922.

Nayek B, Burman K. (2006) Thyrotoxicosis and Thyroid Storm. *Endocrinol Metab Clin N Am* 35 663–686.

Nugent BW. (2005) Hyperosmolar hyperglycaemic state. *Emerg Med Clin Am.* 23(3):629–48,vii.

Perozzi K J, Englert NC. (2004) Amniotic fluid embolism: an obstetric emergency. *Crit Care Nurse* 24(4) 54–61.

Ramaraj R, Sorrell V. (2009) Peripartum cardiomyopathy: Causes, diagnosis and treatment. *Cleveland Clinic J Med* 76 (5) 289–296.

Report of the British Cardiac Society working party (2002) Grown up congenital heart (GUCH) disease: current needs and provision of service for adolescents and adults with congenital heart disease in the UK. *Heart* 88(1):11–14.

Savage MW. (2011) Management of diabetic ketoacidosis. *Clinical Medicine.* 11(2) 154–6.

Savage MW, Dhatariya KK, Kilvert G, Rayman G. *et al* (2011) Diabetes UK Position Statement and Care Recommendations. Joint British Diabetes Societies guideline for the management of Diabetic Ketoacidosis. *Diab. Med* 28:508–15.

Vara KS, Shah VR, Paprikh GP. (2009) Acute fatty liver of pregnancy: A case report of an uncommon disease. *Indian J Crit Care Med* 13:34–36.

Williams D. (2012) Pre-eclampsia. *BMJ* 345:e4437.

CHAPTER 15

Managing major incidents and preparing for pandemics

Introduction

While many critical care staff may never be involved in a major incident or pandemic, the potential certainly exists. If it occurs, it is likely to be one of the most stretching, difficult, and demanding situations they will ever deal with.

In the United Kingdom, the requirement to respond in such situations is governed by the Civil Contingencies Act 2004 which requires organizations at the core of the emergency response (i.e.Designated Category 1 responders, see Table 15.1) to:

- assess the risk of emergencies occurring, and to use this to inform contingency planning
- put in place emergency plans
- put in place business continuity management arrangements
- put in place arrangements to make information available to the public about civil protection matters and maintain arrangements to warn, inform, and advise the public in the event of an emergency
- share information with other local responders to enhance coordination
- cooperate with other local responders to enhance coordination and efficiency.

What this means is that an organization such as an acute hospital will need to form a group of appropriate personnel—emergency department staff, critical care staff, facilities staff, security staff, managers, ICT staff, communications and information teams, etc.—to develop a clear understanding of the risk from such events and put a plan for managing them in place.

Table 15.1 Organizations categorized as responders

Category 1 responders (core responders)	Category 2 responders (cooperating responders)
Emergency services • Police forces • British Transport Police • Fire authorities • Ambulance services • Maritime and Coastguard Agency Local authorities • All principal local authorities (i.e. metropolitan districts, shire counties, shire districts, shire unitaries) • Port Health Authorities Health bodies • Acute Trusts • Foundation Trusts • Local Health Boards (in Wales) • Any Welsh NHS Trust which provides public health services • Health Protection Agency Government agencies • Environment Agency • Scottish Environment Agency	Utilities • Electricity distributors and transmitters • Gas distributors • Water and sewerage undertakers • Telephone service providers (fixed and mobile) Transport • Network Rail • Train operating companies (passenger and freight) • London Underground • Transport for London • Airport operators • Harbour authorities • Highways Agency Health bodies • Regional Health Authorities Government agencies • Health and Safety Executive

The types of event that could occur are classified by location and extent of impact.

A. Single location:

- fixed site—industrial plant, school, airport, train station, sports stadium
- town or city centre
- corridor railway, motorway, air corridor, fuel pipeline
- unpredictable bomb, chemical tanker, random shooting.

B. Multiple locations:

- multiple locations linked, possibly simultaneously, to explosions at different sites

C. Wide area:

- large area toxic cloud; loss of electricity, gas, water, telephone supply
- River or coastal flooding, dam or reservoir failure
- Whole area severe weather, health emergencies (including influenza pandemic, foot-and-mouth disease).

D. Outside area:

- external emergency—residents local to your area involved in an emergency elsewhere, e.g. coach or plane crash; passenger ship sinking; incident at football stadium
- evacuees into your area from another UK area
- refugees from an emergency overseas.

Plans must include generic and specific responses to ensure that the infrastructure to maintain service provision is maintained while dealing with the additional impact of whatever has caused the major incident and the ensuing casualties/patients.

Definitions

Major incident

This is any emergency that requires implementation of special arrangements by at least one emergency service and will generally include involvement, either directly or indirectly, of large numbers of people (e.g. rescue and transportation of a large number of casualties), mobilization and organization of emergency services and support services (e.g. the local authority to cater for the threat of death, serious injury, or homelessness to a large number of people), and handling a large number of enquiries likely to be generated from both public and media.

Major incident within the NHS

This is any occurrence that presents serious threat to the health of the community, disruption to the service, or causes (or is likely to cause) such numbers or types of casualties as to require special arrangements to be implemented by hospitals, ambulance trusts, or primary care organizations (NHS Commissioning Board Emergency Preparedness Framework 2013).

Scale of major incidents

The types of incident for which emergency preparedness plans (and business continuity plans) are required vary in scope and size. These incidents are considered to be over and above the daily fluctuations of demand for the service and constitute a real threat to the organization's ability to deliver their service. The levels of incident for which NHS organizations are required to develop emergency preparedness arrangements are defined by the NHS Commissioning Board Emergency Preparedness Framework (2013).

The NHS Commissioning Board (NHSCB) incident levels are defined as follows:

1. A health-related incident that can be responded to and managed by local health provider organizations that requires coordination by the local Clinical Commissioning Group (CCG).
2. A health-related incident that requires the response of a number of health provider organizations across an NHSCB area team boundary and will require an NHSCB Area Team to coordinate the NHS local support.
3. A health-related incident, that requires the response of a number of health provider organizations across and NHSCB area teams across an NHSCB region and requires NHSCB regional coordination to meet the demands of the incident.
4. A health-related incident, that requires NHSCB national coordination to support the NHS and NHSCB response.[1]

In addition, pre-arranged major events (e.g. public demonstrations with potential for disorder, high profile sports fixtures, air shows, etc.) will also require planning for a response.

Types of incident

Categories of specific hazards include bioterrorism, chemical emergencies, radiation emergencies, outbreaks and incidents, severe weather, natural disasters, and mass casualty events caused by terrorism or war.

- **Bioterrorism**—the deliberate release of biological agents such as viruses, bacteria, and spores to cause illness or death in people, animals, or plants.
- **Chemical emergencies**—these occur when a hazardous chemical has been released with the potential for harm. Release can be unintentional (e.g. an industrial accident) or intentional (e.g. a terrorist attack).
- **Radiation emergencies**—these occur when release of radiation (either intentionally or by accident) is likely to prove harmful.
- **Mass casualty events**—these are events caused by explosions, bomb blasts, or other serious widespread attacks.
- **Outbreaks and incidents**—for example, pandemic influenza, SARS, salmonella gastroenteritis
- **Severe weather and natural disasters**—these include earthquakes, extreme heat, floods, hurricanes, landslides and mudslides, tornadoes, tsunamis, volcanic eruptions, wildfires, and extreme winter weather.

Role of critical care units and specialist staff in a major incident

Between 5% and 15% of patients presenting to hospital following a bomb blast or terrorist-based mass casualty incident will require intensive care (Avidan *et al.* 2007). The demands on critical care resource for other incidents, such as large fires or natural disasters, are less

[1] Reproduced from NHS Commissioning Board, NHS England Core Standards for Emergency Preparedness, Resilience and Response, p. 9, 2013. Available under the Open Government Licence 3.0 (https://www.nationalarchives.gov.uk/doc/open-government-licence/version/3/).

well documented. However, following the aftermath of Hurricane Katrina in New Orleans, the Charity Hospital had to manage increased demand without the opportunity to evacuate for many days (deBoisblanc *et al.* 2005).

In 2007 the US Task force for Mass Critical Care suggested that critical care units should plan to provide emergency mass critical care at three times the existing capacity for up to 10 days (Rubinson *et al.* 2008). However, critical care beds and staff are a limited resource which is usually fully utilized; in the event of a major incident, releasing beds or expanding the resource requires good planning and organization. As critical care resources will often represent the major limiting factor in being able to deal with large numbers of casualties, it is also important that early links with other hospitals are made so that transfer of more stable patients can be undertaken in the safest way possible. Therefore it is vital that critical care leaders are involved in planning for major incidents across healthcare communities.

The CHEST Task Force for Mass Critical Care (Christian *et al.* 2014) have suggested that there are different levels of capacity expansion required by different levels of incident.

Critical care resources need to increase for:

(a) conventional response—able to expand immediately by at least 20% above baseline ICU maximum capacity

(b) contingency response—able to expand rapidly by at least 100% above baseline ICU maximum capacity by accessing local and regional resources

(c) crisis response—able to expand by at least 200% above baseline ICU maximum capacity with support from local, regional, national and international agencies.[2]

The minimum requirements for critical care suggested by the EMCC taskforce (Rubinson *et al.* 2008) are:

- mechanical ventilation
- IV fluid resuscitation
- vasopressor administration
- antidote or antimicrobial administration for specific disease processes, if applicable
- sedation and analgesia
- strategies to reduce adverse consequences of critical care and critical illness
- optimal therapeutics and interventions, such as renal replacement therapy and nutrition for patients unable to take food by mouth, if warranted by hospital or regional preference.[3]

It is suggested that a tiered response should be set up, allowing increasingly high risk management practices to be considered as the impact of the incident increases. Ultimately, triage of patients for access to scarce critical care resources would also be included.

Preparation to manage such an incident includes:

- a degree of stockpiling or identification of alternative sources of equipment (e.g. use of NIV machines and anaesthetic ventilators to supply ventilatory support)
- identification of staff with transferable skills such as respiratory nurses and recovery nurses, and previous critical care nurses
- training and education of staff.

Planning

The critical care consultant and nursing leads must ensure that preparation for a major incident is thorough and well considered. Unlike the emergency department, where the focus is on the initial first few hours, critical care patients may remain in the unit for days to weeks, often placing enormous pressure on the staff. Any expansion of critical care capacity would also dilute the number of skilled staff available, placing further demands on them.

Therefore the critical care unit plan requires:

(1) clear identification of who is in charge

(2) strategies for immediate management of casualties requiring critical care

[2] Reprinted from *Chest*, volume 146, issue 4, Christian M.D, Debereaux A.V, Dichter J.R *et al*, Introduction and Executive Summary Care of the Critically Ill and Injured During Pandemics and Disasters: CHEST Consensus Statement, pp. 8S–34S. Copyright (2014), with permission from Elsevier.

[3] Data from Rubinson, L., Hick, J.L., Hanfling, D.G., *et al.*, Definitive Care for the Critically Ill during a Disaster: A Framework for Optimizing Critical Care Surge Capacity From a Task Force for Mass Critical Care Summit Meeting, January 26–27, 2007, *Chest*, volume 133, pp.18S–31S. 2008, Elsevier.

(3) strategies for increasing capacity if needed (identification of overflow areas, use of critical care outreach, links with other critical care units, access to and maintenance of increased supplies of equipment, disposables, burns dressing and wound care materials, protective clothing, etc.)
(4) strategies for ongoing management (over days)
(5) structure for staff support (counselling, time off, peer support, etc.)
(6) effective communication systems for all staff.

Once the plan is agreed, it must be communicated effectively to all staff. Action cards, which outline the actions required by each role, provide an effective aide-memoire. Training in individual roles and testing of the plan, using either table-top exercises or mock incidents, will ensure that any planning gaps are identified, and that all staff understand what is required of them.

The critical care plans should be part of a hospital-wide major incident response plan; in turn, the hospital plan should be part of a sector-wide response plan. This ensures that silo thinking does not occur, with the consequent potential for serious systems failures

Immediate response

Initial reports of a major incident are often confused and difficult to fully understand. Normal communication links are often affected (e.g. mobile phone networks may be overladen, or shut down to prevent triggering of further explosive devices). Therefore it is important that standard preparations are put in place so that when casualties are known and admissions are imminent, much of the preparatory work has been completed.

Critical care admissions will usually occur at a later point after the incident. Many may arrive via the operating theatre or after resuscitation in the emergency department. This gives much needed time to triage and, if possible, move existing patients, to access additional equipment and stores, and to call in additional staff. Suspension of elective operations and discharge of any patients fit for the ward must be carried out in order to clear beds for admissions (Carter 2014). Clear command and control style leadership is crucial. The short timescales, confusion, and stress make the situation difficult to manage. There is a real danger of chaos unless clear direction, actions, and leadership are maintained. Training and practice responses focus on this; many systems use action cards to direct the actions required by each command role.

The initial response should focus on the following.

1. Contacting appropriate senior staff to ensure adequate leadership and support.
2. Senior review of all current patients to designate those who can be moved, i.e.
   (a) movement of stable patients who do not require ventilation or inotropic support to ward beds
   (b) designation and set-up of an additional critical care area where stable longer-term patients requiring less intensive support can be moved
   (c) movement to neighbouring hospitals, if possible.
3. Preparation of bed areas for admissions, catering for special needs (e.g. burns).
4. Senior intensivist to be based in emergency department.
5. Senior intensivist to be based in critical care working with senior critical care nurse to triage patients and direct junior staff.
6. Senior critical care nurse to be based in additional critical care area (if opened).

Immediate management of patients

In a mass casualty event the general principle is to move patients appropriately from the emergency department through to the operating theatre and critical care wards (or discharge) as quickly and safely as possible. Details of initial patient assessment and management can be found in Chapter 11.

Primary triage of casualties at the site is essential to ensure that the correct level of care is provided to all casualties. The US core criteria for primary triage (Lerner *et al.* 2011) state that triage should take place after initial life-saving interventions are performed only if the equipment is readily available, the intervention is within the provider's scope of practice, the intervention can be performed quickly (i.e. in less than 1min), and the intervention does not require the provider to stay with the patient. Life-saving interventions include the following:

- controlling life-threatening external haemorrhage
- opening the airway using basic manoeuvres (for an apnoeic child, consider two rescue breaths)
- performing chest decompression
- providing auto-injector antidotes.

Table 15.2 Primary triage categories for mass casualties from blast injuries

Category (tag colour)	Category definitions (Lerner *et al.* 2011)	Interventions and care	Examples of injuries (Bridges 2006)
Minimal (green)	Able to follow commands or make purposeful movements, AND they have peripheral pulse, AND they are not in respiratory distress, AND they do not have a life-threatening external hemorrhage, AND their injuries are considered minor	Remove from triage area—assign to 'buddy' care	Minor wounds, psychological trauma, minor auditory trauma
Delayed (yellow)	Able to follow commands or make purposeful movements, AND they have peripheral pulse, AND they are not in respiratory distress, AND they do not have a life-threatening external hemorrhage, AND they have injuries that are not considered minor	Simple care required within next few hours	Isolated extremity trauma or injury without vascular compromise Superficial or partial thickness burns Stable after thoracic drain insertion
Immediate (red)	Unable to follow commands or make purposeful movements, OR they do not have a peripheral pulse, OR they are in obvious respiratory distress, OR they have a life-threatening external haemorrhage, provided that their injuries are likely to be survivable given available resources.	Highly likely to survive, requiring procedures of moderately short duration, or rapid intervention to prevent death such as relief of airway obstruction or placement of chest drain	Airway compromise Haemorrhage, Hypotension, Vascular trauma Major limb deformity Deep partial- thickness or full-thickness burns
Expectant (grey)	Unable to follow commands or make purposeful movements, OR they do not have a peripheral pulse, OR they are in obvious respiratory distress, OR they have a life-threatening external haemorrhage, AND they are unlikely to survive given the available resources.	Treatment would require significant resource and survival is unlikely Comfort measures	Amputation by blast wave of major parts of body Open skull fracture with protruding brain tissue
Dead (black)	Patients who are not breathing after one attempt to open their airway (in children, two rescue breaths may also be given) must be classified as dead	CPR would require consistent resource and attention and is associated with a low survival	Pulseless and unresponsive after immediate life-saving interventions (CPR is not recommended in the field)

CPR, cardiopulmonary resuscitation.

Data from: Lerner *et al.*, Disaster Med Public Health Preparedness. Volume 5, pp. 129-137, 2011; Bridges, E.J., Blast Injuries: From Triage to Critical Care. Critical Care Nursing Clinics of North America, Volume 18, pp. 333–348, 2006.

Five triage categories are identified (see Table 15.2) with treatment interventions depending on what is immediately available and achievable. The priority for transfer and treatment is patients categorized as 'immediate' followed by those categorized as 'delayed' and 'minimal'. Patients categorized as expectant should be provided with treatment and/or transport as resources allow (Lerner *et al.* 2011). Further secondary triage will take place when the patients arrive in the emergency department.

Ongoing management in critical care

Patients

Most of the patients admitted to critical care after a mass incident are likely to require ventilation, surgery and burn management (see Box 15.1). Most will have already undergone 'damage control' or 'injury stabilization' surgery rather than definitive procedures which are often prolonged and would take up too much theatre and

Box 15.1 Injuries sustained by the 512 victims of the 2004 Madrid train bombings admitted to hospital

AIS body region injuries

Head–neck (including basal skull fracture, C-spine fracture, inhalation injury, subdural haematoma, subarachnoid haemorrhage, contusion, infarct, etc.)

Face (including **tympanic perforation**, **eye injuries**, facial injuries, **maxillofacial fracture**)

Chest (including T1–6 segment fracture, **lung contusion**, **blast lung injury**, **rib fracture**, **pneumothorax**, haemothorax, spinal cord trauma)

Abdomen (including liver, spleen, kidney, stomach, small and large bowel injury, lumbar spine fracture)

Extremities (including **long bone**, ankle, metacarpal and clavicle fractures, lower limb and finger amputations, 'mangled' limbs, arterial contusions, vascular and nerve damage)

External (including **shrapnel wounds** to head–neck, torso, limbs, **first-, second-, and third-degree burns**)

*Injuries in bold were more frequent and commonly associated with blasts.

Data from Turégano-Fuentes, F., Caba-Doussoux, P., Jover-Navalón, J.M., Injury Patterns from Major Urban Terrorist Bombings in Trains: The Madrid Experience. *World J ournal of Surgery*, Volume 32, pp.1168–75, 2008 Springer.

surgeon time (Bridges, 2006). Routine laboratory studies and X-rays or more advanced diagnostics are unlikely to have been carried out in the Emergency Department and will be required once the patients are settled and stabilized in critical care. Patients with head injuries will have received a CT scan if they have a low or deteriorating GCS and many patients will have required a FAST (Focused Assessment With Sonography for Trauma) exam for suspected blunt abdominal injury. A FAST scan will detect the presence of free fluid in the abdomen with 93% accuracy and 97% specificity (Beck-Razi *et al.* 2007). If ultrasound is not available, then a diagnostic peritoneal lavage (DPL) can be carried out (see p. 418 for details) immediately in the Emergency department but CT scan with contrast is a more definitive diagnostic tool. Some patients with a negative FAST but clinical symptoms of abdominal injury will require this to confirm or rule out abdominal trauma. If life-threatening, they may require immediate laparotomy without a prior scan.

Blast injuries

The predominant injuries seen following explosive blasts are pulmonary, abdominal, orthopaedic (including soft tissue injuries), neurological, otological and opthalmic.

Pathophysiology

Explosions result in rapid expansion of gas outwards from the point of detonation, displacing the surrounding medium. The wave of high pressure in air creates high velocity winds which propel people and objects causing a range of blast injuries. Injury patterns vary according to the cause and distance from the blast epicentre (Dennis and Kochanek 2007). Several other factors affect the magnitude of the blast, the speed of the blast wave and the likelihood of injury (Wolf *et al.* 2009):

- the medium in which the explosion takes place (i.e. air or water)—water is non-compressible so blast waves move rapidly and dissipate slowly, causing greater potential for injury
- distance from the explosion—blast energy decreases in proportion to the distance cubed
- solid surface amplification—in a confined space (e.g. bus or room) the pressure wave is amplified and prolonged, resulting in increased mortality and injury

Blast injuries directly related to the pressure wave are termed primary blast injuries, those created by debris are secondary blast injuries, while those caused by physical displacement of the individual or damage from surrounding structures are tertiary blast injuries. Additional injuries such as burns, radiation and poisoning have been categorised into quaternary injury. More recently, a hyperinflammatory state seen after a bombing in Israel has been proposed as quinary injury, though this category has yet to be fully accepted. (Wolf *et al.* 2009)

Primary blast injuries

These are most likely to happen at interfaces between air and tissue in the body. The lungs, gastrointestinal tract, and ears are therefore most susceptible to primary blast injury. Pulmonary injury is seen in up to 71% of those who are critically ill and hospitalised after a blast (Wolf 2009).

Assessment should follow the ABCDE approach but should pay particular attention to the clinical signs associated with blast pathology (see Table 15.3).

Table 15.3 Assessment of blast injuries

Type of injury	Pathology	Clinical signs
Primary blast injury	Blast lung (alveolar rupture, pulmonary contusion, pneumothorax and haemorrhage)	Tachypnoea Hypoxaemia Cyanosis Wheezing Decreased breath sounds Haemoptysis Cough Chest pain Dyspnoea Haemodynamic instability
	Tympanic membrane rupture and damage	Deafness Bleeding from the ear
	Abdominal haemorrhage and perforation	Abdominal pain, Rectal bleeding Liver or spleen lacerations Rebound tenderness Guarding Absent bowel sounds Signs of hypovolaemia Nausea and vomiting
	Traumatic brain injury	Loss of consciousness Headache Fatigue Poor concentration, lethargy Amnesia

Management of primary blast injuries

Primary blast lung injury

The underlying pathology is due to alveolar overdistension and rupture with multifocal small haemorrhages, contusions, and arterial air embolism (Wolf *et al.* 2009). In the 12–24 hours following trauma, there is progressive vascular leak and inflammatory changes. The patient will exhibit dyspnoea, cough, and hypoxaemia related to vascular shunting and ventilation/perfusion mismatch. There may also be pneumo- and/or haemothoraces, and where shearing forces disrupt the bronchopulmonary tree there may be bronchopulmonary fistulae and arterial air emboli (NB: this can also occur as a result of positive pressure ventilation). Chest X-rays will show signs of bilateral pulmonary infiltrates which may develop over a number of hours after the blast.

Management is complicated by the conflicting demands from managing other injuries. For instance, the fluid resuscitation required for haemodynamic support may lead to increased pulmonary oedema, while the normocapnia required to reduce cerebral oedema in head injuries may require increased ventilatory pressures or volumes which may increase the risk from barotrauma. Blast lung injury should be managed, where possible, without positive pressure ventilation or PEEP because of the risk of exacerbating barotrauma and air emboli. However, if needed, ventilation settings that employ the lowest level of inspiratory pressure and PEEP should be used. In severe cases, pressure control and inverse ratio ventilation (aiming for oxygen saturations of 90% and tidal volumes of 5–7 ml/kg) with permissive hypercapnia has been used successfully, albeit not for patients with head injuries.

Gastrointestinal blast injury

Diagnosis can be difficult as symptoms are often non-specific, including nausea and vomiting, haematemesis, pain, diarrhoea, and melaena. Bowel wall injuries are difficult to detect on CT or ultrasound, so continued assessment and a high level of suspicion for perforation as a cause of any sudden deterioration are essential. Maintenance of a permissive level of hypotension (e.g. systolic pressure 80–90 mmHg) where there is no concomitant head injury may help to manage volume resuscitation associated with intestinal injury without exacerbating pulmonary blast injury (Wolf *et al.* 2009).

Neurological injury

Secondary and tertiary blast injuries were originally thought to constitute the main central nervous system trauma but, more recently, research has suggested that primary concussive forces resulting from the blast are linked with concussive brain injury without overt head trauma. Patients may present with symptoms ranging from subtle neurocognitive dysfunction to unconsciousness.

Traumatic amputation/limb avulsion

These occur as a result of primary blast injury in 1–3% of victims and have a high associated mortality, often because the patient was very close to the blast itself. Treatment is surgical, aiming to remove necrotic tissue, preserving limb length and viable tissue as much as possible. In some cases, completion of amputation is the only alternative. Daily wound debridement is performed until healthy tissue predominates and all foreign material is removed. Fractures associated with the injury should be externally fixated at an early stage. Compartment syndrome is a risk, and the limb should be observed regularly for signs of swelling, distal temperature change, and loss of pulses; fasciotomy may be required (Plurad 2011).

Burns

Burns are associated with blast injury in 27% of patients, most of whom will have primary blast injury. The hands and face are most commonly affected; such patients should be examined carefully for primary blast and inhalational injuries. Management of burns with a coexisting blast lung injury will require very careful fluid resuscitation with close monitoring of intravascular volume.

Wound management

Wounds are initially cleaned of gross contamination with saline irrigation and debridement. A moist sterile dressing is applied, which should only be removed for further irrigation, debridement, or assessment. Wounds are not usually closed immediately as this is associated with increased wound infection (Bridges 2006). The use of vacuum-assisted closure (VAC) therapy to aid wound healing is effective in reducing infection and improving time to closure (Hinck *et al.* 2010).

Supportive care

Patients will require antibiotic prophylaxis and a tetanus toxoid booster.

Staff

Although the natural response in the immediate aftermath of a major incident is for staff to work over and above their usual hours and duties, it is important to ensure that everyone gets breaks, has access to food and drink, and are relieved before they become too exhausted. The staff rota must be adjusted to ensure that sufficient staff are available both to care for the patients and to relieve existing staff for ongoing shifts. It is also important to ensure that senior staff are also released to allow time off. As exposure to such an event is highly traumatic for staff and emotionally very draining. It is important to secure support from counselling, psychologists, and peers/mentors.Post-traumatic stress disorder may also develop. Debriefing of staff may be useful in preventing this.

Pandemics

The word pandemic comes from the Greek (*pan*—meaning 'all', and *demos*—meaning 'people'). It describes an outbreak of infectious disease which affects a widespread population, usually across a continent or similar-sized area.

The World Health Organization lists conditions for an outbreak to be labelled a pandemic (World Health Organization 2009):

- new pathogen emerges in humans
- minimal or no population immunity
- causes serious illness—high morbidity/mortality
- spreads easily from person to person.

There is some doubt whether the H1N1 influenza outbreak in 2009 should have been labelled a pandemic (Doshi 2011) as the consequences of the disease were, in the main, less severe than expected. Pandemics tend to be associated with a need for a slower but ongoing and increasing requirements for healthcare, the so-called 'rising tide' scenario. Although easier to plan for, and put contingencies in place, it is often more difficult to manage because of its longer duration. It can also have a far greater social and economic impact.

The phases associated with pandemics are outlined in Table 15.4.

Influenza pandemics

There are two types of influenza virus which cause significant illness in the human population—influenza A and influenza B. Influenza A viruses are currently the

Table 15.4 WHO pandemic phase descriptions

Phase 1	No animal influenza virus circulating among animals has been reported to cause infection in humans
Phase 2	An animal influenza virus circulating in domesticated or wild animals is known to have caused infection in humans and is therefore considered a specific potential pandemic threat
Phase 3	An animal or human–animal influenza reassortant virus has caused sporadic cases or small clusters of disease in humans, but has not resulted in human-to-human (H2H) transmission sufficient to sustain community level outbreaks
Phase 4	Human-to-human transmission of an animal or human–animal influenza reassortant virus able to sustain community level outbreaks has been verified
Phase 5	The same identified virus has caused sustained community level outbreaks in two or more countries in one WHO region
Phase 6	In addtion to the criteria defined in Phase 5, the same virus has caused sustained community level outbreaks in at least one other country in another WHO region
Post-peak period	Levels of pandemic influenza in most countries with adequate surveillance have dropped below peak levels
Possible new wave	Level of pandemic influenza activity in most countries with adequate surveillance rising again
Post-pandemic period	Levels of influenza activity have returned to the levels seen for seasonal influenza in most countries with adequate surveillance

only influenza viruses able to pose a significant pandemic threat to humans. An influenza pandemic occurs when a new influenza A virus that is antigenically different to the circulating influenza strain arises. Most of the population will have little or no immunity to the new strain which spreads easily from person to person. The World Health Organization guidance on pandemic influenza states:

> An influenza pandemic occurs when an animal influenza virus to which most humans have no immunity acquires the ability to cause sustained chains of human-to-human transmission leading to community-wide outbreaks. Such a virus has the potential to spread worldwide, causing a pandemic.
>
> World Health Organization 2009

At the genetic level, pandemic influenza viruses may arise through (i) genetic reassortment—a process in which genes from animal and human influenza viruses combine to create a human–animal influenza reassortant virus—or (ii) genetic mutation whereby genes in an animal influenza virus change, allowing the virus to infect and be easily transmissible between humans.

Only four influenza pandemics have occurred in the recent past, the 1918–1919 'Spanish flu', the 1957–1958 'Asian flu', the 1968–1969 'Hong Kong flu', and the 2009–2010 'H1N1 swine flu'. These were all caused by subtypes of the influenza A virus. Avian influenza (H5N1) has also emerged as a threat, although mainly through transmission of the virus from poultry to humans who have close association with either living or dead birds> There has only been very limited human-to-human transmission.

Global health threats

The outbreak of SARS (severe acute respiratory syndrome) in 2003 is an example of a global health threat which spread quickly due to global travel, but was limited and confined before it became a pandemic. It affected approximately 8000 people with 750 dying as a result. It was first identified in China and quickly spread across Asia to Australia, North and South America, Europe, and Africa. It caused widespread disruption, particularly in Asia. The virus causing SARS is a member of the coronavirus family and is thought to have originally spread from small mammals in China. Another coronavirus, the Middle East respiratory syndrome coronavirus (MERS-CoV), was first identified in Saudi Arabia in 2012 and has been responsible for deaths worldwide. There are particular concerns that this virus may be transmitted rapidly worldwide due to the large numbers attending the Haj.

Managing and preparing surge capacity and infrastructure in critical care for pandemics

Although the 2009 H1N1 (swine flu) pandemic turned out to be less of a threat than predicted, a number of valuable lessons were learnt from the process of planning, including the development of contingency arrangements at a local and national level. In Australia, where intensive care units dealt with a significant number of patients, key learning was around the need for preparation and training of staff, as well as the development of triage protocols to guide admission and adequate fit testing for PPE masks (Leen *et al.* 2010). Coordination across all components of the healthcare sectors, including primary and social care, was needed to manage numerous unanticipated knock-on effects. For instance, the proposal to discharge non-affected patients early from hospitals into the community to free up beds would have placed a huge strain on community nursing and support services. The use of staff from non-critical care areas to support enhanced critical care capacity required extensive update training, which there was little time to provide.

The European Society of Intensive Care Medicine has published recommendations for hospitals to prepare for increased critical care capacity (Hick *et al.* 2010).

1. Critical care bed numbers should be increased by expanding existing ICU capacity, and also by locating ICUs in other areas. Suitable locations should be identified, using post-anaesthesia care units and emergency departments, then stepdown units, large procedure suites, and telemetry units, and finally hospital wards.
2. Appropriate beds and monitors should be available for these expansion areas; contingency plans should be developed at hospital and government (local, regional, national) levels to provide additional ventilators.
3. A phased staffing plan should exist that provides sufficient patient care supervision during contingency and crisis situations.
4. Expert input should be provided to the emergency management personnel, both during planning for surge capacity as well as during the response to a pandemic
5. An adequate infrastructure support should be present to support critical care activities.[4]

All of these components should be actively addressed in a local pandemic plan document which ensures that trigger points are identified for initiating responses and planned actions are clearly outlined.

Specialist equipment

It is essential to wear personal protective equipment (PPE). Standard universal precautions are used in most cases, but where respiratory-borne pathogens are involved, especially those to which staff have little or no immunity, increased levels of protection are essential.

In the case of respiratory-borne disease such as SARS or influenza, an important additional component to the universal precautions discussed in Chapter 4 is the respirator or filtering face piece (FFP) mask. During the 2009 H1N1 outbreak the Health Protection Agency (HPA) made the following recommendations.

1. All healthcare workers (HCWs) in contact with a patient with a flu-like illness or a probable/confirmed case should wear a facemask, plastic apron, and gloves. If a risk assessment indicates that eye splashing is likely, then eye protection should be considered. However, if the patient is wearing a mask, this risk is reduced.
2. HCWs caring for a patient with a flu-like illness or a probable/confirmed case and where aerosol- generating procedures are being undertaken should use an FFP3 respirator, gown, gloves, and eye protection.
3. HCWs caring for a patient who is suffering from a serious respiratory illness and where influenza is suspected, should wear the personal protective equipment as for aerosol-generating procedures. Such patients may have a high viral load and be shedding large quantities of virus.

Reports following both the SARS (2003) and the H1N1 (2009) outbreaks found that insufficient preparation, such as fit testing and training around the use of specialist masks, added pressure to the staff caring for the patients (Rankin 2006).

[4] Reproduced from *Intensive Care Medicine*, Chapter 2. Surge capacity and infrastructure considerations for mass critical care. Volume 36 (Suppl 1), S11–S20, pp. 1761–1764, 2010, Hick, J.L., Christian, M.D., Sprung, C.L. With permission from Springer.

Box 15.2 Levels of filtering face piece (FFP) protection (compared with no protection)

- FFP1—offers a nominal protection factor of up to four times the respiratory protection
- FFP2—offers a nominal protection factor of up to 12 times the respiratory protection
- FFP3—offers a nominal protection factor of up to 50 times the respiratory protection

Filtering face piece (FFP) masks/respirators

There are three levels of filtering capability available, offering increasing protection (see Box 15.2). These respirators require a very snug fit to work effectively; all staff using them should be trained on fitting and testing their fit to ensure full protection. Disposable masks should only be worn once; the length of time they can be worn varies according to the procedures being undertaken.

Reusable respirators that have been correctly sized for the wearer should be adjusted using the head straps over and behind the head to provide a snug fit, and after preventing inflow of air through the filters the wearer should perform a sharp inhalation. If the mask is well-fitted it should collapse slightly due to the negative pressure produced; if this does not occur, the mask should be readjusted. An alcohol or detergent wipe can be used to clean the exterior and interior of the mask between use. Illustrations of fit testing use and cleaning can be found at: http://solutions.3m.co.uk/3MContentRetrievalAPI/BlobServlet?lmd=1247237084000&locale=en_GB&assetType=MMM_Image&assetId=1180615338521&blobAttribute=ImageFile. The recommended level for staff who are caring for patients in critical care is an FFP3 mask.

Aerosol-generating procedures

The risk associated with aerosol-generating procedures is due to the greatly increased presence of pathogens in the air and the associated risk of inhalation for all staff involved. When such a procedure is required, it should take place within an isolation room. All staff should wear the required level of PPE and the number of staff involved should be limited to those who are absolutely essential (HPA 2012).

Procedures likely to produce high levels of respiratory pathogen contamination are:

- intubation, extubation, and related procedures (e.g. manual ventilation and open suctioning)
- cardiopulmonary resuscitation
- bronchoscopy
- surgery and post-mortem procedures in which high speed devices are used
- non-invasive ventilation (NIV)
- high frequency oscillatory ventilation (HFOV)
- induction of sputum.

In addition to the use of FFP3 masks/respirators, eye protection such as goggles or a face visor, fluid-repellent gowns, and gloves should be worn.

Triaging patients for critical care during a pandemic

Pandemics are likely to produce a significant rise in the requirement for critical care. Additional capacity allows for some increase in access, but ultimately restrictions may have to be put in place. The ethical and moral foundations for making decisions about restricting access to critical care were discussed extensively during preparations for the pandemic flu outbreak in 2009. The Department of Health (2007) had previously produced an ethical framework for planning and allocating resource which suggested the following principles to underpin decisions:

- respect
- minimizing the harm the pandemic could cause
- fairness
- working together
- reciprocity (meaning potentially receiving benefit for taking risks)
- keeping things in proportion
- flexibility
- good decision-making, which includes (i) openness and transparency, (ii) inclusiveness, (iii) accountability, and (iv) reasonableness.

While these are well-accepted foundations for decision-making, they do little to help in determining how a scarce resource, which could mean the difference between life and death, can be allocated.

Use of an organ dysfunction score such as SOFA or APACHE could give some indication of the likelihood of survival, but is more geared to prognosticating for populations than for individuals. Therefore it is likely that triage will be based on an organ dysfunction scoring system combined with clinical judgement from senior clinicians.

Supporting and maintaining staff

Critical care staff will be under considerable pressure during any period of high intensity demand for critical care. However, the additional stresses of concern for their own health, the health of their loved ones, dealing with the loss of a family member or colleague, the inevitable difficult decisions that may be demanded of them, and the risks associated with potentially working outside their normal field of practice make a pandemic situation much more psychologically traumatic.

Staff should be offered the opportunity to discuss the ethical issues and the management proposed, and be supported in understanding what may be demanded of them. Taylor *et al.* (2010) identify six key factors likely to impact on staff confidence and ability to deliver:

- inability to deliver normal standards of care due to restricted resource/capacity
- necessity to limit patient admissions or escalation of care
- limitation of care interventions that would normally be ongoing
- excessive workload and prolonged working hours
- potential disagreements with colleagues over treatment restriction decisions
- pressure to work or provide interventions outside normal working domains.

Critical care management planning should include consideration of these situations, including development of plans for management and documentation of support by the organization for staff asked to work in these situations. An example can be seen in the paper by Taylor *et al.* (2010). The use of training exercises which help staff to understand the situation and to plan for it will also be useful.

Debriefing and pyschological support for staff

Staff should be offered the opportunity to collectively review the management of the pandemic process on a daily basis. An end-of-shift overview will allow immediate concerns and worries to be picked up, and these can be responded toimmediately, if needed, or logged for discussion at a later date once recovery is in place. A formal overview debrief should be set up which allows all staff an opportunity to contribute once recovery is underway.

Staff will require considerable psychological support which should be offered at a range of levels, from group therapy to individual counselling and psychotherapy. Post-traumatic stress disorder is seen in up to 30% of those involved in traumatic situations such as a mass casualty incident

Summary

The key features for managing major incidents or pandemic/infectious outbreaks producing high demand for critical care are planning, staff education, and staff support. While many of the issues staff will face will be unexpected, a strong, well thought out plan based on clear underlying ethical principles with a culture of review, learning, and communication will ensure that patients receive the best care that can be given within the constraints of the event.

References and bibliography

Adam, S.K., Osborne, S. (2009). *Oxford Handbook of Critical Care Nursing*, p.44. Oxford: Oxford University Press.

Avidan, V., Hersch, M., Spira, R., *et al.* (2007) Civilian hospital response to a mass casualty event: the role of the intensive care unit. *Journal of Trauma, Injury, Infection and Critical Care*, **62**, 1234–9.

Beck-Razi, N., Fischer, D., Michaelson, M., *et al.* (2007) *Journal of Ultrasound Medicine*, **26**, 1149–56.

Bridges, E.J. (2006). Blast injuries: from triage to critical care. *Critical Care Nursing Clinics of North America*, **18**, 333–48.

Carter, C. (2014) Managing a major incident in the critical care unit. *Nursing Standard*, **28**, 31, 39–44.

Christian, M.D., Devereaux, A.V., Dichter, J.R., *et al.* (2014). Introduction and executive summary. Care of the critically ill and injured during pandemics and disasters: CHEST Consensus Statement. *Chest*, **146**(4_Suppl), 8S–34S.

deBoisblanc, B.P. (2005). Black Hawk, please come down: reflections on a hospital's struggle to survive in the wake of Hurricane Katrina. *American Journal of Respiratory and Critical Care Medicine*, **172**, 1239–40.

Centers for Disease Control (2016). *Emergency Preparedness and Response*. https://emergency.cdc.gov/.

Dennis, A.M., Kochanek, P.M. (2007). Pathophysiology of blast injury. In *Yearbook of Intensive Care and Emergency Medicine* (ed. J.L. Vincent), pp.999–1022. Berlin: Springer-Verlag.

Department of Health (2007). Responding to pandemic influenza: the ethical framework for policy and planning. http://www.dh.gov.uk/prod_consum_dh/groups/dh_digitalassets/@dh/@en/documents/digitalasset/dh_080729.pdf

Doshi, P. (2011). The elusive definition of pandemic influenza. *Bulletin of the World Health Organization*, **89**, 532–8.

Hick, J.L., Christian, M.D., Sprung, C.L. (2010). Chapter 2. Surge capacity and infrastructure considerations for mass critical care. *Intensive Care Medicine*, **36** (Suppl 1), S11–S20.

Hinck, D., Franke, A., Gatzka, F. (2010) Use of vacuum-assisted closure negative pressure wound therapy in combat-related injuries—literature review. *Military Medicine*, **175**, 173–81.

Leen, T., Williams, T.A., Campbell, L., *et al.* (2010). Early experience with influenza A H1N109 in an Australian intensive care unit. *Intensive and Critical Care Nursing*, **26**, 207–14.

Lerner, E.B., Cone, DC, Weinstein, E.S., *et al.* (2011). Mass casualty triage: an evaluation of the science and refinement of a national guideline. *Disaster Medicine and Public Health Preparedness*, **5**, 129–37.

NHS Commissioning Board (2013). *Emergency Preparedness Emergency Framework*. http://www.england.nhs.uk/wp-content/uploads/2013/03/eprr-framework.pdf

Plurad, D. (2011). Blast injury. *Military Medicine*, **176**, 276–82.

Rankin, J. (2006). Godzilla in the corridor: the Ontario SARS crisis in historical perspective. *Intensive and Critical Care Nursing*, **22**, 130–7.

Rubinson, L., Hick, J.L., Hanfling, D.G., *et al.* (2008). Definitive care for the critically ill during a disaster: a framework for optimizing critical care surge capacity from a Task Force for Mass Critical Care Summit Meeting, January 26–27, 2007, Chicago, IL. *Chest*, **133**, 18S–31S.

Shirley, P.J., Mandersloot, G. (2008). Clinical review: The role of the intensive care physician in mass casualty incidents: planning, organisation, and leadership. *Critical Care*, **12**, 214.

Taylor, B.L., Montgomery, H., Rhodes, A., Sprung, C. (2010). Protection of patients and staff during a pandemic. *Intensive Care Medicine*, **36** (Suppl 1), S45–54.

Turégano-Fuentes, F., Caba-Doussoux, P., Jover-Navalón, J.M. (2008). Injury patterns from major urban terrorist bombings in trains:the madrid experience. *World Journal of Surgery*, **32**, 1168–75.

Wolf, S.J., Bebarta, V.S., Bonnett, C.J., *et al.* (2009). Blast injuries. *Lancet*, **347**, 405–15.

London Emergency Services Liaison Panel (2007). *LESLP Major Incident Procedure Manual* (7th edn). London: Stationery Office.

Health Protection Agency (2007). *Pandemic influenza. Guidance for Infection Control in Hospitals and Primary Care Settings*, p.19. http://www.hpa.org.uk/webc/HPAwebFile/HPAweb_C/1238055328357

Health Protection Agency (2012). *Infection Control Precautions to Minimise Transmission of Respiratory Tract Infections (RTIs) in the Healthcare Setting*. http://www.hpa.org.uk/webc/HPAwebFile/HPAweb_C/1317131892566

World Health Organization (2009). *Pandemic Influenza Preparedness and Response*. WHO Guidance Document. http://apps.who.int/iris/bitstream/10665/44123/1/9789241547680_eng.pdf

CHAPTER 16
Evaluating evidence and quality of care in the critical care unit

Introduction

Critical care is an expensive service for relatively small numbers of patients who experience significant morbidity and mortality.

- A critical care bed-day is expensive, ranging from €900 to €3302 in an analysis encompassing eight European countries (Bittner *et al.* 2013). In the UK, the typical cost is up to £1642 (approximately €2000) (benchmark data from Department of Health Payment by Results Team 2013).
- Numbers of adult critical care beds vary markedly across Europe (Rhodes *et al.* 2012), ranging from 4.2 (Portugal) to 29.2 (Germany) per 100,000 population, with an average of 11.5 per 100,000.
- Mortality rates vary depending on bed availability. Countries with fewer critical care beds can in general only admit sicker patients in whom mortality is higher. In the UK (average 6.6 beds per 100,000 population), critical care unit mortality is 14.9% and hospital mortality is 21.9% (Intensive Care National Audit & Research Centre 2013).
- Of those patients who do survive critical care, 25% still need care assistance a year after discharge, 44% are anxious or depressed, and 73% have significant pain (Griffiths *et al.* 2013).
- Even 5 years after discharge from critical care, there are still more deaths and a worse quality of life for survivors of critical care than for matched controls (Cuthbertson *et al.* 2010).

These issues are not trivial. It is the responsibility of the entire critical care team to use the most appropriate methods to treat their patients, to continually evaluate the effectiveness and value of the care they give, and to aim for continuous improvement of the service. This chapter will address the following topics:

- evidence-based practice
- auditing care and assuring clinical quality
- quality improvement
- costing and monitoring outcomes
- ethical issues.

Evidence-based practice

Using the most appropiate up-to-date evidence to guide the delivery of nursing and medical interventions has become established as a central tenet of healthcare practice, i.e. taking 'an approach to practice and teaching that is based on knowledge of the evidence upon which practice is based, and the strength of that evidence' (Cook *et al.* 1996). Critical care practitioners must be able to critically evaluate research so that there is 'conscientious and judicious use of current best evidence in making decisions about the care of individual patients' (Sackett *et al.* 1996). They need to decide whether or not published study findings can be generalized to the individual patients that they are caring for.

Being sure about the right management strategy can be very difficult. The traditional view is that randomized controlled trials (RCTs), or systematic reviews and meta-analyses of RCTs, represent the 'gold standard' of evidence (Ho *et al.* 2008). RCTs generally compare and contrast *average* values of demographic, physiological, treatment, and outcome data from groups of patients. However, these studies often occur in somewhat artificial situations as researchers seek to minimize potentially confounding variables. For example, trial entry will often be restricted to patients fulfilling often demanding inclusion and exclusion criteria. Study patients will usually be from a different location (or country) where healthcare practices vary markedly. Data may be historical and clinical practice may well have subsequently evolved. Patient outcomes are influenced by different organizational approaches, staff characteristics, varied working practices, and treatment methods, as well as differences between patients themselves. Such factors are impossible to completely standardize. Therefore a wide range of quantitative and qualitative investigative procedures are needed to gain a more complete understanding. Qualitative research methods such as phenomenology, grounded theory, and action research also have limitations in terms of generalizability and application across different groups of patients. However, these can be used to examine important institutional, staff, and patient variables, and to generate new theoretical constructs and frameworks which can then be tested in local settings.

The most appropriate research method depends on the nature of the research question, the objectives of the researcher, and the resources available. In real-life practice, much more information than quantitative data collected during RCTs is used to inform decision-making, although clincial staff may not always appreciate that fact. For example, personal—often tacit—knowledge of the local context (e.g. the systems and resources available in the instituition), individual patients' values and preferences, and clinicans' experience are key factors that must be integrated with published evidence (Eizenberg 2011).

Application of research to practice

The main requirements for making sense of research are to be familiar with the methodology used to understand the study data, conclusions, and recommendations, and to carefully consider any limitations of the techniques used and the applicability of the results to one's own practice. Different types of research have different levels of importance; for example, results obtained from RCTs are considered high-grade evidence, whereas observational studies are deemed less useful (Ho *et al.* 2008). However, the concept of a strict 'hierarchy of evidence' is not always applicable and may devalue some valuable work. Nevertheless, it does emphasize the need to critically examine the credibility of any research output. The difficulty is that practitioners may not always be equipped with all the required skills and resources for appraisal of all the different forms of research. Furthermore, when evaluating the quality of published research, it is also necessary to have insight into personal biases and, ideally, to sometimes test different approaches in the local setting (see Box 16.1).

Box 16.1 Reviewing research

The approach used to appraise research depends on the type of work under review. Consideration of the following points may help clarification.

- Justification for the research: are the background and rationale of the study clearly established?
- Scientific content: is there a specific question/hypothesis being addressed?
- Originality: is it a new idea, or a re-examination of a long-standing issue that is different or better than before?
- Methodology and study design: are the methods appropriate and likely to produce an answer to the question? For example:
  - comparisons of different treatments generally require quantitative measurements of particular end-points (e.g. dose of a drug needed to achieve a target physiological variable)
  - understanding how an individual thinks or feels usually involves analysis of qualitative material (e.g. data from interviews with patients and families).
- Is the research method described in a way that can be readily understood, and replicated?
- Are the relevant results shown? Are data given that provide details of the individuals under investigation, and details of how representative these might be of a larger population?
- Is the analysis appropriate and is the power of the study adequate? (This is determined by the numbers involved and the size of the difference being examined.)
- Interpretation and discussion: are the conclusions and comments reasonable in the light of the results? Do the conclusions follow from the analysis?
- Are any references to background literature comprehensive and appropriate?
- What can be taken from the study; that is, what value does the study have in terms of supporting or developing clinical practice?
- What is the overall impression of the work? Is it credible? Is the presentation clear and informative?
- If evaluating a paper, has the work undergone proper peer review?

Outcome measurement and prediction

Outcome measurement is the process of collecting and analysing data that reflect the effects of interventions. When evaluating the ability of a study to prognosticate, the following points should be considered (Randolph *et al.* 1998).

1. Is the sample of patients representative?
2. Are patients homogeneous with respect to prognostic risk?
3. Is follow-up sufficient to minimize the possibility that missing patients could alter the interpretation of the results?
4. Are the outcomes evaluated using objective and unbiased criteria?

Risk adjustment

This technique is used to compare outcomes of patients with different levels of acuity, comorbidity, and other factors that can influence the course of illness. It is a means of 'levelling the playing field' by allowing meaningful comparisons of outcomes across critical care units, hospitals, and diagnoses. For example, the predicted risk of death based on severity scores such as APACHE II (see Table 16.1) can be used to compare mortality rates in different groups of patients. Risk adjustment can also be used to ensure that patient groups are similar for the purposes of evaluation when the effects of treatments are being studied. However, it should be stressed that no risk adjustment model can take into account every factor influencing outcome as some variables are either unrecorded or unrecognized.

Use of statistical tools for evaluating the ability to predict accurately

The receiver operating characteristic (ROC) curve can be used to describe the discriminating ability of a predictive tool. An example is shown in Figure 16.1. The ROC plots true-positive predictions (sensitivity) against false-positive predictions (1-specificity). The closer the area under the curve is to a value of 1.0, the more accurate the tested model. Pure chance will result in a ROC area of 0.50. The minimal clinically acceptable ROC area is typically taken to be ≥0.704 but often needs to be higher (e.g. for biomarkers).

Table 16.1 APACHE II Severity of Disease Classification System

Variable	+4	+3	+2	+1	0	+1	+2	+3	+4
Temperature (rectal) (°C)	≥41	39–40.9		38.2–38.9	36–38.4	34–35.9	32–33.9	30–31.9	≤29.9
Mean BP (mmHg)	≥160	130–159	110–129		70–109		50–69		≤49
Heart rate (bpm)	≥180	140–179	110–139		70–109		55–69	40–54	≤39
Respiratory rate (breaths/min)	≥50	35–49		25–34	12–24	10–11	6–9		≤5
If FiO_2 ≥0.5: A–a DO_2 (mmHg)	≥500	350–499	200–349		<200				
If FiO_2 < 0.5: PO_2 (mmHg)					>70	61–70		55–60	≤55
Arterial pH	≥7.7	7.6–7.69		7.5–7.59	7.33–7.49		7.25–7.32	7.15–7.24	≤7.15
Serum Na (mmol/L)	≥180	160–179	155–159	150–154	130–149		120–129	111–119	≤110
Serum K (mmol/L)	≥7	6–6.9		5.5–5.9	3.5–5.4	3–3.4	2.5–2.9		<2.5
Serum creatinine (μmol/L) (double score if acute renal failure)	≥300	171–299	121–170		50–120	<50			
Haematocrit (%)	≥60		50–59.9	46–49.9	30–45.9		20–29.9		<20
White cell count (mm³)	≥40		20–39.9	15–19.9	3–14.9		1–2.9		<1

Neurological score = 15 minus measured Glasgow Coma Score.

Age points: age ≤44 years = 0 points; 45–54 years = 2 points; 55–64 years = 3 points; 65–74 years = 5 points; ≤75 years, 6 points.

Chronic health points: 2 points for elective post-operative admission or 5 points if emergency operation or non-operative admission, if patient has cirrhosis, heart failure (NYHA Grade 4), respiratory failure, or dialysis-dependent renal disease, or is immunocompromised.

Quality of care, clinical audit, standards of care, and benchmarking

Monitoring the quality of care provided in practice has become an essential part of healthcare (see Box 16.2). The traditional, generally professionally decided (particularly medical) focus of what should and should not be done has been supplanted by more of a partnership model between healthcare users (patients), their relatives, and healthcare staff. Six dimensions can be used to structure reviews of quality of healthcare: (1) access, (2) equity, (3) relevance to need, (4) social acceptability, (5) efficiency, and (6) effectiveness (Maxwell 1992). This approach emphasizes that quality healthcare and particularly quality nursing care are very much socially defined. There is an imperative to involve healthcare users in developing services that are genuinely responsive to patient and family needs. The views of critically ill patients and

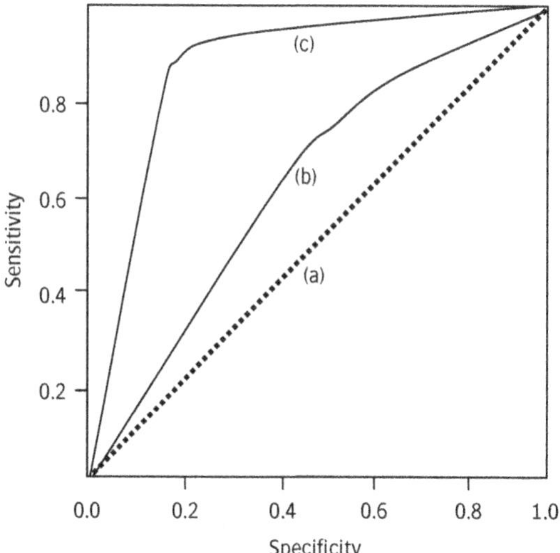

(a) = area under the curve of 0.5 and a discrimination that is no better than chance
(b) = small area under the curve and a poor discrimination
(c) = large area under the curve and a good discrimination

Figure 16.1 Diagram showing negative feedback control of thyroid hormones.

their relatives must be actively sought, but this also presents challenges as there may be different patient requirements in different circumstances. For example, a patient's desired outcome may change from recovery when first admitted, to peaceful dignified death if it becomes apparent that recovery is not possible.

Clinical audit

Audit is an explicit systematic continuous process aimed at improving and then maintaining the quality of care to an agreed, or better, standard. The process requires:

- deciding what is expected in everyday practice by agreeing specific measurable evidence-based standards or goals of care with both relevant members of the healthcare team and patients or their representatives involved in the process
- measuring and monitoring the actual care that is given, assessing (a) structures, (b) processes and (c) outcomes
- evaluating the quality of practice, i.e. comparing actual performance with the expected standard
- making any improvements required to bring practices up to the agreed standards
- sustaining and continuing to improve the quality of care, primarily by developing a culture and systems that promote continuous improvement throughout the organization (see Figure 16.2).

> **Box 16.2 Quantitative indicators of quality**
>
> - Rates of nosocomial infection: cannulae, urinary tract (especially associated with an in-dwelling catheter), wound infection, chest infection (e.g. ventilator associated pneuomina)
> - Incidence of pressure sores evaluated against severity of illness and chronic health problems
> - Patients' or relatives' complaints and/or satisfaction
> - Achievement of pain relief using visual analogue scoring
> - Amount of time spent on non-nursing duties
> - Number of medication errors
> - Incidence of sharps injuries, back injuries, etc
> - Critical incident analysis

Quantitative and qualitative measurements

Effective measurement of quality encompasses both objective quantitative measurement of care criteria and a qualitative analysis of caring. Quantitative data such as indicators of structure and outcome are usually relatively easy to collect. However, these may be problematic to use for evaluation of nursing practice as many care processes are associated with value judgements based on socialization that are difficult to quantify. Analysis of qualitative data obtained by methods such as survey or interview will enable a greater understanding of the quality of nursing care and where improvements are needed. If the whole range of factors is measured, comparisons can be made between levels of quality and cost in different units and hospitals. More importantly, individual areas can identify the strengths and weaknesses of their practices. By measuring performance of key processes every week or month, the effectiveness of any initiatives employed to improve care can be tracked.

Standard of care

This is an agreed achievable level of performance appropriate to a specified population, with most standards incorporating a systematic review of published research that provides support for the standard. Donabedian's seminal paper on evaluating quality in medical care

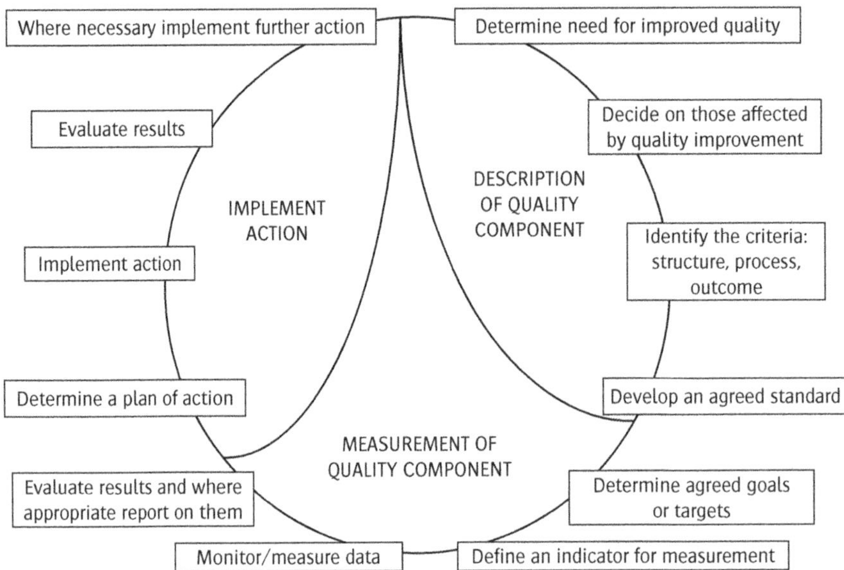

Figure 16.2 The quality assurance cycle.
Data from Healthcare Quality Improvement Partnership, Criteria and indicators of best practice in clinical audit, 2009.

(Donabedian 1966) laid out a framework for standard setting and the writing of descriptors of quality, i.e. a categorization of (i) structure, (ii) process, and (iii) outcome, that is still useful.

Structure includes the fabric and facilities of the instituition, the environment, staffing and organization, and the resources. Process includes the delivery of care, the values and philosophy of the caregivers, and the way care is managed. Outcome includes survival, the quality of life of survivors, and family satisfaction with care.

Outcome is probably the easiest and most frequently audited area; but outcomes are highly dependent on structural and process factors.

Process can be investigated by comparing actual practices with agreed standards such as nursing quality assessment tools (usually based on expert professional opinion).

Critical care has some particular features which make audit challenging. These include the lack of an agreed detailed definition of what constitutes critical care both around the world and within individual countries, the heterogeneity of the patients involved, and the difficulty of establishing links between specific therapies or modes of care and survival. However, there are considerable data available to inform numerous aspects of critical illness and responses to interventions. This wealth of information could provide important insights into many facets of patient care, including more clarity about the effectiveness of treatments, although it needs to be collated and analysed in a structured format. This approach may be particularly useful if standardized data from many sites were amalgamated (see Box 16.3). This use of 'big data' is already occuring in critical care (Celi *et al.* 2013). The increasing use of computerized clinical information systems is likely to make such complex data analysis relatively commonplace in the near future.

Benchmarking

Benchmarking is another approach involving measurement of actual care and comparison with agreed standards based on published evidence and expert opinion (see Box 16.4). However, the process of benchmarking is distinguished by the aim of developing standards of excellence 'to which all should aspire' (Ellis 2006), as illustrated by the paper 'Benchmarking to identify top performing critical care units ... their policies and practices' (Zimmerman *et al.* (2003). Benchmarking can be used to promote comparison and sharing of methods of care delivery across different critical care units. Unfortunately, the lack of definitive research data about many everyday practices can make it difficult to agree upon a benchmark standard (see Table 16.2).

Box 16.3 Sources of data for quality criteria

- Patient observation
- Patient interview
- Environmental observation
- Nurse interview
- Patient record review
- Allied health professional and ancillary staff interview
- Family and relatives interview

Critical incident reporting and risk management

The prevalence of adverse events (AEs) resulting from medical/nursing treatments is a marker of the safety and quality of care in a department. AEs are incidents that could have caused or did cause harm, i.e. outcomes with negative effects. Most can be attributed to human error. AEs can occur in any setting—with a high frequency in critical care—and often have very serious consequences; there are an estimated 98,000 patient deaths per year due to human error in American hospitals each year (Drews *et al.* 2008).

In an observational study conducted on just one day, 20% of critical care patients around the world experienced one or more AEs, such as endotracheal tube displacement, obstruction or leakage of airway devices, displacement or disconnection of lines/catheters/drains, medication errors, and other equipment failures (Valentin *et al.* 2006). While many of these events are related to nursing activities, nurses also have an important role in detecting and rectifying AEs; in one study, critical care nurses reported recovering 18,578 'medical errors', of which 23% were judged potentially fatal (Dykes *et al.* 2010). Staffing factors are significant; having more consultants and more nurses per bed are both associated with improved survival in critical care, with nursing numbers having a particular impact on outcomes of very high risk patients (West 2014). Investing in teamworking and training also improves clinical outcomes (West *et al.* 2006).

Box 16.4 Published British critical care standards/benchmarks

Critical care units: planning and design

Guidance on the location, layout, and design of the critical care unit: what is required in the bed space, facilities for visitors, staff spaces, etc. (Department of Health 2013a).

Core Standards for Intensive Care Units: 'what is necessary to ensure the best care and outcome'

Required and advisable standards of (i) staffing (e.g. availability of senior staff, staff–patient ratios, frequency of ward rounds, training requirements), (ii) operational aspects (e.g. management of admissions, transfers, rehabilitation, discharges), (iii) equipment, (iv) data collection (Faculty of Intensive Care Medicine/Intensive Care Society 2013).

Table 16.2 Perceived impact of benchmarking over other quality initiatives

Quality initiatives	Benchmarking
Fit for purpose	Best possible practice
Traditional practice	Evidence-based practice
Internal focus	External focus
Professional fragmentation	Patient-focused care
Internal efficiency	Recognized excellence
Management led	Practitioner led with management support
Pockets of good practice	Dissemination of good practice
Outcome measurement	Process improvement to outcome improvement
What is done	How it is done
Achieving agreed standards	Continuous improvement
Repetition of effort	Sharing
Competitive protectionism	Open comparison and sharing

Box 16.5 Examples of risk management responses to critical incidents

1. The incidence of contamination through eye splashes from ventilator tubing disconnections may be reduced by instigating mandatory safety goggles when approaching the patient.
2. The likelihood of medication error may be reduced by altering the number of drugs given as intravenous boluses at the same time.
3. The education of staff about specific drug interactions may reduce the incidence of adverse interactions.

There is a need for a systems approach to reducing clinical risk. Reporting of AEs should be positively encouraged and incidents examined in order to identify any educational needs, additional safety processes, or even extra resources to reduce the risk of recurrence (see Box 16.5). Pronovost's group have developed a safety scorecard for use in critical care that utilizes standard process and outcome measures but also incorporates structural measures such as the learning from AEs and context measures such as the extent to which there is a safety culture in a particular critical care unit (Barenholtz *et al.* 2007).

Illness severity scoring systems in critical care

These scoring systems allow objective quantification and comparison of the severity of various disorders and disease states in critical care. Most were designed to define the extent of deviation from normal ranges of acute and chronic physiological, functional, and psychosocial variables related to the risk of adverse outcomes, particularly death. More recently, some systems have also taken into account the effects of timespans and interventions preceding admission to critical care as well as different ways of working in the critical care unit, both of which impact upon outcomes.

Outcome prediction

While scoring systems are used to predict the probability of particular outcomes, such predictions apply only to patient populations and not to individuals. Nonetheless, these methods are useful for comparing predicted outcomes with actual measured outcomes and therefore can be used to assess the efficacy of treatments and other factors such as the environment, organization, staffing, etc.

Various scoring systems have evolved in critical care to provide:

- an index of disease severity—either general, e.g. APACHE, Simplified Acute Physiology Score (SAPS), Sequential Organ Failure Assessment (SOFA), or specific, e.g. Glasgow Coma Score, Trauma Score.
- an index of workload and consumption of resources, e.g. Therapeutic Intervention Scoring System (TISS)).
- a means of comparison for (i) audit of performance (either in the same unit over time or between units) and (ii) research (e.g. evaluation of new products and treatment regimens)
- patient management objectives (e.g. sedation, pressure area care).

Severity scoring systems

These systems have been devised either for specific conditions, e.g. trauma (Trauma Score), pancreatitis (Ranson Score), head injury (Glasgow Coma Score), or for the general critical care patient (e.g. APACHE). Most systems use clinical assessments and physiological measurements, often complemented by laboratory measurements such as white blood cell count and haematocrit.

APACHE

The Acute Physiology and Chronic Health Evaluation (APACHE) system was originally developed in 1981, based on data from 805 patients in two US critical care units. The APACHE classification enables calculation of a score derived from the degree of abnormality of various physiological and biochemical variables, as well as age and chronic health status (e.g. the presence of conditions such as severe heart failure, cirrhosis, or immunosuppression). The first version required measurement of 33 physiological measurements but this proved unwieldy in practice. The simplified APACHE II score was developed by Knaus in 1985. This score uses the most extreme values of the 12 most commonly measured physiological and biochemical variables recorded in the first 24 hours following admission to critical care, in addition to age and chronic health grading (Table 16.1). The risk of subsequent death from a range of admission disorders was computed and this risk stratification was then validated using data from 5815 patients in 13 US units (with burns and cardiac surgery patients excluded). This validation study was repeated in 26 UK and Irish critical care units to determine its applicability to UK patients (Rowan *et al.* 1993). While it generally provided a satisfactory fit, there some significant differences; for example, APACHE II over-predicted deaths in surgical patients and under-predicted deaths in older patients. A UK-specific model developed by the Intensive Care National Audit & Research Centre (ICNARC) created a more accurate system. This undergoes development and periodic recalibration of the 'ICNARC risk prediction model' for UK patients (Harrison *et al.* 2007).

Further refinements of the APACHE system have come in the forms of APACHE III (1991) and APACHE IV (2006), aiming to improve their statistical predictive power by various means. These have included (i) adding new physiological variables (e.g. albumin, bilirubin, glucose), (ii) changing the thresholds and weighting of existing variables, (iii) using both admission and 24-hour scores, (iv) incorporating the source of admission (e.g. emergency department, ward) and length of hospital stay before admission to critical care, and (v) reassessing the effects of age, chronic health, and specific diseases. However, as APACHE III and APACHE IV are proprietary and have to be purchased, this has limited their widespread usage.

SAPS

SAPS (Simplified Acute Physiology Score) was first devised in 1984, effectively as a simplified form of APACHE incorporating 14 readily measured clinical and biochemical variables. It has also been modified over time as SAPS II (1993) and SAPS III (2005), using data from European, US, and, most recently, Australian, Central American, and South American critical care units (Moreno *et al.* 2005). SAPS III highlights the importance of factors that take effect even before entry to the critical care unit, such as the source of admission, the length of hospital stay beforehand, and the use of vasoactive drugs prior to admission. The diversity of the database used to develop SAPS III has also enabled the formulation of region-specific versions.

MPM

The MPMs (Mortality Probability Models) use the logistic regression statistical technique on databases of critical care patients. This was initially taken from just one critical care unit in 1987, from the SAPS II database in the second version in 1993 (MPM II), and from analyses of patients from one Brazilian and 134 North American units in 2007 (MPM_0III) (Higgins *et al*). MPM_0III allows for the decision not to attempt resuscitation in calculating the risk of mortality.

No scoring system is infallible; the individual patient prognosticated to do poorly can defy the odds, while an expected survivor may still die. Thus outcome prediction systems cannot be used to justify either early withdrawal or refusal of critical care treatments. Nonetheless, increasing rationalization of healthcare resources may eventually force the use of these tools as part of the decision-making process. At this point in time, there is no universally accepted system practised by all critical care units other than the Glasgow Coma Score. Competing systems have often been developed simultaneously; APACHE and SAPS are both widely used for scoring disease severity, with APACHE being the predominant system in the USA and UK, while SAPS is more popular in mainland Europe. Each system has its devotees who are not inclined to shift allegiance. Owing to the considerable financial implications, a common system is unlikely to be agreed upon any time soon.

Scoring nursing workload

The Therapeutic Intervention Scoring System (TISS) and its variants provide an index of workload by giving a score to different procedures and techniques performed in the care of individual patients; for example, the use and number of vasoactive drug infusions, renal replacement therapy, and administration of enteral nutrition. The first version (1974) included 57 possible interventions, later increased to 76, but was then simpified to 28 items (TISS-28) by Miranda *et al.* (1996). TISS has been used to cost individual patients by attaching a monetary value to each TISS point scored. A discharge TISS score can also be used to estimate the amount of nursing work required for a patient in step-down facilities or on the general ward. A simple user-friendly tool based on just nine variables from TISS-28 Nine Equivalents of Nursing Manpower Use (NEMS)).was described by Miranda *et al.* (1997). However, TISS does not capture all nursing activities as it fails to take account of tasks and duties such as coping with the irritable or confused patient or dealing with grieving relatives. The TISS Working Group subsequently published the Nursing Activities Score which adds aspects of indirect care (e.g. care of relatives and administrative work) to the TISS-28 variables (Miranda *et al.* 2003).

Specific scoring systems

Trauma

Trauma scoring systems have been utilized for a variety of purposes:

- performing rapid field triage to direct the patient to appropriate levels of care
- quality assurance
- developing and improving trauma care systems by categorizing patients and identifying problems within the systems
- making comparisons between groups from different hospitals, in the same hospital over time, and/or undergoing different treatment strategies.

The Injury Severity Score (ISS) is a severity scoring system for trauma patients based on the anatomical injuries sustained. The Revised Trauma Score (RTS) utilizes measures of physiological abnormality (breathing, circulation, consciousness) to predict survival. The Trauma Injury Severity Score (TRISS)—a combination of ISS and RTS—has been developed to overcome the shortcomings of anatomical or physiological scoring alone. This score incorporates ISS, RTS, patient age, and whether the injury was blunt or penetrating to provide a measure of the probability of survival.

A challenge for all scoring systems is that both the case mix of patients and methods of treatment vary and evolve over time. Thus the data on which systems are based become outdated and/or do not match the characteristics of patients in a particular area. The Trauma Audit and Research Network (www.tarn.ac.uk) regularly collects data from hospitals across England and Wales, and has used statistical modelling of these data to update and further refine the prediction of outcomes following traumatic injury. The probability of survival (P_s) from trauma is scored with calculations of the influences and interactions of patient age, gender, Glasgow Coma Score, and ISS. This method is currently considered to be the most accurate in this group of patients (Woodford 2014).

Head injury

The Glasgow Coma Score, first described by Teasdale and Jennett (1974), utilizes eye opening, best motor response, and best verbal response to categorize the severity of head injury. It is probably the only system used universally in critical care. Apart from its ability to prognosticate, GCS is also frequently used for therapeutic decision-making (e.g. elective ventilation in patients presenting with a GCS score of 8 or less).

Sepsis, ARDS, and multiple organ dysfunction

Descriptors and definitions of the systemic inflammatory response syndrome (SIRS), sepsis, and the acute respiratory distress syndrome (ARDS) have evolved over several decades. Recently published definitions are set out in Chapter 10. The PIRO model takes account of patients' **P**redisposition to sepsis, **I**nfective organisms involved, different **R**esponses, and the nature of subsequent **O**rgan dysfunction, and can be used as a method of staging severe sepsis (Rubulotta *et al.* 2009).

Various systems for scoring severity of multiple organ dysfunction in critical care are available (Vincent and Moreno, 2010). These include the widely-used Sequential Organ Failure Assessment (SOFA), which was initally developed as the Sepsis-related Organ Failure Assessment, the Logistic Organ Dysfunction System (LODS), and the Multiple Organ Dysfunction Score (MODS). Each uses measures of respiratory, circulatory, neurological, kidney, liver, and haematological dysfunction which can be calculated each day to provide a crude indicator of the patient's progress over time.

Sedation

Several subjective, relatively simple scoring systems have been developed for gauging and recording the level of sedation of critically ill patients, particularly for use with those who are mechanically ventilated. The aim is usually to titrate the dose of sedative agents so that the patient is generally aware but calm and cooperative, while also feeling comfortable and able to sleep when appropriate. Assessments should be performed at regular intervals (typically every hour) using a structured sedation scoring system. A recent review of 10 such systems concluded that the Richmond Agitation–Sedation Scale and Sedation–Agitation Scale had the highest inter-rater reliability in a range of settings (see Chapter 3), and also had reasonable correlation with more sophisticated monitors such as the electroencephalogram (EEG) or bispectral (BIS) index monitor (Barr *et al.* 2013).

Cost versus outcome

Critical care is costly and is becoming even more expensive, with the annual costs of critical care rising by 44% in just 5 years in the USA (Halpern and Pastores 2010). This escalation in expenditure reinforces the

Table 16.3 Long-term outcomes of critical care patients

	Unit mortality	Hospital mortality	One-year mortality
1989 Danish data (same patient cohort)	18%*	29%*	42%† 26% of admissions to critical care survived for one year and returned to 'normal activity', i.e. the same as before admission
2013 UK data (two different cohorts)	15%‡	22%‡	48%§ 18% of survivors to one year had 'no problems' with 'usual activity'

*Dragsted *et al.* 1989.
†Dragsted and Qvist 1989.
‡Intensive Care National Audit & Research Centre 2013.
§Griffiths *et al.* 2013 (the 48% mortality figure is an extrapolated value that may overestimate one-year mortality in all critical care patients).

need to scrutinize the finances of critical care services in relation to their effectiveness, assessing the benefits of prolonging meaningful quality of life against the considerable costs of treatment. In particular, length of survival following discharge and the quality of life for survivors are key factors. Many patients admitted to critical care do not survive beyond 12 months and/or are unable to manage normal activity. This pattern of outcome has changed little in 25 years: see Table 16.3.

It is important to note that marked differences exist between definitions of what constitutes critical care, how it is delivered, and the populations served in different locations in different countries. These services and patient characteristics may also change over time. The context of any data must be conisdered when making comparisons between different studies/countries (Murthy and Wunsch 2012).

Critical care costs are heavily weighted towards the small group of patients who have a prolonged length of stay: a Scottish study found that just 4.4% of critical care patients were ventilated for 3 weeks or more, but these cases accounted for 29% of critical care bed-days and also had a hospital mortality of 40.3% (Lone and Walsh, 2011). Not surprisingly, non-survivors of critical care have a higher severity of illness and usually require more organ support and a longer stay than those who survive (Harrison *et al.* 2004).

Quality of life

Follow-up studies of patients after critical illness have used different criteria to define quality of life but have still generated relatively consistent results. Quality of life is generally linked to the patient's ability to resume the usual activities and employment that existed when they were previously working. Patients admitted to critical care who are already frail or suffering from some long-term condition—usually in older age groups and often with a reduced quality of life—are less likely to survive and are also less likely to return to their previous level of function (see Box 16.6).

Not surprisingly, the other patients most likely to have significant problems are those who were the most severely ill. Herridge *et al.* (2011) reviewed 109 critical care patients with ARDS for up to 5 years after discharge, at which point 74 were still alive. These survivors were relatively young, with a median age of 45 years on enrolment. Their lung function had returned to normal or near normal at 5 years after discharge, and they had no gross physical weakness on examination. However, their exercise limitation was 25% worse than that of matched controls and they had an array of of physical and psychological conditions linked to social isolation and sexual dysfunction. Over half the patients experienced significant anxiety and depression, and so did more than a quarter of their family members. Some 52% of patients had not returned to work a year after discharge; even at 5 years, 23% were not working (Herridge *et al.* 2011).

A profile of a wide range of critical care patients from 22 different UK units who survived for at least a year was recently reported by Griffiths *et al.* (2013). Their median age was 62 years and, on average, they had spent 8 days in critical care and 29 days in hospital. Approximately a third had problems with usual activities before critical care, but this proportion doubled on review 12 months later. A quarter needed 50 hours or more of care per week. Family members were meeting most of the increased care needs, but this was associated with a negative impact on their employment and income. Three-quarters reported

Box 16.6 Factors influencing outcome from critical illness

- Age
- Chronic disease/previous health status
- Previous functional level
- Severity of acute illness
- Diagnosis

moderate or extreme pain, and an overall poorer quality of life compared with population norms.

A UK single-centre study monitored 300 general critical care patients for 5 years after ICU discharge, though 105 were lost to follow-up at various points (Cuthbertson *et al.* 2010). If all the cases described as lost were assumed to have remained alive, 17% of those patients discharged from the critical care unit died within three months, 23% within a year, 28% within 30 months, and 33% withinin 5 years. While the cohort of patients experienced significant mortality throughout the 5 years after critical care, most deaths occurred in the first months. A focus on care in this period may possibly improve outcomes. Survivors also had worse physical quality of life and quality adjusted life-years compared with population norms, but nonetheless only 12% of the 97 survivors interviewed at 5 years said that they were dissatisfied with their quality of life (Cuthbertson *et al.* 2010). Managing the aftermath of critical illness may be similar to living with other chronic diseases.

Long-term problems associated with prolonged critical care

The effects of critical illness are devastating and there are few patients who spend more than 2–3 days in critical care who do not suffer significant physical and psychological complications over the medium to long term.

Physical problems

Weight loss and muscle wasting Skeletal muscle loss during illness is due to inactivity, catabolism, and frequently inadequate nutrition. In many patients, this loss will take months to recover. Other pathology may limit the patient's ability to exercise and rebuild muscle bulk.

Reduced respiratory function Diaphragmatic and intercostal muscle loss may contribute to reduced respiratory function on top of any residual pulmonary pathology from infection or other problems. Patients may remain short of breath on exertion due to either respiratory problems or cardiac insufficiency.

Complications of endotracheal intubation or tracheostomy Patients may experience vocal disturbance due to vocal cord damage or stridor and wheezing due to tracheal stenosis.

Neurological problems Sensory and motor neuropathies may occur and there may be disturbances of fine motor control. Some patients experience visual deficits and auditory problems such as tinnitus.

Psychological problems

These can be severe and are often associated with low mood (and symptoms such as nervousness, anger, and confusion), hallucinations, sleep disturbance, and nightmares. A recent UK follow-up study of high acuity critical care patients showed that 55% had psychological morbidity, including anxiety and depression, and a 27% rate of post-traumatic stress disorder (Wade *et al.* 2012). These conditions can persist for many months (Davydow *et al.* 2013) or even years.

As recovery from physical illness progresses, the adjustment of their role from total dependence to relative independence can be challenging, with adjustment to the experience of critical illness and sometimes near-death also being difficult. Some patients have complete memory loss with regard to time spent in critical care; this may lead to false expectations of their ability to recover rapidly. Patients may also suffer loss of concentration, mental fatigue, and difficulty in following a line of reasoning. Short-term memory may be affected, and there may also be abrupt mood swings.

General problems

Issues such as altered taste sensation, loss of appetite, altered body image, and sexual dysfunction can all cause problems in the long term. The extent of problems experienced by these patients requires a broad range of professional expertise in providing advice and support.

Social factors

Relationships with family and friends may suffer as a result of the patient's experience of critical care and associated psychological problems. Patients may have what are perceived as personality changes and difficulty in connecting to others, including those who were previously close friends or relations.

Recovery and follow-up

The growing understanding of the many medium and long-term complications of critical illness has led to the realization that a structured programme of recovery and rehabilitation of physical and psychological function is likely to be beneficial for many patients.

In the UK, the National Institute for Health and Care Excellence (2009) recommended that all critical care patients are assessed for their risk of physiological and psychological morbidity while in critical care. At discharge, specific problems should be clearly identified, with goals of rehabilitation being detailed. The patient's progress in relation to these goals is monitored after ward transfer and discharge home. Critical care outreach and similar services, where they exist, can support patients discharged to general wards. These services, with staff who understand critical illness and its aftermath, can both identify risks and prevent significant harm to patients recovering from critcal illness (Park *et al.* 2003), and also reduce hospital length of stay and mortality (Harrison *et al.* 2010).

Many hospitals run outpatient follow-up clinics for patients who have spent a period of time in critical care. The purpose of these clinics is twofold. One function is to allow reassessment, diagnosis of problems, treatment, counselling, and support of the individual patient and their family in the first months after hospital discharge. The other purpose is to allow collection of data regarding specific problems associated with critical care treatments and the overall experience of the critical care unit. Former critical care patients value these services highly, and suggest that they enhance recovery and rehabilitation (Prinjha *et al.* 2009). However, these effects have not yet been demonstrated in a quanitative prospective study.

Follow-up service for bereaved relatives

Most critical care units offer a high degree of support, information, and advice in the event of patient death, but few offer a formal follow-up service for relatives. Coming to terms with loss is often very difficult, especially after the period of (sometimes false) hope offered by admission to critical care; and particularly if the patient was young and/or death was sudden. There may also be difficulty leaving what is in some ways a safe supported environment (the critical care unit) to face the challenges of going home and dealing with the aftermath of death.

Voisey *et al.* (2007) reported the uptake of a critical care bereavement follow-up service offered to all relatives of patients who had died. Approximately 6% of families wanted to use the service, to ask specific questions about the patient, to review information in the patient records, to address complaints, to clear up misunderstandings, and to communicate with other health professionals. The service was most requested by relatives of younger patients that had died within a week of admission.

At the very least, most units ought to be able to provide a telephone follow-up service where an appropriately skilled nurse speaks to bereaved families, and offers condolences, information, and further support where necessary (see Box 16.7).

Box 16.7 Sources of further help

- Bereavement support groups
- Chaplains or ministers of other religions
- Bereavement counsellor (if available)
- Citizens Advice (for assistance with practical difficulties)

Ethics

The definition of 'ethics' is the philosophical study of the moral value of human conduct and the rules and principles that govern it. However, it has come to be regarded as the morals or code of conduct of particular social groups such as the professions.

Morals are the principles of behaviour actually held or followed by individuals or groups in accordance with standards of right and wrong.

Ethics are an important issue in critical care partly due to the increasing sophistication of medical science and technology concurrent with an increasing emphasis on the autonomy of the individual. The effects of financial constraints on resources also contribute to ethical dilemmas in this expensive area of care.

Among the many ethical challenges facing staff in critical care, several are encountered with reasonable frequency. These are:

- determining the point of withdrawal of treatment
- withholding resuscitation measures
- deciding when the burdens of further therapeutic measures outweigh the benefits
- when resources are limited, deciding which patient will receive critical care
- evaluating when critical care is an appropriate measure.

Ethical decision-making is complex, stressful, and often extremely difficult. Guidelines can only provide a general framework to apply in specific cases. Although use of a structured process may help in clarifying the different features of a particular case, individual issues must be reappraised in each instance.

Ethical decisions depend on moral judgements. These will be influenced by personal values and social pressures. Nonetheless, a well-written department philosophy can be helpful in setting out the broad attitudes, values, and beliefs held by the whole critical care team. Knowledge of accepted ethical principles can also help provide a foundation on which to base decisions.

Ethical theories

There are two main approaches to determining whether an action is right or wrong. The first refers to the consequences of the action (consequentialist) and the second to the moral rules or guidelines governing that action (deontological).

Consequentialist theory

Moral or ethical dilemmas are resolved by calculating the good over the harm that can be expected to result from any particular choices. Utilitarianism is the best known consequentialist philosophy, detailed by John Stuart Mill (1863). It is based on the need for human beings to act in bringing about the best outcome for all concerned.

Deontological theory

Moral or ethical dilemmas are resolved by considering each action in itself according to certain duties, rights, and justice. The act itself is judged right or wrong, not the consequences. The ultimate proponent of this approach was the German philosopher Immanuel Kant, who advocated using the individual's moral sense to judge each act.

The philosopher Jacques Thiroux described five principles that might be used to guide ethical behaviour and as a means of highlighting the key issues in ethical decision-making, but not to make the decision itself (Thiroux and Krasemann 2014) (see also Figure 16.3).

1. The value of life—humans should revere life and accept death.
2. Goodness or rightness—promote good over bad, cause no harm, prevent harm.
3. Justice or fairness—egalitarianism over scarce resources.
4. Truth-telling or honesty—there may be circumstances when this is not always best.
5. Individual freedom—freedom to choose and to choose what may not always be best.

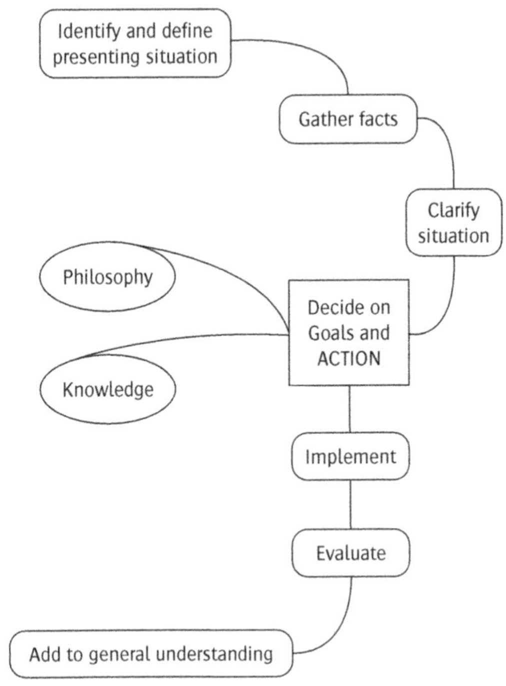

Figure 16.3 The ethical decision-making process.

Withdrawing treatment

One of the most difficult decisions in critical care is deciding the point at which a patient's illness is terminal and that none of the technological and pharmacological interventions that have been used to support him or her are providing benefit in terms of either symptom relief or recovery. As Thiroux indicates, it is then appropriate to accept the inevitability of death. This may sometimes be more of a problem to medical than nursing staff because of the values and ethos inherent in each profession.

Nursing staff may raise the possibility of withdrawing treatment as they are usually most involved with the patient and family through giving continuous care and having a close view of the burden of treatment. This means that they can gain an understanding of when the patient's quality of life is at a level likely to be unacceptable to him or her, both in the critical care unit and projecting forward to the future. In these circumstances, nurses can advocate on the patient's behalf if needed, aiming to ensure that the patient is enabled to have control over his or her own affairs as far as that is possible. This sort of care is very important but requires considerable skill; it is about supporting patients so that their needs and rights are addressed, that unnecessary and unproductive treatments are stopped, that the emphasis is moved from cure to care, and that the goals are redefined to allow death within a comfortable, humane, and peaceful environment.

Although the final decision in most cases will generally rest with the consultant involved, the situation should usually be discussed among the multidisciplinary team, with the patient's relatives, and, where appropriate, with the patient (see Box 16.8). The establishment of a consensus view is an important part of acceptance of a

Box 16.8 Criteria to be considered when discussing withdrawal of treatment

- Prognosis
- Age
- Chronic health status
- Attainable quality of life
- Family
- Social support
- Cultural and religious background

final decision. There may be a loss of trust in the validity of the decision and resentment about the decision-making process if those closely involved in the patient's care have no opportunity to explore and express their feelings. The VALUE mnemonic can be useful in planning and structuring discussions in these situations (Truog *et al.* 2008):

Value statements made by family members.
Acknowledge emotions.
Listen to family members.
Understand who the patient is as a person.
Elicit questions from family members.[1]

Expanding critical care nursing

If critical care nursing is to continue to progress and improve, there must be a concerted effort to increase the understanding of the effects of critical illness and the critical care environment on the patient. Alternative designs and methods of configuring the unit, organising and delivering care must be explored. This can only be achieved with a structured programme of research which is replicated and validated in a variety of settings and institutions. The multidisciplinary approach which is so important in the delivery of care must also encompass the approach to research. At present, relatively few institutions offer the facility for nursing involvement in research at every level: the studies that are performed are usually undertaken by individuals with a specific commitment to research or as part of a thesis leading to a higher education award. There is an urgent need for a structure that promotes collaborative research examining all aspects of care in different situations, with a coordinated approach to testing a whole range of conventional and sometimes unconventional treatments and methods of care.

References and bibliography

Barr, J., Fraser, G.L., Puntillo, K., *et al* (2013). Clinical practice guidelines for the management of pain, agitation, and delirium in adult patients in the intensive care unit. *Critical Care Medicine*, **41**, 263–306.

Berenholtz, S.M., Pustavoitau, A., Schwartz, S.J., *et al* (2007). How safe is my intensive care unit? Methods for monitoring and measurement. *Curr Opin Crit Care*, **13**, 703–8.

Bittner, M.I., Donnelly, M., van Zanten, A.R., *et al* (2013). How is intensive care reimbursed? A review of eight European countries. *Annals of Intensive Care*, **12**, 37.

Celi, L.A., Mark, R.G., Stone, D.J., *et al.* (2013). 'Big data' in the intensive care unit. Closing the data loop. *American Journal of Respiratory and Critical Care Medicine*, **187**, 1157–60.

Cook, D.J., Sibbald, W.J., Vincent, J.L., *et al* (1996). Evidence based critical care medicine. What is it and what can it do for us? Evidence Based Medicine in Critical Care Group. *Critical Care Medicine*, **24**, 334–7.

Cuthbertson, B.H., Roughton, S., Jenkinson, D, *et al.* (2010). Quality of life in the five years after intensive care: a cohort study. *Critical Care*, **14**, R6.

Davydow, D.S., Zatzick, D., Hough, C.L., *et al.* (2013). A longitudinal investigation of posttraumatic stress and depressive symptoms over the course of the year following medical-surgical intensive care unit admission. *General Hospital Psychiatry*, **35**, 226–32.

Department of Health (2013a). *Health Building Note 04-02: Critical Care Units*. Department of Health, London.

Department of Health (2013b). *Reference Costs 2012–13*. Department of Health: London.

Department of Health Payment by Results Team (2013). *Payment by Results Guidance for 2013–14*. Department of Health, Leeds.

Donabedian, A. (1966). Evaluating the quality of medical care. *Milbank Memorial Fund Quarterly*, **44**(Suppl),166–206.

[1] Reprinted from Chest, 134, 4, Curtis J.R., White D.B, Practical guidance for evidence-based ICU family conferences, pp. 835–843.

Dragsted, L., Qvist, J. (1989). Outcome fra.om intensive care. III: A 5-year study of 1308 patients: activity levels. *European Journal of Anaesthesiology*, **6**, 385–96.

Dragsted, L., Qvist, J., Madsen, M. (1989). Outcome from intensive care. II: A 5-year study of 1308 patients: short-term outcome. *European Journal of Anaesthesiology*, **6**, 131–44.

Drews, F.A., Musters, A., Samore, M.H. (2008). Error producing conditions in the intensive care unit. In *Advances in Patient Safety: New Directions and Alternative Approaches*. Vol. 3, *Performance and Tools* (eds K. Henriksen, J.B. Battles, M.A. Keyes). Rockville, MD: Agency for Healthcare Research and Quality.

Dykes, P.C., Rothschild, J.M., Hurley, A.C. (2010). Medical errors recovered by critical care nurses. *Journal of Nursing Administration*, **40**, 241–6.

Eizenberg, M.M. (2011). Implementation of evidence-based nursing practice: nurses' personal and professional factors? *Journal of Advanced Nursing*, **67**, 33–42.

Ellis, J. (2006). All inclusive benchmarking. *Journal of Nursing Management*, **14**, 377–83.

Faculty of Intensive Care Medicine/Intensive Care Society (2013). *Core Standards for Intensive Care Units*. Report, Faculty of Intensive Care Medicine/Intensive Care Society, London.

Griffiths, J., Hatch, R.A, Bishop, J., *et al*. (2013). An exploration of social and economic outcome and associated health-related quality of life after critical illness in general intensive care unit survivors: a 12-month follow-up study. *Critical Care*, **17**, R100.

Halpern, N.A., Pastores, S.M. (2010). Critical care medicine in the United States 2000–2005: an analysis of bed numbers, occupancy rates, payer mix, and costs. *Critical Care Medicine*, **38**, 65–71.

Harrison, D.A., Brady, A.R., Rowan, K. (2004). Case mix, outcome and length of stay for admissions to adult, general critical care units in England, Wales and Northern Ireland: the Intensive Care National Audit & Research Centre Case Mix Programme Database. *Critical Care*, **8**, R99–111.

Harrison, D.A., Parry, G.J., Carpenter, J., *et al*. (2007). A new risk prediction model for critical care: the Intensive Care National Audit & Research Centre (ICNARC) model. *Critical Care Medicine*, **35**, 1091–8.

Harrison, D.A., Gao, H., Welch, C.A., *et al*. (2010). The effects of critical care outreach services before and after critical care: a matched-cohort analysis. *Journal of Critical Care*, **25**, 196–204.

Health and Social Care Information Centre (2014). *Summary Hospital-level Mortality Indicator October 2012–September 2013*, Health & Social Care Information Centre https://indicators.ic.nhs.uk/webview/.

Healthcare Quality Improvement Partnership (2009). *Criteria and Indicators of Best Practice in Clinical Audit*. Report, Healthcare Quality Improvement Partnership, London.

Herridge, M.S., Tansey, C.M., Matté, A., *et al* (2011). Functional disability 5 years after acute respiratory distress syndrome. *New England Journal of Medicine*, **364**, 1293–1304.

Higgins, T.L., Teres, D., Copes, W.S., *et al*. (2007). Assessing contemporary intensive care unit outcome: an updated Mortality Probability Admission Model (MPM0-III). *Critical Care Medicine*, **35**, 827–35.

Ho, P.M., Peterson, P.N., Masoudi, F.A. (2008). Evaluating the evidence. Is there a rigid hierarchy? *Circulation*, **118**, 1675–84.

Intensive Care National Audit & Research Centre (2013). *Key Statistics from the Case Mix Programme Database, 1 April 2011 to 31 March 2012*. Report, Intensive Care National Audit & Research Centre, London.

Keegan, M.T., Gajic, O., Afessa, B. (2011). Severity of illness scoring systems in the intensive care unit. *Critical Care Medicine*, **39**, 163–9.

Knaus, W.A., Draper, E.A., Wagner, D.P., *et al* (1985). APACHE II: a severity of disease classification system. *Critical Care Medicine*, **13**, 818–29.

Le Gall, J.R., Lemeshow, S., Saulnier, F. (1993). A new Simplified Acute Physiology Score (SAPS II) based on a European/North American multicenter study. *JAMA*, **270**, 2957–63.

Levy, M.M., Fink, M.P., Marshall, J.C., *et al* (2003). 2001 SCCM/ESICM/ACCP/ATS/SIS International Sepsis Definitions Conference. *Critical Care Medicine*, **31**, 12506/*Intensive Care Medicine*, **29**, 530–8.

Lone, N.I., Walsh, T.S. (2011). Prolonged mechanical ventilation in critically ill patients: epidemiology, outcomes and modelling the potential cost consequences of establishing a regional weaning unit. *Critical Care*, **15**, R102.

Maxwell, R.J. (1992). Dimensions of quality revisited: from thought to action. *Quality in Health Care*, **1**, 171–7.

Miranda, D.R., de Rijk, A., Schaufeli, W. (1996). Simplified Therapeutic Intervention Scoring System: the TISS-28 items. Results from a multicenter study. *Critical Care Medicine*, **24**, 64–73.

Miranda, D.R., Moreno, R., Iapichino, G. (1997). Nine Equivalents of Nursing Manpower Use Score (NEMS). *Intensive Care Medicine*, **23**, 760–5.

Miranda, D.R., Nap, R., de Rijk, A., *et al*. (2003). Nursing activities score. *Critical Care Medicine*, **31**, 374–82.

Moreno, R.P., Metnitz, P.G., Almeida, E., *et al*. (2005). SAPS 3—From evaluation of the patient to evaluation of the intensive care unit. Part 2: Development of a prognostic model for hospital mortality at ICU admission. *Intensive Care Medicine*, **31**, 1345–55.

Murthy, S., Wunsch, H. (2012). Clinical review: International comparisons in critical care—lessons learned. *Critical Care*, **16**, 218.

National Institute for Health and Clinical Excellence (2009). *CG83: Rehabilitation After Critical Illness*. Clinical Guideline, National Institute for Health and Clinical Excellence, London.

Park, G.R., McElligot, M., Torres, C. (2003). Outreach critical care—cash for no questions? *British Journal of Anaesthesiology*, **90**, 700–1.

Prinjha, S., Field, K., Rowan, K. (2009). What patients think about ICU follow-up services: a qualitative study. *Critical Care*, **13**, R46.

Randolph, A.G., Guyatt, G.H., Richardson, W.S. (1998). Prognosis in the intensive care unit: finding accurate and useful estimates for counseling patients. *Critical Care Medicine*, **26**, 767–72.

Rhodes, A., Ferdinande, P., Flaatten, H., *et al*. (2012). The variability of critical care bed numbers in Europe. *Intensive Care Medicine*, **38**, 1647–53.

Rowan, K.M., Kerr, J.H., Major, E., *et al*. (1993). Intensive Care Society's APACHE II study in Britain and Ireland. II: Outcome comparisons of intensive care units after adjustment for case mix by the American APACHE II method. *British Medical Journal*, **307**, 977–81.

Rubulotta, F., Marshall, J.C., Ramsay, G., *et al* (2009). Predisposition, insult/infection, response, and organ dysfunction: a new model for staging severe sepsis. *Critical Care Medicine*, **37**, 1329–35.

Sackett, D.L., Rosenberg, W.M., Gray, J.A., *et al.* (1996). Evidence based medicine: what it is and what it isn't. *British Medical Journal*, **312**, 71–2.

Teasdale, G., Jennett, B. (1974). Assessment of coma and impaired consciousness: a practical scale. *Lancet*, **2**, 81–4.

Thiroux, J.P., Krasemann, K.W. (2014). *Ethics: Theory and Practice* (11th edn). Pearson Education: Harlow.

Truog, R.D., Campbell, M.L., Curtis, J.R., *et al.* (2008). Recommendations for end-of-life care in the intensive care unit: a consensus statement by the American College [corrected] of Critical Care Medicine. *Critical Care Medicine*, **36**, 953–63.

Valentin, A., Capuzzo, M., Guidet, B., *et al.* (2006). Patient safety in intensive care: results from the multinational Sentinel Events Evaluation (SEE) study. *Intensive Care Medicine*, **32**, 1591–8.

Vincent, J.L., Moreno, R. (2010). Clinical review: scoring systems in the critically ill. *Critical Care*, **14**, 207.

Vincent, J.L., Martinez, E.O., Silva, E. (2011). Evolving concepts in sepsis definitions. *Critical Care Nursing Clinics of North America*, **23**, 29–39.

Voisey, S., Davies, J., Parry-Jones, J., *et al.* (2007). Five years experience of critical care bereavement follow-up. *Critical Care*, **11**(Suppl 2), P494.

Wade, D.M., Howell, D.C., Weinman, J.A., *et al.* (2012). Investigating risk factors for psychological morbidity three months after intensive care: a prospective cohort study. *Critical Care*, **16**, R192.

Welch, J. (2014). Critical care nursing. In *Oh's Intensive Care Manual* (7th edn) (eds A.D. Bersten, N. Soni). Oxford: Butterworth-Heinemann.

West, E., Barron, D.N., Harrison, D., *et al.* (2014). Nurse staffing, medical staffing and mortality in intensive care: an observational study. *International Journal of Nursing Studies*, **51**, 781–94.

West, M.A., Guthrie, J.P., Dawson, J.F. (2006). Reducing patient mortality in hospitals: the role of human resource management. *Journal of Organizational Behaviour*, **27**, 983–1002.

Woodford, M. (2014). Scoring systems for trauma. *BMJ*, **348**, g1142.

Zimmerman, J.E., Alzola, C., von Rueden, K.T. (2003). The use of benchmarking to identify top performing critical care units: a preliminary assessment of their policies and practices. *Journal of Critical Care*, **18**, 76–86.

Further reading

Curtis, J.R., Vincent, J.L. (2010). Ethics and end-of-life care for adults in the intensive care unit. *Lancet*, **376**, 1347–53.

Jackson, W.L., Jr, Sales, J.F. (2014). Potentially ineffective care: time for earnest reexamination. *Critical Care Research and Practice*, **2014**, 134198.

Appendix

Appendix Table 1 Normal ranges of monitoring parameters

Term	Abbreviation	Normal range
Central venous pressure	CVP	3–10 mmHg
Right atrial pressure	RA or RAP	3–8 mmHg
Mean right atrial pressure	MRAP	4–6 mmHg
Right ventricular systolic pressure	RVSP	15–25 mmHg
Right ventricular diastolic pressure	RVDP	3–8 mmHg
Pulmonary artery systolic pressure	PASP	15–25 mmHg
Pulmonary artery diastolic pressure	PADP	8–12 mmHg
Pulmonary artery wedge pressure (also known as pulmonary artery occlusion pressure or pulmonary capillary wedge pressure)	PAWP or PAOP or PCWP	6–12 mmHg
Left atrial pressure	LA or LAP	6–12 mmHg
Mean arterial pressure	MAP	70–105 mmHg
Stroke volume	SV	60–100ml
Cardiac output	CO	4–8 L/min
Cardiac index	CI	2.4–4.0 L/min
Ejection fraction	EF	55–70%
End-diastolic volume	EDV or LVEDV	120–150 ml
End-systolic volume	ESV	50–70 ml
Systemic vascular resistance	SVR	800–1200 dyn sec/cm^5
Pulmonary vascular resistance	PVR	<250 dyn sec/cm^5
Corrected flow time	FTc	330–360 msec
Peak velocity	PV	90–120 cm/sec (at 20yr) 60–90 cm/sec (at 50yr) 50–80 cm/sec (at 70yr)

Appendix Table 2 Normal ranges of laboratory results

Measurement	Abbreviation	Normal range
Potassium	K	3.5–5.1 mmol/L
Urea	U	2.5–8.3 mmol/L
Sodium	Na	135–145 mmol/L
Creatinine	Cr	55–125 umol/L (varies with age and sex)
Calcium	Ca	2.15–2.65 mmol/L
Ionized calcium	iCa	1.1–1.4 mmol/L
Glucose (fasting)	Gluc	4.4–6.1 mmol/L (79.2–110 mg/dL)
Inorganic phosphate	P	0.87–1.45 mmol/L
Amylase		28–100 IU/L
Urate		155–357 µmol/L
Uric acid		110–420 µmol/L males 110–360 µmol/L females
C-reactive protein	CRP	0–5.0 mg/L
Brain natriuretic peptide *N*-terminal pro-brain-naturetic peptide	BNP (NT-proBNP)	0–99 ng/L (varies with age)
Erythrocyte sedimentation rate	ESR	0–12mm/h
Troponin T Troponin I High-sensitivity troponin T	TnT TnI HSTn	<14 ng/L < 50 ng /L* <14 ng/L
Estimated glomerular filtration rate (for African Caribbean patients multiply by 1.21)	eGFR	>90 ml/min/1.73 m^2
International normalized ratio	INR	0.9–1.2
APTT	APTT	22–41 sec
Thrombin time	TT	9–15 sec
Prothrombin time	PT	10.0–12.0 sec
Iron	Fe	6.6–26 µmol/L
Total iron-binding capacity	TIBC	41–77 µmol/L
Serum cholesterol	SC	2.5–5.0 mmol/L
HDL-cholesterol	HDL	0.0–1.5 mmol/L
LDL-cholesterol	LDL	0–3.5 mmol/L
Triglycerides	TRIG	0.4–2.3 mmol/L
Cholesterol:HDL ratio	CHDLR	<3.0
Lactate dehydrogenase	LDH	240–480 IU/L
Creatine kinase	CK	26–140 IU/L

Albumin	ALB	34–50 g/L
Globulin		20–40 g/L
Total protein		60–83 g/L
Alanine aminotransferase	ALT	10–50 IU/L
Alkaline phosphate	ALP	40–129 IU/L
Aspartate aminotransferase	AST	13–35 IU/L
Gamma-glutamyl transpeptidase	GGT	5–39 IU/L
Bilirubin (total)	BIL	0–20 µmol/L
Thyroid stimulating hormone	TSH	0.27–4.2 mU/L
Free T_4	FT_4	12.0–22.0 pmol/L
Free T_3	FT_3	4.0–6.8 pmol/L
Serum vitamin B_{12}	VB_{12}	191–663 pg/ml
Platelets	PLTS	150–400 × 10^9/L
Haemoglobin	Hb	Adult males 130–170 g/L (13–17 g/dl) Adult females 120–150g/L (12–15g/dl)
Red blood cells	RBCs	4.4–5.8 × 10^9/L
White blood cells	WCCs	3.0–10.0 × 10^9/L
Mean cell haemoglobin concentrate	MCHC	320–360 g/L (32–36 g/dl)
Mean cell haemoglobin	MCH	27.0–33.5 pg
Mean cell volume	MCV	80–99 fL
Neutrophils absolute count	NEA	2.0–7.5 × 10^9/L
Lymphocytes absolute count	LYA	1.2–3.65 × 10^9/L
Monocytes absolute count	MOA	0.2–1.0 × 10^9/L
Eosinophils absolute count	EOA	0.0–0.4 × 10^9/L
Basophils absolute count	BAA	0.0–0.1 × 10^9/L
Neutrophils %	NEP	40–75%
Lymphocytes %	LYP	20–45%
Monocytes %	MOP	2–10%
Eosinophils %	EOP	1–6%
Basophils %	BASOP	0–2%
Haematocrit	HCT	40–50%

NB: normal ranges may vary bertween different laboratories.

* Several different assays are available for measuring troponin I; therefore normal values may vary.

Index

N